World Health Organization

Strategizing national health in the 21st century: a handbook

Edited by

Gerard Schmets

Dheepa Rajan

Sowmya Kadandale

WHO Library Cataloguing-in-Publication Data

Strategizing national health in the 21st century: a handbook / Gerard Schmets ... [et al].

Contents: 13 individual chapters

1.Health Policy. 2.National Health Programmes. 3.Health Planning. 4.Handbooks. I.Schmets, Gerard. II.Rajan, Dheepa. III.Kadandale, Sowmya. IV.World Health Organization

ISBN 978 92 4 154974 5 (NLM classification: WA 540)

The document has been produced with the financial assistance of the European Union and the Grand Duchy of Luxembourg. The views expressed herein can in no way be taken to reflect the official opinion of the European Union nor the Grand Duchy of Luxembourg.

Graphic design by Valerie Assmann.

Suggested citation: Schmets G, Rajan D, Kadandale S, editors. Strategizing national health in the 21st century: a handbook. Geneva: World Health Organization; 2016.

Printed in Italy

Contents

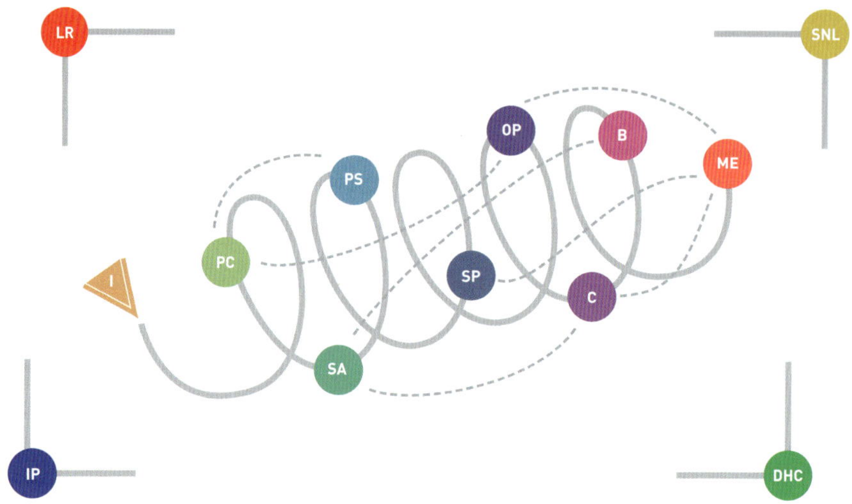

Cross-cutting topics relevant to national health planning

Acknowledgements

The editors would like to give special thanks to Agnes Soucat for overall guidance.

Thanks are also due to Alyssa Muggleworth Weaver for overall background research support, and to the many authors, reviewers and other contributors who made this publication possible.

English language editing was undertaken by Dorothy van Schooneveld and Thomson Prentice.

This publication was produced with the financial assistance of the European Union and the Grand Duchy of Luxembourg.

Chapter 1. Introduction (Gerard Schmets, Sowmya Kadandale, Denis Porignan and Dheepa Rajan)

Information and graphs for boxes were provided by Maryam Bigdeli, Jim Campbell, David Clarke, Carmen Dolea, Edward Kelley, Marie-Paule Kieny and Nuria Toro Polanco.

Chapter 2. Population consultation on needs and expectations (Katja Rohrer and Dheepa Rajan)

Background research support was provided by Olaitan Awonusi and the annex tables were provided by Elisabeth Paul.

This chapter was reviewed by Mohamed Lamine Drame, Jane Dyrhauge, Ann-Lise Guisset, Sowmya Kadandale, T headora Koller, Joe Kutzin, Franziska Meier, Elisabeth Paul, Paolo Piva, Denis Porignon and Gerard Schmets.

Comments and insights on the first draft were provided by the following reviewers in June 2014: Kodzo Mawuli Rene Adzodo, Osman Niyazi Cakmak, Claudia Castillo, Ayesha de Lorenzo, Amalia del Riego, Tessa Edejer, Mounir Farag, Johana Hanefeld, Xu Ke, Martin Ekeke Monono, Daniel Rodriguez, Archana Shah, Alaka Singh, Maria Skarphedinsdottir, Juan Tello, Phyllida Travis, Prosper Tumusiime, Soledad Urrutia and Pushpa Wijesinghe.

The following participants of a retreat in August 2015 provided valuable comments on a revised draft of the chapter: Olaitan Awonusi ,Maryam Bigdeli, David Clarke, Casey Downey, Sowmya Kadandale, Thomas O'Connell, Denis Porignon, Finn Schleimann, Gerard Schmets, Archana Shah, Karin Stenberg, Frank Terwindt and Kavitha Viswanathan.

Chapter 3. Situation analysis of the health sector (Dheepa Rajan)

Olaitan Awonusi and Romain Oguey contributed to the development of this chapter.

Frank Terwindt provided information for Table 3.2, Box 3.6, Box 3.12 and Fig. 3.3. and Elisabeth Paul provided information for Box 3.1 and Box 3.2.

This chapter was reviewed by Qaiser Pasha, Humayun Rizwan, Gerard Schmets and Frank Terwindt.

The following participants of a retreat in August 2015 provided valuable comments on a revised draft of this chapter: Olaitan Awonusi, Maryam Bigdeli, David Clarke, Casey Downey, Sowmya Kadandale, Thomas O'Connell, Denis Porignon, Finn Schleimann, Gerard Schmets, Archana Shah, Karin Stenberg, Frank Terwindt and Kavitha Viswanathan.

Chapter 4. Priority-setting for national health policies, strategies and plans (Frank Terwindt, Dheepa Rajan and Agnes Soucat)

Research on priority-setting methods, approaches and tools was conducted by Marpessa Arnault and Victoria Bakare, under the supervision of Denis Porignon. Sowmya Kadandale provided information for Box 4.1 on Sierra Leone.

This chapter was reviewed by Jordi Carbonell, Annie Chu, Luke Elich, Rochelle Eng, Xu Ke, Eun Gyo Kim, Jeremy Lauer, Yeiji Lee, Lachlan McDonald, Elisabeth Paul, Gerard Schmets, Marlon Sison and Ronald Tamangan.

Chapter 5. Strategic planning: transforming priorities into plans (Frank Terwindt and Dheepa Rajan)

A background literature review was undertaken by Oriane Bodson and information on the national planning cycle database was provided by Casey Downey.

This chapter was reviewed by Hermes Karemere, Denis Porignon and Gerard Schmets.

Chapter 6. Operational planning: transforming plans into actions (Dean Shuey, Maryam Bigdeli and Dheepa Rajan)

Oriane Bodson conducted a background literature review for this chapter.

This chapter was reviewed by Mohamed Lamine Drame, Anne Johansen, Tolib Mirzoev, Denis Porignon and Gerard Schmets.

Chapter 7. Estimating cost implications of a national health policy, strategy or plan (Karin Stenberg and Dheepa Rajan)

This chapter was reviewed by Helene Barroy, Melanie Bertram, Elina Dale, Tessa Edejer, Odd Hanssen, Sowmya Kadandale, Joseph Kutzin, Tania Lourenco, Laurent Musango, Gerard Schmets, Susan Sparkes, Jean-Marc Thome and Andre Zida.

Valuable input for country example boxes was provided by Kahsu Bekuretsion, Nejmudin Bilal, Tania Lourenco and Andre Zida.

Chapter 8. Budgeting for health (Dheepa Rajan, Hélène Barroy and Karin Stenberg)

This chapter was a collaboration between the following units in the Department of Health Systems Governance and Financing: Health Systems Governance, Policy and Aid Effectiveness; Health Financing; and Economic Analysis and Evaluation. Guidance and input on budgeting for health were provided by Tessa Edejer, Joseph Kutzin and Gerard Schmets.

This chapter was reviewed by Benoit Mathivet and Jacky Mathonnat.

Chapter 9. Monitoring and evaluation and review of national health policies, strategies and plans (Kathryn O'Neill, Kavitha Viswanathan, Eduardo Celades and Ties Boerma)

This chapter was extracted from the document "Monitoring, evaluation and review of national health strategies: a country-led platform for information and accountability" (http://www.who.int/classifications/ME_component_national-healthplans_prepub_july2011. pdf); an updated version is currently in press. Major health partners and selected experts from country level contributed to developing the original document.

The following provided valuable comments on this chapter: Jun Gao, Derege Kebede, Mark Landry, Juliet Nabyonga, Sam Omar and Hongy Xu. Valuable input for country example boxes was provided by Hillary Kipchumba Kipruto and Isabel Maina (Kenya); Issac Dambula, Francis Magombo, Rhino Mchenga, Maganizo Monawe and Simon Ndira (Malawi); Catherine Flag-othier, Nelitta Nassone, Siv Nygaard and Daisy Trovoada (Mozambique); and Claud Kumalija (United Republic of Tanzania).

This chapter was reviewed by Denis Porignon, Dheepa Rajan and Gerard Schmets.

Chapter 10. Law, regulation and strategizing for health (David Clarke)

Additional background research was carried out by Olaitan Awonusi and valuable contributions on contracting were provided by Riku Elovainio.

The following participants of a retreat in August 2015 provided valuable input into the chapter: Olaitan Awonusi, Maryam Bigdeli, Casey Downey, Sowmya Kadandale, Thomas O'Connell, Denis Porignon, Dheepa Rajan, Katja Rohrer, Finn Schleimann, Gerard Schmets, Archana Shah, Karin Stenberg, Frank Terwindt and Kavitha Viswanathan.

A revised draft of the document was reviewed in early 2016 by Gwen Dhaene, Luke Elich, Sowmya Kadandale, Benn McGrady, Dheepa Rajan and Gerard Schmets.

Chapter 11. Strategizing for health at sub-national level (Katja Rohrer)

This chapter received valuable input from Maryam Bigdeli, Tarcisse Elongo, Sowmya Kadandale, Denis Porignon, Dheepa Rajan, Gerard Schmets and Frank Terwindt.

Maryam Bigdeli provided Box 11.10 on the decentralization process in Pakistan. Inke Mathauer provided valuable information on strategic purchasing in decentralized settings.

Chapter 12. Intersectoral planning for health and health equity equity (Erik Blas, Nathalie Roebbel, Dheepa Rajan and Nicole Valentine)

Additional background research was carried out by Kawselyah Juval.

This chapter was reviewed by Patricia Frenz, Denis Porignon, Gerard Schmets and Eugenio Villar.

Chapter 13. Strategizing in distressed health contexts (Enrico Pavignani and Sandro Colombo)

The following participants of a retreat in August 2015 provided valuable comments on this chapter: Olaitan Awonusi, Maryam Bigdeli, David Clarke, Casey Downey, Sowmya Kadandale, Thomas O'Connell, Denis Porignon, Dheepa Rajan, Katja Rohrer, Finn Schleimann, Gerard Schmets, Archana Shah, Karin Stenberg, Frank Terwindt and Kavitha Viswanathan.

LE GOUVERNEMENT
DU GRAND-DUCHÉ DE LUXEMBOURG
Ministère des Affaires étrangères
et européennes

Direction de la coopération
au développement et
de l'action humanitaire

Chapter 1

Introduction

Gerard Schmets
Sowmya Kadandale
Denis Porignon
Dheepa Rajan

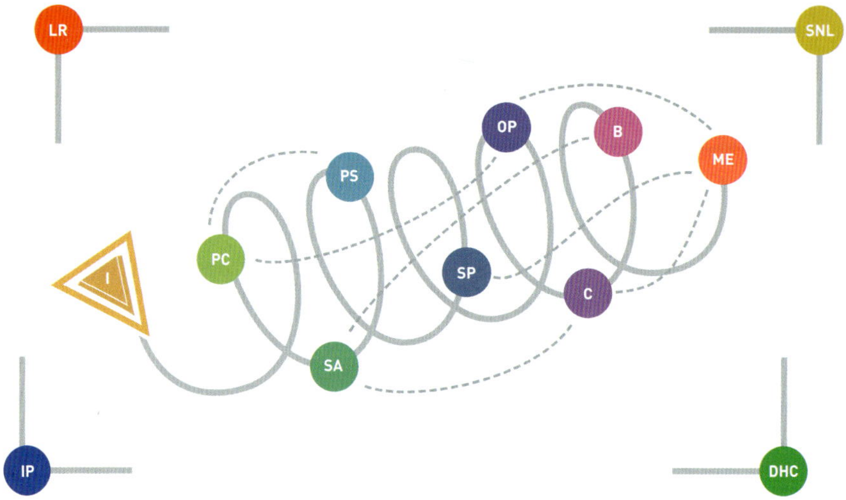
LR
SNL
OP
B
ME
PS
PC
I
SP
C
SA
IP
DHC

1.1 Rationale for this handbook

The global health environment is becoming increasingly complex. Social, demographic and epidemiological transformations fed by globalization, urbanization and ageing populations pose challenges of a magnitude that was not anticipated three decades ago. In addition, recent global health security threats such as the Ebola virus disease or Zika virus outbreak, and the growing mismatch between the low performance of health systems and the rising expectations of societies, are increasingly becoming a cause for political concern. This often leads to countries prioritizing, or re-prioritizing, efforts towards strengthening health systems, moving towards universal health coverage (UHC) and implementing the idea of health in all policies.[1]

Countries recognize that these calls for efficiently strengthening health systems and improving health security must be translated into robust, realistic, comprehensive, coherent and well balanced health policies, strategies and plans. In the post-Millennium Development Goals (MDGs) era, they also recognize that in pluralist, mixed, public-private health systems, these policies, strategies and plans have to relate to the entire health sector and cannot be limited anymore to "command-and-control" plans for the public sector.

Functional health systems that deliver high quality services to the population are the main priority for governments. Achieving this requires permanent, well-structured and dynamic processes, with a true consensus between the demand and supply of services, as well as between governments, services providers and the population. A solid, evidence-informed *policy dialogue* is the only real way to achieve this in the 21st century.[2,3,4]

Furthermore, it is now widely understood that national health policies, strategies and plans (NHPSPs[I]) extend much beyond "health care", i.e. clinical personal services, and cover the broad public health agenda, including disaster preparedness, risk management and the International Health Regulations, encompassing action on the social determinants of health and the interaction between the health sector and other sectors in society.

In the face of both these gradual and acute changes over the past decade, NHPSPs, and more importantly the process of developing the NHPSP, need to be adapted and given a different focus. This handbook attempts to address that need.

In the context of the Paris, Accra and Busan principles of effective development cooperation, it is also widely recognized that in countries that receive significant external aid, NHPSPs are increasingly seen as crucial for making aid more effective.

It is recognized that, during the MDGs era, plans or policies did not always fulfill their promises; this was often because of design deficiencies or implementation failures. It was common to observe that national plans were not inclusive, not comprehensive enough, often imbalanced and incoherent with the wide variety of health problems to be tackled. Often, there was a disconnect between national plans and the broader national development policies or policy frameworks, health financing strategies and macroeconomic policies.

I The terms "policy", "strategy" and "plan" are used interchangeably by WHO, following a WHO Global Policy Group meeting and decision in 2009.

1.2 Context in the 21st century

1.2.1 Sustainable development goals, strengthening health systems and universal health coverage

Strategizing means designing plans and policies to achieve a particular goal related to the health of a nation.

This handbook aims to make the case that strategizing – meaning designing plans and policies to achieve a particular goal related to the health of a nation – is absolutely critical in the 21st century. It is not only recommended by the Member States of the World Health Organization (WHO), but is also feasible for all countries in all settings.

This handbook builds on the experiences gathered by WHO and its partners during the MDGs era. It presents the way of developing NHPSPs from a new pluralistic perspective, and it advocates for policy dialogue as a means to ensure inclusiveness and the participation of both service providers and the population in debates and the decision-making process with the government, as well as in the follow-up, monitoring and evaluation of NHPSP implementation.

As the world shifts from the MDGs to the Sustainable Development Goals (SDGs), governments are afforded a tremendous opportunity to better engineer the development of their countries. This is particularly relevant in the health sector, as countries make progress towards universal health coverage (UHC), i.e. *ensuring that all people have access to needed promotive, preventive, curative and rehabilitative health services, of sufficient quality to be effective, while also ensuring that people do not suffer financial hardship when paying for these services.*[5] In other words, this entails reducing the gap between access, need for and use of services, improving quality, and improving financial protection (see Fig. 1.1).

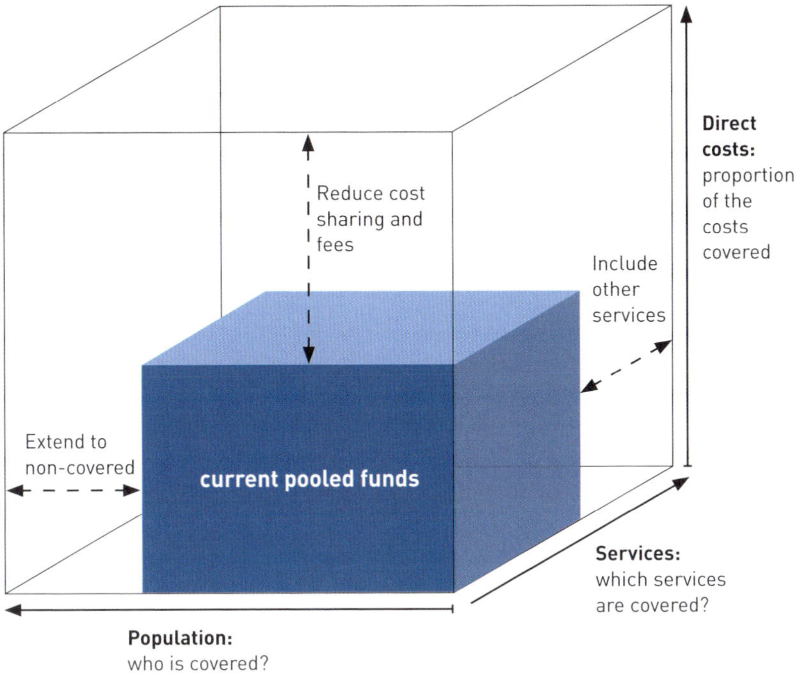

Fig. 1.1 Moving towards UHC[6]

UHC will only be achieved by its target date of 2030 if consistent and comprehensive health systems are developed, ones which are able to deliver on health outcomes and the well-being of the populations they serve. In particular, strong health systems are essential to ensure both individual and global public health security. As sharply illustrated during recent health emergencies in West Africa, or natural disasters in Nepal and the Philippines, health systems must also be prepared to guarantee the health security of the population and the resilience of societies.

Health system strengthening (HSS) efforts thus must be scaled up immediately. HSS is the process of identifying and implementing the changes in policy and practice in a country's health system (institutions, people and actions), so that the country can respond better to its health and health system challenges.[7] HSS implies mobilizing or better prioritizing the allocation of financial resources for health, as well as building the capacities of health systems in a variety of institutional, economic, fiscal, and political contexts.

Strategizing for health relates to SDG 3 but also to other SDGs such as SDG 1 (Poverty), SDG 4 (Education, SDG 5 (Gender equality) or SDG 8 (Inclusive economic growth and decent jobs).

Health systems and their strengthening are seen as the foundational set of policies, institutions, actions, approaches and tools, required to achieve the goals of UHC and the SDGs. Attaining these goals will, in turn, make essential contributions to global health security and resilient societies, equitable health outcomes and well-being, and inclusive economic growth —a dynamic further illustrated in Fig. 1.2 below. Realistically, strategizing for health needs to build on solid financial evidence and a stable financial perspective, as discussed in the next section.

Fig. 1.2 A framework for UHC as part of the SDGs

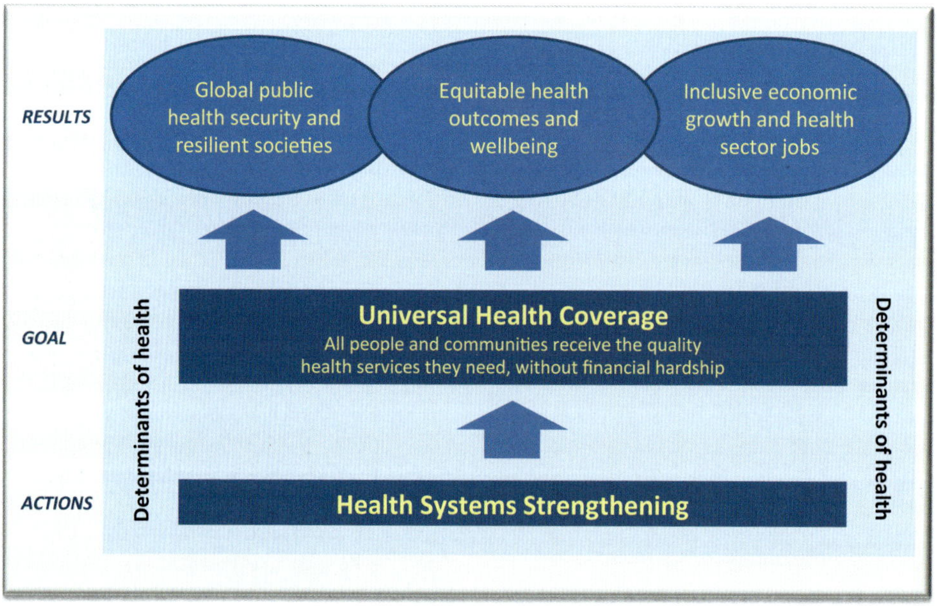

Adapted from a presentation by Kieny, MP, Category Network Meeting, Geneva, January 2015

Box 1.1

Key concepts for the HSS agenda

- **A health system** is the aggregate of all public and private organizations, institutions, and resources mandated to improve, maintain or restore health. This includes both personal and population services, as well as activities to influence the policies and actions of other sectors to address the political, social, environmental, and economic determinants of health.
- **Health system strengthening** is the significant and purposeful efforts to improve the performance of existing health systems.
- **Resilience** reflects the ability of health systems and institutions and societies to absorb disruptions, adapting and responding as needs evolve and the wider context changes. Resilience is a dynamic objective, captured over time as systems progressively build capacities to effectively respond to future shocks.
- **Health security** has two separate dimensions—individual and collective. Improving individual health security aims at reducing individual vulnerability to health risks through trusted access to safe and effective health services, products, and technologies. Collective health security at the global level involves reducing the vulnerability of societies to health threats that spread across national borders.
- **Universal health coverage** is the goal that all people and communities receive needed quality health services (including prevention, promotion, treatment, rehabilitation, and palliation) without financial hardship.

1.2.2 The fiscal gap and the importance of domestic resources

NHPSPs need to be guided by better and more efficient use of existing domestic resources, and by a very strategic and very well reflected allocation of the expected additional future domestic resources. This requires increased accountability of all concerned stakeholders, with strong policy dialogue at the highest level.

Estimates of the resources required to strengthen health systems point to a stark financial gap. In 2015, WHO estimated that the minimum investment required in the health sector for countries to attain the SDGs by 2030 is USD 55 billion per year.[II] Of this annual amount, according to the The Taskforce on Innovative International Financing for Health Systems, between two thirds and three quarters— USD 40 billion—must be spent on HSS efforts.[8]

The global HSS gap of USD 40 billion per year demands additional resources, as well as a realignment of existing resources. One cannot expect that this gap, mainly located in low and middle income countries, will be covered by external aid. Indeed, in 2013, the total combined amount of funding for HSS from all international sources was just over USD 2.3 billion, whereas funding for disease-specific programmes such as HIV/AIDS, tuberculosis or malaria amounted to USD 34 billion.[9] It is unrealistic to expect a twenty-fold increase in external aid for HSS to reach the required annual funding targets. Consequently, this gap will need to be covered by domestic funding (government and household contributions).

As echoed in the 2015 Addis Ababa Action Agenda,[10] the growing use of domestic resources for financing the health sector signifies that governments must make smart choices in determining how and where investments are made. In 2013, domestic resources represented 75% of total health spending in fragile states and low-income countries, and more than 95% in middle-income countries.[11] Notably, however, these domestic resources are often not optimally distributed, neither geographically nor among various income quintiles. Out-of-pocket expenditures remain unacceptably high.[III] This trend also suggests the need to reduce fragmentation and duplication among the different programmes, thereby increasing efficiency within and outside the health sector.

These issues of misallocation and inefficient use of domestic resources in many low- and middle-income countries underline the crucially-important role of better strategizing and planning domestic resources in order to improve the health and well-being of populations. NHPSPs need to be guided by a better and more efficient use of existing domestic resources, and by a very strategic and very well reflected allocation of the expected additional future domestic resources. This requires increased accountability of all concerned stakeholders, with strong policy dialogue at the highest level. As discussed in the next section, to achieve these objectives, strategizing national health in the 21st century clearly needs to be inclusive of all relevant actors and sectors.

II WHO estimates 2016, based on the 2009 Financing for Development Conference.

III In 2013, out-of-pocket expenditures represented 49% of total health expenditures in this group of countries, while public expenditures represented only 39% of total health expenditures.

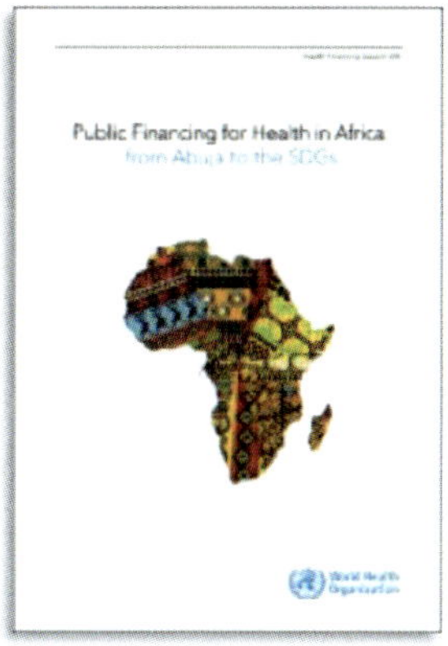

Box 1.2

Why are sound NHPSPs so important? The evidence from Africa

In the 2016 WHO report Public financing for health in Africa: from Abuja to the SDGs,[12] WHO concluded that **"For every USD 100 that goes into state coffers in Africa, on average USD 16 is allocated to health, only USD 10 is in effect spent, and less than USD 4 goes to the right health services."** The authors assessed that four key areas need to be addressed to overcome this situation:

1. the de-prioritization of health in the context of increasing revenues;
2. funding inconsistency and the lack of predictability of both domestic and external resources for health;
3. budget underspending;
4. misallocation of resources.

The development of sound health policies and strategies through intersectoral (whole-of-government) and intrasectoral inclusive policy dialogue with all health stakeholders (whole-of-society) is the way forward. In other words, to address the above-mentioned key issues, robust NHPSPs that reflect the vision, formalize the agreements, and put implementation aspects down on paper, need to be developed. They must be well prioritized and reflect the needs and the demand for health services, with resource allocation orientated towards UHC objectives. They need to clearly specify health sector goals and be anchored in strong political agreements to improve consistency and predictability. NHPSPs must be well translated into operational plans and budgets that will allow for full implementation. They also need to be well monitored and transparently evaluated for increased accountability and transparency.

1.2.3 A whole-of-government and a whole-of-society approach to policy dialogue (see Box 1.3)

Linked to the evolution of democratic and human right values in national debates, and supported by more rapid, real-time communication offered by the media in the age of the internet, governance has evolved towards a whole-of-government and a whole-of-society approach: improving health and well-being is no longer the role of the public health sector only, and no longer only under the purview of the ministry of health (MoH) (see Box 1.4). In other words, all sectors are part of the UHC road to success, and all stakeholders, beneficiaries, providers and the state must be involved in its design, implementation and follow-up. By thus taking on an increased role in defining the "what" and the "how", health actors accept increased responsibility and accountability for delivering results on agreed targets.

Fig. 1.3 Structuring the policy dialogue[14]

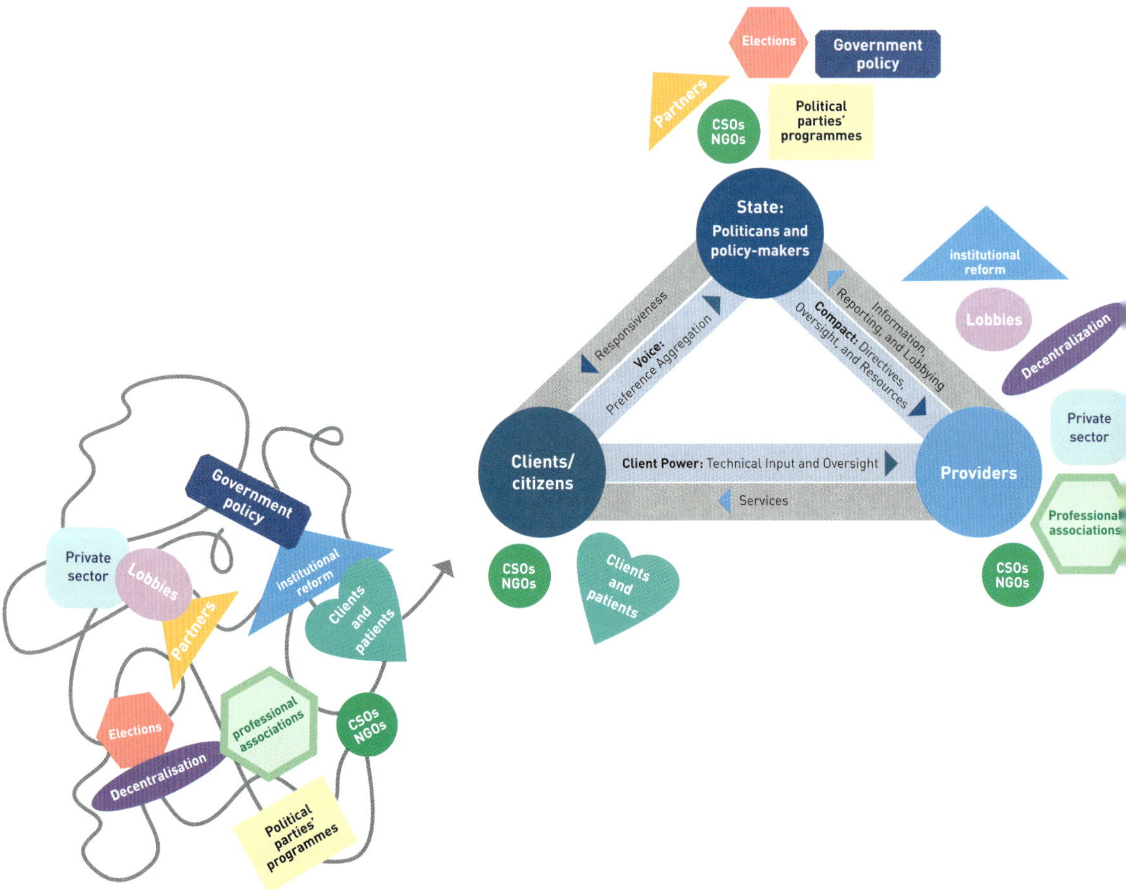

Box 1.3

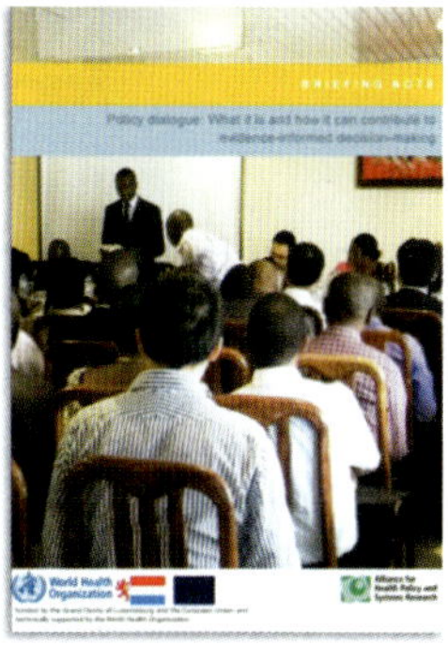

Policy dialogue: a fundamental process for the development of truly "whole-of-society" and "whole-of-government" NHPSPs?[13]

Policy dialogue can be defined as the "set of formal and informal exchanges aimed at facilitating policy change, influencing policy design and fostering further processes for decision-making where stakeholders of the different health system levels participate and contribute". It is an iterative inclusive process connecting the technical to the political, addressing the aspirations of the people, involving multiple stakeholders aimed at questioning and changing formal or informal policy, strategy and plans or addressing specific health issues to have maximum (public) health impact through a face-to-face and interactive discourse.

In the health sector, the entry points for policy dialogue can be very diverse. The entry point may be an issue that has arisen in the course of a policy process that provokes dialogue, often (but not always) due to the sensitivity or the wide-reaching consequences of the policy. It can be the emerging need for reforms, national or sub-national political debates, technical challenges, or even operational problems related to health systems or disease control activities. Examples of such entry points are health system reform, fiscal policy, health financing strategies, coordination of stakeholders within and outside of the health sector, health accounts, human resources for health, service delivery models, and drug pricing strategy, among many others.

Ideally, a robust policy dialogue leads to key policy decisions with the buy-in and ownership of a wide range of stakeholders – this is crucial because policy implementation is directly dependent on buy-in from at least those stakeholders who are involved in implementation. Stakeholder ownership is invaluable and is, among other things, a consequence of having a voice in the policy process. It includes any communication (informal consultations, electronic correspondence, corridor meetings, among others) or contact between people who are ultimately contributing in some way, shape, or form to a process which culminates in a policy decision. Policy dialogue provides a means to enhance mutual understanding of problems and to expand trust between partners by providing a platform to clarify expectations and agree on commitments. Policy dialogue also offers a way to increase accountability, more effectively implement policies, and more rapidly respond to barriers or challenges that are ideally addressed in a collective and collaborative manner.

Ensuring continued participation of all the actors necessitates innovation to allow dialogue outside the formal frameworks and spaces that constitute formal dialogue processes.

Recent policy dialogue processes at country level have demonstrated that flexibility is key to supporting strategic interventions. A MoH should be capable to adapt its policy orientations to the evolution of the national situation as well as to the transformation of the outside world.

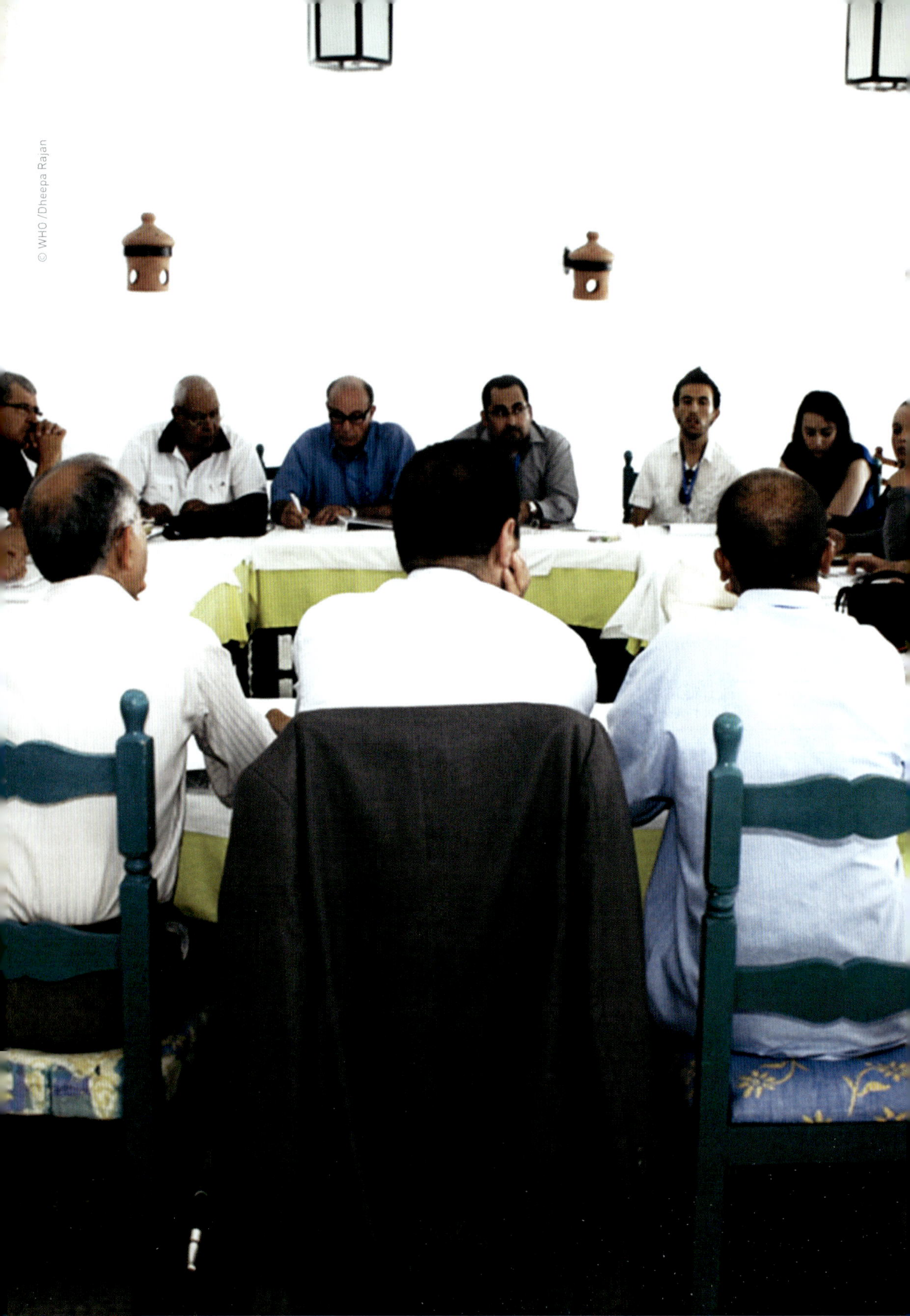

© WHO /Dheepa Rajan

Box 1.4

Overview of health system governance in Cabo Verde 2016[14]

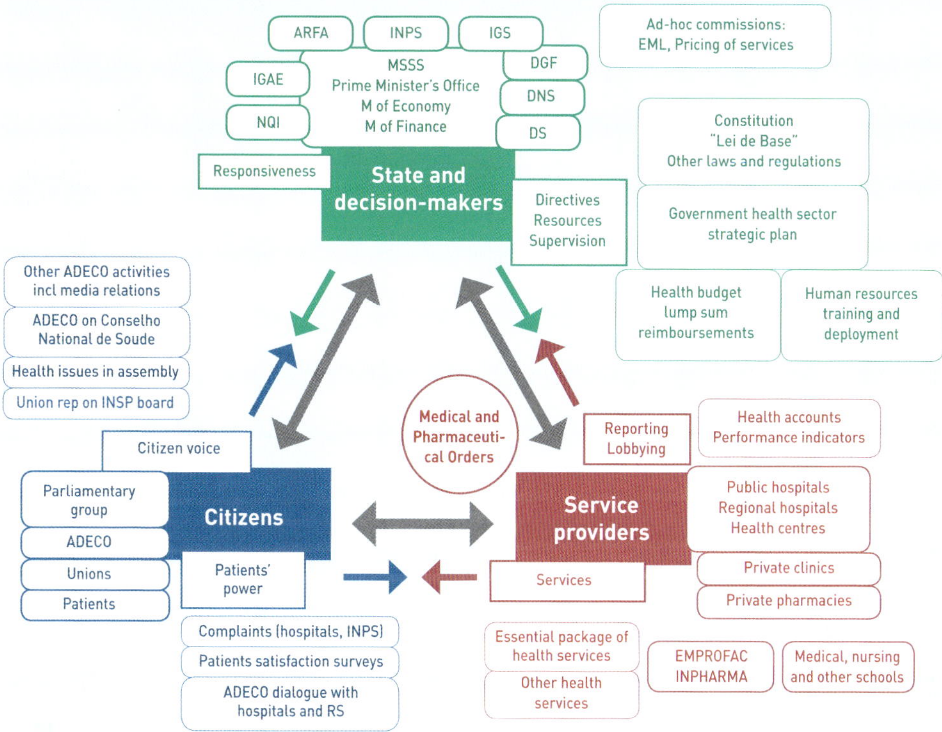

How do participation and inclusiveness play out in practice? A recent analysis of health stakeholders and major health governance issues in Cabo Verde demonstrates the sheer plethora of actors involved in the health sector. The graphical and visually "busy" representation above makes it strikingly clear how overwhelming the health policy arena can be. The illustration elucidates how complex a simple stakeholder analysis can be, with multiple actors, multiple interests and a multiplicity of relationships and connections between them. It also drives home the point that the health policy playing field is no longer necessarily dominated by the public sector, and that participation and inclusiveness must be structured and managed.

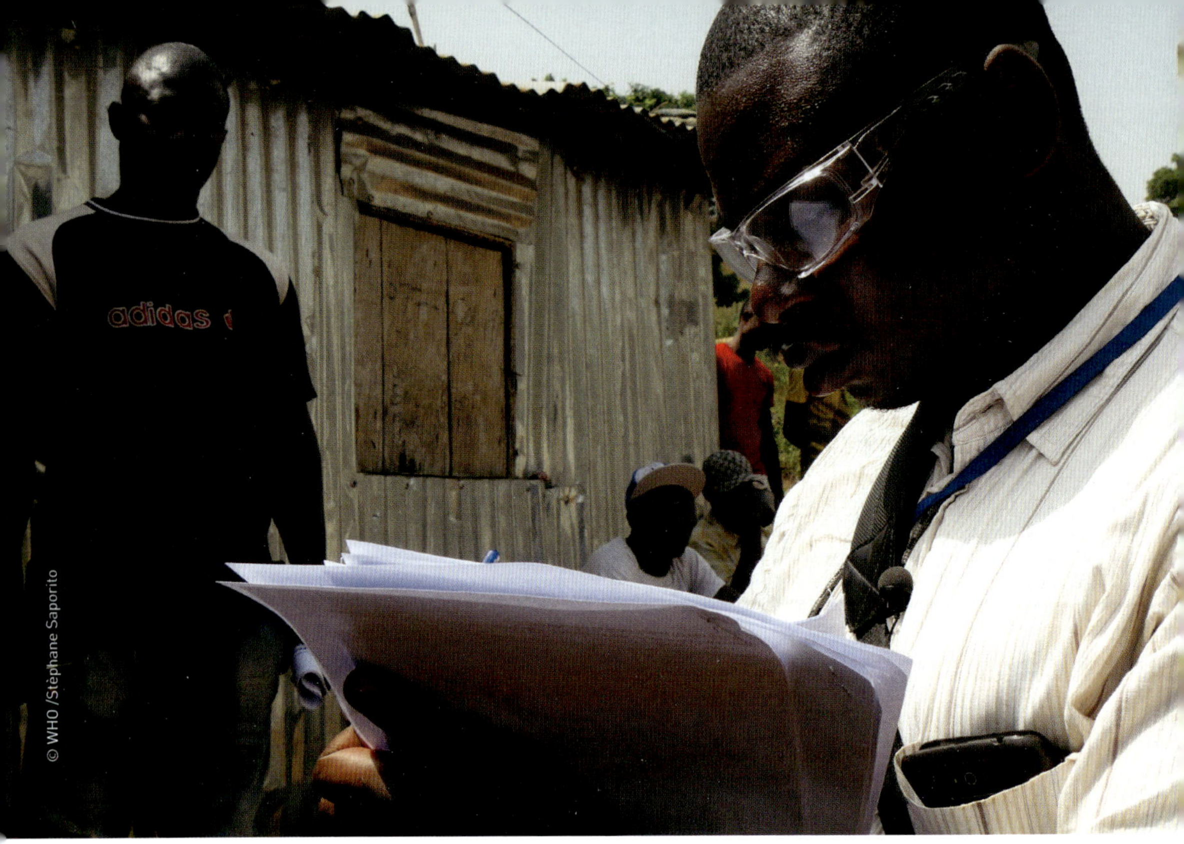

© WHO /Stéphane Saporito

The national and in some cases international stakeholders need to agree on baselines and targets, on methods and strategies to achieve the targets, on plans to implement the strategies, on mechanisms and process to monitor and correct strategies in a dynamic environment where external conditions will guide and reshape initial strategies to keep the objectives on track all along the journey.

They will need to be present at all levels, wherever a decision-making process is needed. In highly decentralized countries, it may mean a pluralistic participation in various facility boards or other steering, management or health committees. In all cases, it is clearly a dynamic process that needs to be sustained: in order to be effective and ensure accountability, this policy dialogue is not a "one shot" exercise; it is a permanent process to guide countries towards UHC (Box 1.5).

Box 1.5

Using crises to improve health planning

The 2014-15 Ebola Virus Disease (EVD) outbreak in West Africa exposed significant gaps in the health systems of the affected countries. Prior to that period, Sierra Leone had embarked on a series of efforts to improve national health planning: the National Health Sector Strategic Plan 2010-2015, which provided the overarching framework for informing the strategic orientations of the country; the Joint Programme of Work and Funding 2012-2014, which aligned interventions to key sector priorities; the Basic Package of Essential Health Services 2010-2015, which provided the platform for guiding delivery of health services and a Results and Accountability Framework 2010-2015, which articulated the monitoring and evaluation requirements to support health services management. With the EVD epidemic, the implementation of many of these measures was hindered. However, the post-Ebola environment has provided a fertile ground for improved national health planning, incorporating the lessons learnt from the past as well as during the outbreak to enhance the health and well-being of the population. The Government of Sierra Leone, with support from partners, has identified a series of targeted, prioritized interventions across all sectors to revitalize the country. In health, this has meant a sustained effort in the 6-9 month period following Ebola to tackle patient safety and revive essential services, while in the medium term 10-24 months, there have been identified key result areas to reduce maternal and child mortality, maintain a 'resilient zero' – i.e. no new cases of Ebola, and provide care to EVD survivors. These prioritized interventions have enabled the Government and partners to rationalize limited resources, allowing for focused planning, budgeting and monitoring.

Similarly, the lessons from Tunisia illustrate the impetus crises can provide to strengthen planning processes. During the post-revolution period, in 2012, the Government launched a "societal dialogue", which was instrumental in providing the basis for sector's health priorities.[IV]

These two experiences – from Sierra Leone and Tunisia – highlight the growing recognition by countries to move towards innovative ways of better planning for health, particularly, as they emerge from challenging situations.

IV For more information, please see chapter 2 "Population consultation on needs and expectations" in this handbook

1.2.4 Different contexts, different countries, different strategies for strengthening a health system

In national planning and policy dialogue, context is of prime importance and thus blueprint approaches are unlikely to provide sufficient support. Fortunately, enough knowledge has been accumulated to identify good practice elements. Experience shows that the policy dialogue for building comprehensive NHPSPs is as much a political process as a technical one. The balance between vision and policy, and operational detail and implementation arrangements, varies considerably from country to country, as well as within the same country over time.

Context is of prime importance in national planning and policy dialogue.

Some countries are more advanced in the process, while others are still facing fatal gaps that need to be addressed in order to improve population health. The way systems are strengthened will be different in every country context, and subsequently reflected as such in each NHPSP. WHO has categorized three broad country contexts from the specific vantage point of strengthening health systems as a means to achieve UHC (see Fig. 1.4).

These are further described below, and are pertinent with regard to the NHPSP content.

1. Strategy 1: "F": Strengthening health systems **foundations** in least-developed and fragile countries with poor health system performance and negligible fiscal space to increase public spending on health.

2. Strategy 2: "I": Strengthening health systems **institutions** in least-developed countries where the health system foundations are in place.

3. Strategy 3: "T": Supporting health systems **transformation** in countries with mature health systems where reaching UHC and health security is still challenging.

Fig. 1.4 Health systems contexts and the WHO FIT strategies[16]

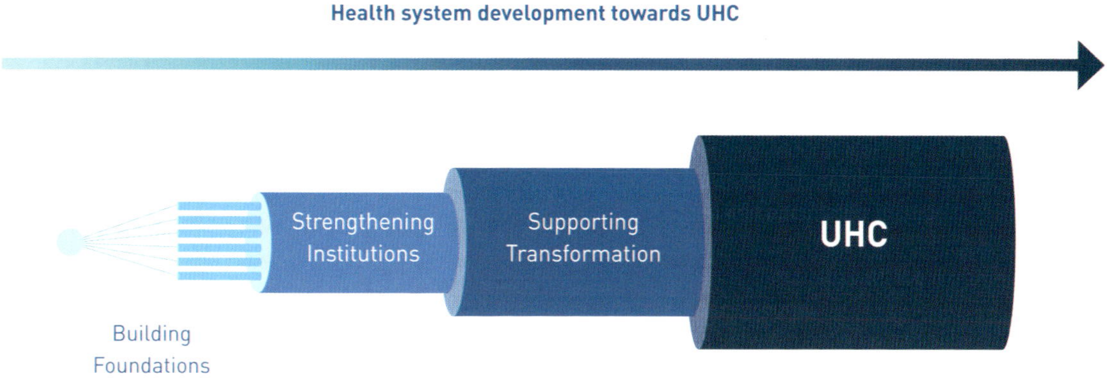

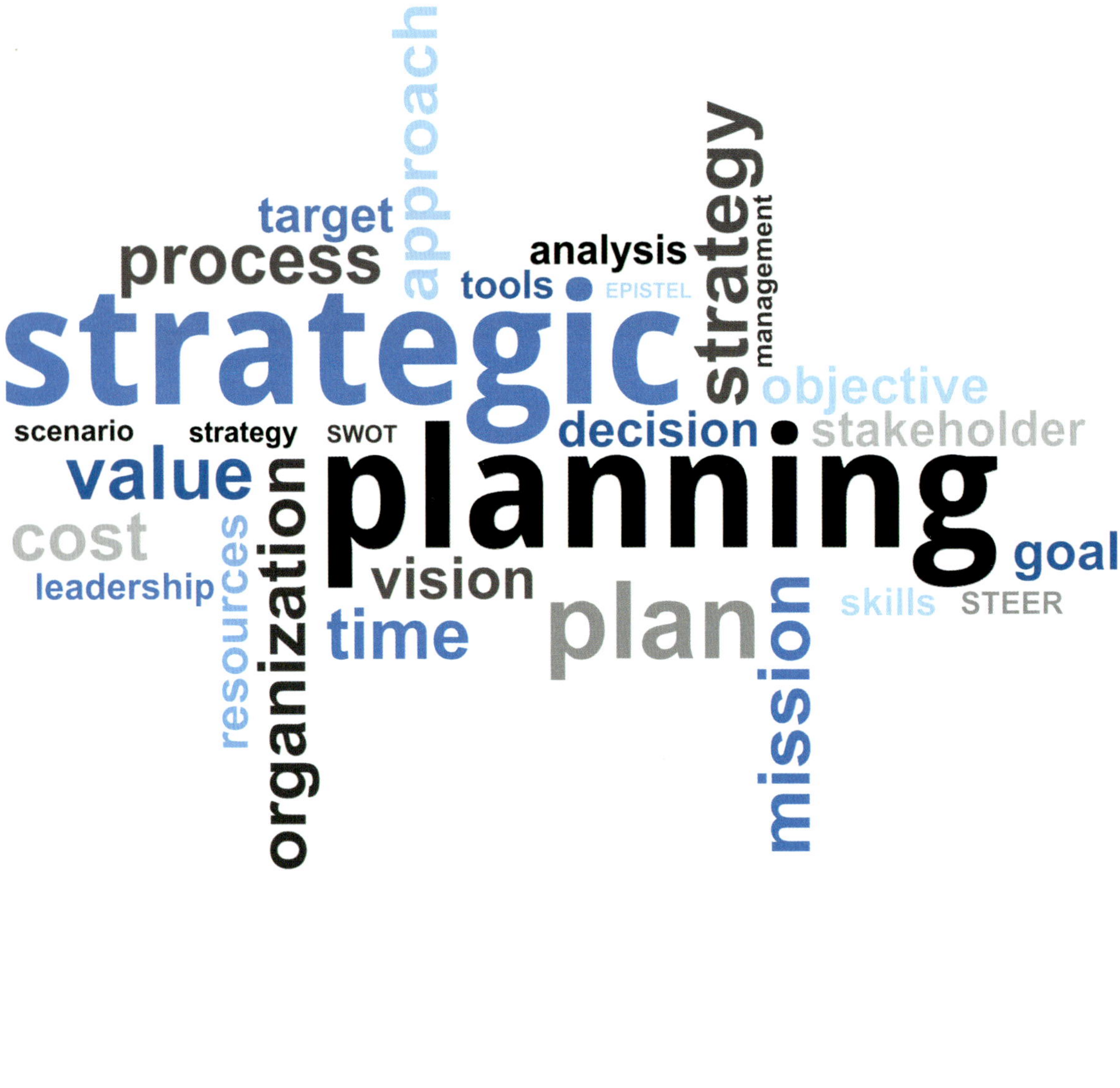
approach
target
process
analysis
tools
EPISTEL
strategy
management
strategic
objective
scenario
strategy
SWOT
decision
stakeholder
value
planning
cost
goal
leadership
resources
organization
vision
time
plan
mission
skills
STEER

1.3 NHPSPs in the 21st century

1.3.1 Good practice for the development of robust NHPSPs

The various contextual factors summarized above have translated into a renewed focus on strengthening countries' capacity to strategize their health and develop robust, efficient, evidence-informed NHPSPs that can:

- respond to growing calls for strengthening health systems as a means towards achieving UHC;
- guide and steer the entire pluralist health sector rather than being limited to command-and-control plans for the public sector alone;
- go beyond the boundaries of health systems, addressing the social determinants of health and the interaction between the health sector and other sectors in society;
- be used as the key element for governmental negotiations regarding fiscal space and budget execution;
- be used, mainly in countries with "foundational" problems, where external aid plays a significant role, as the key element to improve development effectiveness.

The current context favours getting more value from NHPSPs, with a growing expectation that they will be informed by a realistic assessment of capacities and a bold vision of the future, with much more emphasis on stakeholder accountability. In addition, in a globalized world, expectations are growing that NHPSPs will support the development of resilient health systems leading to more security, more equity and more health.

Based on this, elements of good practice for developing robust national health policies, strategies and plans are outlined below.[17]

A robust, efficient, evidence-informed NHPSP should be able to guide and steer the entire pluralist health sector, and form a key element for fiscal space and budget negotiations in government.

(a) UHC as an overarching vision

While UHC is generally accepted as an overall objective to strive for, in practice this means that all debates and discussion take place with the following in mind:

- ensuring coverage of the population – leaving no one behind;
- ensuring financial health protection and avoiding catastrophic expenditures;
- providing a comprehensive package of high-quality integrated and people-centred health services (see Box 1.6).

Box 1.6

Framework on integrated people-centred health services

Globally more than 400 million people lack access to essential health care. Longer lifespans and the growing burden of long-term chronic conditions requiring complex interventions over many years are also changing the demands on health systems.

Adopted by Member States at the World Health Assembly in May 2016, the Framework on integrated people-centred health services (IPCHS) aims to address these issues by calling for a fundamental shift in the way health services are funded, managed and delivered. The Framework presents a compelling vision of a future in which all people have access to health services that are provided in a way that is coordinated around their needs, respects their preferences, and is safe, effective, timely, affordable, and of acceptable quality. It proposes five interdependent strategies:

1. empowering and engaging people and communities;
2. strengthening governance and accountability;
3. reorienting the model of care;
4. coordinating services within and across sectors; and
5. creating an enabling environment.

Developed as a universal vision – the Framework can be adapted to all countries whether high-, medium- or low-income, with mature or fragile health systems.

Related links:
WHO Website on IPCHS:
http://www.who.int/servicedeliverysafety/areas/people-centred-care/en/

Integratedcare4people web platform:
http://www.integratedcare4people.org

Box 1.7

The International Health Regulations

The International Health Regulations (IHR (2005)) represent a binding international legal agreement involving 196 countries, including all the Member States of WHO. The purpose and scope of the IHR (2005) is to prevent, protect against, control and provide a public health response to the international spread of disease in ways that are commensurate with and restricted to public health risks, and which avoid unnecessary interference with international traffic and trade.

The IHR (2005), which entered into force on 15 June 2007, establish the procedures that WHO and States Parties must follow to uphold global public health security. Under the IHR (2005), States Parties are required to assess and notify to WHO public health events that may constitute a public health emergency of international concern, on the basis of defined criteria, which include the seriousness of the event, its unusual or unexpected features, the risk of its international spread and the risk of international travel or trade restrictions. WHO is obliged to request verification of events that it detects through its surveillance activities with the countries concerned, who must respond to such requests in a timely manner. Notifications and information are communicated by a National IHR Focal Point to a WHO IHR Contact Point which, together, establish a unique and effective communications network between countries and with WHO. States Parties are further required to ensure that their national health surveillance and response capacities meet certain functional criteria, and to report annually to the World Health Assembly on the implementation of the IHR.

Building synergies between IHR core capacities, strengthening health systems and essential public health functions is key to ensure a coordinated and effective response to global public health threats.

WHO website on IHR: http://www.who.int/topics/international_health_regulations/en/

(b) The international context

An NHPSP should be compliant with the International Health Regulations[18] (Box 1.7), the Global Framework Convention on Tobacco Control[19] as well as other WHO recommendations or UN resolutions.

One recent example is the United Nations Secretary-General's 2016 High-Level Commission on Health Employment and Economic Growth (see Box 1.8); the co-chairs, French President Francois Hollande and South African President

Box 1.8

High-Level Commission on Health Employment and Economic Growth

The High-Level Commission on Health Employment and Economic Growth was launched by the UN Secretary-General in March 2016 with the aim of stimulating and guiding the creation of 40 million new jobs in the health and social sector, and to reduce the projected shortfall of 18 million health workers, primarily in low- and lower-middle income countries, by 2030. The Commission, chaired by the Presidents of France and South Africa, submitted its report *Working for health and growth: Investing in the health workforce* to the UN Secretary-General on 20 September 2016. The Commission is a strategic political initiative that lends momentum to implementation of the WHO Global Strategy on Human Resources for Health: Workforce 2030.

The Commission's vision is an expanded, transformed and sustainable health workforce that will deliver benefits across the Sustainable Development Goals (e.g. poverty elimination, good health and well-being, quality education, gender equality, and decent work and economic growth). The Commission proposes six recommendations to transform the global health workforce to address SDG needs, focusing on the following areas: job creation, gender equality, education training and competencies, health service delivery and organization, technology, and crisis and humanitarian settings. An additional four recommendations, in the areas of financial and fiscal space, partnerships, international migration, and data, information and accountability, are presented as enabling factors for this transformation.

Stressing the urgency for action, the Commission identifies five immediate actions to be taken between October 2016 and March 2018, aligned with national, regional and global processes. These include accelerated actions on technical and vocational education and training, labour mobility, national health workforce accounts, and enhanced accountability. Moreover, ILO, OECD, and WHO, the Vice-Chairs of the Commission, are tasked with bringing together relevant stakeholders by the end of 2016 to develop a five-year implementation plan to give effect to the Commission's ten recommendations. All stakeholders are invited to integrate the Commission's recommendations in their national, regional and international plans.

WHO website on the Commission: http://www.who.int/hrh/com-heeg/en/

Jacob Zuma, in their speech to the UN General Assembly in September 2016, invited "all stakeholders to join ... in implementing ... [the] ten recommendations [of the Commission's final report] and to integrate these in their national, regional and international plans. We need to align our efforts with other related plans if we are to achieve the Sustainable Development Goals."

(c) Comprehensive, balanced and coherent NHPSP content

The emphasis given to policy, strategy formulation and planning must be based on a broad and inclusive consultation on what affects the health sector, in order to ensure balanced and coherent choices of what to address and what not to address in the given context. The following range of elements and structures deserve consideration.

- A comprehensive analysis should be undertaken of current and future challenges in the health sector, ideally covering: stakeholder positions; social determinants of health and health needs; demand for services and social expectations; health system performance and shortfalls, including the system's ability to respond and anticipate.
- NHPSP content should be well-balanced in terms of finances and inputs, as well as depth of analysis on the principal health issues of the country. In other words, each strategic direction needs to be developed with the same level of detail as the others, and with a level of resources that rightly corresponds to its extent and scope. On finances, this implies that the resources and costs necessary to implement the NHPSP is reasonable and within the given fiscal space for health.
- Coherence should be assured with: other sectors and the national development plan; with programme-specific or sub-sector plans; with the epidemiological and socioeconomic context; and with the available current and estimated future resources.
- Scenarios and policy directions should move towards universal coverage, shifting health-care delivery towards integrated people-centred health services,[20] protecting and promoting the health of communities and building capacity to deal with future challenges.
- Intersectoral mindset should be fostered, implying that governments and other stakeholders proactively address the determinants for health inequities by identifying and promoting intersectoral action as an integral and vital component of the national health planning process.
- The associated costs and resource mobilization implications should be carefully considered.
- Attention should be devoted to the leadership and governance arrangements for implementing the strategy in terms of the role of various institutions and stakeholders, regulatory and legal frameworks to ensure sustainability, working with other sectors, dealing with the donor community and monitoring performance.

Policy formulation must be based on broad and inclusive consultation in order to ensure balanced and coherent choices of what to address by priority in the given context.

(d) Sound process

As explained in Box 1.3, policy dialogue is more likely to lead to better results, such as improved service delivery and better outcomes, if it is inclusive of all relevant social, technical and political stakeholders in and beyond the health sector. The quality of the process of policy dialogue is crucial to formulating the goals, values and overall policy directions that will guide strategy formulation, planning and decision-making. The process must support consensus building at different stages of the planning process, including situation analysis, priority-setting, NHPSP design, implementation and review. A sound process encompasses mechanisms for obtaining feedback on implementation, and initiating corrective measures, as well as high-level endorsement of these policy directions. Smart timing is crucial for alignment with broader development frameworks and country political and institutional cycles.

(e) Realism

NHPSPs are more likely to be implemented if they are realistic and compatible with the health sector's capacities, resources and constraints. They are more likely to lead to sustained results if political commitment and policy directions are translated into legal frameworks. They are more likely to be effective if the link between strategic and operational planning is sufficiently flexible to allow for adaptation to unforeseen economic, political and health events. Finally, greater commitment is likely to be achieved if the concerns of the people who are at the forefront of implementation are adequately reflected.

(f) Linkage with operational plans

NHPSPs must be linked to regional or district-level operational plans.

NHPSPs must be linked to regional or district-level operational plans. The extent of linkage depends on the level of detail in the NHPSP and the degree of autonomy at decentralized level. Some countries choose a more centralized approach with explicit, tight links between the national and sub-national plans; the advantage is coherence between the plans at different levels, but this may be at the price of being overly controlling and insufficiently adaptable to context. Other countries opt for a more decentralized approach leaving much more freedom of interpretation at decentralized levels; this allows for flexibility and creativity, but may affect coherence. Many countries link the national strategic plan with operational plans through rolling medium-term plans and expenditure frameworks.

(g) Linkage with programmes

The extent to which NHPSPs address the concerns and operational plans of the country's disease-specific or life-cycle programmes varies greatly. In many countries the disconnect to the NHPSP leads to imbalance or lack of coherence between health sector planning efforts and subsequent problems in implementation. The causes are complex and include: (i) inadequate situation analysis and priority-setting; (ii) the programme's operational planning is often conducted in a different arena, with different constituencies and with different planning cycles; and (iii) donors' earmarking of funds, leading to fragmentation, competition for scarce resources, and imbalances in national priority-setting. Balance and coherence can be improved by ensuring realistic assessments of how programmes can draw on shared resources and capacities, and of the impact they will have on these shared resources and capacities, and by adequate reflection of programme concerns in the comprehensive NHPSP. Ideally, the integration of programmes in the national planning need to be fully harmonized and aligned, as expressed in Fig. 1.5.

Fig. 1.5 Integration of programmes in NHPSPs

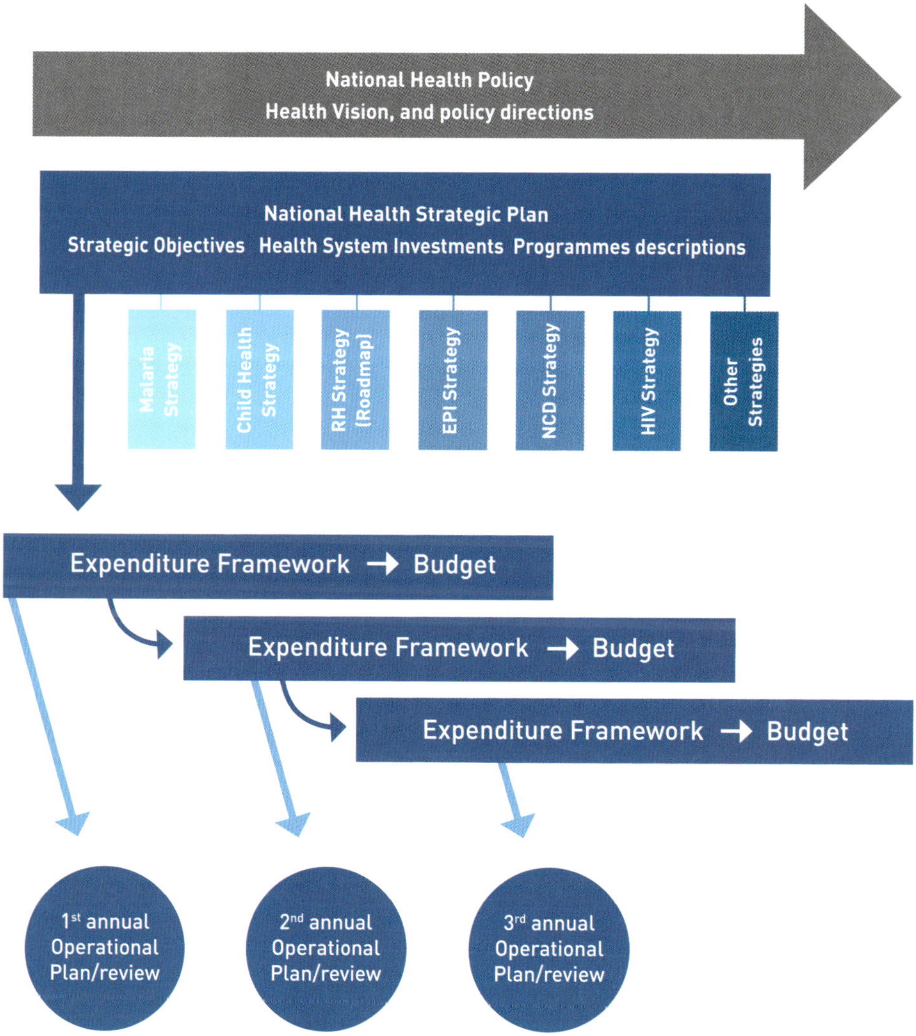

(h) Linkage with the political agenda

The policies, strategies and plans for the health sector have major political and budgetary implications, well beyond their direct implications for the public sector. Eventually they have to be endorsed as part of the government programme. As health takes increasing political space in how

Box 1.9

Health Data Collaborative

The Health Data Collaborative (HDC), launched in March 2016, is an inclusive partnership of international agencies, governments, philanthropies, donors and academics, with the common aim of improving health data. The approach is to ensure that different stakeholders in national, regional and global health are able to work together more effectively to make better use of resources, and by doing so help to accelerate impact of investments and improvements in country health information systems. The Health Data Collaborative aims to put the IHP+ principles of country ownership and alignment into practice by translating them into a joint operational plan that specifies concrete collective actions at country and global levels.

The work of the Collaborative is facilitated by a small core team hosted within WHO with dedicated focal points within key partner institutions.

One of the first countries where this is being operationalized is Kenya. In to support of the health ministry's leadership in integrating monitoring and evaluation (M&E) systems into a unified, more efficient framework, global health partners are now working together to harmonize their financial and technical resources to ensure they are in line with country priorities.[V] During a four-day meeting in Nairobi in May 2016, various stakeholders signed a joint statement of commitments to support a unified "One M&E Framework" and launch the Kenya Health Data Collaborative.

The MoH has drafted a detailed costed roadmap to be implemented by technical working groups focused on data analytics, quality of care, a new national health data observatory, civil registration and vital statistics, and informatics. This collaborative approach is expected to strengthen Kenya's health information system through a united front supporting and investing in one national M&E plan.

HDC Website:
http://www.healthdatacollaborative.org/

HEALTH DATA COLLABORATIVE
DATA FOR HEALTH AND SUSTAINABLE DEVELOPMENT

V Please see chapter 9 "Monitoring, evaluation and review of national health policies, strategies and plans' in this handbook

countries view their future, the legitimacy of, and political commitment to, the sector's policies, strategies and plans depends on integration with the broader national development dialogue. In order for arguments to carry the most weight, they need to make the linkage by insisting on the role of health as a factor of development, rather than relying solely on statements about expected health benefits.

(i) Strong accountability

Strengthening the institutional base for progress and performance review, information use and accountability is essential. This requires considerably improving the quality of the situation analysis on which policies, strategies and plans are based; bringing coherence and balance to priority-setting; facilitating the adoption of a single country-led monitoring and evaluation framework; facilitating alignment of international partners (see Box 1.9); and ensuring accountability through progress and performance reviews integrated with country planning processes.

(j) Sustainability

Some countries have been striving to develop more inclusive approaches to policy dialogue. However, in most countries, the process remains largely unsystematic. In some cases, this situation is partly due to a high turnover of planners, which constrains the skill base and the institutional memory. In others, this relates to successive waves of externally driven priorities and reform agendas. There is a need to increase the robustness of the process through a combination of: investing in institutional and individual capacities for conducting meaningful policy dialogue; promoting the framework for guiding the policy dialogue process; assisting with better synchronization of planning cycles and better guidelines for programme planning; and helping to broaden the policy dialogue beyond the public sector and to align national health strategies with national development plans and financial policy cycles.

(k) Redefining the role of the Department of Planning, Ministry of Health

In the 21st century, the role and functions of the MoH Department of Planning needs to evolve from a pure planner's role to a planning and brokering role, from a top-down approach to a bottom-up approach and from a monolithic to an inclusive pluralistic approach.

This department must have adequate human resources and budget to fulfill its new role, to enable the regular convening of different stakeholders for a true bottom-up and pluralistic process.

This department must also be well-connected to all modern forms of media to ensure transparency and proper communication to the citizens. Regular communication requires dedicated staff time and a budget as well which must be foreseen. In countries where resources are scarce, this might need additional support from donors.

The EU-Luxembourg-WHO Universal Health Coverage Partnership is an example of a targeted approach to support ministries of health to more smoothly transition to its more modern convening & brokering role (see Box 1.10).

In the 21st century, the role and functions of the MoH Department of Planning needs to evolve from a pure planner's role to a planning and brokering role, from a top-down approach to a bottom-up approach and from a monolithic to an inclusive pluralistic approach.

Box 1.10

EU-Luxembourg-WHO UHC Partnership

The focus on national health planning and universal health coverage has gained momentum on the global agenda during the last few years, leading to more intensified WHO country support for health planning, health financing and policy dialogue.

In 2011-2012 the European Union, the Government of Luxembourg and the World Health Organization entered into a collaborative agreement to support policy dialogue on national health policies, strategies and plans (NHPSP) and UHC.

The Partnership was made operational in 28 countries by 2016, with a diverse and numerous set of activities directly supporting health policy, health financing and effective development cooperation at country level. Seed monies are provided to all countries to actively foster inclusive policy dialogue and ensure a stronger convening and brokering role for ministries of health.

The Partnership is an integral part of WHO's support to countries' endeavours to steer towards UHC, with a lucid recognition that it can only happen if ministries of health take on their new and changing role with confidence. The Partnership provides dedicated WHO Country Office staff to accompany MoH in this ambition, acknowledging that the new MoH role will take time to become the norm.

For example, in Moldova, the WHO Country Office and MoH jointly organized a series of policy dialogue events over the course of 5 years 2012-2016. These events focused on specific topics highly relevant to UHC. The topics were pushed high on the policy agenda through the inclusive dialogue process supported by the Partnership. Examples of some of these topics are: strengthening public health services, performance-related pay and service delivery access.

Currently, the Partnership targets the following countries: Burkina Faso, Burundi, Cape Verde, Chad, Democratic Republic of the Congo, Guinea, Guinea-Bissau, Kyrgyz Republic, Lao PDR, Liberia, Mali, Morocco, Mozambique, Niger, Republic of Moldova, Senegal, Sierra Leone, South Africa, South Sudan, Sudan, Tajikistan, Timor-Leste, Togo, Tunisia, Ukraine, Viet Nam, Yemen, Zambia.

UHC Partnership web site:
www.uhcpartnership.net

1.3.2 Dynamic 21st century process

The renewed interest in using NHPSPs to enhance health sector performance and improve the health and well-being of populations differs substantially from the planning approaches employed in the 1980s and 1990s (see Fig. 1.6). Indeed, the poor performance of health systems in many countries, as well as the rising expectations of citizens regarding their health, are increasingly becoming causes of political concern, which in many countries lead to reforms to put in place integrated and people-centered health services, UHC and health in all policies.

That being said, this handbook advocates for a final element of good practice: moving away from a command and control planning process towards a process focused on dialogue and debate (Fig. 1.7), and from a more static planning cycle mainly owned by department of planning of the ministry of health towards a dynamic, flexible, open and pluralist planning process towards UHC, owned by the community of stakeholders.

This handbook advocates for a planning process focused on dialogue and debate which is dynamic, flexible, open and pluralist.

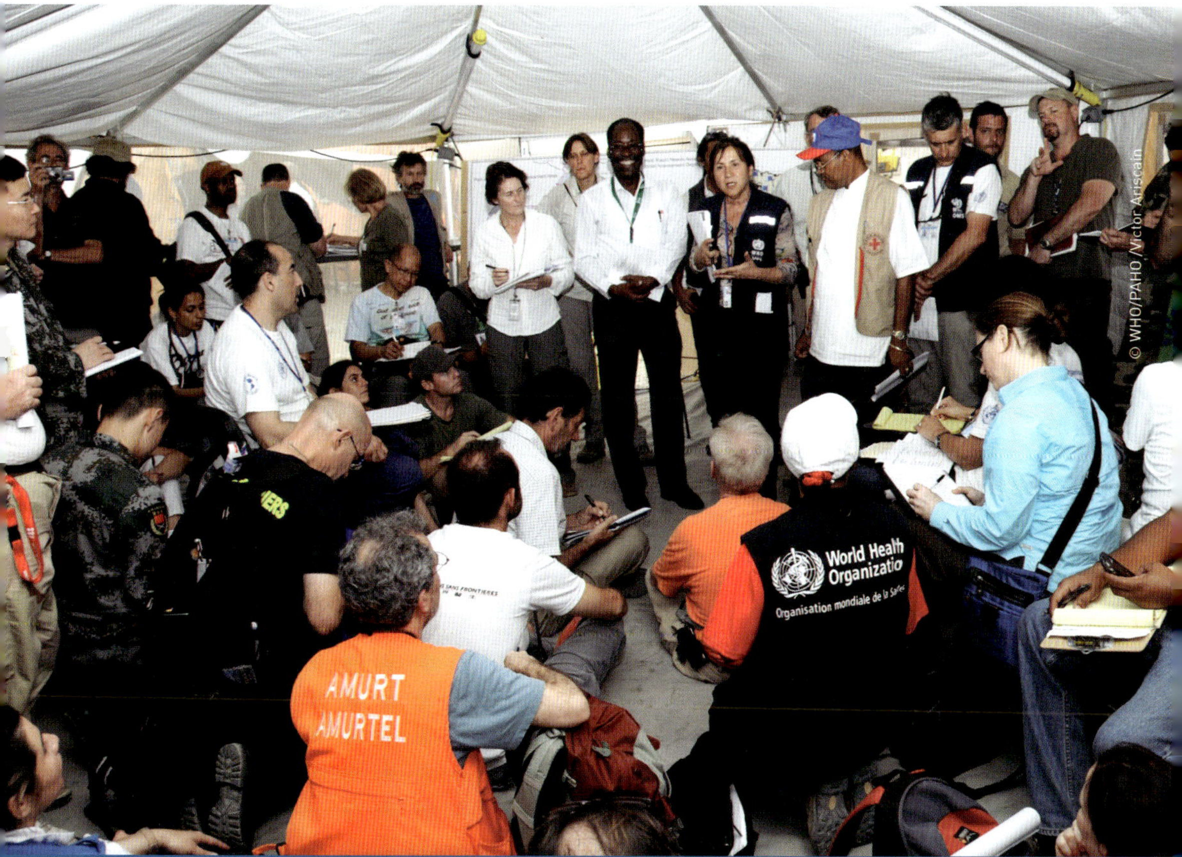

Fig. 1.6 1980s and 90s technocratic planning process

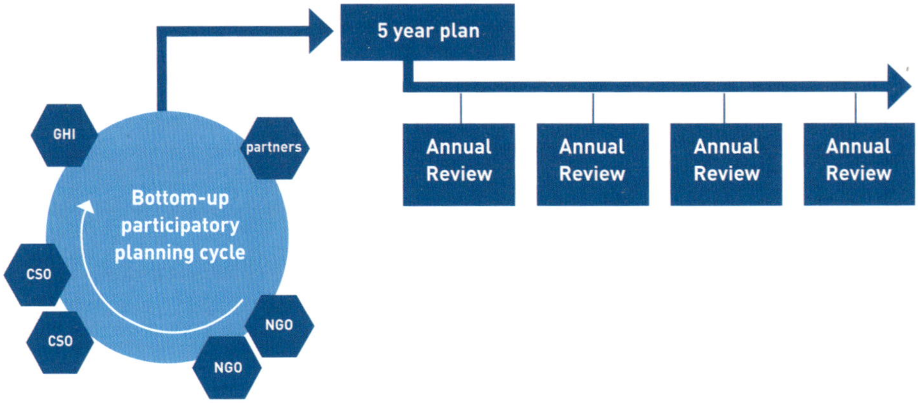

Fig. 1.7 A dynamic policy dialogue-led process

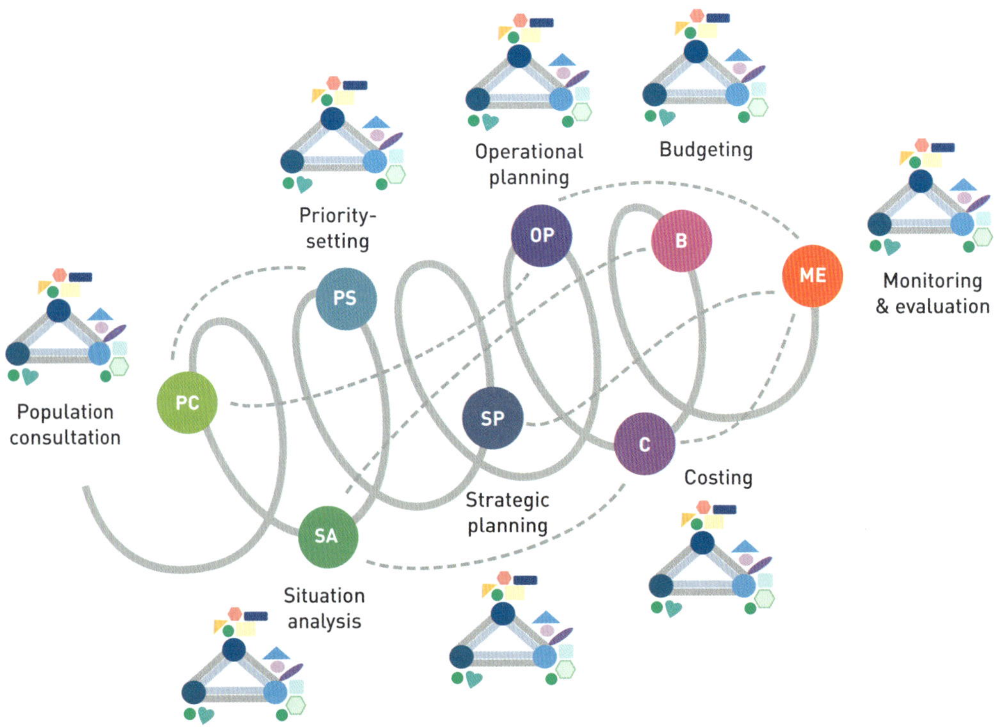

1.4 The handbook scope and content

1.4.1 Scope

The handbook covers the main steps of a **national health plan**, defined for the purposes of this book as a medium-term national strategic plan of approximately 3–7 years. The handbook is not intended to serve as a classical technical planning textbook, but rather seeks to capture the **innovative realities** of national planning at the country level, taking into account the **policy dialogue process** in ensuring the success of the plan. It takes the health plan as a living, dynamic document, with all its associated sub-plans, that guides overall strategic reforms in a country rather than as a static, monolithic paper.

Furthermore, the handbook provides a concrete, **practical** picture of the different aspects of planning and develops on existing work, literature reviews and country experiences. By building on **multisectoral** participatory approaches, while covering all the key elements of national health planning, the handbook links the conceptual with the pragmatic – thereby, for the first time, consolidating essential guidance to countries in one place. It emphasizes the role of democratic structures and the importance of political will, while reflecting the significance of international legally binding treaties.

Lastly, recognizing the prominence of vertical disease programmes and global health initiatives in certain settings, the handbook gives feasible advice in tackling such issues, drawing on country case studies.

The target audience of the present handbook is health ministries and other relevant stakeholders involved in national health planning.

This handbook links the conceptual with the pragmatic by building on multisectoral participatory approaches, consolidating essential guidance to countries in one place.

1.4.2 Content

Although national health planning is often viewed as linear or cyclic in nature, in reality, it is a complicated, difficult, challenging process (as illustrated in Fig. 1.8). Therefore, the handbook can be read in its entirety, but each chapter is also stand-alone, so it can be easily understood and used by relevant stakeholders. There is a clear conducting line among the chapters, with the main concepts reinforced.

Fig. 1.8 National health planning in action

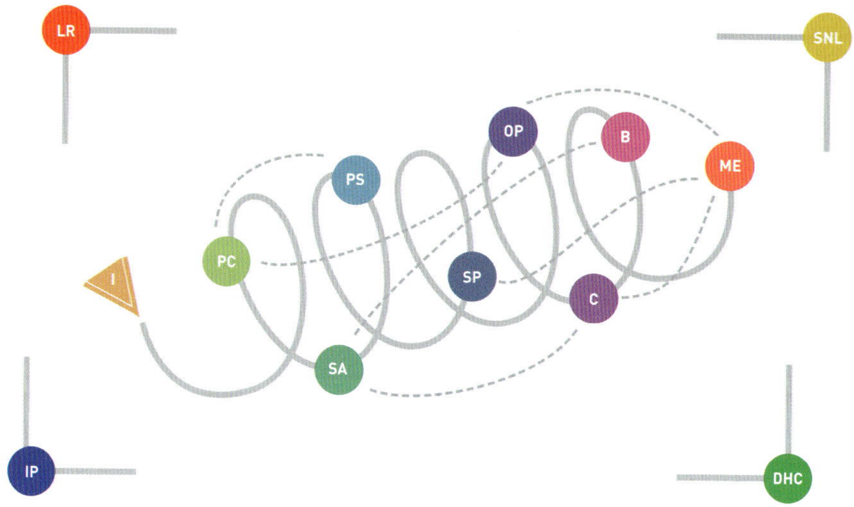

In Chapter 2 "Population consultation on needs and expectations **(PC)**", Rohrer and Rajan make a strong case for including citizens' voices in planning processes, providing concrete ways in which people can be engaged during the development of a national health plan. The chapter outlines the aims of a population consultation, its specific added value to national health planning, and how to undertake a consultation from the methodological and conceptual perspectives.

In Chapter 3 "Situation analysis of the health sector **(SA)**", Rajan emphasizes the comprehensive nature of undertaking a detailed health sector assessment, taking into account different methodological options while ensuring broad stakeholder input. The latter is especially highlighted, since a balanced analysis will include technical analysis as well as opinions, viewpoints and experiences of health system users.

Similarly, in Chapter 4 "Priority-setting for national health policies, strategies and plans **(PS)**", Terwindt, Rajan and Soucat guide the reader through the critical choices that must be made to determine the strategic directions of the national health plan. Priority-setting being a shared responsibility between the MoH and the entire health stakeholder community, a case is made for a structured and inclusive exercise elaborated upon in the chapter.

In Chapter 5 "Strategic planning: transforming priorities into plans **(SP)**", Terwindt and Rajan provide guidance on developing a relevant NHPSP that is referred to, consulted and used. Steps are proposed to manage the NHPSP development process, and common challenges and mistakes are pointed out with suggested solutions.

This leads to "Operational planning: transforming plans into action **(OP)**", Chapter 6, by Shuey, Bigdeli and Rajan, where implementation issues linked to strategic planning are explored. They make the case that operational plans should not be under the sole remit of professional planners or managers. The best operational plans, and certainly the ones most likely to be implemented, are those that are developed with the people who will carry them out.

In Chapter 7 "Estimating cost implications of a national health policy, strategy or plan **(C)**", Stenberg and Rajan provide guidance on costing options for a NHPSP. They advocate for a process of estimating costs as a crucial step within the NHPSP formulation process, as it allows decision-makers to consider the extent to which policy objectives and strategic orientations are feasible and affordable.

In Chapter 8 "Budgeting for health **(B)**", Rajan, Barroy and Stenberg examine health budgets, national budgeting processes and fiscal space for health. This chapter discusses the specific role of the MoH and other health sector stakeholders within the budgeting process and examines how they can provide timely inputs.

The main "cycle" of national health planning concludes with Chapter 9 "Monitoring, evaluation and review of national health policies, strategies and plans **(ME)**" by O'Neill, Viswanathan, Celades and Boerma. This chapter outlines how monitoring, evaluation and review require an integrated approach that builds on a single country-led monitoring and evaluation platform.

In addition, four cross-cutting chapters provide guidance on critical issues that influence all stages of national health planning.

In Chapter 10 "Laws, regulation and strategizing for health **(LR)**", Clarke explores how regulation represents a key means by which a government gives effect to its health policy preferences, especially through the exercise of a government's law-making powers.

Given the significance of sub-national structures and functions in health planning, Rohrer unpacks the key elements of "Strategizing for health at sub-national level **(SNL)**" in Chapter 11, going through each step in the health policy and planning cycle. The chapter aims at supporting policy-makers with specific recommendations strategizing for health in a decentralized system.

Blas, Roebbel, Rajan and Valentine tackle the work across sectors to address health determinants in Chapter 12 "Intersectoral planning for health and health equity **(IP)**". They outline the need and practical action for including intersectoral planning for health and health equity as a mindset within the overall process of strategizing for health.

Finally, in Chapter 13 "Strategizing in distressed health contexts **(DHC)**", Pavignani and Colombo consider the challenges posed by policy and strategy formulation in health systems under stress, highlighting the main differences with these processes in more stable environments.

The chapters contain country illustrations throughout the document along with, where relevant, annexes on relevant tools, documents and references.

References

1 See resolution WHA62.12, Primary health care, including health system strengthening (http://www.who.int/hrh/resources/A62_12_EN.pdf?ua=1, accessed 11 October 2016).

2 Rajan D, Adam T, El Husseiny D, Porignon D, Ghaffar A, Schmets G. Policy dialogue: what it is and how it can contribute to evidence-informed decision-making. Geneva: WHO; 2015 (Briefing Note; https://www.researchgate.net/publication/297698707, accessed 11 October 2016).

3 Nabyonga-Orem J, Dovlo D, Kwamie A, Nadege A, Guangya W, Kirigia JM. Policy dialogue to improve health outcomes in low income countries: what are the issues and way forward? BMC Health Serv Res. 2016;16(4):217 (https://www.ncbi.nlm.nih.gov/pmc/articles/PMC4959394/, accessed 11 October 2016).

4 Dovlo D, Nabyonga-Orem J, Estrella Y, Mwisongo A. Policy dialogues: the "bolts and joints" of policy-making: experiences from Cabo Verde, Chad and Mali. BMC Health Serv Res. 2016;16(4):216 (https://www.ncbi.nlm.nih.gov/pmc/articles/PMC4959380/, accessed 11 October 2016).

5 Universal health coverage. In: Health systems (website). Geneva: WHO; 2016 (http://www.who.int/healthsystems/ universal_health_coverage/en/, accessed 11 September 2016).

6 World Health Report 2010, (http://www.who.int/whr/2010/en/, accessed 11 September 2016).

7 Health Systems Strengthening Glossary G-H. In: Health systems (website). Geneva: WHO; 2016 (http://www.who.int/healthsystems/hss_glossary/en/index5.html, accessed 11 September 2016).

8 Taskforce on Innovative International Financing for Health Systems. Constraints to scaling up and costs: working group 1 report. Geneva: International Health Partnership; 2009 (http://www.internationalhealthpartnership.net/fileadmin/uploads/ihp/Documents/Results___Evidence/HAE__results___lessons/Working%20Group%201%20Technical%20Background%20Report%20%28World%20Health%20Organization%29.pdf, accessed 11 October 2016).

9 Flows of global health financing. Seattle (WA): Institute for Health Metrics and Evaluation; 2015 (http://vizhub.healthdata.org/fgh/, accessed 11 October 2016).

10 United Nations General Assembly. Resolution 69/313. Addis Ababa Action Agenda of the third international conference on financing for development. 27 July 2015 (http://www.un.org/en/ga/search/view_doc.asp?symbol=A/RES/69/313, accessed 11 October 2016).

11 Global health expenditure database (GHED). [online database] Geneva: WHO; 2016 (http://apps.who.int/nha/database, accessed 11 October 2016).

12 Public financing for health in Africa: from Abuja to the SDGs. Geneva: World Health Organization; 2016 (Health Financing toward UHC; http://www.who.int/health_financing/documents/public-financing-africa/en/, accessed 11 October 2016).

13 Rajan D, Adam T, El Husseiny D, Porignon D, Ghaffar A, Schmets G. Briefing Note: Policy dialogue: What it is and how it can contribute to evidence-informed decision-making. Geneva: World Health Organization; 2015 (Briefing Note; https://www.researchgate.net/publication/297698707, accessed 11 October 2016).

14 Original design, adapted from World Development Report 2004: Making services work for poor people. World Bank; 2004. and Brinkerhoff D, Bossert T. Governance: concepts, experience and program options. Bethesda: Health Systems 20/20 Project; 2008.

15 adapted by Bigdeli M and Clarke D, from World Development Report 2004: Making services work for poor people. World Bank; 2004. and Brinkerhoff D, Bossert T. Governance: concepts, experience and program options. Bethesda: Health Systems 20/20 Project; 2008.

16 Foundations Institutions Transformation. World Health Organization; 2016.

17 Health systems strengthening: improving support to policy dialogue around national health policies, strategies and plans: report by the Secretariat to the Sixty-fourth World Health Assembly. Geneva: WHO; 2011 (Document A64/12; http://apps.who.int/gb/ebwha/pdf_files/WHA64/A64_12-en.pdf, accessed 12 October 2016).

18 International Health Regulations (2005), Second Edition. Geneva: WHO; 2008 (http://www.who.int/ihr/publications/9789241596664/en/, accessed 11 October 2016).

19 WHO Framework Convention on Tobacco Control. Geneva: WHO; 2005 (http://www.who.int/fctc/en/, accessed 11 October 2016).

20 Framework on integrated, people-centred health services: report by the Secretariat. Sixty-ninth World Health Assembly. Geneva: WHO; 2016 (Document A69/39; http://apps.who.int/gb/ebwha/pdf_files/WHA69/A69_39-en.pdf?ua=1, accessed 12 October 2016).

Chapter 2

Population consultation on needs and expectations

Katja Rohrer
Dheepa Rajan

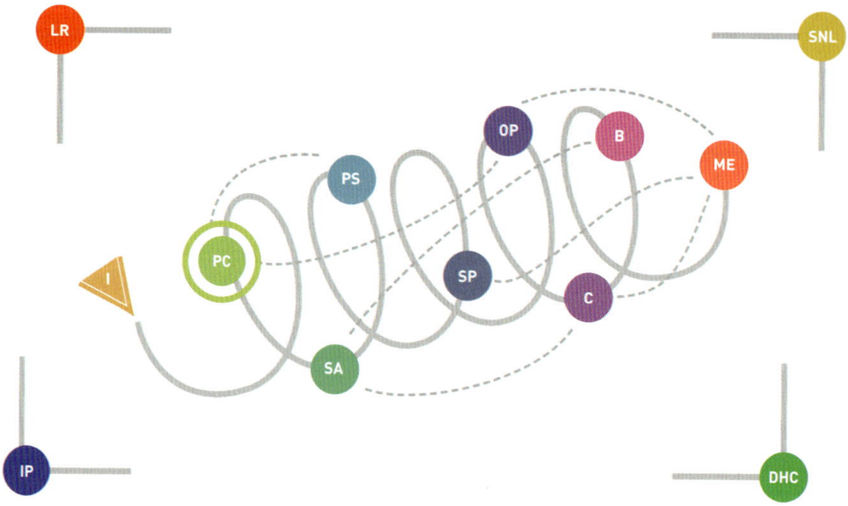

Cross-cutting topics relevant to national health planning

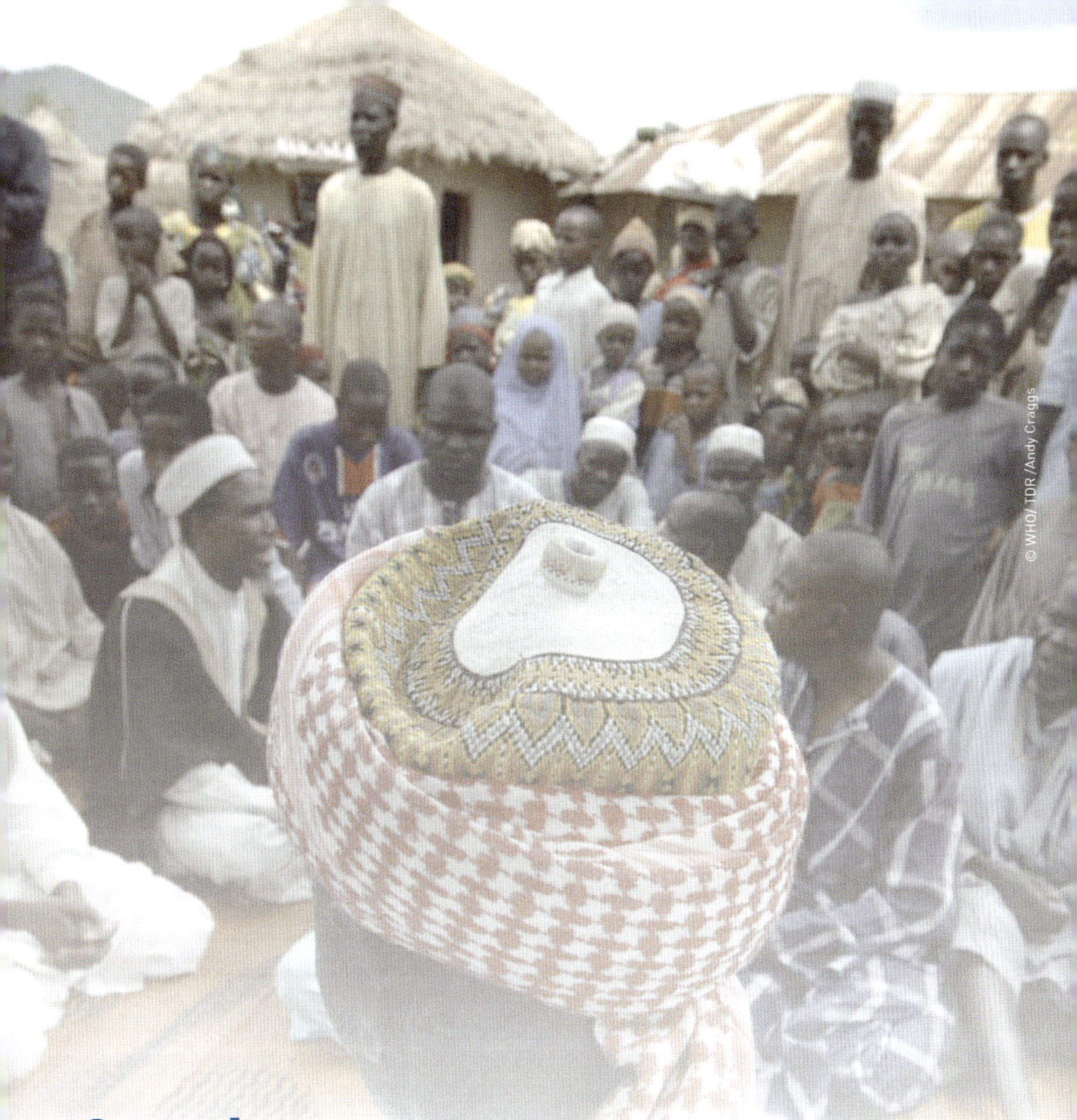

© WHO/ TDR /Andy Craggs

Overview

This chapter outlines the aims of a population consult ation, its contribution to national health planning, and how to undertake a consultation from the methodological and conceptual perspectives.

Summary

What is the purpose of a population consultation?

It is to capture the population's demands, opinions and expectations on health-related matters, in order to improve policy responses.

Why is it important?

The reasons a population consultation is important are:

- to obtain feedback from the population on the current health situation and proposed reforms will enlarge the information base for health policy-making;
- to increase consultation with the ownership and engagement of the population – especially marginalized groups – and to transform the population into active stakeholders;
- to provide essential information on the population's opinions and expectations for improved health outcomes;
- to strengthen monitoring and evaluation;
- to strengthen government policy decisions and resource allocation;
- to improve accountability and transparency.

When should a population consultation be done?

A population consultation can be undertaken at any stage of the health planning cycle. Ideally, it should be one of the first steps of the whole process, so the results can feed into the development of a new national health policy or strategy. It can also be done in the middle of the planning cycle to monitor progress or at the end of the policy development process, in order to get the population's opinion on what has been done.

Who could undertake a population consultation or could be engaged in one?

- government departments and ministries;
- independent research institutions and think tanks;
- foundations;
- political parties;
- civil society organizations (CSOs) and non-governmental organizations (NGOs);
- community leaders and community institutions;
- market research institutions;
- media.

How should a population consultation be done?

1. Choose the methodological approach that is suited to the national context:
   - face-to-face dialogue;
   - consultative methods;
   - survey types and survey tools;
   - referendum.

2. Adapt the methodology chosen to your country's circumstances and planning cycle context;

3. Conduct the consultation, and analyse the results;

4. Ensure a sustainable and transparent follow-up to the consultation (develop a road map including the different institutions involved and their roles and responsibilities, processes and follow-up mechanisms).

Anything else to consider?

- decentralized environment;
- fragile environment;
- highly aid-dependent context.

2.1 What do we mean by "capturing population needs and opinions" on health issues?

2.1.1 What is a population consultation?

Based on the varying degrees of involvement of the population, the Organisation for Economic Co-operation and Development (OECD) identifies a spectrum of interaction between the public and government institutions.

Notification: communication of information

Consultation: actively seeking the opinions of interested and affected groups

Participation: active involvement of interest groups in the formulation of regulatory objectives, policies and approaches

Based on the definition of the OECD, we refer to a consultation as:

[...] a two-way flow of information, which may occur at any stage of [the planning process], from problem identification to evaluation of existing regulation. It may be a one-stage process or, as it is increasingly the case, a continuing dialogue. Consultation is increasingly concerned with the objective of gathering information to facilitate the drafting of higher quality regulation.[1]

In line with this definition, the objectives of a population consultation may include:

- to gauge the population's expectations and opinions on health-related matters;
- to get a sense of people's prevailing thoughts of – and experiences with – the health system;
- to facilitate the inclusion of public opinion in decision-making processes, in policy design and in policy implementation modalities;
- to assess possible unintended consequences of policy decisions.

In this handbook, we refer to a population consultation, even when undertaken regularly, as a special event outside any regular interaction between population and policy-makers. It focuses on seeking information directly from interested and affected parts of the population, rather than referring to institutionalized mechanisms of representation (such as elected, selected or appointed individuals) or using institutionalized forms of participation to express opinions (e.g. local health committees[I] or parliamentary health groups). It is also distinct from consultation mechanisms used by advocacy patient groups, where the purpose of the consultation is to seek support for their respective advocacy cause.

Population consultations are designed to gauge the population's expectations and opinions on health-related matters, get a sense of people's thoughts about the health system, include public opinion in the decision-making process, and/or assess possible unintended consequences of policy decisions.

I Health committees are usually seen as the link between the community (or the district) and the health facility or clinic. Depending on the context and the country, they consist of community members, health personnel, community health workers and local government representatives. They usually serve the community (or the district) by informing them and including them in discussions around the provision of health services. See: UNICEF (United Nations Children's Fund). Evaluation report of the community health strategy implementation in Kenya. 2010 (http://www.unicef.org/evaldatabase/files/14_2010_HE_002_Community_Strategy_Evaluation_report_October_2010.pdf, accessed 29 December 2015).

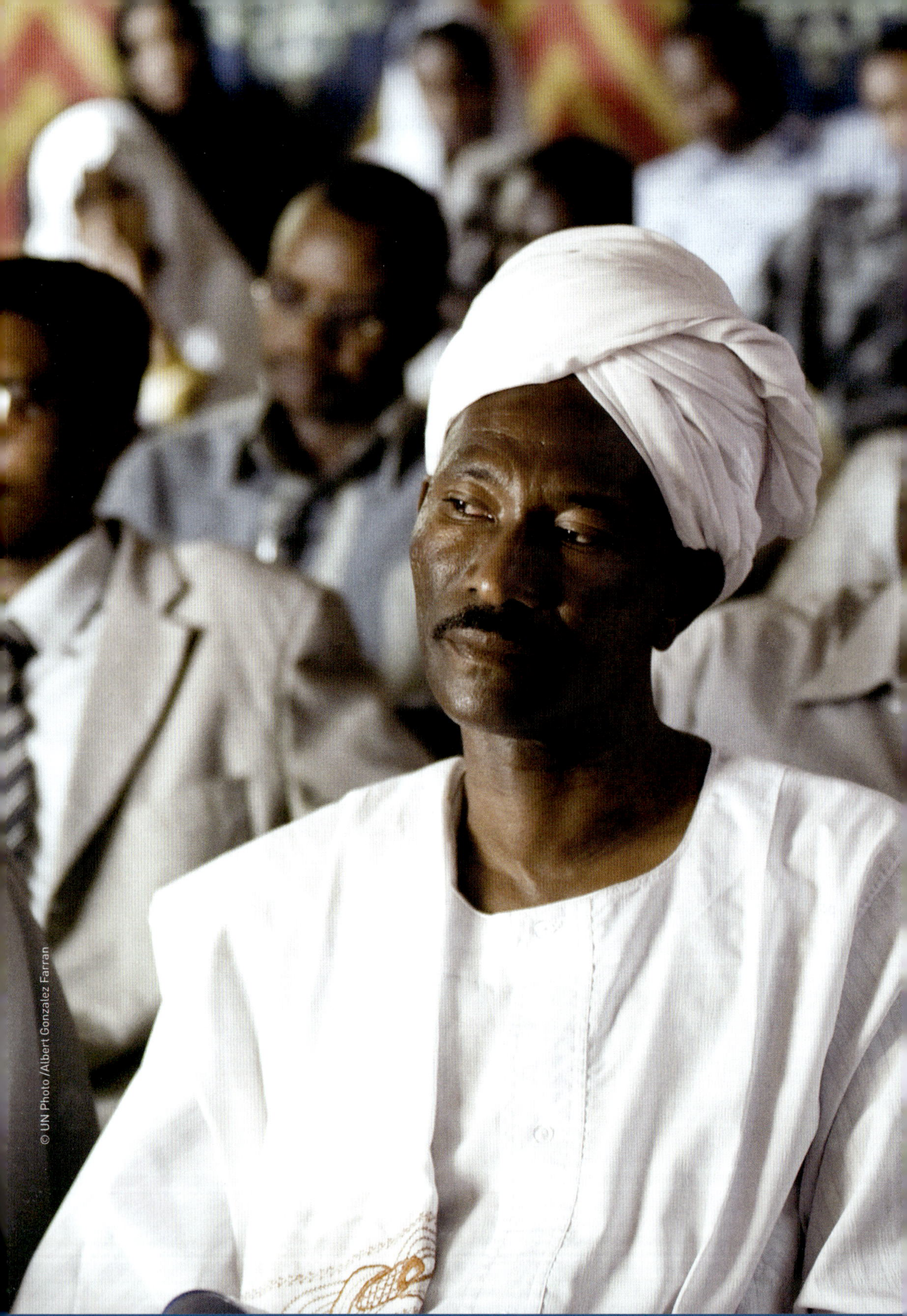

© UN Photo /Albert Gonzalez Farran

2.1.2 The spectrum of population consultation

A population consultation should constitute an essential element of the continuous dialogue between the government, decision-makers, other stakeholders' representatives and the population.

A population consultation can happen:

(a) at any stage of the national planning process;

(b) at any level of the state (national, province/region, district);

(c) on varying themes and scopes, for example:
- service delivery modalities;
- policy design and reform processes;
- implementation and management modalities;
- problems and challenges regarding access to health care;

(d) with all parts of the population or just certain groups, for example:
- social categorization: old, young, vulnerable, income, education;
- geographical categorization: urban, rural, population groups that live in hard-to-reach locations or have been affected by natural disasters or civil unrest.

This list is not exhaustive and there are multiple possibilities for its combination.

When discussing population in this chapter, we are referring to the simple Oxford dictionary (2015 edition) definition of population, meaning "a particular group or type of people living in a place",[2] i.e. country, state or district.

When discussing only certain parts of the population, we will identify and specifically name those (e.g. low-income groups of the population).

However, the term population should not be confounded with civil society, which is the "sphere of social interaction between economy and state, composed above all of the intimate sphere (especially family), the sphere of associations (especially voluntary associations), social movements, and forms of public communications."[3]

Population consultations should be undertaken to improve national health planning processes and increase the responsiveness of the health system to population needs and expectations.

2.2 Why do we want to capture population expectations?

The main motivation for undertaking a population consultation should be to improve national health planning processes and consequently increase the responsiveness of the health system to the needs and expectations of the population. Therefore, the basic questions decision-makers should ask themselves when developing a new strategy or a reform are: Will this policy or reform correspond to the population's expectations? Will it be accepted? Will it be used? How can we ensure population buy-in? This section will consider the different reasons for consulting the population, principally from a policy-maker's perspective.

Consultation and participation are cross-cutting principles enshrined in the human rights-based approach to health.

From an international perspective, consultation and participation are cross-cutting principles embodied in international human rights treaties and are enshrined in the human rights-based approach to health.[4,5] In the long term, a regularly conducted and methodologically sound consultation may serve as an entry point for the establishment of more institutionalized participatory processes.

2.2.1 A key source of information for policy-making

(a) **Governments and ministries of health (MoHs)**, usually have high technical expertise and good technical information and evidence on normative needs. They may, however, have limited knowledge of the expectations and demands of the population they serve. A population consultation allows for better situation assessment and performance improvement.

For example, if a MoH is aware of low coverage rates, a population consultation might provide insights into the challenges some population groups face when trying to access facilities. Those challenges might not lie uniquely within the sphere of the health sector. A consultation might provide a more holistic view of the social and economic burden the population is facing, thus encouraging the MoH to build bridges to other sectors.

(b) **Parliamentary health committees and health groups** are positioned at the interface of legislative and executive powers. They are accountable to the population and heavily involved in possible health reform and decision-making processes. For this group, a population consultation is an essential instrument in the policy dialogue process,[6] providing evidence on the demand side and of people's expectations.

(c) **Political parties** would find an expression of the people's need and demands useful to have it better reflected in political programmes.

(d) **Ministries of finance and planning** will be more inclined to fund a national strategy or reform that demonstrates that it takes into account population opinions, expectations and demand.

2.2.2 An essential component for influencing policy

(a) **Media** generally welcome population consultations, as they indicate transparency and accountability on the part of government.

(b) **Professional (medical and union) associations** represent the health workforce in charge of providing services and implementing national strategies and reforms. For them, consulting the population is key to improving performance, understanding demand and adapting services. It may help them to take appropriate public-health promotion or prevention measures when deemed appropriate (for example, in case of excessive demand for non-essential services).

(c) **Civil society organizations** represent non-profit-making and/or faith-based partners engaged in health service delivery, health promotion, or advocacy programmes and other interventions. For this group, better understanding of people's demands and expectations through sound consultation methods is essential: it brings evidence to the policy dialogue that they are facilitating in many cases,[II] and captures opinions and expectations of disadvantaged population groups for whom they are advocating.

If a consultation has taken place, international partners supporting national health priorities within the framework of International Health Partnership (IHP+)[III] principles of aid effectiveness can better assess if the given national strategies and reforms are in line with population demands and expectations – and where appropriate, can better formulate their own programmes.

2.2.3 Increasing population's ownership

The population is both the recipient of services provided by the health system and the group affected by health policy decisions and health reforms. Engaging in a consultation can help strengthen the voice of the population or of certain population groups (such as marginalized population groups, or people living in remote areas), thus supporting the policy objective of improving health equity. It could enable policy-makers to adjust the services offered, thanks to a better understanding of the population's needs and demands.

It is important for the population to be involved in policy-making as it is both the recipient of services provided by the health system and the group affected by health policy decisions and reforms.

Likewise, it might increase acceptance of policy decisions based on public opinion. Tough reforms or restructuring exercises might be accepted more easily when built on a dialogue between decision-makers, service-providers and service users.[7]

II One example is the role of CSOs in the European Union. The European Commission (EC) has clearly identified them as important stakeholders and facilitators for policy dialogue and actively encourages their involvement in consultation processes (European Commission; 2001; https://www.usaid.gov/evaluation/policy, accessed 14 January 2016).

III For more information, see www.internationalhealthpartnership.net, accessed 14 January 2016.

2.2.4 Increasing accountability and transparency

A national health planning process might not be transparent or even visible to the population. By organizing a population consultation that enhances people's input to and understanding of national health priorities, and by capturing opinions and expectations, the government or the MoH will de facto increase transparency and accountability, especially if the chosen strategy or decisions are in line with population expectations.[8]

Undertaking a consultation is an indication of government accountability and transparency towards its citizens.

It should be recognized that a consultation may expose the government to criticism and objections. However, undertaking a consultation is an indication of government accountability and transparency towards its citizens. How the consultation is organized (including with appropriate measures for more socially-disadvantaged populations), who is involved in its design and implementation, how it is explained to the population, and how consultation outcomes are fed back to the population are key factors in increasing trust and reducing the risk of criticism. It is important that the consultation be seen as unbiased, if it is to be effective and credible.[9] One way some countries ensure that a consultation, or indeed the policy-making process as a whole, is unbiased, is by periodically monitoring the process of participation in health policy development (for example, through human rights institutions).[10]

2.2.5 Support monitoring and evaluation

A population consultation, especially when leading to sustainability of interaction between policy-makers and population, can support the monitoring and evaluation of a strategy or a reform process. For example, a cross-sectional survey undertaken in Turkey to gauge people's opinion on recent healthcare reforms (see section 2.5.3) showed that increased patient satisfaction with quality and responsiveness of health services was well reflected through this exercise.

2.2.6 Support for resource allocation decisions to MoH

Using accrued information and evidence that reflects the population's opinion and expectations can strengthen the position of the MoH in national resource allocation negotiations by providing the requisite backing through evidence-based lines of argumentation.

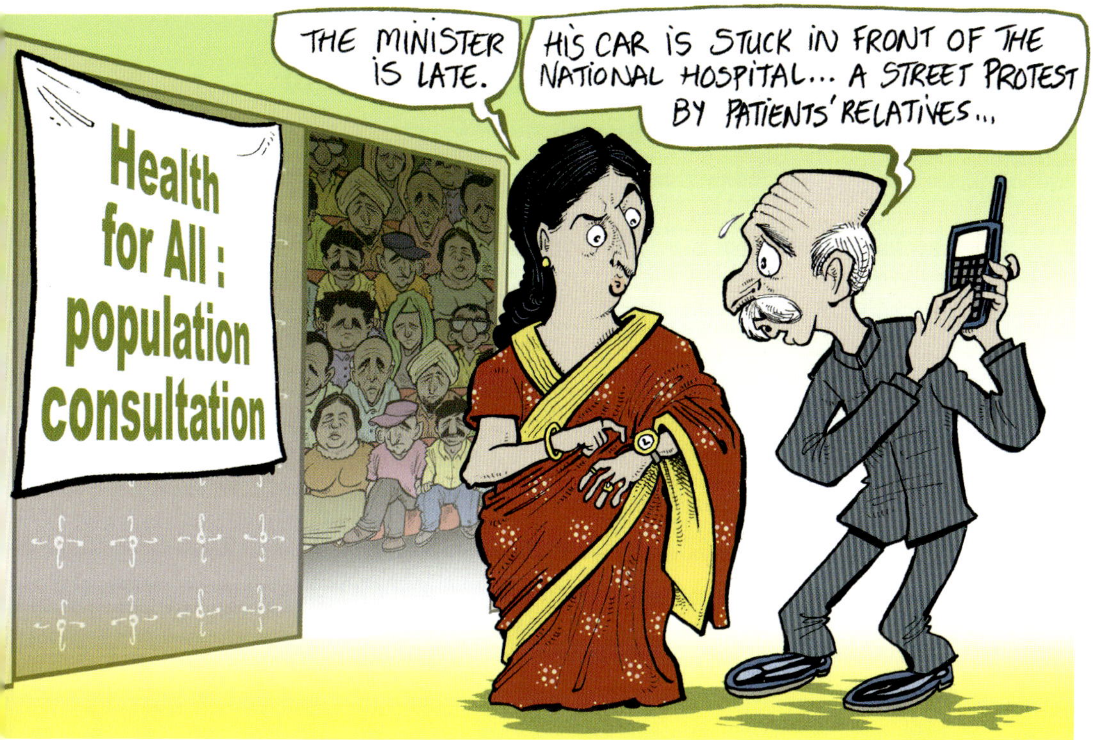
THE MINISTER IS LATE.
HIS CAR IS STUCK IN FRONT OF THE NATIONAL HOSPITAL... A STREET PROTEST BY PATIENTS' RELATIVES...
Health for All : population consultation

Fig. 2.1 Population consultation

Damian Glez; scenario by Bruno Meessen

2.3 When to conduct a population consultation

Although there is no set timing for a population consultation in regard to national health planning, it is useful for it to take place during the preparation phase of a new plan (even before the situation analysis) or at the beginning of the planning period, since it might heavily influence priority-setting decisions.[IV] To avoid instrumentalization of the results of the consultation, it is best not to undertake a population consultation during a national or local election or pre-election period.[11]

Population consultation involves a certain periodicity; it should be done once per cycle to be able to feed into regular processes like the Joint Annual Review (JAR) and the Mid-Term Review (MTR). Although a costly process, periodicity of the population consultation will increase the ability to trace population needs and expectations over time, and strengthen the relationships built between policy-makers and population. Periodicity also allows for measuring the trend in people's perceptions of the impact of strategies and reforms on their conditions, thus complementing established monitoring and evaluation activities.[12]

For population consultations to be most useful and influence priority-setting decisions, they should take place during the preparation phase of a new plan or at the beginning of a planning period.

IV It is important to ensure that supply of health system services is analysed in parallel to the demand

2.4 Who should be involved – roles and responsibilities

Determining who should be involved in a population consultation depends on the objectives as well as on the level (national, sub-national, district level) and the subject of the consultation.

2.4.1 Multiplicity of stakeholders

Stakeholders who may organize or be actively involved in conducting a population consultation include:

While a multiplicity of stakeholders may organize or be involved in conducting a population consultation, it is important that, regardless of differing views, the consultation be impartial and unbiased.

- government departments, such as the MoH, other ministries (e.g. planning, social welfare, education), and the prime minister or president's office;
- independent research institutions (e.g. universities) and think tanks;
- foundations;
- political parties;
- CSOs and NGOs (including faith-based organizations);
- community leaders and community institutions;
- market research institutions;
- professional associations;
- media.

For the results of the population consultation to be considered legitimate, it is important that it be impartial and unbiased. Some of the listed stakeholders have different views and positions by definition (e.g. political parties). Therefore it is important to make explicit from the beginning that stakeholders should not attempt to influence the process of the consultation or use the results for their own political purposes.

A possible bias and conflicts of interest can also be avoided by involving stakeholders from different political parties and backgrounds in the preparatory phase and in the organizational committee of the consultation:[V]

- to increase the credibility of the consultation, it is important to communicate openly who participated in the process.
- to increase transparency and fairness, the interests behind a consultation should always be communicated to the population.

V See also Commission of the European Communities (2002): Communication from the Commission: towards a reinforced culture of consultation and dialogue – general principles and minimum standards for consultation of interested parties by the Commission, COM 704 final, Brussels (http://ec.europa.eu/governance/docs/comm_standards_en.pdf, accessed 29 December 2015).

2.4.2 Role of the MoH

In many cases, a population consultation is coordinated and conducted by the MoH at national or sub-national level, or by another public entity. However, in some cases, for instance when the ministry is not equipped with the necessary quantitative or qualitative expertise or personnel, it may be preferable for an independent institution (e.g. a research institute) to support the MoH or even actually conduct the consultation. Transparency in the selection process of the independent institution is key. When the MoH is not involved in a public consultation related to health matters and organized by other actors (media, CSO, international organizations, etc.), the organizers should ensure that the MoH is properly informed of the scope and objectives of the consultation, as well as its transparency.

It would also be the MoH´s role to potentially link-up with other ministries to ensure a more holistic approach for conducting the consultation. Especially in regard to concerns of access and affordability of health care, intersectoral collaboration during and in the follow-up to the consultation might be useful (e.g. sectors like social welfare, environment, and finance). At the same time, the MoH should be aware that responses to the consultation might be influenced by service delivery challenges other sectors might be facing.

2.4.3 Role of independent facilitators

When the MoH is the initiator or main organizer of a population consultation, it can be helpful to seek independent facilitators from other stakeholders or agencies. The design of the consultation (content and methodology) should always be led by individuals with expertise in appropriate fields such as:

- technical experts for the specific topics;
- independent experts for survey methods and data analysis.

If an institution external to the MoH is to support or even conduct the population consultation, it is crucial that this third party selection process is transparent.

CSOs can have an important role during a consultation process, as they are often spokespeople for certain population groups. This is a valuable and often necessary way to engage with population groups that have specific needs or might be difficult to include in the consultation. Collaborating with other sectors – such as the social welfare or environmental sectors – may provide entry points for joint coordination on common challenges.

2.4.4 Role of the media

The traditional media – like newspaper, radio and television – will most likely have a dual role during a population consultation, at least in settings where the media enjoys some level of independence from government and other parties.

The media can critically accompany a consultation and also be useful in disseminating information.

On one hand, as part of their self-concept of being free of the influence of the government, the media will monitor and critically accompany all stages of the consultation. They might serve as a neutral actor, reporting on background information and analytical evidence that might be useful for the population when responding to the questions.

On the other hand, even though the media should not be compromised during a consultation, it needs to be recognized that traditional media, and especially television, are accessible to large parts of the population and might be used as means for disseminating information regarding the consultation (see Box 2.1).

The media are a good way to announce publicly that the consultation will happen and inform the population of specificities they need to know.

The MoH (or whoever is leading the consultation process) might need to use the media to pass on relevant information needed to respond to the consultation in an understandable, open and critical way.

The media could be used to disseminate information on the outcomes and the follow-up of the consultation.

Box 2.1

The media as crucial partners contributing to the success of the Societal Dialogue in Tunisia

The Societal Dialogue in Tunisia depended heavily on trust from the population that their feedback and input would be taken seriously and valued. The Steering Committee for the Societal Dialogue, and WHO, which was technically supporting this work, took great care to work closely with the media to spread this message in a sincere way to the population. Measures taken are listed below.

1. A member of the media was invited to be a part of the Technical Committee on Societal Dialogue that was tasked to organize all of the dialogue events. This media member, a television journalist, organized short clips and longer, more informative TV programmes around the societal dialogue, which were widely viewed.

2. Regional radio aired societal dialogue-themed programmes and interviews in the lead-up to various Societal Dialogue events in the regions. These radio programmes were absolutely critical to encouraging people to come to the events and reassuring the populace in a somewhat tense post-revolution context that their voice was truly needed and valued. The Steering Committee on Societal Dialogue initially invited the radio stations to listen to their objectives and aims in order to better understand what was envisaged with the population's input.

3. Newspaper articles and special newspaper supplements were published, mainly to raise visibility and interest in the Societal Dialogue programme but also to underline its aims and objectives in a transparent way.

China, Hong Kong, Special Administrative Region (SAR): an unexpected outcome from a public consultation process

Health policy development in China, Hong Kong SAR during the last decade is characterized by proposals submitted for population consultation, after which the proposals are modified and re-submitted for consultation. Especially for issues where there are several options and conflicting views, this method has helped the Bureau for Food and Health to obtain a sense of agreement as to the direction in which health sector reform goes.

In 2008, for example, the Bureau for Food and Health launched an effort at health service delivery and financing reform with the publication of a consultation document: Healthcare service and financing reform.[13] The document offered different financing options that the public could comment upon, without an explicit government recommendation for any one of the options. This being said, many accompanying reference materials provided on the Bureau for Food and Health website demonstrated a government preference for a compulsory medical savings account. Several thousand comments were received, including official analyses and commentaries by professional associations, hospitals, and insurance companies. The public consultation resulted in strong opposition to any scheme requiring mandatory contributions, individual savings account or insurance. Instead, the public clearly showed its preference for voluntary schemes subsidized by the government.

Following this consultation, the Bureau for Food and Health drafted a reform proposal and a second consultation paper, entitled My Health, My Choice,[14] was submitted for a second round of consultation in 2010.

The document is based on the feedback on the 2008 paper, results from several focus group discussions, and a government-commissioned consultancy report.[15] The crux of the document is a proposal for a private voluntary health insurance scheme called the Health Protection Scheme (HPS). The public consultation results showed support for the scheme; the China, Hong Kong SAR government is thus currently developing a voluntary, government-regulated health insurance system.

Despite the long and careful consultation process, implementation of the new system is not easy, with the devil being in the details. Angry reactions to various aspects of the proposed scheme from special interest groups have led to further internal consultations and re-drafts of the HPS. However, it is to be emphasized that the Bureau for Food and Health has the basic backing of its population to move forward with reform, which gives it a legitimacy to continue working towards a successful HPS that many other MoHs would envy. It is also to be lauded that the Bureau for Food and Health set aside its preference for a mandatory medical savings account once the public voiced its strong opposition to it.

The China, Hong Kong SAR example demonstrates that a public consultation can end up going in unexpected directions. Especially when a MoH is coordinating such a consultation, it is important to accept that internal plans may steer off-course and that the public may not accept a government recommendation.

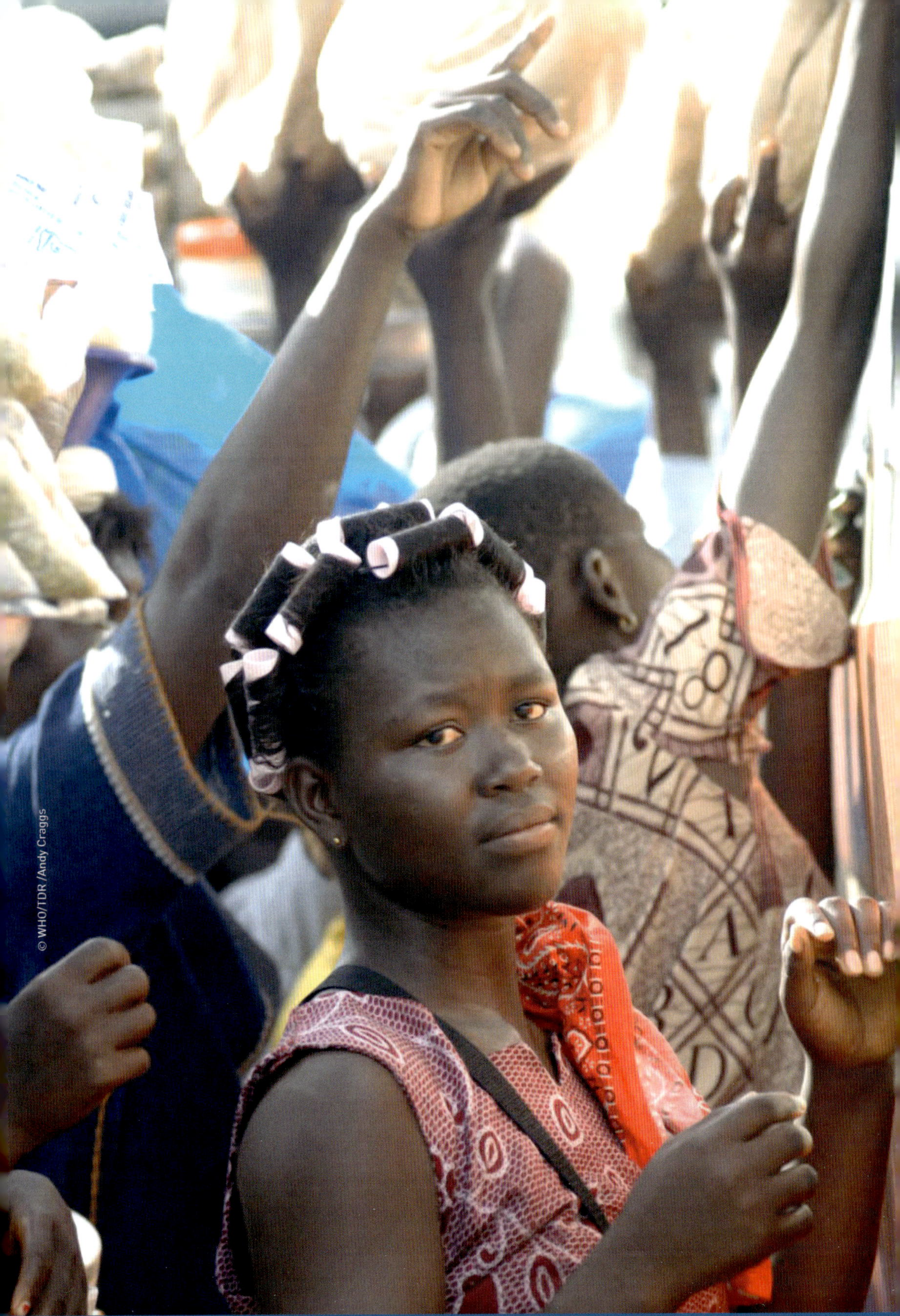

© WHO/TDR /Andy Craggs

2.5 Methodological approaches

The methodological approaches to a population consultation vary considerably, depending on the scope and aims of the consultation. Each approach requires country-specific preparation, which may involve evidence and information gathering, targeted dialogue with special population groups, or a variety of other activities.

In this handbook, the most common approaches to a population consultation will be discussed:

1. face-to-face dialogue with large population sample(s);
2. consultative methods with invited participants from different population groups;
3. survey types and survey tools with invited/selected population groups;
4. one-on-one individual survey types and tools.

Please note that it is always best, if possible, to use several approaches in order to triangulate findings and ensure good representativeness. Each approach will give information about a specific subject in a different way and from different population groups.

- The first approach, a face-to-face dialogue with a large population sample, aims at capturing the views, opinions and expectations of a large cross-section of the population, with the objective to both inform the decision-making process and get widespread participation and buy-in from the population.
- Consultative methods and surveys also aim to inform decisions – the former fosters participation and buy-in as well – albeit with a limited sample size, since participants are usually carefully selected from different population groups.
- A very unique and specific method, which is usually used for the decision-making per se and is only possible within a specific legal context, is the referendum. This method will be presented for information only as it is an interesting way to capture population opinion. However, putting it in place requires a specific cultural, historical, institutional and legal framework which most countries may not have.

The methodological approach to a population consultation depends on the scope and aims of the consultation.

Table 2.1 briefly summarizes the different population consultation methods and gives a practical overview of each method type.

Table 2.1 A practical overview of different population consultation methods

TYPE	MODE	PURPOSE	WHEN	PREPARATION
Face-to-face dialogue with large population sample(s)	Face-to-face – open debate – open forum for exchange with the population at large	To capture population opinion and expectations, to get widespread participation and buy-in from the population	Before a priority-setting exercise or decision-making process	Good technical situation analysis in terms of content, organization and sampling; media coverage and information/communication campaign

TIMING*	COSTS	ADVANTAGES	CHALLENGES
Between 6 and 12 months; several months of preparation and several months of implementation and analysis	Expensive – face-to-face meetings, facilitation, long-term process, etc. Costs vary with size of the sample, number of events, etc.	Face-to-face debates are normally richer and deeper than individual questionnaires (better information from participants and constructive debates) Priorities are built by participants (versus priorities developed by experts in survey questionnaires or referendum questionnaires) Large-scale events enjoy wide media coverage – importance of health sector issues is given a boost Direct population involvement and later ownership of policy/plan Greater accountability and transparency demonstrated	Face-to-face debates are normally richer and deeper than individual questionnaires (better information from participants and constructive debates) Long lead time necessary for sound technical preparation, planning of face-to-face events and their organization Resource- and time-intensive event(s) Due to the large-scale and labour-intensive nature, it could be easily postponed in favour of more urgent tasks; outsourcing such a process might be a solution

* The timings indicated are very rough-guess estimates. Timing is highly dependent on the amount of financial and human resources available to undertake the consultation. Large countries with large populations will clearly need more time than small countries with small populations.

	TYPE	MODE	PURPOSE	WHEN	PREPARATION
2.	Consultative methods with invited participants from different population groups	Face-to-face – open debate – open forum for exchange with a closed number of representatives of population groups and technical experts	To inform decisions and foster participation and buy-in	Before a priority-setting exercise or decision-making process	Stakeholder analysis is important to ensure good representativity. Good technical situation analysis in terms of content, organization and sampling; media coverage and information/communication campaign play a less important role
3.	Survey types and survey tools with invited/ selected population groups	Individual opinion	To capture population opinion and expectations	To inform priority-setting exercise or decision-making process	Brief information sheets and survey questionnaires preparation (by professionals)
4.	One-on-one individual survey types and tools	Individual	To capture population opinion and expectations	To inform priority-setting exercise or decision-making process	Brief information sheets and survey questionnaires preparation (by professionals)

TIMING*	COSTS	ADVANTAGES	CHALLENGES
Usually several smaller consultations are necessary before the large consultation – this could take 2–4 months; in addition, 2–4 months preparation and 1 month to analyse results	Much less expensive than face-to-face dialogue with large population sample. However, this method is resource intensive in terms of human resource time	Face-to-face debates are normally richer and deeper than individual questionnaires (better information from participants and constructive debates), even if the consultations are limited in size compared to dialogue with a large population sample Possibility to go more in-depth on the technical side of the discussion due to limited number of participants and more technical expertise present More buy-in and ownership of policy/plan Greater accountability and transparency demonstrated Can verify or substantiate information and results in a certain topic area	Ensuring represent-ativity is not easy – a sound stakeholder analysis and good knowledge of the setting is important Resource-intensive especially in terms of human resources – a dedicated person or group of people must work on preparing a consultative meeting or focus group over a period of several weeks Analysis of qualitative methods (especially focus groups) is not straightforward and can be complicated
2-3 months Short period preparation and short period implementation and analysis	Cheap to expensive, depending upon method and sampling	Depends on the type of survey; see Annex 2.1 for more details	Depends on the type of survey; see Annex 2.1 for more details
2-3 months Short period preparation and short period implementation and analysis	Cheap to expensive depending upon method and sampling	Depends on the type of survey; see Annex 2.1 for more details	Depends on the type of survey; see Annex 2.1 for more details

2.5.1 Face-to-face dialogue with large population sample(s)

Face-to-face dialogue with a large cross-section of the population is sometimes termed the "états généraux de la santé" (EGS) in francophone countries. In other settings, it can be called a citizens' assembly, citizens' jury, and/or a citizen forum.

Whatever the term used, the essence of this approach is a large-scale, organized series of public debates. The main characteristic of this method is that it captures the population's opinions and expectations through structured face-to-face debates between the organizers and the population, as well as among citizens themselves. Its purpose is to inform the priority-setting process and/or the decision-making process. Its strength comes from the level of evidence-based technical preparation of the topics to be discussed: from a simple, short and easy-to-understand way of presenting the topics to an excellent structuring of the debates so as to lead to a clear formulation of opinions and expectations.

Large-scale, organized public debates can capture opinions and expectations directly to inform the priority-setting or decision-making process.

The emphasis with this method is on providing the population with an honest, open forum for exchange, with the objective of creating momentum for a particular issue and a better understanding of population views and needs. Volunteer sampling or random sampling can be applied here. Depending on the number of events held, a different sampling approach can be used for different events.

This section contains two examples of face-to-face dialogue with large population samples in two very different settings: France and Tunisia.

Checklist: necessary resources to capture population views

- √ personnel time
- √ consultant time
- √ travel funds
- √ access to office materials such as computer, phone, and copy machine
- √ interview materials
- √ any necessary trainings
- √ governance bodies' meeting space, time, and refreshments

Box 2.3

The 14 cross-cutting themes for France's 1999 Etats généraux de la santé

1. newborn health;
2. the future of our youth's health;
3. ageing;
4. healthy lifestyle;
5. access to care;
6. drug dependence, addictions and risk reduction;
7. preventive health;
8. quality of health care;
9. the patient's right to health;
10. research perspectives;
11. urban hospitals;
12. mental health;
13. palliative care and pain management;
14. cancer screening.

France

Today, the rights of health system end-users and their participation in health system decision-making are anchored in public health laws in France. This is partly the result of the last EGS in France, in 1999. This EGS's aim was to get a better insight on the population's main concerns and expectations with respect to the health system and its principal actors. The objective was underpinned by the philosophy of creating a real public debate for health, in stark contrast to a more traditional position that reserved health debates for professionals or health experts.[16]

The magnitude of the French EGS was considerable: nine months of deliberations, over 1000 meetings, and approximately 200 000 people in attendance. The organization of the EGS was very decentralized in order to get better representation of the population. A National Guiding Committee ("Comité d'Orientation") was set up to guide the overall process, while Regional Steering Committees guided and supported the Citizens' Forums and other regional-level activities.

Fourteen cross-cutting themes were selected by the National Guiding Committee. The themes (see Box 2.3) were explained in simple, easy-to-understand language in written material distributed to participants. In addition, the themes were explained orally in detail without too much technical jargon. A specific effort was thus made to bring home the different health themes to the common understanding of all citizens. The regions were given considerable autonomy and freedom to choose sub-topics relevant to them, and to organize debates as appropriate to their context. All of the regions conducted Citizens' Forums; in some regions, health facilities and private clinics offered "open days"; other regions set up radio debates. Yet other regions conducted surveys and questionnaires before the Citizens' Forums and debated on their results in the Forum itself. The decentralized nature of the EGS created a dynamic that was very local in nature and engendered high levels of interest and participation.

The 1999 EGS in France was judged a success, demonstrating that there is considerable potential to mobilize the population on issues which touch them directly, such as health.[17] The subjects that drew the most attention and participation were: access to care, pain and palliative care, ageing, and adolescent health issues. Most of the key recommendations which fed back to government decision-makers were centred on these topics.

Population consultation in France was a huge undertaking with over 20 000 people in attendance, demonstrating that there is considerable potential to mobilize the population on issues which touch them directly, such as health.

Tunisia

Tunisia is a small, upper-middle income country located on the Mediterranean coast of north Africa. It shot to the headlines when its people engaged in civil resistance, leading to the "Arab Spring" revolution that began in December 2010. The demonstrations were spurred on by decades of a repressive regime in addition to high unemployment, corruption, and poor living conditions. The post-revolution context is thus characterized by a strong reaction against these very issues, especially the past lack of citizen voice in any public policy and reform processes.

Given this backdrop, and the very real changes to the Tunisian public sector and society, it was imperative and generally agreed that a fundamental reorientation of the health sector needed to happen sooner rather than later. An in-depth population consultation was crucial to capture people's views, needs, and daily challenges given the post-revolution circumstances.

A programme called "societal dialogue" was launched in 2012 – the emphasis being on the term "societal" in order to highlight the importance of having all of society's actors involved in reform development.[18] It was clear that the feasibility and acceptability of reforms in the current political and social context was highly dependent on people's participation (or perception of participation). Thus the population consultation in Tunisia was done with the twin aims of capturing population opinion, and of giving people a platform to express themselves in ways that they had never done before.

The first-ever "Citizens' Meetings on Health" were organized in each governorate, where input was gathered on the key challenges in the health sector but also on values and attitudes of the population for sector reforms. On this occasion, citizens also shared their views on how health services could be improved. Simultaneously, focus groups were facilitated for vulnerable populations in different parts of the country (see Box 2.6).

Following the citizens' meetings and focus groups, complemented by several literature reviews and technical studies, several major themes began to emerge as needing urgent reform. With these issues in mind, approximately 100 people selected by lottery from each of the governorates formed a "citizens' jury" with the task of pronouncing a verdict on specific questions around the themes listed below:

- Solidarity and health system financing mechanisms.
- "Neighbourhood health services" and coordination and integration of care.
- Health promotion and health culture.
- Confidence and revitalization of the health sector.[19]

The feedback from these population consultation events has been overwhelmingly positive, even with several obstacles faced (see Box 2.5). The huge popularity of these events has led to the government explicitly recommending this methodology to other sectors such as education and social services. In addition, it has helped citizens' groups to focus on key issues and strengthen their own capacity.

Box 2.4

Principal challenges to Tunisia's population consultation

- There was initial lack of trust that the consultation was 'real', as Tunisia has a history of consultations which were undertaken in name only; most people assumed that this was the same.
- Diverging interests between different population groups, especially between health professionals and lay people, very often led to tensions during the consultations.
- It was difficult to get participation from marginalized groups, especially in the Citizen's Meetings on Health. This was overcome by organizing specific focus group sessions for vulnerable and marginalized populations.
- Lack of trust and deep-rooted misunderstandings between professionals, ordinary citizens, and government administration posed challenges.

Box 2.5

Population consultation in Tunisia: some numbers[20]

- 96 lottery-selected jury members represented at the Citizens' Jury for Health from 24 governorates
- 120 hours of audio and video recorded material of citizens' voicing their concerns
- 3 424 citizens participated in the Citizens' Meetings on Health
- 20 556 kilometers travelled by facilitators for the various population consultation events

2.5.2 Consultative methods with invited participants from different population groups

This section describes two predominant types of consultative methods, the *consultative meeting* and the *focus group*. Two examples of consultative meetings, which were called "états généraux de la santé" in their respective countries, are chronicled, as well as one example of the focus group method being used as part of a larger effort to capture population opinion. The examples are meant to inspire reflection on possible ways to conduct such events, with all its modalities, challenges, and successes.

Please note that the terminology used in various countries for their population consultation methods is anchored in the countries' histories and traditions. Hence, for example, the term "états généraux de la santé" may be used for an event which resembles a face-to-face dialogue with large population sample(s) in one country. In another setting, the same term could be used for a consultation which resembles a consultative workshop or meeting. The same holds true for "policy dialogue", "citizens' jury", etc.

(a) Consultative meetings

Consultative meetings bring together stakeholders who are informed about, have a view on, and/or are experienced in a particular area, for the purpose of voicing their opinions and assessments for a particular objective. These workshops are also called 'états généraux de la santé' in some (francophone) countries; other terms used are 'policy dialogue' and 'stakeholder consultation'. Whatever the term, these meetings are smaller in number than the larger face-to-face consultations mentioned above. Usually, the participants are carefully selected from different population groups to ensure adequate representativity – for example, professional associations, patient groups, district health authorities, and others are typical participants of these types of gatherings. Technical experts from government, development partners, and civil society are usually present as well and may provide specific technical inputs on an issue.

The advantage of consultations with invited participants is that a smaller group can provide greater depth to a discussion. In general, dialogue with a restricted number of invited participants can be more intense, especially when they are well prepared for the discussion. A dialogue in this type of setting can verify or substantiate information and results in a certain topic area, precisely because there is space to present study results and discuss more technically than in a consultation with a general cross-section of the population. Participants must, however, be carefully selected with no conflicts of interest vis-à-vis the issues at hand.

The advantage of consultations with invited participants is that a smaller group can provide greater depth to a discussion.

A caveat to note here is that consultative meetings are heavily dependent on the agenda set, the preparation taken, the facilitator's skill, and the honest effort of the event organizers to be objective and neutral. The intention must sincerely be to gather input on a topic of importance and/or interest and to listen to participants' thoughts and views.

Guinea

In Guinea the 'Etats Généraux de la Santé', as its consultative meeting was called, was held on 23–25 June 2014, and is seen as one of the key preparatory steps in the development of the new 10-year National Health Development Plan (NHDP). To prepare the EGS,[21] a sound technical analysis of the health system was undertaken by thematic groups gathering experts from various backgrounds (including civil society, development partners and other ministries). One of the outcomes of this analysis was a series of suggestions for a new health sector vision statement as well as the identification of a number of key, transversal issues important for framing the future of the sector.

The EGS in Guinea combined a technical analysis with expert opinion, bringing in other points of view and a more system-wide perspective. It enabled a wide range of external stakeholders to contribute to the debate in a political and personal way, rather than in a technical way.

The EGS meeting in Guinea deliberated on the vision statement and on other key questions coming out of the technical analysis. The EGS in Guinea has brought together some 250 participants coming from all sections of society. The meeting was not intended to duplicate or "validate" the technical analysis, but to go beyond and complement it by bringing in other points of view and a more system-wide perspective. The EGS enabled a wide range of external stakeholders to contribute to the debate in a political and personal way, rather than in a technical way. In addition, it provided a forum whereby the population could express their expectations of the health sector, and produce useful recommendations to be included in the NHDP. Expectations are high for a successful reorientation of the health sector to be reflected in the NHDP.

Haiti

In Haiti, the impetus for conducting a consultative workshop, which was also termed an 'Etats Généraux de la Santé', in 2012 was to prepare for a new overarching National Health Plan which would serve as a reference document for the health sector. The EGS was preceded by intense organized debate and deliberation within the ten administrative departments (akin to states or regions) of the country – these discussions were more technical in nature and were conducted mainly by health and/or policy experts. Following this, a three-day EGS took place on the basis of the results of the departmental discussions. Suggestions and proposals from these two events helped to steer the development of a new National Health Policy and a National Strategic Health Plan 2012–2022.

During the three days, guided group discussions with selected themes were interspersed with plenary sessions, which allowed different groups to present their work to the rest of the participants and then debate upon it. The five key themes which were decided during the departmental discussions were: governance; decentralization; human resources for health; service provision and health service financing; and monitoring and evaluation.

The high-level representation and wide media coverage of the EGS impressed upon the Haitian population the importance their government was placing in the health sector. Results of the EGS discussion directly fed into the formulation phase of the National Strategic Health Plan 2012–2022.

(b) Focus groups

Focus group interviews are usually done with small, relatively homogeneous groups (6–12) of people with similar backgrounds and experience. The homogeneity and the much smaller size of the groups are the main differences from consultative workshops. The group interviews provide a platform to discuss a specific topic freely and interactively, with the help of a moderator. The moderator uses general guidelines and protocol such as introducing the subject, keeping the discussion flowing while using subtle probing techniques, and preventing a few participants from dominating the discussions. Note-takers record comments and observations. A session generally lasts one to two hours.

Focus group discussions allow a more in-depth exploration of stakeholder opinions, similar or divergent points of view, judgements, as well as information on behaviours, understanding and perceptions of an initiative. They are also extremely useful for gathering information on tangible and intangible changes resulting from an initiative.

Generally, several sessions are held on the same specific topic. Data should be adequately recorded (e.g. audio-taped), and discussed jointly by the moderator, observers and note-takers at the end of each session. Discussions should start with very general issues, then continue with topics of ever-increasing specificity. A skilful facilitator is required to ensure balanced participation of all members.

Focus groups represent a fairly low-cost, quick, and reliable way to obtain a broad range and depth of qualitative information, notably overall impressions from diverse stakeholders. The flexible format allows the facilitator to explore unanticipated issues and encourages interaction among participants. In a group setting, participants provide checks and balances, thus minimizing false or extreme views and providing a quality control mechanism.

This method is particularly adapted for complex issues as it helps uncover perceptions, attitudes, feelings and customers' preferences in a more in-depth, focused way. Focus groups are also good for testing the acceptability of and/or possible resistance to specific development initiatives, as well as in developing effective communication strategies to gain acceptance for new ways of doing things.

Potential drawbacks to this method include its time-intensiveness and potential difficulty to schedule. Qualitative data is generally more challenging and time-consuming to analyse. A discussion guide should be carefully prepared and pre-tested/adapted if possible. Finding a skilled moderator who facilitates rather than acts as an authoritative figure can be difficult.

Focus groups differ from consultative meetings in that they involve less people at a time and the groups are generally fairly homogeneous.

The discussions are also susceptible to facilitator bias, which can undermine the validity and reliability of findings; discussions can be side-tracked or dominated by a few vocal individuals as well. Many of these bias issues can, however, be solved with a well-trained facilitator.

In order to be able to generalize focus group findings, it is important to corroborate information (triangulation) with further focus group discussions or other methods. If not, the findings may only relate to specific communities or localities – they thus risk being less valid and reliable than formal surveys.

Tunisia

In Tunisia, the focus groups were used as a tool to go more in-depth into barriers to healthcare access faced particularly by vulnerable and marginalized population groups.

In Tunisia, the focus groups were used as a tool to go more in-depth into barriers to healthcare access faced particularly by vulnerable and marginalized population groups. Within the context mentioned earlier, a concerted effort to capture population opinion for purposes of redefining the health sector vision into a new National Health Policy was the general backdrop for this work. The focus groups were hence only one of a series of methods used to capture population opinion.

The Citizens' Meetings on Health gave extremely valuable feedback on perceptions of the Tunisian health system by the vast majority of the population. However, it was felt that challenges specific to vulnerable groups were not adequately captured. The focus groups were thus organized in several governorates, each focus group being for one homogenous marginalized group (see Box 2.6 below for list of groups targeted for focus group discussions). The focus group discussions allowed for a much more in-depth insight into very real healthcare difficulties faced by vulnerable groups which were not expressed by others. In addition, the groups' main expectations and hopes for an improved health system were teased out during these discussions. This would have been difficult and potentially distracting in the larger Citizens' Meetings.

A central challenge in conducting the focus groups in Tunisia was identifying and training facilitators – not an unusual challenge in any setting. Due to tensions between anything perceived as coming from the central government in some of the more interior regions of the country, extensive preparation on the ground was necessary beforehand. Alliances were forged with local media and allies sought to spread the message as to the true aims and objectives of the focus groups. Facilitators' backgrounds were carefully taken into consideration during the selection process. Three facilitators and one observer conducted all focus group discussions. They received detailed scripts and were trained by an external focus group expert from Canada.

The main facilitator came with a civil society background, displayed excellent empathy with the focus group, and was very popular. The drawback with a facilitator who identifies with the focus group participants is becoming too involved and taking up much of the talking time. The second facilitator was a retired higher-level governorate official who was appreciated by focus group participants for his calm professionalism. He inspired confidence. The drawback was that participants had side meetings with him, sometimes during the focus group, to discuss personal issues. The third facilitator did not intervene in the discussions and was mainly present to take notes.

The findings from the focus groups were triangulated with data coming from other population consultation events in Tunisia. Therefore, it is safe to say that the focus group facilitator issues that may have led to any type of bias in the findings were largely cancelled out. However, this example demonstrates that finding skilled facilitators, or facilitating a group oneself, is a tall order which should not be underestimated.

Box 2.6

Vulnerable and marginalized populations targeted for focus group discussions in Tunisia

- patients living in remote areas;
- patients living in poor urban; zones
- single mothers;
- families living in impoverished regions;
- isolated senior citizens; families living in polluted industrial areas.

2.5.3 Survey types and survey tools with invited/selected population groups

One-on-one individual survey types and tools

Like the face-to-face dialogue with large population samples and consultative workshops, the purpose of a survey is to capture the opinion of the population and its expectations. However, the methodology is different and leads to different results: in surveys, debates do not take place; randomly selected citizens answer questionnaires prepared by technical experts and statisticians, or answer interviews guided by professional interviewers.

A multiplicity of methods exists to survey the population, with specific advantages and challenges presented in the tables in Annex 2.1. In addition, two examples of capturing population opinion via surveys are outlined: one on health sector reform in Turkey and the other, on physical activity levels in the 28 European Union (EU) member states.

Turkey

Population opinion on Turkey's health system reform (Health Transformation Programme)

Turkey began major health sector reforms, the Health Transformation Programme (HTP), in 2003, with the aim of increasing access, availability, and patient satisfaction with health care. The principal pillars of the reform were:

- accessibility: all public health facilities were transferred to the MoH as the principal public provider of care;
- financing: the "Social Security and Universal Health Insurance Law" extended insurance coverage to the entire population and established the Social Security Institute as the principal purchaser of health services;
- people-centred primary care: the family practitioner is given a clear gatekeeper role, with every Turkish resident assigned to one or a group of family practitioners;
- healthcare quality: quality units have been established at the ministerial, provincial, and organizational levels;
- patient's rights: special units within healthcare institutions that investigate complaints by patients and providers.

Several initiatives were used to gauge population opinion and satisfaction with the ongoing reforms. The Turkish Statistics Institute's (TURKSTAT) Life Satisfaction Survey reported 39.5% overall population satisfaction with health services in 2003, just before the launch of the HTP. In 2010, that number had dramatically increased to 73%.[22] In 2013, Ali Jadoo et al. surveyed almost 500 households spread across seven regions with regard to population views on the Turkish health system before and after the HTP reform.[23] The closed-ended questionnaire delivered personally to households specifically requested respondents to compare their views on health services before the reform and at

In surveys, randomly selected citizens answer prepared questions from technical experts or answer interviews guided by professional interviewers.

the present time. Over three quarters of the respondents preferred the current health system and were more satisfied with health services now than previously.

Eurobarometer structured interview: physical activity in the European Union

The Eurobarometer is both a tool designed and used by political institutions and a database created with the help of researchers in social sciences, who are its main users.

The standard Eurobarometer,[24] or public opinion surveys, was established in 1973 with the aim of gauging population views on various topics. Internationally recognized survey research institutes, on behalf of the European Commission (EC), monitor public opinion in the Member States, mainly for use in policy-making and for better communication with EU citizens. In the EU political and institutional context, opinion polls are not merely seen as a simple instrument to collect information, but as a source of legitimacy. Despite some critique on its methodology (notably regarding the use of closed-ended questions), the Eurobarometer is now widely seen as an effective investigative instrument for the EU and European research institutions. In addition, the Eurobarometer has contributed to European leaders' taking the opinion of EU citizens more seriously.[25]

The Eurobarometer is a hybrid instrument: it is both a tool designed and used by political institutions – mainly the EC – and a database created with the help of researchers in social sciences, who are its main users. Indeed, in addition to internal use by the EC, primary data is placed at the disposal of the scientific community for research and training.

Each survey consists of approximately 1000 face-to-face interviews per Member State. When needed, in-depth thematic studies are carried out for various services of the European Commission or other EU institutions and integrated into standard Eurobarometer's polling waves. One such example is a series of recent studies (2002, 2009, 2014) on physical activity levels in Europe. EU member state residents aged 15 and over took part. A multi-stage, random sampling technique was applied. All interviews were based on a structured questionnaire and carried out face-to-face in the respondent's home and in the appropriate national language.

Results showed that the overall trend in physical activity remained unchanged over the last 12 years in the EU. In general, citizens in the northern part of the EU remain more active in sport and physical activity than the citizens in the southern part.[26] Almost half (47%) of the inhabitants of the 28 EU Member States were active physically at least once a month, while 42% were not active at all in sports or other physical activities. The main reason stated by citizens for participating in a sport or to be physically active is to improve one's health. The main reason for not practicing a sport more regularly is a lack of time.

One of the decisions resulting from the survey data was an EC plan to launch a European Week of Sport from 2015 onwards, with a view to encouraging people to engage more in sport and physical activity.[27]

2.5.4 Referendum

Contrary to surveys and consultative meetings or face-to-face consultations, a referendum is a political decision-making process. It is a vote by the population on various options for a particular topic, which leads to a decision/endorsement by parliament. Even if it effectively captures the population opinion and expectations, it is much stronger than the two other ways of consulting the population presented earlier. Also, its preparation is different and normally more in-depth: sound technical consultations have taken place, as well as costing of options, discussion of advantages and challenges of the different options, the way the options fit with the political programmes of the different parties, etc. Since only a few countries, including Switzerland, incorporate use of the referendum as part of their legal system, this interesting way of consulting the population should be considered as an exception.

Switzerland

Switzerland has a unique system of direct democracy whereby any Swiss citizen can initiate a popular referendum with the requisite number of signatures gathered within a certain time frame. Within the last 10 years, many such popular referenda have been initiated on health-specific issues, with health financing and insurance funds being the most frequently contested topic. Population consultation thus takes on a very different meaning in Switzerland, as people are not only consulted but also called upon to make health-sector decisions.

One of the key issues dividing Swiss public opinion is the financing of the costly health system and the role of health insurance funds. Residents of Switzerland choose their health insurance from a plethora of private not-for-profit funds.[VI] A popular referendum in 2007 sought to change this landscape with a single government-operated health insurance fund. Following heavy campaigning by the pro- and contra- groups, 72% of the population voted against the single health insurance fund. Critics denounced the heavy political influence and lobbying by insurance companies and professional associations. Swiss citizen groups complained that both sides' calculations of hypothetical insurance premiums with the proposed single fund were faulty and conflicting.

What are the consequences of the population deciding regularly through referenda on health sector issues? Those in favour argue that direct democracy is a powerful instrument, which ensures that all decisions are widely debated. In addition, extreme laws and measures have little chance of being passed. On the other hand, the decision-making process can be very slow and any major change or reform, often necessary in the health sector, can be arduous or blocked altogether. It should be noted that most popular referenda in Switzerland uphold the status quo.[28-30]

A referendum is a vote by the population on various options for a particular topic. Referenda are usually preceded by technical discussions, a costing of options, debates on advantages and challenges, and a clear stand taken by different political parties.

VI Swiss residents can purchase health insurance coverage from private insurers, who are not allowed to earn profits on the mandated benefit package but may earn profits on supplemental insurance only.

2.6 Factors for success: translating the theoretical approaches into practical realities

As seen in the previous parts of this chapter, a successful population consultation can allow health policy-makers to:

In preparing for population consultations, policy-makers should pay special attention that methods and measures capture the views of all groups of the population, including the "hard-to-reach".

1. engage with different socioeconomic groups;

2. increase people's understanding of and engagement in the policy-making processes; and

3. assess people's opinions and expectations, and better inform the decision-making process.

To all the three layers of a population consultation, there are issues that one would need to take into consideration because they might cause more concern than others, depending of the context of the country in question.

Issues of concern which policy-makers will need to pay special attention to:

1. the methods and measures should be able to capture the views of all groups of the population, including the so-called "hard-to-reach";

2. findings should be relevant as opinions and expectations of the population.

2.6.1 Reaching the hard-to-reach

When undertaking a population consultation, particularly in the context of moving towards universal health coverage, it is important to design a methodology which addresses the full social and political spectrum of the country. Issues that one might be confronted with and which might cause special concern are linked to gauging the opinion of those who are not well represented. One of the main conceptual and logistical challenges is to capture opinions and expectations of marginalized minority groups, who are "hard-to-reach"[VII] due to geographical and/or social barriers. To this end, it is important to understand who these population groups are and why they are hard-to-reach.

VII This handbook uses the term "hard-to-reach", bearing in mind its limitations and risks, since the main idea is to provide an idea of how to overcome the challenges.

Box 2.7

Romanian health sector reform: what do the more vulnerable and hard-to-reach think?

The 2002 assessment of population opinion on the health sector reforms which took place in the decade following the fall of the Berlin Wall in 1989 and the consequent dissolution of the Soviet Union in 1991 highlighted that involving the population in (reform) decisions leads to better acceptance of the changes (e.g. when introducing co-payments). The assessment surveyed roughly 600 adults from Dolj district and demonstrated that one third of the respondents believe that the reforms have affected the quality of care in a negative way; half of the respondents had a contrasting opinion. The majority of the respondents preferred the new health care system over the old one.

An interesting sub-analysis, however, showed that those who use health services more frequently believe that they have less access to health services than before the reforms. The elderly, the chronically ill, and the poor consistently expressed their belief that quality of care and accessibility of services have decreased over time. This category of respondents is usually the target of health sector reforms under the principle of providing care to those who need it most – but according to the study in Romania, this is the very category of people who seem to prefer the previous health care system.

The study authors advance the problematic of Romania's health reform decisions being non-participatory as a key reason for vulnerable groups' distrust in and negative evaluation of the reforms. The study results underline the need to particularly target hard-to-reach and vulnerable groups when seeking population opinion and when designing reform, especially since they will likely be the most affected by it and the ones who have the most decided opinion on it.[31]

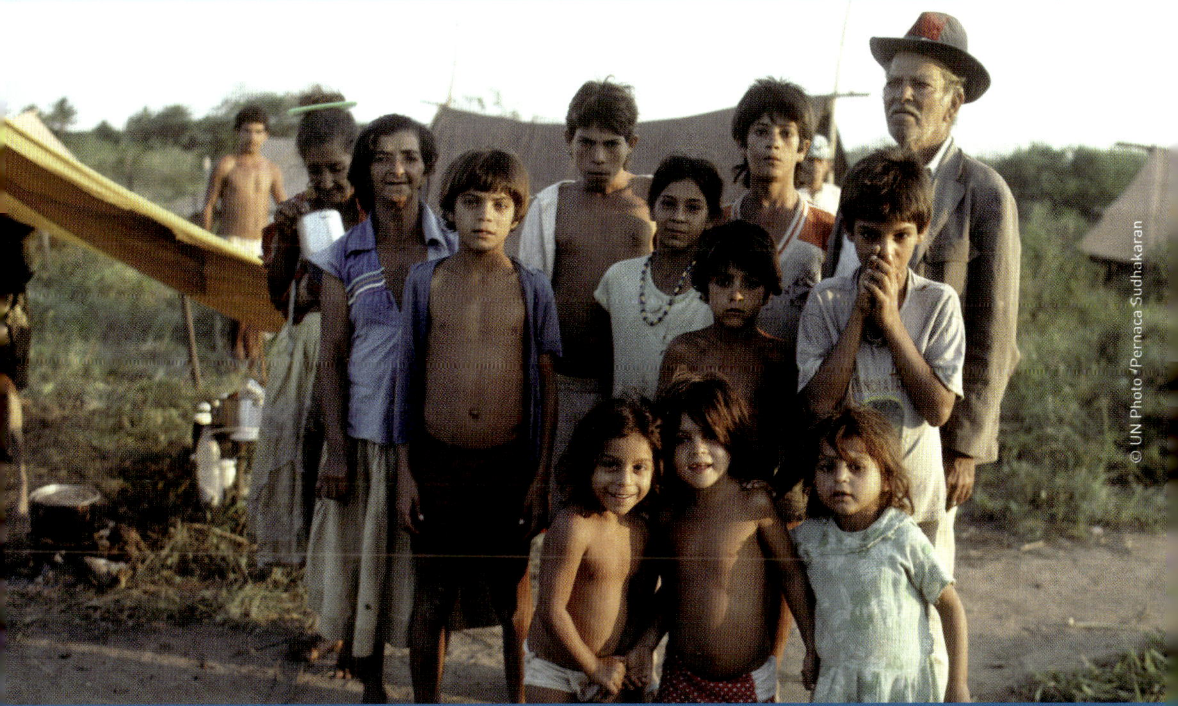

Who is hard-to-reach for a population consultation and why is it important to reach them?

There is no homogenous definition of hard-to-reach population groups. "Hard-to-reach" as a term is problematic itself since it is used inconsistently, can be misleading and might even be stigmatizing.[32] Therefore it is important to have a closer look at the structure of hard-to-reach groups to be able to allow for some differentiation and hence, more suitable consultation methodologies.

When studying the literature, we can see that there are two perceptions of "hard-to-reach" groups:

"Hard-to-reach" groups are most commonly perceived as those who might be difficult to access when providing services and those who are unable or might not feel comfortable engaging in the consultation process.

- those who might be difficult to access when providing services (service delivery perspective); and
- those who are unable or might not feel comfortable engaging in the consultation process (a so-called "sociological perspective").

It is the sociological perspective (or lens) that we need to take into consideration, in addition to the aspect of being unable to receive health services (e.g. economically disadvantaged), when discussing population consultation. For this specific group of people to be included in a population consultation, it might be necessary to design tailored approaches that are adjusted to their needs and living conditions, and that can manage to capture their input.

People who are hard-to-reach for a population consultation could be:

unresponsive: time-poor, hard-working, commuting between job and home;

silent: illiterate, not enough formal education to be able to answer surveys;

uninterested: the consultation could not be of interest because it is not perceived as useful to them;

travelling: no identification with local area/district (migrants, nomads);

not travelling: people who might lack transportation to the consultation venues;

averse: disappointed with political processes or previously rejected by political authorities (e.g. single parents) or difficult to influence (e.g. strong religious beliefs);

young: people who might not have the age to vote or actively participate in political process yet (not registered), but still might be a good source of information.

The two perspectives of "hard-to-reach" groups ("service delivery perspective" and "sociological perspective") might not be mutually exclusive. Persons difficult to be approached from a service delivery perspective ("underserved"), might also be silent or unresponsive. People who are not visible in public or formal space might not have adequate access to health services.

Each country will need to define its hard-to-reach population according to its own context and characteristics, and tailor its approaches to consulting the broad spectrum of population accordingly.

Designing tailored approaches to gather needs and opinions of hard-to-reach population groups

Context-specific tailored approaches to design an inclusive consultation process including hard-to-reach groups need to be developed, for example:

- printing materials in different/local languages/dialects and even considering illiteracy, working with visual techniques or simply adjusting methodologies to the skills of participants;
- interviewers speak local dialect and/or are from the community themselves;
- methodologies (questionnaires, interviews, etc.) chosen depending on the community context;
- design of interview questions to be chosen according to the context of the community;
- involving community leaders, or peer-group leaders, in the design and logistical arrangements of the consultation to increase comprehensiveness of the consultation materials or processes and reliability of the participants;[33]
- when intending to create relationships between policy-makers and population groups, a face-to-face methodology might be more helpful.

Any methodology chosen will have effects on the short-term arrangements as well as on the long-term goals of the consultation. Including qualitative components (e.g. personal interviews, group brainstorming) will also allow for more flexibility towards people in marginalized living conditions, and will enable the interviewer to capture information regarding the context of these living conditions – and might therefore be more appropriate for consultation of the hard-to-reach.[34]

Potential risks

When tailoring approaches for hard-to-reach groups, it might be worthwhile using supporting documentation (e.g. community health records, statistical information) and also trying to draw from the knowledge and experience of health workers. However, a certain caution might be necessary, since health workers may only have information on those who actually use health services, which may be biased towards people who can afford health services (most likely homeless or very poor/destitute might not be able to do so) and believe that the available health services can help them. Also, information gathered through supporting documentation might not necessarily represent the opinions and expectations of the hardest-to-reach.

Supporting data and information that is drawn from health workers might be biased towards those who can afford health services.

Positive effects of consulting hard-to-reach

- It might increase the sentiment of recognition of their specific problems by the MoH and the social/political system.
- Consultation processes can pave the way of better involving marginalized and hard-to-reach communities in policy and decision-making processes.
- It enables policy-makers to design specific, tailored policies better accepted by these groups and potentially improving the equity orientation of health systems performance.
- Strategies and plans tailored to these groups are more likely to be supported by the communities, which might increase the likelihood of success of these strategies.

2.6.2 Ensuring relevance of the findings

Understanding and correctly interpreting the replies to a consultation is essential to drawing the right conclusions. It also increases the legitimacy of the policy decision that will (hopefully) build on its findings. At the same time, making most use of the results of the consultation for the ensuing situation analysis and priority-setting processes is essential for it to be successful. This section explores when a consultation can be considered relevant and useful in terms of participants and contents.

Relevance in terms of participation

The inclusion of marginalized or hard-to-reach groups in the overall sample is a key criterion to assess representativeness. In addition, even though the information drawn from the survey (or any other method that was used) seems to be correct, there might still be some caveats regarding the relevance of the information sought. A few examples are listed below.

Hard-to-reach population groups are not homogenous, they vary from country to country and sometimes even within a country, based on political context and social living conditions.

Was the methodological approach chosen (e.g. culturally and socially) acceptable to the consulted groups? Would a different methodology have a different return of information?

Were the levels of knowledge and understanding of the participants high enough to be able to give well-thought-out replies to the questions?

Were the questions phrased simply enough to ensure that every participant was able to provide an answer that is useful to the consultation?

Is it possible to assume that the needs and opinions expressed by the chosen participants are characteristic for the whole population of the assessed district or country?

Were the formats for consultation appropriate for the circumstances/living conditions and capacities of more disadvantaged and marginalized populations (e.g. in case of lack of IT connectivity, illiteracy, opportunity costs of engagement).

It is important to keep in mind that consultation (as outlined on section 2.1.1) consists of a "two-way flow of information" and it is part of the responsibility of the MoH when undertaking a consultation to pass on all relevant information in an understandable and open way to the concerned population, in order for them to be able to give informed answers.[35] There is a danger that people might not be knowledgeable enough to give well-thought-out answers.[36]

Pure participation of marginalized groups does therefore not automatically increase relevance or representativeness.[37] When looking at the population consultations that were undertaken to assess opinions on changes in the Romanian healthcare system[38] as well the Turkish health care reform,[39] it becomes apparent that opinions might vary greatly among individuals wand among socioeconomic groups. The participation of a variety of (sub-)groups is therefore extremely important and cannot be limited to those who are most easily accessible and available.

Sometimes, including the full population might not be possible. In this case, recruitment criteria for participants will need to be established, keeping in mind that any sort of recruitment criteria and methodology will introduce some bias into the consultation, given that the criteria will be based on preferences of the institution undertaking the consultation.

A common challenge regarding participation is the management of expectations. A Canadian study specifically looking into public consultation challenges highlighted this issue:

> *Officials anticipate large numbers of participants; fewer citizens participate than expected, creating the impression of public apathy. Officials expect citizens to have a solid grasp on the issues if they are offering them up as input to the policy-making process; some participants have limited policy knowledge, engendering scepticism about the practical value of their contributions.*[40]

Policy-makers and other stakeholders who are engaged in the consultation should be aware of their expectations beforehand; this can help put into perspective the relevance of the exercise and facilitate an increased level of participation.

Assessing the gaps between expectations and status quo as the main objective of a consultation – a difficult exercise

One of the main goals of a population consultation is to capture the gaps between population expectations and the current situation or, in other words, the difference between what the population perceives to get with the current system versus what the population would like to get (in the future). Some attention needs to be given to some aspects of the consultation process that might hinder capturing these gaps.

Gathered information should always be contextualized. As an example, the population consultation in Turkey on the health reform process showed that people with lower education levels where less satisfied with the Turkish health system than people with higher education levels. In this regard, it was essential to contextualize these findings, and acknowledge that people with low(er) education levels are exposed to higher chances of out-of-pocket expenditure which leads to lower levels of satisfaction.[41]

It is important to contextualize the data and information collected.

Also, individual views and experiences might differ from community views. It is almost impossible to include whole communities in nationwide consultation processes, but it should always be remembered to put extreme individual views in context.

Opinions and needs addressed to policy and decision-makers without them actively seeking it

This chapter has mainly focused on discussing population consultation based on the understanding that a public institution is actively seeking population opinion and an expression of their needs. However, in some cases, it is not a public institution that is asking for information; it might as well be the population, or groups of the population, trying to pass a message to policy-makers in other ways. Capturing needs and opinions expressed by the population or groups of the population through "conventional forms" (e.g. demonstrations, protests, strikes, petitions) or "unconventional forms" of public engagement (e.g. viral campaigns via Internet) might be equally as important as an organized consultation. MoHs, parliamentary health groups, or any other public stakeholder engaged in health, should always be open-minded towards spontaneous or organized forms of expression of public opinion.

Public stakeholders engaged in health should always be open-minded towards expressions of public opinions, whether they be officially organized consultations, conventional forms of expression through demonstrations or protests, or unconventional forms such as viral internet campaigns or on social media.

It is also important to recognize that social media has an increasing role in expression of public opinion. Population (groups) may find easy access to platforms of communication and possible ways of distributing their interests through the Internet. A MoH might want to take advantage of that and make use of social media to interact with the population.

However, it is important to keep in mind that the increasing role of mass media, which usually purports to echo public opinion, might not necessarily reflect representativeness. There is a risk that the most visible will be heard loud and clear whereas the invisible (hard-to-reach) might not have access to those functionalities.

Examples of forms of engagement for policy-makers

Protests

The health care reform ("ObamaCare") in the USA has led to a wide array of demonstrations and protests, both from supporters and from opponents. Both political camps used these protests to further nurture their campaigns and arguments. The decision-making process during the health care reform was heavily influenced and shaped by forms of spontaneous expression of public opinion.

Public consultation session

In Germany, most parliamentarians (including Ministers and Chancellor) offer public consultation sessions in their electoral districts. Anyone can attend those sessions and discuss whatever they feel important. Some of the parliamentarians even provide online chat sessions to interact with the public.[42]

Using social networks to communicate with the population

The Health Promotion Board of the MoH of Singapore[43] and the Ontario MoH and Long-Term Care (Canada)[44] use Facebook to disseminate information on health issues and to communicate with the public. People can leave comments, ask questions and interact with the Board.

The MoH of New Zealand[45] and the United Kingdom Department of Health[46] use "Twitter" to disseminate information and react to comments.

2.6.3 Ensuring communication and feedback

Feedback and visible follow-up are two key elements to develop the dynamics of a virtuous circle between the population and the policy level that will have positive implications on accountability and ownership.

A crucial issue when interacting with the public is the management of expectations. It should be communicated from the beginning what the aim of the consultation is, why people are consulted and how their input to the consultation and the results of the consultation will be used.[VIII] In this sense, it is also essential to provide feedback to the population on the outcomes of the consultation. In addition, it is necessary to show that the consultation was followed-up, fed the decision-making processes and led to concrete actions.

Ensuring feedback to the population

Providing feedback is essential. It demonstrates to the communities both the value that is given to their opinion, views and expectations, and the importance of the consultation to policy-makers. Good communication regarding the translation of the population´s input to policy decisions is essential. This type of feedback to the population can also be done during another stage of the planning process, likely during or after the priority-setting exercise.

Another reason for providing feedback is to allow for continuity in the interaction and relationships built during the consultation process between the state and the population. If no feedback is provided, the population might resist undertaking another consultation at a later point in time. This feedback process must be thought through, planned and budgeted from the very beginning, during the initial planning phase of the consultation.

One step in the feedback process could be a verification of the results by the community at hand. This may or may not be feasible, depending on the heterogeneity of the community – it may be difficult for various community members to find themselves and their points of view in the synthesis document, which may lead to resentment. In such a case, an effort to dialogue with the community and adequately explain how the findings were derived might make more sense.

Feedback can be provided in various forms, with different degrees of interaction. The most direct form would certainly be providing feedback directly to the people that were surveyed or to the whole community. Another, less direct method, could be to use media, like newspaper, television or radio, including press releases or mailings to disseminate information on the outcomes and the follow-up of the consultation. The least direct version would be through a formal review process, for example during the MoH's annual sector review.[47]

Finally, and regardless of how feedback is provided, it is important to create mechanisms or transparent discussion platforms through which the findings from the consultation can be disseminated, discussed, and questioned afterwards.

Feedback after the population consultation is crucial; it shows communities that value is given to their opinion, views and expectations and allows for continuity in the interaction and relationships built during the consultation process between the state and population.

VIII Giving people the chance to opt-out and not participate in the consultation should also be ensured. Obviously, the preferred option is for the whole/consulted part of the population to participate. Nevertheless, communication with the population and preparation of the consultation should highlight the voluntary aspects of the consultation and that people might chose not to participate, without fearing restrictions or sanctions. Especially poor parts of the population depending on public services should be reassured that the (non-)participation as well as their replies to the consultation will not have any effect on their ability to benefit from public services.

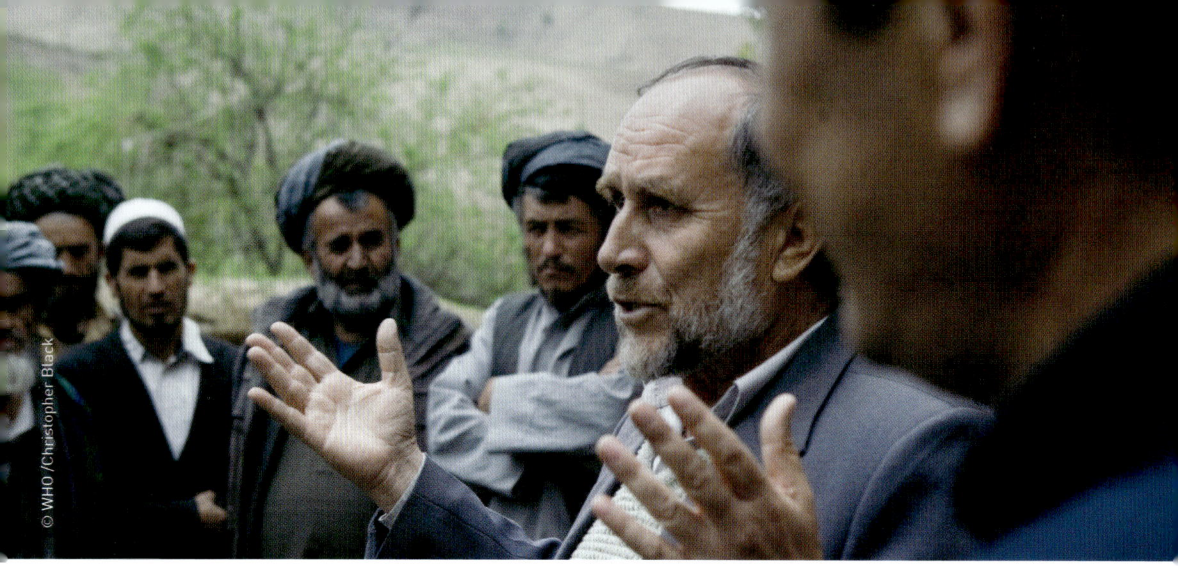

Ensuring follow-up and sustainability of the dynamic created among and between population groups and stakeholders

Equally important as providing feedback is the actual follow-up of activities post-consultation that need to be timely and transparently communicated to the population.

Follow-up to the consultation mainly consists of translating consultation results into priorities and finally into policy decisions.

Follow-up to the consultation is mainly organized around the translation of the results into priorities and finally into policy decisions. As discussed above, feedback to the population and validation of their input – respective to the results of the consultation – is a first step in this process. Subsequent steps would include the translation of the population´s input into policy recommendations and then into policy design.

It is important to realize that the population consultation per se raises expectations. Those expectations need to be addressed, and communication on actions is key. These expectations may even create dynamics leading to better sustainability and further engagement, an opportunity that should not be missed by policy-makers. In some consultations an unexpected positive side-effect occurs due to continuing interaction with the population: communities and population groups find creative and innovative ideas themselves through discussions and debates, leading to local solutions to their own problems.[48]

A consultation might also serve as an entry point for introducing a permanent link for exchange between the public sector and the population, for instance through the establishment of an ombudsperson.[IX]

Whichever way to ensure follow-up is chosen, a population consultation without follow-up (just for the sake of the consultation) should be avoided. The follow-up process as well as the communication plan should be thought through, planned and budgeted at the planning stage of the consultation process.

IX An example for a well-established system of ombudspersons, in the public sector as well as in the private sector, is Canada. See: Forum of Canadian Ombudsmen, www.ombudsmanforum.ca

2.7 How to measure the success of a population consultation

To summarize, for a population consultation to be successful, it is important to:

design a satisfactory methodological approach to assess a population's needs and opinions;

make sure to adequately translate and adapt the chosen methodological approaches to in-country reality;

ensure optimal utilization of the results as well as sustainability of the consultation through responsible follow up action;

incorporate the priorities that were identified through the consultation into the planning process and create a demand-oriented strategy/plan/policy;

introduce a regularity of the consultation for it to credibly feed into national review process (JAR, MTR) and inform policy-makers on a regular basis.

Fig. 2.2 Measuring the success of a population consultation

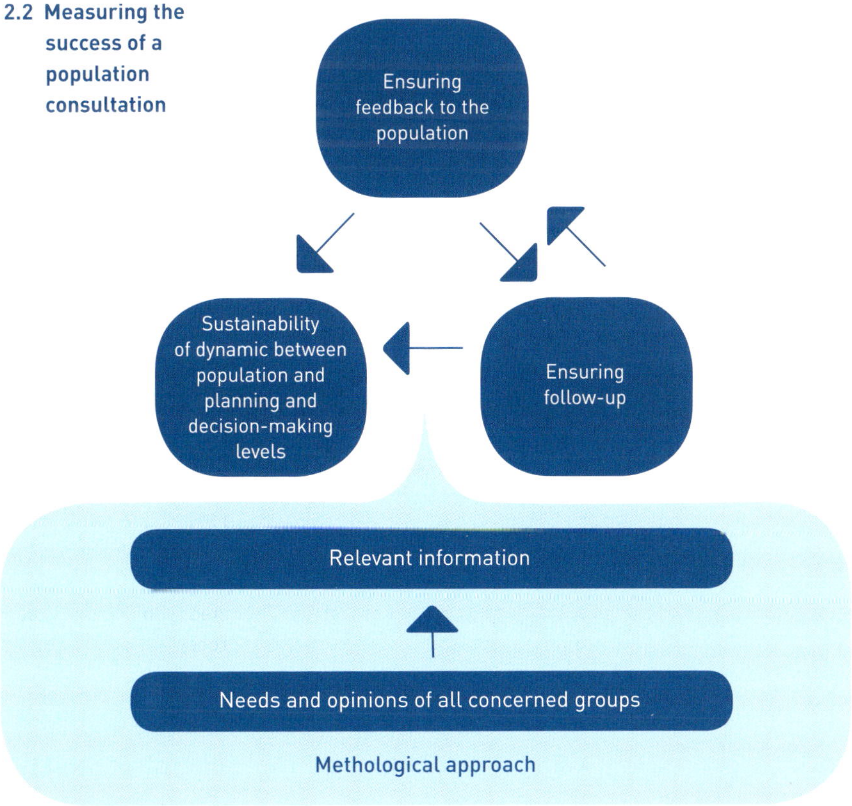

One of the main aims of the population consultation is to feed into the situation analysis, the priority-setting and decision-making processes, as well as to support monitoring and evaluation efforts. A successful and effective consultation should go one step further and provide feedback, create a sense of follow-up action and introduce some regularity in regard to interaction between public institutions and the population. Providing feedback to the population is a very powerful mechanism to integrate population opinion and needs into the policy decision-making process. At the same time, it has the potential to build a degree of sustainability of the relation between policy-makers and population.

The population consultation should ideally be followed by the situation analysis, with both feeding into the priority-setting of the national (health) planning exercise. Of course, national planning processes are not linear. In some cases it might be very useful to carry out some analytical work before engaging in the consultation to have a better understanding of the questions to be raised.

A successful and effective consultation should provide feedback, create a sense of follow-up action and introduce some regularity in regard to interaction between public institutions and the population.

In the long term, the consultation would be a point for reflection and policy correction. Every consultation exercise should demonstrate that the results were actively incorporated into the planning process.

Most population consultations in the health sector so far were seen as one-off exercises, which might not lead to the expected outcomes. Repetition or regularity should be sought, as it creates a knowledge base which helps to interpret the data correctly. It also allows participants get used to the process and increases their learning curve.

To summarize: Did we do a good job?

- √ The methodology chosen was adequately used and translated to the national context to assess the needs and opinions of the whole (targeted parts of the) population.
- √ Feedback was provided to the population after the consultation and a well-thought-out and responsible plan for follow-up action was developed and implemented.
- √ The priorities identified through the consultation were incorporated into the planning process and the strategy/plan/policy is demand-oriented.
- √ The consultation will happen on a regular basis and will feed into national review process (JAR, MTR) and inform policy-makers on a regular basis.

2.8 What if ...?

Some countries might be facing challenging and difficult situations where it might not be easy to undertake a population consultation or where certain conditions might require more flexible approaches. Subsequently, we are introducing "what if..." scenarios to highlight some of the most common concerns while planning or undertaking a population consultation.

2.8.1 What if your country is decentralized?

For decentralized[X] countries – political decentralization (federal system) as well as geographical (e.g. islands) – to undertake population consultations, it is necessary to look at their constitutional backgrounds and legal frameworks. Usually there is a clear understanding and regulation regarding the feasibility and responsibility concerning population surveys and referenda at national versus sub-national level (see box 2.8).

Box 2.8

Swiss example of rules and regulations between national and sub-national entities and how they are influencing the health landscape

Switzerland is one of the few countries where referenda are regularly undertaken. In addition, Switzerland is an interesting example due to the high degree of decentralization: the cantons have a strong autonomy and are heavily engaged in all phases of the political decision-making process at national level. Even though the cantons are responsible for health care, including for its financing, the health insurance law deals with healthcare policy at the national level.

In 2007 as well as in 2014, the population was called upon to decide whether to reform the health insurance system and abolish private not-for-profit funds, and introduce a single government-operated health insurance fund.

In both instances, the Swiss population voted against the reform. It is now up to the cantons (sub-national level) to bear the financial and managerial consequences of this decision; in most other countries, the reform would have had implications for the regulations and laws at national level.

X For a more detailed discussion regarding the dimension, degree and range of decentralization affecting the content and process of health planning, see Chapter 10 of this handbook.

From a consultation perspective, decentralization can be seen as an asset to engaging the population and especially to the consultation follow-up.

From a consultation perspective, decentralization can be seen as an asset to engaging population through a consultation and especially to the follow-up. Sub-national entities (e.g. states) tend to be closer to the reality and living conditions of the population. There is an assumption that a bottom-up planning approach, favoured by a decentralized system, which includes participation in planning and political debate through a consultation, will increase the responsiveness of a government/ MoH to local needs and expectations.[49] National policies that need to be adaptable to different sub-national (local) contexts will benefit from consultations at sub-national level.

At the same time, remote areas could be integrated better into the prioritization process when the design of the consultation itself is taking a decentralized approach. Sub-national institutions could be strengthened during resource allocation negotiations on national level by providing informed evidence of needs and demands.

Laws and regulations in regard to roles and responsibilities between national and federal level will need to serve as the primary guidance. However, even if one of the two levels can overrule the other, it is important to keep in mind that a population consultation might generate useful evidence and information that would ideally feed into policy-making and subsequently into implementation, which is a matter of all levels of government. Therefore, it might still be worth informing and updating all levels regarding the consultation, and including all levels in all stages of the consultation and the subsequent follow-up process. In this case, the coordination between different stakeholders will be more complicated, as not just the horizontal level will need to be coordinated (different stakeholders), but also the vertical level (different levels of government).[50]

Sometimes it might not even be necessary for a consultation to be undertaken for the full country, but only certain groups of the population. In this case, it should be established before the consultation if the region, area or group of population that will be consulted is part of just one federal state or if it might be spread across different states. In the latter case, administrative boundaries should not stand in the way of capturing the views of the entire population concerned.

Table 2.2 gives an indication on what would need to be considered when undertaking a population consultation in a decentralized context, following the framework for a population consultation that was developed during the course of this chapter.

Table 2.2 Issues to consider when undertaking a population consultation in a decentralized setting

RECOMMENDED ACTION	IMPLICATIONS FOR A DECENTRALIZED SYSTEM
Design a satisfactory methodological approach to assess a population's needs and opinions	▸ The inclusiveness of national as well as sub-national levels in the design of the methodology is ensured. ▸ Actors that only exist on sub-national (e.g. state MOH, grass-root organizations, professional associations), or only exist on national level (e.g. federal MoH, parliamentary groups, ministries of finance and planning, professional associations) are informed and adequately included.
Make sure to adequately translate and adapt the chosen methodological approaches to in-country reality	▸ The survey method chosen is compliant with legal framework and constitutional background. ▸ Roles and responsibilities between national and sub-national levels have been clarified. ▸ National and sub-national levels are adequately represented during the preparation and follow-up to the consultation. ▸ The methodological design of the consultation was tailored towards the differing characteristics of the population (e.g. different languages, different living conditions due to differences in services and entitlements per state).
Ensure sustainability of the consultation results through feedback and responsible follow-up action	▸ The results of the consultation were made available to all concerned levels. ▸ Follow-up on the results is demonstrated by national as well as sub-national levels – there is clear understanding of which level is responsible for implementation of the follow-up plan.
Incorporate the priorities that were identified through the consultation into the planning process and create a demand oriented strategy/plan/policy	▸ National and sub-national planning processes are equally benefiting from the results of the consultation. ▸ Sub-national as well as national level are accountable towards the population regarding the results of the consultation, regardless at what level the consultation was undertaken.
Introduce a regularity of the consultation for it to credibly feed into national review process (JAR, MTR) and inform policy-makers on a regular basis	▸ Review processes at national level are designed in a way that allows for the results of sub-national consultation processes to be included, and vice versa.

2.8.2 What if fragmentation and/or fragility is an issue in your country?

This section looks at how to undertake population consultations in fragile scenarios. "Fragility" refers to a country that includes certain areas of limited statehood, "where the state does not have the administrative capacity (either material or institutional) to exercise effective control over activities within its own borders".[51]

Countries in crises especially require national health planning approaches tailored to their dynamic context – a population consultation can be very helpful in this regard.

Countries in crises especially require health strategy and plan approaches that are tailored to their dynamic context – a population consultation can be very helpful in this regard. However, fragile contexts are usually highly aid-dependent, with donors influencing the political debate and prioritization processes. Needs and expectations identified through the consultation might have to be defended against donor priorities.

Nevertheless, in a context where efforts must be concentrated and financial and human resource capacities are low, a population consultation could be a good way to not just support the identification of priority areas, but also to realistically measure the resources that might be needed.

Consider whether a population consultation would be possible and what prerequisites would be needed

It might be possible to conduct a population consultation in a country with:

- politically-legitimate but technically-weak government, with a MoH willing to lead health care developments;
- absent, uninterested or resource-less government, leaving both policy formulation and health care provision to other actors.

In such contexts, the MoH might have the ability to conduct the consultation but might need to be supported by other actors.

It might be difficult, but not impossible, to conduct a population consultation in a stable but poor and vulnerable country, with health authorities unable to play a leading role in the health care field (despite their legitimate mandate). The consultation might therefore need to be conducted by a neutral party, supporting the MoH.

It might be impossible to conduct a consultation in a country with a:

- recognized government, formally in charge of the health care field, but opposed by powerful donors on political or human-rights grounds;
- protracted turmoil, with contested government, competing power holders, unresolved conflicts.

Design a satisfactory methodological approach to assess a population's needs and opinions

When designing a methodological approach in distressed situations, it is essential to consider if it is logistically even possible and safe to undertake a population consultation. Fragmented and unstable scenarios can pose an additional burden to the feasibility of the consultation. Additionally, there might be resource and capacity constraints that will need to be tackled with caution.[52]

Due to the political and financial constraints there tends to be a high disconnect between existing policies and plans and realities in fragile/fragmented countries. The focus of the consultation should therefore be around the identification of priorities, to be able to increase government engagement in improving living conditions.

Nevertheless, a population consultation in the face of the highly demanding logistical and political challenges of seeking the population's needs and opinions in these scenarios might be one of the few chances to increase engagement with remote and hard-to-reach population groups. In that regard, a "good governance" approach might even be supported through the consultation.[XI]

Additionally, the consultation could be designed more comprehensively to identify the key contextual factors that need to be considered in the development of health strategies and plans, since those are highly dependent on the current context of the country.

Based on the problem that documentation and quantitative as well as qualitative information regarding the health of the population can be unavailable or difficult to retrieve, the population consultation, if undertaken, can also serve the purpose of putting a firm emphasis on population needs and health status, not just assessing the expectations.

A population consultation in the face of the highly demanding logistical and political challenges in fragile settings might be one of the few chances to increase engagement with remote and hard-to-reach population groups.

XI For a discussion on the inclusion of population (groups) in policy and decision making processes in light of "good governance" see: United Nations Democracy Fund (www.un.org/democracyfund, accessed 4 January 2016).

Make sure to adequately translate and adapt the chosen methodological approaches to in-country reality

The methodological approach used for a population consultation in a fragile setting must be well-thought-out and adjusted to the living conditions of the people.

Adapting methodological approaches to the country context, and especially taking into consideration how to reach all (concerned) parts of the population could be challenging. As discussed, designing context-specific tailored approaches is key in that regard. However, additionally to hard-to-reach groups, political fragility and instability – often going hand-in-hand with a lack of trust in governmental institutions – might decrease a population's interest in participating in this kind of exercise even more.[53] It is therefore important to adjust the methodological approach to the living conditions of the people – hard-to-reach might even be harder to reach when the political and security environment does not offer comfort. Designing a well-thought-out approach and using specifically-tailored methodologies will be critical. Due to the high level of fragility, countrywide generalizations should be avoided when analysing the results of the consultation. It is also important to keep in mind when designing the consultation that violence-affected locations may be better served than peaceful ones, owing to a high representation of donors and aid-backed investments.

It is even more important in these scenarios to be precise and thorough when designing the tailored approach. The approach should be adjusted to the conditions of the (politically and geographically separated) population groups.

- A geographical fragmentation, for example through displacements due to natural disasters, would put an additional logistical burden on a consultation because the population to be consulted might be spread across a huge area.
- If the fragmentation is not geographical, but political, it should take political sensitivities into account. For example, a consultation in a fragmented environment with strong hierarchies could also reinforce those hierarchies and additionally marginalize hard-to-reach groups.[54]

Ensure sustainability of the consultation results through feedback and responsible follow-up action

From a more political perspective, in divided scenarios (either politically and/or geographically) there is, as highlighted before, a danger of using results of a population consultation according to political priorities. In that sense, it is important to be aware that fragmentation in a society might be mirrored in the results of the consultation – depending on the group of population and its relationship with the government/MoH. This will be even more the case in conflict scenarios, where consultations might be used to increase support for one of the conflict groups.

Looking at this from a different angle, a population consultation could also pose an opportunity. Making informed choices during a situation of political fragility could be one of the results of a population consultation and may lead to a more sustainable political scenario. The way decisions are taken could be changed by following-up thoroughly on the results of a population consultation.

Bearing this in mind, follow-up action should be seen as one of the most critical elements of the consultation. Even if the political situation is too difficult to follow-up on a plan right away, feedback to the population should nevertheless be provided.

Even in divid[e]d scenarios, consultations have the potential to help change t[he] dynamics of t[he] situation.

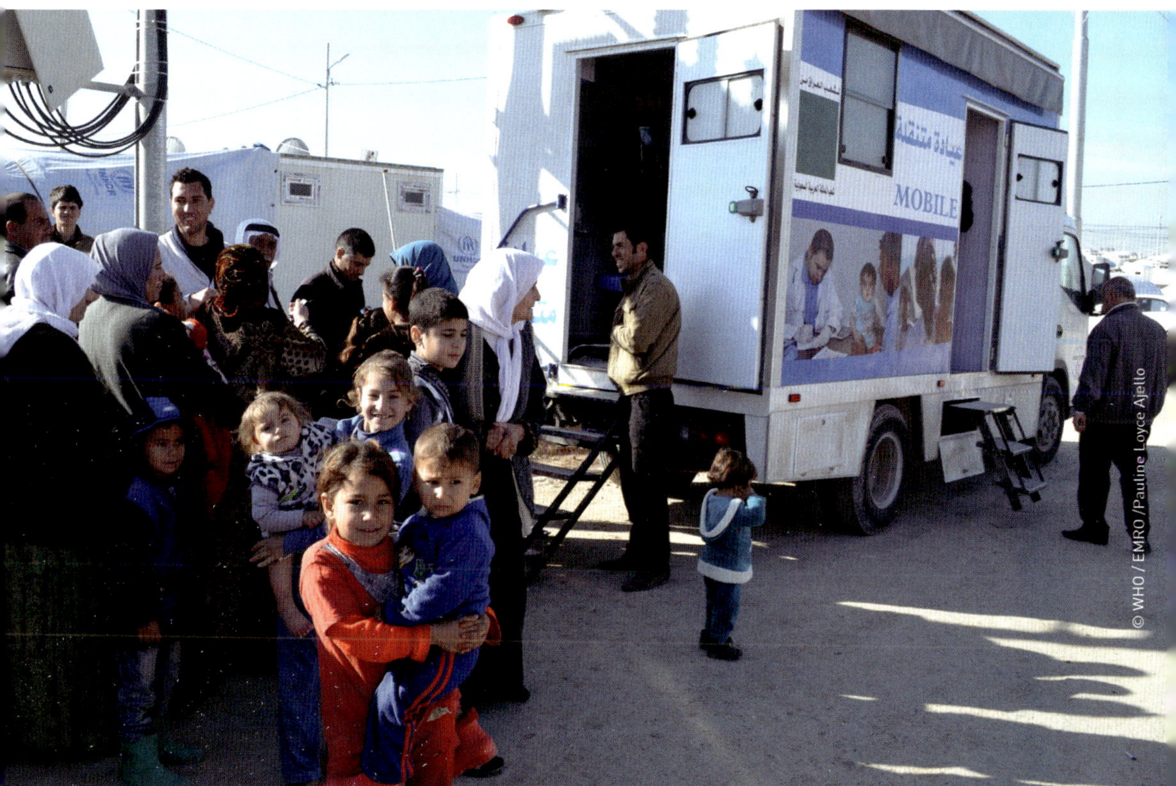

© WHO / EMRO /Pauline Loyce Ajello

Identify priorities through the consultation to support national health planning processes or system-strengthening processes

During a phase of high fragility and instability, designing a new national plan might not be feasible. The results of the population consultation, instead of laying the groundwork for a well-designed national plan, can be used to support bottom-up planning by introducing demands and needs into the process of building up a functional system.

In that case, the methodological design of the consultation would need to be adjusted so that priorities identified are actually supporting a system-building process. They should, therefore, focus on concrete objectives of the process to improve the health of the population, rather than on defining a conceptual vision that might not be useful for the current situation of the country.

In a context where financial and human resource capacities are low, a population consultation can support the identification of priority areas as well as the estimation of the resources that might be needed.

Keeping this in mind, it is also important to consider that the information that will be collected might not be sufficient in the end to support system-building efforts. Political fragility and instability might decrease a population's capacity, interest, and accessibility to participate in this kind of exercise.

In contexts where part of the country is very accessible, conducting a consultation in that limited area might be possible. However, reliability and representativeness of the results might become an issue of concern, since areas that are open to government/MoH initiatives in a (politically) unstable environment, might not be politically neutral. Including an independent facilitator for the consultation (e.g. research institution) could increase legitimacy.

Introduce a regularity of the consultation for it to credibly feed into national review process (JARs, MTRs) and inform policy-makers on a regular basis

Especially in fragmented and fragile scenarios, it will always be essential to consider the transaction costs of the consultation. If the distressed situation of the country is due to a fragile political environment or based on political unrest, the transaction costs might be too high to conduct a population consultation or introduce certain regularity.

However, even in a distressed situation, the potential benefits of the exercise may overweigh the transaction costs. Therefore, a sound analysis of the environment of the consultation will be necessary, as well as a serious consideration of the potential benefits and negative consequences. Although the work might be very resource-intensive, in fragile scenarios, monitoring trends and evaluation of implementation might be particularly important; a regularly undertaken population consultation might help in this regard.

The following table summarizes some of the issues that should be considered when planning for a population consultation in a fragile environment. Countries under stress will most likely not be able to meet all the criteria that we are suggesting. For a consultation to be successful, therefore, it will be essential to weigh all the criteria against each other.

Table 2.3 Issues to consider when undertaking a population consultation in a fragile state setting

RECOMMENDED ACTION	IMPLICATIONS IN A FRAGILE SETTING
Design a satisfactory methodological approach to assess a population's needs and opinions	▸ Would the potential benefits of the consultation outweigh the costs? ▸ Are logistical arrangements feasible and do they not pose an unacceptable burden on the country? ▸ Are financial and human resources as well as capacities sufficient to manage the process of a consultation? ▸ Is the methodology focusing on the identification of priorities to enable increased government engagement in improving living conditions?
Make sure to adequately translate and adapt the chosen methodological approaches to in-country reality	▸ Do political interests or fragility and instability not undermine the effort to reach out to all (concerned) parts of the population (hard-to-reach)? ▸ If only a part of the population can be reached due to political or geographical inaccessibility, can the outcome of the consultation still be considered representative? ▸ Does the population feel comfortable and secure to participate in the consultation? ▸ Does the population feel safe to express their opinion and needs freely, even though their answers might reflect on the difficult political situation that the country is undergoing? ▸ Are political sensitivities that might influence the process and the outcome of the consultation taken into consideration?
Ensure sustainability of the consultation results through feedback and responsible follow-up action	▸ Will results of the consultation be used in a neutral manner and not be subject to arbitrary political interpretation by opposing (political) camps? ▸ Will follow-up action be possible to undertake, even though the security situation and political context of the country might be changing? ▸ Are results of the consultation reliable enough to be representative, despite a possible lack of control of the information-gathering processes?
Identify priorities through the consultation and support national health planning processes or system-strengthening processes	▸ Can priorities identified in the consultation be used to support planning processes and/or system-building processes? ▸ Can priorities be identified and translated into concrete courses of action? ▸ Will information gathered through the consultation be sufficient to support the purpose of the consultation? ▸ Are donors' engagements coordinated and their efforts harmonized to support priority-setting processes based on the consultation results?
Introduce a regularity of the consultation for it to credibly feed into national review process (JAR, MTR) and inform policy-makers on a regular basis	▸ Are the transaction costs of a population consultation too high to introduce regularity? ▸ Will review processes take place that would benefit from the results of the consultation? ▸ Will policy and decision-makers be able to benefit from the consultation?

2.8.3 What if your country is heavily dependent on aid?

A country that is heavily depending on external aid might suffer from two main constraints when discussing population consultation during a health-planning process.

(a) In a heavily aid-dependent context, prioritization and agenda-setting processes might be influenced by donor priorities. Those priorities and strategic preferences might not necessarily reflect the situation in the country, but might be defined by domestic politics of a donor country – be it through direct support through the donor or through indirect support via Global Health Initiatives.[55] This situation could lead to another risk.

(b) Countries that are heavily dependent on foreign aid often suffer from a verticalization in the health sector due to programme-specific approaches or programmatic priorities by external donors.

Donor dependency might not necessarily impact the methodology and feasibility of the consultation, but can influence the process as well as impact the outcomes of the consultation.

The methodology and feasibility of a consultation might not necessarily be linked to a high or low donor dependency. The question is rather whether a high degree of reliance on foreign aid could influence the process as well as impact the outcomes of the consultation. To better understand in what way the consultation could be affected, policy-makers might need to analyse the situation of their country and assess: a) to what extent donors are influencing the policy autonomy and hence the priority-setting of the government, and b) the institutional strength and weaknesses of the health system.

Based on this assessment, it might be easier to understand how the consultation could be undertaken, what the purpose of the consultation could be, and how donors' support could be helpful without distorting the process or the outcomes of the consultation. From the perspective of a MoH it might be important to consider the gains of such a consultation. A population consultation in an aid-dependent context could be used as a means to provide evidence-based information to support negotiations between and among development partners and government to regain the policy autonomy of the government.[56]

The results of the consultation might even be used to hold up national or local needs and opinions against external priorities. External donors' need for justification back at home ("success stories") could be realized through a public consultation. Policy decisions and actions based on the results of a population consultation are more likely to be supported by the communities, which might also increase the likelihood of success. Whether directly or indirectly (through publicity), success of programmes might attract donor funding. External development partners might even be considered as a source for funding, as well as technical and logistical support for the consultation.

A second layer to this is that active participation of concerned groups in the policy formulation process (in this case, through the consultation) could also lead to an improvement of the quality of aid that is provided by external actors. A population consultation could serve as a control mechanism regarding the quality as well as the compliance with local structures.[57] Many international as well as national initiatives (Busan Partnership, IHP+, Paris Declaration) are trying to increase aid effectiveness and efficiency practices as well as individual donor behaviour to align donor engagement with national priorities as outlined in the National Health Strategy or Plan.[58] The MoH should not hesitate to remind the donor community of their commitments (WHO could be a useful companion in this regard).

The Table 2.4 provides some suggestions of what should be considered when undertaking a population consultation in a heavily external aid-dependent context.

Table 2.4 Issues to consider when undertaking a population consultation in an aid-dependent context

RECOMMENDED ACTION	IMPLICATIONS FOR AN AID-DEPENDENT SETTING
Design a satisfactory methodological approach to assess a population's needs and opinions	▸ When establishing the methods and deciding on who is to be involved (stakeholders), it might be necessary to involve and consult external partners, while retaining the independence of the consultation. ▸ The consultation might be used as a tool to hold national or local needs/opinions against external priorities. Therefore, it could be important to make sure not to stumble over any methodological, conceptual or procedural flaws, and to be very precise and accurate in the design of the approach.
Make sure to adequately translate and adapt the chosen methodological approaches to in-country reality	▸ Donor engagement in consultation processes might change the dynamics and reception of the consultation process within the population, which might influence the results of the consultation.
Ensure sustainability of the consultation results through feedback and responsible follow-up action	▸ Demand orientation will be based on priorities identified in the consultation; in some cases this might not be congruent with programme-specific approaches of donors. A follow-up plan will need to take possible discrepancies into consideration.
Incorporate the priorities that were identified through the consultation into the planning process and create a demand-oriented strategy/plan/policy	▸ In addition to the population consultation, external development partners might still conduct their own analysis (or even consultation) of a specific programme or interpreting people's living conditions. This would need to be clarified well in advance. ▸ Donors' engagements can be coordinated and their efforts harmonized to support priority-setting processes based on the consultation results.
Incorporate the priorities that were identified through the consultation into the planning process and create a demand-oriented strategy/plan/policy	▸ It should be taken into consideration that people benefitting from external aid might not see the difference between external and national actors (e.g. service provision). In some cases, this might distort the results of the consultation and might even influence the outcomes of national review processes.

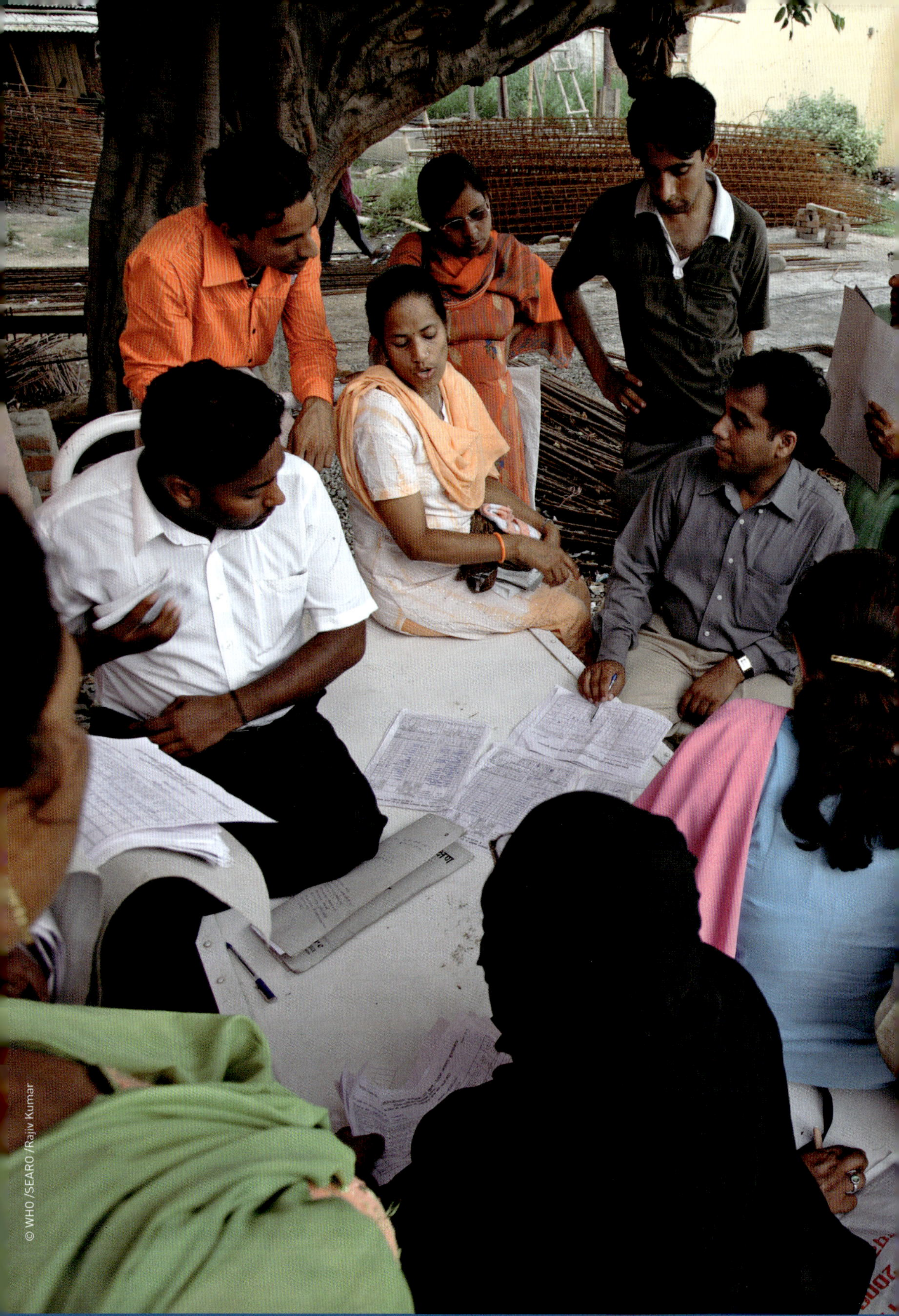

2.9 Conclusion

A population consultation will always have positive effects on the interaction between policy-makers and the population, even if it is just a first step. The political power of a population consultation in influencing the policy dialogue should not be underestimated.

A population consultation is a crucial source of information for policy- and decision-makers and an essential component for non-government actors to influence policy in a way which reflects population's perceived needs. Population consultations serve to increase the population's ownership of policies and plans, thereby increasing the chance of successful implementation. In addition, a government demonstrates itself as transparent and accountable by supporting regular population consultation processes and following up on its results.

The most common population consultation approaches as outlined in this chapter range in complexity, resource needs, and scope: a face-to-face dialogue with a large population sample; consultative methods with invited participants from different population groups; surveys with invited or selected population groups; and individual surveys.

A country may choose one or a combination of these methods, depending on its objective, capacities, and resources.

Optimally, the results of the consultation will feed into the priority-setting exercise of the national health planning process. The population consultation unfolds its full usefulness when it is embedded as an essential step of the process into the planning cycle. Different stages of planning can draw from its results. Given that this would be the only possibility for policy-makers to directly interact with the population to jointly define priorities during the planning process, policy-makers should not hesitate to take advantage of this unique opportunity.

Skilful national health planning is an essential part of the aim to reach universal health coverage. In this regard, a population consultation provides a strong foundation for the planning process, linking factors that are outside the health sector (social determinants of health) back to the arena of the MoH, and strengthening the role of state actors in their aims of providing qualitative and free services to all parts of the population.

References

1 Rodrigo D, Amo PA. Background document on public consultation. Paris: Organisation for Economic Co-operation and Development; 2006 (http://www.oecd.org/mena/governance/36785341.pdf, accessed 30 December 2015).

2 Oxford Dictionaries. Oxford: Oxford University Press; 2015 (http://www.oxforddictionaries.com/definition/english/population, accessed 30 December 2015).

3 Cohen JL, Arato A. Civil society and political theory. Cambridge (MA): Massachusetts Institute of Technology; 1994; 9 (Studies in Contemporary German Social Thought).

4 Potts H. Participation and the right to the highest attainable standard of health. Colchester: Human Rights Centre, University of Essex; 2008 (http://repository.essex.ac.uk/9714/, accessed 30 December 2015).

5 United Nations. Human rights indicators: a guide to measurement and implementation. New York (NY)/Geneva: UN Office of the High Commissioner on Human Rights; 2012 (http://www.ohchr.org/Documents/Publications/Human_rights_indicators_en.pdf, accessed 30 December 2015).

6 For a discussion of the roles of (standing) Health Committees and their role in policy-making processes, see: Neuhold C. The "legislative backbone" keeping the institution upright? The role of European Parliament committees in the EU policy-making process. European Integration online Papers. 2001; 5(10) (http://eiop.or.at/eiop/pdf/2001-010.pdf, accessed 30 December 2015).

7 Brookings Institution; University of Bern Project on Internal Displacement. Moving beyond rhetoric: consultation and participation with populations displaced by conflict or natural disasters. 2008 (http://www.brookings.edu/~/media/research/files/reports/2008/10/internal%20displacement/10_internal_displacement.pdf, accessed 30 December 2015);
Rodrigo D, Amo PA. Background document on public consultation. Paris: Organisation for Economic Co-operation and Development; 2006 (http://www. oecd.org/mena/ governance/36785341.pdf, accessed 30 December).

8 Rodrigo D, Amo PA. Background document on pub- lic consultation. Paris: Organisation for Economic Co-operation and Development; 2006 (http://www. oecd.org/mena/governance/36785341.pdf, accessed 30 December 2015).

9 Handbook on stakeholder consultation and participation in AfDB operations. Tunis-Belvedère: African Development Bank; 2001 (http://www.afdb.org/en/documents/document/handbook-on-stakeholder-consultation-and-participation-in-afdb-opera- tions-17096/, accessed 31 December 2015).

10 Potts H. Participation and the right to the highest attainable standard of health. Colchester: Human Rights Centre, University of Essex; 2008 (http://repos- itory.essex.ac.uk/9714/, accessed 30 December 2015).

11 Government of the UK. Consultation principles. London: Government Digital Service; 2013. (https://www.gov.uk/government/uploads/system/uploads/attachment_data/file/255180/Consultation-Principles-Oct-2013.pdf, accessed 31 December 2015).

12 Communication from the Commission: towards a reinforced culture of consultation and dialogue – general principles and minimum standards for consultation of interested parties by the Commission. Brussels: Commission of the European Communities; 2002 (COM 704 final ; http://ec.europa.eu/governance/docs/comm_standards_en.pdf, accessed 31 December 2015).

13 Documents related to this consultation are archived at: http://www.fhb.gov.hk/beStrong/emain.html, accessed 29 December 2015.

14 http://www.myhealthmychoice.gov.hk/pdf/report/full_report_eng.pdf, accessed 31 December 2015.

15 Local market situation and overseas experience of private health insurance and analysis of stakeholders' views. Hong Kong: Milliman Limited; 2010 (http://www.myhealthmychoice.gov.hk/pdf/studyreport/insurance_background_research.pdf, accessed 31 December 2015).

16 Brücker G, Caniard E. États généraux de la santé: une démarche innovante pour plus de démocratie. Actualité et Dossier en Santé Publique. 1999;27:6–9 (http://www.hcsp.fr/explore.cgi/adsps?ae=adsps&menu=11, accessed 31 December 2015).

17 Ibid.

18 EU-Luxemburg-WHO Universal Health Coverage Partnership: supporting policy dialogue on national health policies, strategies and plans and universal coverage. Year 2 Report: Jan. 2013 – Dec. 2013. Geneva: WHO. 2014 (http://www.uhcpartnership.net/documents/, accessed 31 December 2015).

19 Universal Health Coverage Partnership [website]: (http://www.uhcpartnership.net/citizens-jury-concludes-in-tunisia-with-key-recommendations-for-a-15-year-health-sector-policy-and-plan/).

20 Notre santé un droit une responsabilité: dialogue sociétal sur les politiques, les stratégies, et les plans nationaux de santé. En bref. Tunisie; 2014 (http://www.hiwarsaha.tn/upload/1409230744.pdf).

21 Preparation of the EGS in Guinea was intensively supported by WHO under the EU-LUX Universal Health Coverage Partnership.

22 Turkish Statistics Institution Data base (TURKSTAT); 2013: table 3 (www.tuik.gov.tr/VeriTabanlari.do?ust_id=11&vt_id=30, accessed 31 December 2015).

23 Ali Jadoo SA, Aljunid SM, Sulku SN, Nur AM. Turkish health system reform from the people's perspective: a cross sectional study. BMC Health Serv Res. 2014;14:30. (http://www.ncbi.nlm.nih.gov/pmc/articles/PMC3932508/, accessed 31 December 2015).

24 Eurobarometer surveys are explained at: http://ec.europa.eu/COMMFrontOffice/PublicOpinion/, accessed 12 January 2016).

25 Signorelli S. The EU and public opinions: a love-hate relationship. Paros:Notre Europe – Jacques Delors Institute; 2012 (Studies & Reports 93; http://www.notre-europe.eu/media/eupublicopinionsur-veys-signorelli-ne-jdi-nov12.pdf?pdf=ok, accessed 31 December 2015).

26 Sport and physical activity report. Brussels: European Commission; 2014 (Special Eurobarometer 412; http://ec.europa.eu/health/nutrition_physical_activity/docs/ebs_412_en.pdf, accessed 31 December 2015).

27 Press release. Eurobarometer on sport and physical activity. Brussels: European Commission; 2014 (http://europa.eu/rapid/press-release_MEMO-14-207_en.htm).

28 Kirchgaessner E. The status quo bias in direct democracy: empirical results for Switzerland, 1981–1999. (Preliminary version, January 2007, of paper to be presented at the Annual Congress of the Verein für Socialpolitik, Munich, October 9–12, 2007; https://www.researchgate.net/publication/255596026_The_Status_Quo_Bias_in_Direct_Democracy_Empirical_Results_for_Switzerland_1981_-_1999, accessed 17 February 2016).

29 Krieger J, editor. The Oxford companion to comparative politics. volume 2. Oxford: Oxford University Press; 2012, p.430.

30 Immergut EM. Health politics: interests and institutions in Western Europe. Cambridge: Cambridge University Press; 1992.

31 Bara AC, van den Heuvel WJ, Maarse JA, van Dijk J, de Witte LP. Opinions on changes in the Romanian health care system from people's point of view: a descriptive study. Health Policy. 2003;66(2):123–34. pmid: 14585512.

32 Jones T, Newburn T. Widening access: improving police relations with hard to reach groups. London: Policing and Reducing Crime Unit, Research, Development and Statistics Directorate; 2001 (Police Research Series 138; http://webarchive.nationalarchives.gov.uk/20110220105210/rds.homeoffice.gov.uk/rds/prgpdfs/prs138.pdf, accessed 31 December 2015).

33 Community health needs assessment: an introductory guide for the family health nurse in Europe. Copenhagen: World Health Organization; 2001 (http://www.euro.who.int/__data/assets/pdf_file/0018/102249/E73494.pdf, accessed 4 January 2016).

34 Nicola Brackertz, Who is hard to reach and why? Hawthorn (Victoria); Swinburne University of Technology, Institute for Social Research; 2007 (ISR Working Paper; http://researchbank.swinburne.edu.au/vital/access/manager/Repository/swin:6419?queryType=vitalDismax&query=Nicola+Brackertz&y=0&x=0, accessed 9 January 2016); Brackertz N, Meredyth D. Social inclusion of the hard to reach community – consultation and the hard to reach: local government, social profiling and civic infrastructure. Hawthorn (Victoria): Swinburne University of Technology, Institute for Social Research; 2008 (http://healthissuescentre.org.au/images/uploads/resources/Social-inclusion-of-the-hard-to-reach.pdf, accessed 9 January 2016); Community health needs assessment: an introductory guide for the family health nurse in Europe. Copenhagen: World Health Organization; 2001 (http://www.euro.who.int/__data/assets/pdf_file/0018/102249/E73494.pdf,.accessed 4 January 2016);
Farrell SJ, Reissing E, Evans S, Taylor J. Using community collaboration to develop the first successful needs assessment of the street homeless population in Canada. J Interprof Care. 18(2);2004:197–8 (http://www.tandfonline.com/doi/abs/10.1080/13561820410001686945 [subscription required])DOI:10.1080/13561820410001686945;
Pain R, Francis P, Fuller I, O'Brien K, Williams S. Hard-to-reach young people and community safety: a model for participatory research and consultation. London: Policing and Reducing Crime Unit, Home Office Research, Development and Statistics Directorate; 2002 (Police Research Series Paper152);
Brookings Institution; University of Bern Project on Internal Displacement. Moving beyond rhetoric: consultation and participation with populations displaced by conflict or natural disasters. 2008 (http://www.brookings.edu/~/media/research/files/ reports/2008/10/internal%20displacement/10_internal_displacement.pdf, accessed 30 December 2015).

35 Code of good practice on public consultation. Bristol: Bristol City Council. (http://www.bristol.gov.uk/page/council-and-democracy/code-good-practice-public-consultation, accessed 31 December 2015).

36 Fishkin JS, Luskin RC, Jowell R. Deliberative polling and public consultation. Parliam Aff. 2000;53(4):657–66 (http://pa.oxfordjournals.org/content/53/4/657.citation [subscription required.])

37 De Geoffroy V. ALNAP Global Study on Consultation and Participation of Disaster-affected populations. Country monograph: the case of Colombia. London: Overseas Development Institute; 2003 (http://www.alnap.org/resource/5367, accessed 4 January 2016).

38 Bara AC, van den Heuvel WJ, Maarse JA, van Dijk J, de Witte LP. Opinions on changes in the Romanian health care system from people's point of view: a descriptive study. Health Policy. 2003;66(2):123–34. pmid: 14585512

39 Ali Jadoo SA, Aljunid SM, Sulku SN, Nur AM. Turkish health system reform from the people's perspec- tive: a cross sectional study. BMC Health Serv Res. 2014;14:30. (http://www.ncbi.nlm.nih.gov/pmc/arti- cles/PMC3932508/, accessed 31 December 2015).

40 Ali Jadoo SA, Aljunid SM, Sulku SN, Nur AM. 2014 (see ref. 23); Pain R, Francis P, Fuller I, O'Brien

K, Williams S. Hard-to-reach young people and community safety: a model for participatory research and consultation. London: Policing and Reducing Crime Unit, Home Office Research, Development and Statistics Directorate; 2002 (Police Research Series Paper152).

41 Deutscher Bundestag [website]. Berlin: Deutscher Bundestag - Verfassungsorgan der Bundesrepublik Deutschland. (https://www.bundestag.de/service/faq/abgeordnete/244894, accessed 31 December 2015).

42 Health Promotion Board Singapore [Facebook]. Singapore: Singapore Government. (https://www.facebook.com/hpbsg, accessed 31 December 2015).

43 Ontario Ministry of Health and Long-Term Care [Facebook]. Ontario: Ministry of Health and Long-Term Care. (https://www.facebook.com/pages/Ontario-Ministry-of-Health-and-Long-Term-Care/217753654940869, accessed 31 December 2015).

44 Ministry of Health, New Zealand [Twitter]. Wellington: Ministry of Health, New Zealand. (https://twitter.com/minhealthnz, accessed 31 December 2015).

45 Department of Health [Twitter]. London: Government of the UK. (https://twitter.com/DHgovuk, accessed 31 December 2015).

46 Communication from the Commission: towards a reinforced culture of consultation and dialogue - general principles and minimum standards for consultation of interested parties by the Commission. Brussels: Commission of the European Communities; 2002 (COM 704 final ; http://ec.europa.eu/governance/docs/comm_ standards_en.pdf, accessed 31 December 2015).

47 Communication from the Commission: towards a reinforced culture of consultation and dialogue - general principles and minimum standards for consultation of interested parties by the Commission. Brussels: Commission of the European Communities; 2002 (COM 704 final; http://ec.europa.eu/governance/docs/comm_ standards_en.pdf, accessed 31 December 2015).

48 Pain R, Francis P, Fuller I, O'Brien K, Williams S. Hard-to-reach young people and community safety: a model for participatory research and consultation. London: Policing and Reducing Crime Unit, Home Office Research, Development and Statistics Directorate; 2002 (Police Research Series Paper152).

49 Mullins DR. Accountability and coordination in a decentralized context: institutional, fiscal and governance issues. Washington (DC): American University; 2004 (http://www1.worldbank.org/publicsector/decentralization/June21seminar/LiteratureReview.pdf, accessed 4 January 2016).

50 Krassner S, Risse T. External actors, state-building, and service provision in areas of limited statehood: introduction. Governance. 2014;27(4):545–67 (http://onlinelibrary.wiley.com/doi/10.1111/gove.12065/pdf, accessed 4 January 2016 {subscription required}).

51 Ibid.

52 Diamond L. Building trust in government by improving governance. Stanford's Center on Democracy;2007. (Paper presented to the 7th Global Forum on Reinventing Government; 2007 June 27. UN Headquarters in Vienna, Austria; (http://stanford.edu/~ldiamond/paperssd/BuildingTrustinGovernmentUNGLobalForum.pdf, accessed 4 January 2016).

53 Brookings Institution; University of Bern Project on Internal Displacement. Moving beyond rhetoric: consultation and participation with populations displaced by conflict or natural disasters. 2008 (http://www.brookings.edu/~/media/research/files/reports/2008/10/internal%20displacement/10_internal_displacement.pdf, accessed 30 December 2015); Rodrigo D, Amo PA. Background document on pub- lic consultation. Paris: Organisation for Economic Co-operation and Development; 2006 (http://www. oecd.org/mena/ governance/36785341.pdf, accessed 30 December).

54 Brookings Institution; University of Bern Project on Internal Displacement. Moving beyond rhetoric: consultation and participation with populations displaced by conflict or natural disasters. 2008 (http://www.brookings.edu/~/media/research/files/ reports/2008/10/internal%20displacement/10_internal_displacement.pdf, accessed 30 December 2015); Rodrigo D, Amo PA. Background document on public consultation. Paris: Organisation for Economic Cooperation and Development; 2006 (http://www. oecd.org/mena/governance/36785341.pdf, accessed 30 December 2015).

55 For a discussion on the challenges of aid dependency for policy autonomy and national planning processes, see: Thomas A, Viciani I, Tench J, Sharpe R, Hall M, Martin M, et al. Real aid 3: ending aid dependency. London: ActionAid UK; 2011 (http://www.actionaid.org/sites/files/actionaid/real_aid_3.pdf, accessed 9 January 2016).

56 De Geoffroy V. ALNAP Global Study on Consultation and Participation of Disaster-affected populations. Country monograph: the case of Colombia. London: Overseas Development Institute; 2003 (http://www.alnap.org/resource/5367, accessed 4 January 2016).

57 De Geoffroy V. ALNAP Global Study on Consultation and Participation of Disaster-affected populations. Country monograph: the case of Colombia. London: Overseas Development Institute; 2003 (http://www.alnap.org/resource/5367, accessed 4 January 2016).

58 Aligning for better results [website]. Geneva: Interna-tional Health Partnership. (http://www.international- healthpartnership.net/en/, accessed 4 January 2016).

Further reading

Brookings Institution; University of Bern Project on Internal Displacement. Moving beyond rhetoric: consultation and participation with populations displaced by conflict or natural disasters. 2008 (http://www.brookings.edu/~/media/research/files/reports/2008/10/internal%20displacement/10_internal_displacement.pdf, accessed 30 December 2015).

Culver K, Howe P. Calling all citizens: the challenges of public consultation. Toronto: Canadian Public Administration; 2004. doi:10.1111/j.1754-7121.2004.tb01970.x.

Eurobarometer surveys: methodology – instrument description [website]. Brussels: European Commission; 2015 (http://ec.europa.eu/COMMFrontOffice/PublicOpinion/, accessed 12 January 2016).

Rodrigo D, Amo PA. Background document on public consultation. Paris: Organisation for Economic Co-operation and Development; 2006 (http://www.oecd.org/mena/governance/36785341.pdf, accessed 30 December 2015).

Trochim, WMK. The Research Methods Knowledge Base [online database], 2nd edition. 2006 (http://www.socialresearchmethods.net/, accessed 30 December 2015).

United Nations Development Programme (UNDP). Handbook on planning, monitoring and evaluating for development results. New York (NY): United Nations Development Group; 2009 (http://web.undp.org/evaluation/handbook/documents/english/pme-handbook.pdf, accessed 30 December 2015).

United States Agency for International Development (USAID). Performance monitoring and evaluation tips. Washington (DC): Center for Development Information and Evaluation (https://www.usaid.gov/evaluation/policy, accessed 14 January 2016).

World Bank. Monitoring and evaluation for results: some tools, methods and approaches. Washington (DC), World Bank: 2004 (http://www-wds.worldbank.org/external/default/WDSContentServer/WDSP/IB/2006/02/15/000012009_20060215093620/Rendered/PDF/246140UPDATED01s1methods1approaches.pdf , accessed 30 December 2015).

World Bank. Qualitative methods. Washington (DC): The World Bank [website]. (http://web.worldbank.org/WBSITE/EXTERNAL/TOPICS/EXTPOVERTY/EXTISPMA/0,,contentMDK:20190070~menuPK:412148~pagePK:148956~piPK:216618~theSitePK:384329,00.html, accessed 30 December 2015).

Annex 2.1

Description, advantages and challenges of individual survey tools

INDIVIDUAL SURVEY TOOLS	DESCRIPTION	ADVANTAGES	CHALLENGES
Structured interviews (cf. survey)	▸ Interviews supported by questionnaires. ▸ Standardized approach to obtaining information on a wide range of topics from a large number or diversity of stakeholders. Structured/standardized open-ended interviews consist of a set of open-ended questions carefully worded and arranged in advance. ▸ The interviewer asks each respondent the same questions with essentially the same words and in the same sequence.	▸ Collects detailed data systematically and facilitate comparability among all respondents. ▸ Quickly gathers descriptive data on a wide range of topics. ▸ Easy to analyse. ▸ Relatively low cost. ▸ Gives anonymity to respondents. ▸ Particularly appropriate when there are several interviewers (minimize the variation in the questions they pose); also useful for gathering the same information from each interviewee at several points in time or when there are time constraints for data collection and analysis.	▸ Susceptible to selection and interviewer biases. ▸ Data may provide a general picture but may lack depth; may not provide adequate information on context. ▸ Does not permit the interviewer to have broad understanding and insight, and to pursue topics or issues that were not anticipated when the interview instrument was developed.

INDIVIDUAL SURVEY TOOLS	DESCRIPTION	ADVANTAGES	CHALLENGES
Semi-structured interviews (usually with "key informants")	▸ A series of open-ended questions. ▸ Interviews are qualitative, in-depth, and semi-structured. They rely on interview guides that list topics or questions. ▸ Key informants are usually community experts who can provide particular knowledge and understanding of problems and can recommend solutions. ▸ Involve the preparation of an interview guide that lists a pre-determined set of questions or issues that are to be explored. This guide serves as a checklist during the interview and ensures that basically the same information is obtained from a number of people. Yet, there is a great deal of flexibility. The order and the actual working of the questions are not determined in advance. Moreover, within the list of topic or subject areas, the interviewer is free to pursue certain questions in greater depth. ▸ If informants agree, interviews can be audio-taped.	▸ Low cost, simple and quick to conduct. ▸ Provides flexibility to explore new ideas and issues not anticipated. ▸ Makes interviewing of a number of different persons relatively systematic. ▸ Can provide insight on the nature of problems, a snapshot of the current state of a system, and give recommendations for solutions. ▸ Can provide different perspectives on a single issue or on several issues. ▸ Can be especially useful to highlight the constraints faced by private actors in systems historically dominated by public entities (perception of barriers, systems constraints, and untapped, under-exploited or emerging opportunities).	▸ Susceptible to selection and interviewer biases. ▸ Can be difficult to analyse. ▸ Must have some means to verify or corroborate information (triangulation). ▸ Less valid, reliable, and credible than formal surveys.
Open or informal interviews	▸ Informal conversational interviews rely primarily on the spontaneous generation of questions in the natural flow of an interaction. This type of interview is appropriate when the evaluator wants to maintain maximum flexibility to pursue questioning in whatever direction appears to be appropriate, depending on the information that emerges from observing a particular setting or from talking to one or more individuals in that setting.	▸ The interviewer is flexible and highly responsive to individual differences, situational changes and emerging new information.	▸ Susceptible to selection and interviewer biases. ▸ May generate less systematic data that are difficult and time-consuming to classify and analyse. ▸ Must have some means to verify or corroborate information (triangulation).

INDIVIDUAL SURVEY TOOLS	DESCRIPTION	ADVANTAGES	CHALLENGES
Face-to-face or personal interview	▸ The interviewer works directly with the respondent and has the opportunity to probe or ask follow-up questions. ▸ A special case is the household drop-off survey. In this approach, a researcher goes to the respondent's home or business and hands the respondent the instrument. (In some cases, the respondent is asked to mail it back or the interviewer returns to pick it up.)	▸ Interviews are generally easier for the respondent, especially if opinions or impressions are sought. ▸ Allows personal contact and gestural communication. Allows follow-up questions to explore the answers of the respondents. Facilitates the researcher's understanding of the respondent's answers. ▸ Suitable for locations where telephone or mail are not developed. ▸ The household drop-off survey blends the advantages of the mail survey and the group administered questionnaire: the respondent can work on the instrument in private, when it is convenient; and the interviewer makes personal contact with the respondent, and the respondent can ask questions about the study and get clarification on what is to be done. This is expected to increase the percentage of people willing to respond.	▸ Time-consuming. ▸ Resource intensive. ▸ Susceptible to interviewer bias. The interviewer is considered a part of the measurement instrument and interviewers have to be well trained in how to respond to any contingency. ▸ Easy to manipulate.
Telephone	▸ Questionnaire administered by telephone. Many major public opinion polls are based on telephone interviews.	▸ Enables a researcher to gather information rapidly. ▸ Fairly cost-effective. ▸ Like personal interviews, they allow for some personal contact between the interviewer and the respondent. ▸ Higher response rates ▸ Allows the interviewer to ask follow-up questions.	▸ Many people do not have publicly-listed telephone numbers. Some do not have telephones. ▸ May be perceived as intrusive. ▸ Interviews have to be relatively short or people will feel imposed upon. ▸ Susceptible to interviewer bias. ▸ Cannot be used for non-audio information.

INDIVIDUAL SURVEY TOOLS	DESCRIPTION	ADVANTAGES	CHALLENGES
Mail-out	‣ The questionnaire may be handed to the respondents or mailed to them, but in all cases they are returned to the researcher via mail.	‣ Relatively inexpensive to administer; more cost effective than face-to-face interviews, especially for studies involving large sample sizes, large geographic areas and large number of questions. ‣ Ideal for asking closed-ended questions; can send the exact same instrument to a wide number of people and thus reduce bias, and is easy to analyse. ‣ Allows the respondent to fill it out at his/her own convenience and is thus less intrusive than telephone or face-to-face surveys. ‣ Possible to obtain large amount of information.	‣ Response rates are often very low. ‣ Long delays, often of several months, before the surveys are returned and statistical analysis can begin. ‣ Not suitable for issues that may require clarification. ‣ Little flexibility left to the respondent (nuances easily lost). ‣ Lack of personal contact; limited researcher understanding of the respondent's answers. ‣ Uncertainty about the respondent's identity. ‣ Subject to levels of literacy.
Online	‣ Questionnaires are now commonly administered online, as in the form of web surveys. Different types of survey software exist to help design, administer and analyse online surveys.	‣ Similar to mail-out; faster, simpler, and cheaper. ‣ Ease of data gathering. ‣ Flexibility in design; more dynamic interaction between the respondent and the questionnaire. ‣ Quicker response and analysis time. ‣ Less intrusive. ‣ Suffer less from social desirability bias.	‣ Similar to mail-out; response rate higher. ‣ Subject to reading and PC/ internet equipment. ‣ Susceptible to survey fraud.
Mobile	‣ Survey tool available on a device such as a smart phone or a tablet.	‣ Not subject to constraints relative to time and location of the respondent. ‣ In places with high mobile phone penetration, possibility to reach previously hard-to-reach target groups. ‣ Quicker response times.	‣ Subject to reading and appropriate equipment/ software.

Annex 2.2

Checklist: Selecting the most appropriate type of survey for my setting

Checklist: Selecting the most appropriate type of survey for my setting

Selecting an appropriate survey is a critical decision which should be guided by a number of factors.

- ✓ Population issues: Can the population be enumerated? Is the population literate? Are there language issues? Will the population cooperate? What are the geographical restrictions?
  For example, If the population is not literate or there are language barriers, telephone or face-to-face interviews may be considered.

- ✓ Sampling issues: What data is available? Can respondents be found? Who is the respondent? Can all members of population be sampled? Are response rates likely to be a problem?
  If the population to be surveyed is small, you can survey them all, for example. Otherwise, you are likely to need to go through sampling techniques.
  Qualitative studies can rely on less restrictive sampling techniques, for example convenience sampling and interviews until information saturation.

- ✓ Question issues: What types of questions can be asked? How complex will the questions be? Will screening questions be needed? Can question sequence be controlled? Will lengthy questions be asked? Will long response scales be used?
  Closed (multiple choice) questions are easy to administer through written questionnaires. Open-ended questions are often better administered through interviews.
  Mail-out or online questionnaires are probably better if there are a lot of questions. Telephone interviews should rather be short. Face-to-face interviews may be longer but it is preferable to plan them in advance.

- ✓ Content Issues: Can the respondents be expected to know about the issue? Will respondent need to consult records?
  If respondents cannot answer directly, written (mail-out or online) questionnaire is better.

- ✓ Bias issues: Can social desirability be avoided? Can interviewer distortion and subversion be controlled? Can false respondents be avoided?
  If there is a strong potential for social desirability (respondent wanting to please interviewer) and/or topics which will not be discussed due to the characteristic of the interviewer (for instance women vis-à-vis male interviewers), avoid face-to-face and telephone interviews.

- ✓ Administrative Issues: costs; facilities; time; personnel

Source: Trochim WMK. The research methods knowledge base (see Further reading, above).

Annex 2.3

Questionnaire vs. interviews

ISSUE	QUESTIONNAIRE			INTERVIEW	
	Group	Mail	Drop-Off	Personal	Phone
Will visual presentations be possible?	+	+	+	+	-
If you prefer short, closed-ended survey responses...	+	+	+	+/-	-
If privacy is an issue which needs to be considered...	-	+	-	+	+/-
If flexibility in administering the questionnaire is important...	-	-	-	+	+
If you wish to increase your likelihood of good open-ended responses...	-	-	-	+	+
Reading and writing are necessary for...	+/-	+	+	-	-
The quality of the response can be evaluated	+	-	+/-	+	+/-
Are high response rates likely?	+	-	+	+	-
If you wish to be able to explain the study in person...	+	-	+	+	+/-
The lower-cost options are...	+	+	-	-	-
Resource requirements such as staff/facility are low	+	+	-	-	-
Are you seeking to target a sub-section of the population which is hard-to-reach?	-	+	-	-	-
If you want to ensure ample time for respondents to answer...	-	+	+	-	-
If potential interviewer bias could be a problem...	-	+	-	-	+
If you wish to undertake a longer, open-ended survey...	-	-	-	+	-
If quick turnover time is important...	-	+	-	-	+

+ : Yes	- : No	+/- : it depends on several factors and context

Sources:

Kumar, K, editor. Rapid appraisal methods. Washington (DC): The World Bank; 1993 (World Bank Regional and Sectoral Studies).

Handbook on planning, monitoring and evaluating for development results. New York (NY): United Nations Development Group (UNDP); 2009 (http://web.undp.org/evaluation/handbook/documents/english/pme-handbook.pdf, accessed 30 December 2015).

United States Agency for International Development (USAID). Performance Monitoring and Evaluation Tips. Washington (DC): Center for Development Information and Evaluation: Conducting a participatory evaluation, n°1, 2011 printing (http://pdf.usaid.gov/pdf_docs/pnadw101.pdf, accessed 30 December 2015)

Conducting key informant interviews, n°2, 2011 printing (http://pdf.usaid.gov/pdf_docs/pnadw102.pdf, accessed 30 December 2015)

Using rapid appraisal methods, n°5, 2nd edition 2010 (http://pdf.usaid.gov/pdf_docs/pnadw105.pdf, accessed 30 December 2015)

Conducting focus group interviews, n°10, 2011 printing (http://pdf.usaid.gov/pdf_docs/pnadw110.pdf, accessed 30 December 2015)

Monitoring and evaluation for results: some tools, methods and approaches. Washington (DC): World Bank; 2004 (http://www-wds.worldbank.org/external/default/WDSContentServer/WDSP/IB/2006/02/15/000012009_20060215093620/Rendered/PDF/246140UPDATED01s1methods1approaches.pdf, accessed 30 December 2015).

World Bank [website]. Qualitative methods. Washington (DC): The World Bank; 2004 (http://web.worldbank.org/WBSITE/EXTERNAL/TOPICS/EXTPOVERTY/EXTISPMA/0,,contentMDK:20190070~menuPK:412148~pagePK:148956~piPK:216618~theSitePK:384329,00.html, accessed 30 December 2015).

WHO evaluation practice handbook. Geneva: World Health Organization; 2013 (http://apps.who.int/iris/handle/10665/96311, accessed 30 December 2015).

Chapter 3

Situation analysis of the health sector

Dheepa Rajan

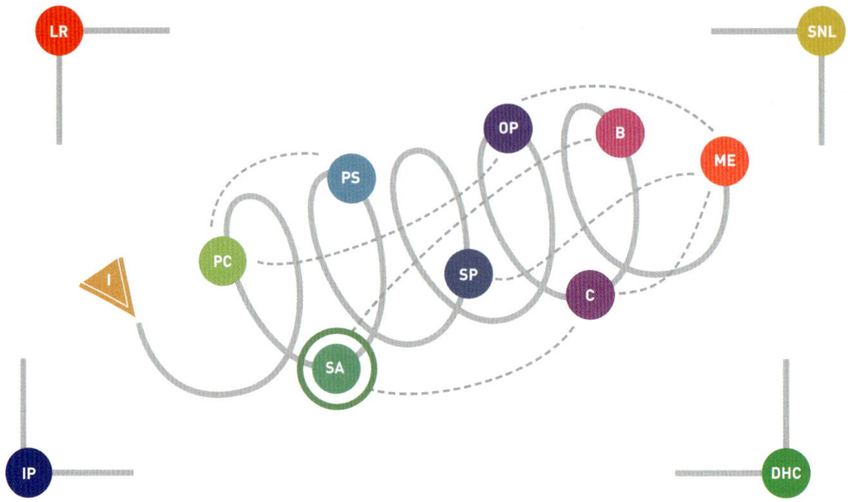

Cross-cutting topics relevant to national health planning

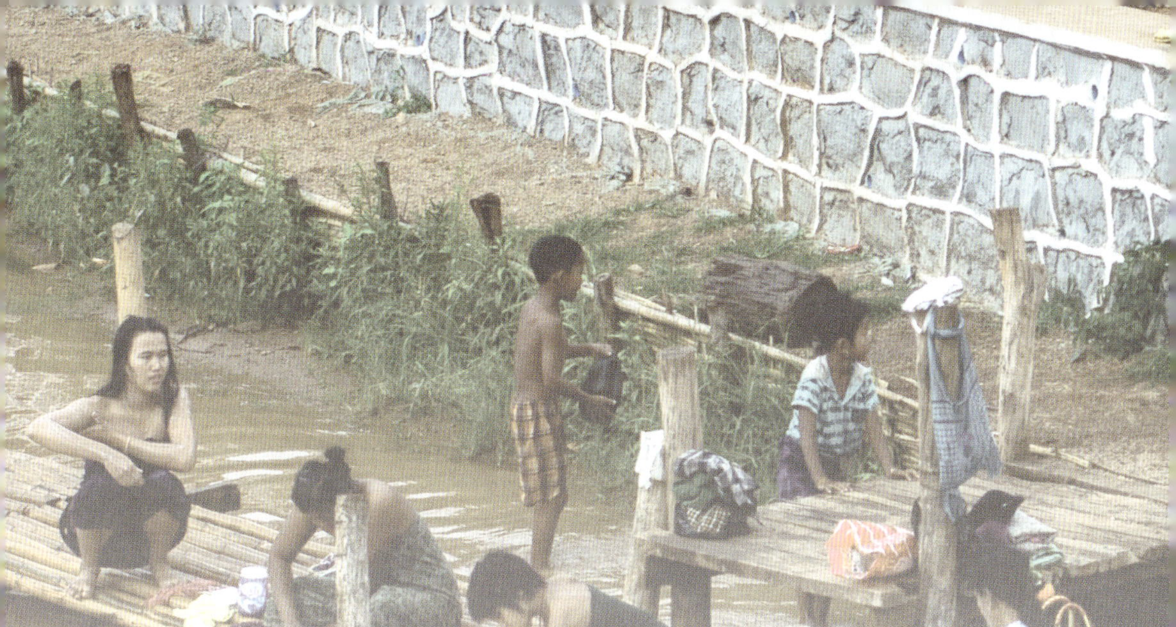

Overview

The strategic directions and the principal orientation of a national health policy, strategy or plan (NHPSP) need to be grounded in a sound understanding of the status of the health sector. This chapter aims to elaborate on a participatory, inclusive health sector situation analysis methodology to address that simple but very basic need of obtaining a realistic snapshot of the strengths and weaknesses of a country's health system, as well as a more profound understanding of the reasons behind those strengths and weaknesses, so as to better enable a viable alternative (or successful scale-up).

Summary

What is a situation analysis of the health sector?

A health sector situation analysis should aim:

(a) to realistically assess the current health sector situation, with all its strengths, weaknesses opportunities and threats, including their root causes and effects;

(b) to provide an evidence-informed basis for responding to health sector needs and expectations of the population;

(c) to provide an evidence-informed basis for formulating future strategic directions for the health sector.

Several characteristics of a sound health sector situation analysis are elaborated upon in this chapter. These are:

- participatory and inclusive;
- analytical;
- relevant;
- comprehensive;
- evidence-based.

Why should a situation analysis be done?

A whole-of-sector situation analysis is important because:

- it is a crucial step in the planning cycle;
- it gives a voice and a platform to all health sector stakeholders, including the population;
- it increases accountability and transparency;
- it supports and strengthens monitoring and evaluation;
- it contributes to concretizing roles and responsibilities; and
- it helps to establish consensus on the status of health in the country.

When should a situation analysis take place?

It should be done as a key initial step in the development of a NHPSP. Ideally, it should be undertaken at least once during the health policy and planning cycle, and updated every few years, because an updated, in-depth technical analysis that includes stakeholder viewpoints is an invaluable resource for the whole health sector.

Who should be involved in a health sector situation analysis?

When examining the roles and responsibilities of the various health sector stakeholders, it is important to keep in mind the three main functions which are needed for a successful situation analysis: active and inclusive multi-stakeholder participation, decision-making, and organization and coordination. Some health actors will be active on all three fronts, while others will only be involved in one or another function, as described in more detail in this chapter.

How should it be conducted?

It is recommended to go for an approach which is as participatory and inclusive as possible, with a core team coordinating working groups. The working groups should be comprised of relevant experts and health stakeholders who are given adequate space and time for dialogue. This process is a crucial investment, whose potential to unite together those who have a stake in health into a common understanding of health sector challenges and solutions should not be underestimated. This methodology is elaborated upon in more detail in this chapter.

Anything else to consider?

- decentralized setting;
- fragile environment;
- aid-dependent environment.

3.1 What do we mean by "situation analysis" of the health sector?

3.1.1 What is a situation analysis?

No one disagrees with the fact that the strategic directions and the principal orientation of a NHPSP need to be grounded in a sound understanding of the status of the health sector. However, a myriad of options exist on how to go about the situation analysis, depending on the setting and objectives. In this chapter, the focus is on a situation analysis of the full health sector for purposes of developing a NHPSP. However, even for this same purpose, it may be necessary to go more in-depth into certain key areas – for example, health financing or human resources for health – depending on the country setting. The principles and approach as described in this chapter can still be used, although we specifically address an overarching whole-of-sector situation analysis here.

This chapter aims to elaborate on a participatory, inclusive methodology to address that simple but very basic need of obtaining a realistic snapshot of the strengths and weaknesses of a country's health system, as well as a more profound understanding of the reasons behind those strengths and weaknesses, so as to better enable a viable alternative (or successful scale-up).

WHO defines a health-specific situation analysis as "an assessment of the current health situation ... [that] is fundamental to designing and updating national policies, strategies and plans".[1] The World Bank proposes the term "health systems analysis" with the following definition: "Health systems analysis includes evidence on health system inputs, processes, and outputs and the analysis of how these combine to produce the outcomes. It considers politics, history, and institutional arrangements. Health systems analysis proposes causes of poor health system performance and suggests how reform policies and strengthening strategies can improve performance."[2]

This chapter elaborates on a participatory, inclusive methodology to obtain a realistic snapshot of the strengths and weaknesses of a country's health system.

Based on the above definitions, the objectives of a situation analysis in this handbook are:

(a) to realistically assess the current health sector situation, with all its strengths, weaknesses, opportunities and threats, including their root causes and effects;

(b) to provide an evidence-informed basis for responding to health sector needs and expectations of the population;

(c) to provide an evidence-informed basis for formulating future strategic directions for the health sector.

A health sector situation analysis can begin as a one-off activity, but parts of the analysis can be updated and revisited on a regular basis for programming and monitoring purposes.

Several characteristics are recommended to ensure a sound health sector situation analysis.

- **Participatory and inclusive**—include all relevant stakeholders in the health sector, including the population.
- **Analytical**—base it on a causal framework of how inputs, processes, and outputs interact with each other and with other important environmental factors. It is critical to make a distinction here between being descriptive, i.e. narrating the state of the current situation, and analytical, i.e. attempting to understand the current situation based on past decisions, choices, and plans, as well as underlying causal factors.
- **Relevant**—focus on issues that ultimately affect the health status of the population, and consider solutions to ongoing challenges.
- **Comprehensive** — cover all aspects related to the health sector, including health systems, programmes, the full range of (personal and non-personal) health services, intersectoral action for health, etc.
- **Evidence-based**—utilize a wide range of information and data, both quantitative and qualitative, as well as, where relevant, other countries' experiences.[3]

3.1.2 The spectrum of a situation analysis

A situation analysis can happen:

(a) at any stage of the national planning process, from priority-setting to monitoring and evaluation;

(b) at any level of the state (national, province/region, district);

(c) on varying themes and scopes (i.e. for the health sector in general or for health financing in particular, for example);

(d) with the lead taken by ministry of health (MoH).

Please note that for the purposes of this chapter, the focus will be an overall health sector situation analysis.

3.2 Why do we want to undertake a situation analysis?

3.2.1 It is a crucial step in the planning cycle

Coherent and needs-oriented health sector planning cannot take place without an adequate base of information, data, and evidence on the current state of the health system. Is the health system responding to population needs? Is the health status of the population improving? Is the current national health plan being implemented well? What are the challenges faced? These are just some of the crucial queries whose answers are imperative to better plan for and orient the future. Taking stock of existing knowledge is the first step towards decision-making.

3.2.2 In order to give a voice and a platform to all health sector stakeholders, including the population

(a) Stakeholder buy-in can lead to better policy implementation

Even the most ingeniously-designed health policies will not be implemented without the buy-in from health sector stakeholders (which includes stakeholders from other sectors who work in and with health), because they are precisely the ones who will be involved in the launching and practical implementation of the policy. In order to have adequate buy-in, stakeholders must be involved in all crucial steps of the planning cycle, starting with the situation analysis.

(b) A wide range of expertise and viewpoints, in particular the views of citizens, leads to better-designed policies

Policy-makers at the central level may not be aware of all the details and challenges faced in other sectors and at the level of implementation – therefore, the input of those who are in other sectors and those who are close to the "field" is necessary in order to ensure that a situation is reflecting the true status of the health system.

The first step towards decision-making is taking stock of existing knowledge about the health sector.

It is important to note here that "input" may not solely be from technical experts. Policy-making is a complex process that clearly should be guided by scientific knowledge and experts' views. However, the views and opinions of end-users and the population at large add a demand-side dimension that highly influences success in implementation. For instance, experts are well-placed to identify high-mortality diseases in the country and the most cost-effective ways to reduce their incidence. However, the most cost-effective ways may be ignoring some dire realities and barriers to access at the population level, which will only emerge when hearing population views.[I] Examples include some ethnic groups' beliefs preventing women from delivering in health facilities because health staff do not respect traditional rituals; social norms which are contrary to health experts' message for health prevention; health centres not being used because the opening hours are not convenient for the local population's schedules. These few examples evince the bias that a situation analysis can take if populations' points of view are not taken into account.

I Please see Chapter 2 "Population consultation on needs and expectations" in this handbook.

3.2.3 In order to increase accountability and transparency

A situation analysis done properly, with the characteristics mentioned above, allows governments to account for health sector activities and results in a transparent way. The more participatory and honestly open the situation analysis is, the more accountable and transparent the government shows itself to be. This is not to say that the types of participation and representativeness of those participating should not be thought through in detail and care given to practical considerations for fair participation (see Boxes 3.2 and 3.4).

Conducting a situation analysis in a participatory manner implies making data and information available and accessible to different health sector stakeholders who may not have the opportunity to look at, discuss, and understand this information otherwise – thus promoting transparency. Transparency also means giving stakeholders a voice by providing information and explanations on issues that matter to them most and affect them directly. Accountability entails enabling stakeholders to influence decision-making and hold those making decisions to account. A participatory situation analysis is the first step to joint decision-making and monitoring progress on those decisions.

In some settings, the MoH may fear that if a sector analysis is done in a genuinely participative way, the outcome may point out weaknesses at their level which can become politically burdensome. However, experience shows that

Box 3.1

Expert views and population opinion in West Africa: two sides of the same coin

If one asks most health staff in rural West Africa what are the major problems impeding the performance of health services, they will probably mention the following: lack of sufficient and timely resources; poor staff motivation due to low salaries and no recognition of merit; and poor working conditions. At the same time, a socio-anthropological study performed in five of these countries shows that the main complaint of patients about the local health system is the bad reception and rude behaviour of health staff towards them.[4] The two are very likely interconnected, but the latter would certainly not have emerged as a major problem if the situation analysis only took into account views of experts and health professionals. Thus the solutions to the first set of problems alone (e.g. raising salaries and upgrading equipment) would probably not be an appropriate solution to the problem in its full complexity.

Experience shows that if stakeholders' well-founded critical views are taken into account in the situation analysis, their willingness to align, harmonize and contribute resources increases. On the other hand, if a sector analysis is perceived to be biased, obscuring obvious system weaknesses, the MoH may have difficulties obtaining a consensus with stakeholders.

Fig. 3.1 Situation Analysis: getting a good understanding of a country's health system

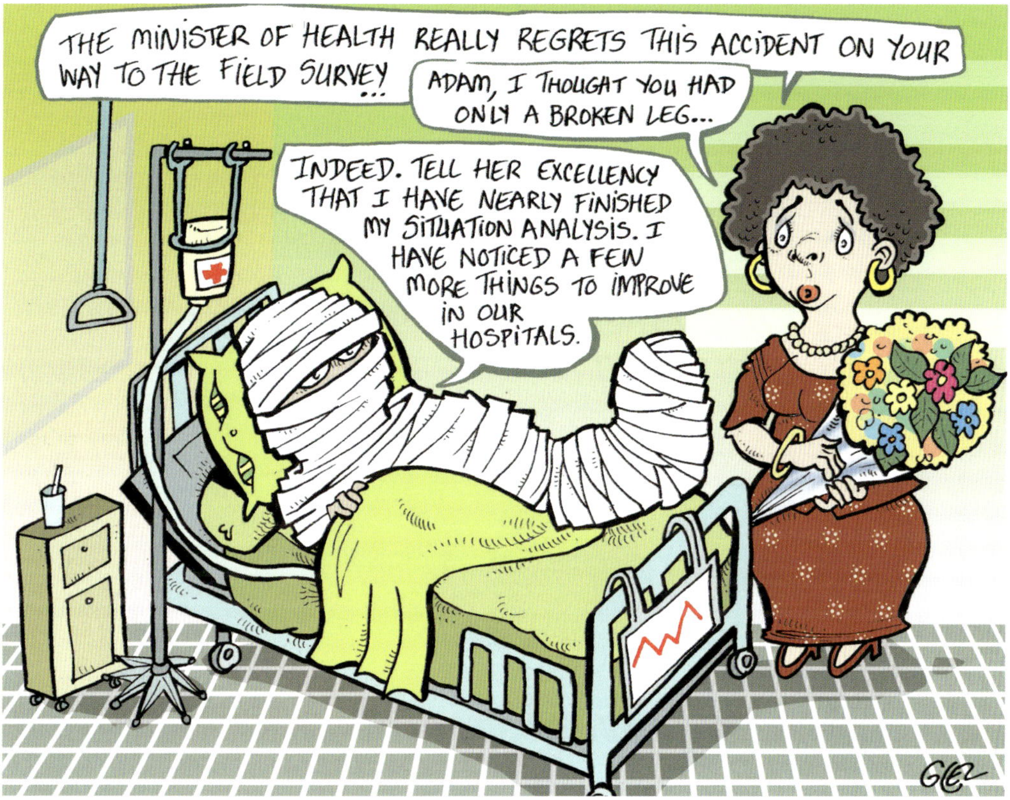
THE MINISTER OF HEALTH REALLY REGRETS THIS ACCIDENT ON YOUR WAY TO THE FIELD SURVEY...
ADAM, I THOUGHT YOU HAD ONLY A BROKEN LEG...
INDEED. TELL HER EXCELLENCY THAT I HAVE NEARLY FINISHED MY SITUATION ANALYSIS. I HAVE NOTICED A FEW MORE THINGS TO IMPROVE IN OUR HOSPITALS.
GLEZ

Damian Glez; scenario by Bruno Meessen.

if stakeholders' well-founded critical views are taken into account in the analysis, their willingness to align, harmonize and contribute resources increases. On the other hand, if a sector analysis is perceived to be biased, obscuring obvious system weaknesses, the MoH may have difficulties obtaining a consensus with stakeholders. Subsequently, overall adherence to new policies may end up being weak.

Box 3.2

What do we mean by "voice and accountability" and by "participation"? What are some of the common challenges to ensuring widespread participation?

"Voice and accountability" is a driving concept in strategizing for health in the 21st century. It signifies that those in charge of developing national health plans need to include all concerned stakeholders, giving them the space and opportunity to freely express their views. In particular, the population (and their representatives) should be explicitly included as "concerned stakeholders" in the debates that lead to strategies which affect them.

The word "participation" in the context of a health sector situation analysis implies a meaningful participation, i.e. the stakeholder who is requested to participate is prepared and informed in an objective way and is allowed an adequate platform to express his/her voice. Participation by a greater number of people and a wider cross-section of society can be reached by linking a participatory situation analysis to a population consultation. Many countries may not conduct a population consultation with every situation analysis due to time and cost constraints but it is necessary to capture population demands and expectations with some level of periodicity.[II]

Ensuring widespread participation often necessitates good and early preparation – this is because, depending on the political context of the country, dialogue and consensus must be sought at an early stage. This often means reaching out to actors one is less comfortable with, and potentially facing confrontation. This is an extra effort and its importance is not to be underestimated in view of achieving broad adherence and alignment.

Ideally, the stakeholders who participate in a situation analysis should have sufficient understanding of the issue, have sufficient communication skills so as to claim their voice (including being socially "allowed" to speak), and be representative of all the categories of population that should participate. In practice, however, it is not always easy to identify those representative stakeholders and enable them to participate. The following dilemmas require careful consideration but should not be seen as deterrents – rather, by thinking these issues through beforehand, they can be more easily resolved.

- The greater the number of participants there are in the consultative event, the more difficult it is to allow fair participation of all points of view, to reach a consensus on situation analysis, and to take decisions. It is important to strike a balance between casting the net wide to include as many stakeholders as possible and having a fair number of participants who are really able to have a say.
- Even when all relevant categories of stakeholders have been identified (e.g. civil society, religious communities, women, labour unions, other line ministries, etc.), it is not easy to identify those organizations or individuals which are most appropriate and legitimate to represent those stakeholders. In many countries, civil society organizations (CSOs) are federated into national platforms, but these are not always viewed as legitimate by all organizations. It can thus be extremely difficult to know who constitute

II For more information, see Chapter 2 "Population consultation on needs and expectations" in this handbook.

adequate representatives of the whole. A similar situation can be found with non-profit organizations: there may be hundreds of them, varying greatly in size, coverage and expertise, while effective coordination, and therefore representativity, can be unclear. A careful analysis and understanding of stakeholder groups, as well as engagement with them, can help to identify the right people.

- As for representatives of other sectoral line ministries the MoH may wish to involve, it is not straightforward whether the "right" representatives will be sent by their ministry. Very often, ministries send medium-grade staff, who do not have decision-making power (and sometimes even do not know the issues to be discussed). Specifying the person who should attend the event may be against protocol (but if it is not, this is one way to overcome this challenge). In countries where official "health focal points" have been nominated in non-health ministries, this problem occurs much less frequently.
- Even when the appropriate stakeholders are represented, they may not feel empowered to effectively participate in the dialogue – be it due to lack of technical skills or due to social norms. Particular care should be given to supporting the participation of representatives from rural and hard-to-reach populations. It may even be appropriate to organize separate consultative events to allow these groups to freely express their opinions.
- In the case of NHPSPs, it is important that the government leads the consultative process, especially in aid-dependent contexts where donors may unduly influence debates.

3.2.4 In order to support and strengthen monitoring and evaluation

A health sector situation analysis is an in-depth look at all aspects related to inputs, processes, and outputs of the health sector, i.e. a full snapshot of the sector. This information is extremely relevant and useful to compare and contrast with existing data and information, to assess trends, and monitor progress. If existing data and information are sparse, a situation analysis can serve as a baseline to inform future monitoring and evaluation rounds.[III] In addition, sector situation analyses provide essential and accessible documentation in a concise, analytical format for all stakeholders interested in the health system, giving a common overview of the situation, using the same language and definitions for all, thus improving the quality of policy dialogue.

A situation analysis can serve as a baseline to inform future monitoring and evaluation rounds.

III Please see Chapter 9 "Monitoring, evaluation and review of national health policies, strategies and plans" in this handbook.

3.2.5 It contributes to concretizing roles and responsibilities

A situation analysis is the basis for planning health sector activities, often making it the first step towards a new national health plan or health sector reform.

A situation analysis is often the first step towards a new national health plan or health sector reform. It is the basis for planning of activities which will take place in the health sector over the following few years. Successful implementation of these activities is highly dependent on a clear definition of roles and responsibilities between all types of stakeholders, especially including those who are on the ground, in districts, in more remote areas, and closer to or representing the population, the citizens and/or the patients. A situation analysis is a key step for all relevant stakeholders to understand which strategic orientations and linked activities need to happen in the health sector – and based on this, which concrete roles and responsibilities each stakeholder has.

It is highly recommended that a stakeholder analysis forms an integral component of the health sector situation analysis (see Box 3.3). Such an analysis can help elucidate how the characteristics of the various stakeholders influence the NHPSP development process. By better understanding the stakes of each actor, roles and responsibilities can be better distributed and managed to the benefit of all.

Fig. 3.2 Analysis of health sector actors, their relationships and interests, in Cape Verde

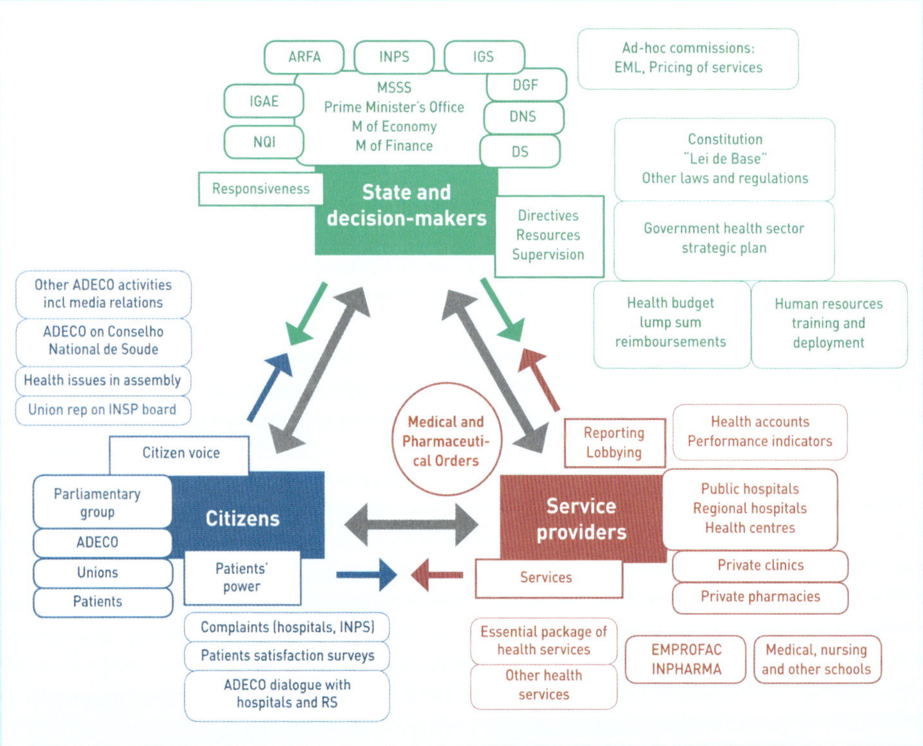

adapted by Bigdeli M and Clarke D, from World Development Report 2004: Making services work for poor people. World Bank; 2004. and Brinkerhoff D, Bossert T. Health governance: concepts and program options. Bethesda: Health Systems 20/20 Project; 2008

Box 3.3

Stakeholder analysis

A stakeholder analysis is frequently used in health system management, development, and health policy-making.[5] It aims to evaluate and understand stakeholders from the perspective of a certain organization or their relevance to a specific policy or project based on information from stakeholder surveys and interviews, supplemented by in-country experiences, literature reviews, expenditure data, and reports or publications.[6] Stakeholder analyses can address important questions such as: Who are the key players, formal and informal, in this field? What are the relationships between the actors? Who has the power or influence in this situation? How do the actors influence the policy process? (see example of an analysis of health actors, their relationships and interests, from Cabo Verde)

One of the results of a stakeholder analysis is a net map or a stakeholder movement map. A net map visually displays the actors in the health field and their relationships to each other using labels and arrows indicating the flow of resources versus action. A stakeholder movement map, on the other hand, can visually display a comparison of past, present, and future projected influence of a stakeholder, graphing level of influence in the health sector versus level of support over time. Visual representation of stakeholder analysis results provides an easy way to grasp a wealth of information about stakeholders' relative positions – i.e. in support, neutral, or opposed – to policy goals.

Knowledge of the actors present in the health system, their interests, and positions can allow policy-makers to interact more effectively with key stakeholders for health reform.[7] In the health sector, a stakeholder analysis can be used as a tool to inform project planning, implementation, and evaluation and is most useful when incorporated into a larger policy analysis process.[8] For instance, the role of CSOs and donors in health policy is vast – through stakeholder analysis, policy-makers can best understand which ones have the largest stake in a policy and be prepared for future funding opportunities or for potential barriers to passing a policy. While this specific type of analysis is useful in managing actors in the health field and identifying opportunities for stakeholder support or mobilization, a degree of caution is necessary in applying analysis results due to biases or uncertainties in data retrieved from stakeholders.[9]

Net map

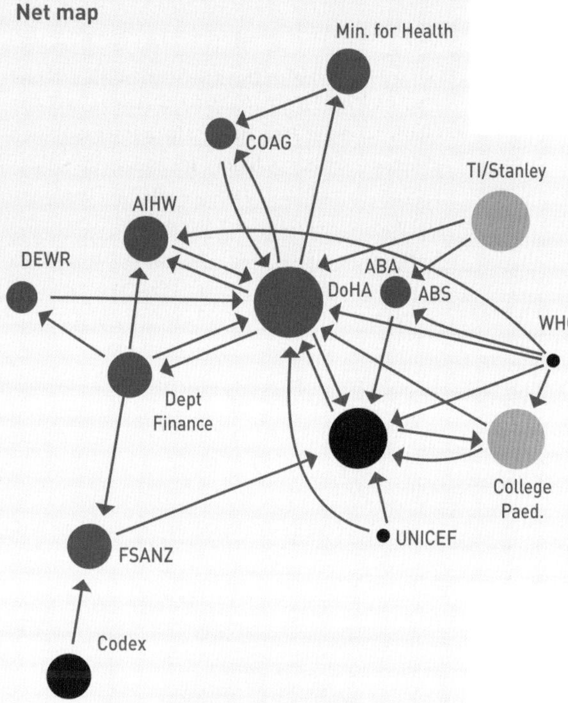

Source: Thow AM. Stakeholder analysis for health policy research. Sydney Health Policy Network and Qualitative Health Research Collaboration Forum; May 2013 (http://sydney.edu.au/health-policy-network//news-events/Thow.pdf, accessed 14 October 2016).

3.2.6 It helps to establish consensus on the status of health in the country

Different stakeholders will probably have diverging interests and varying points of view. This is precisely why information sharing and a jointly-undertaken situation analysis are essential to building trust between different players and negotiating a consensus among them. A situation analysis is often the principal first step in establishing trust by having stakeholders work together to agree upon the health sector status quo.

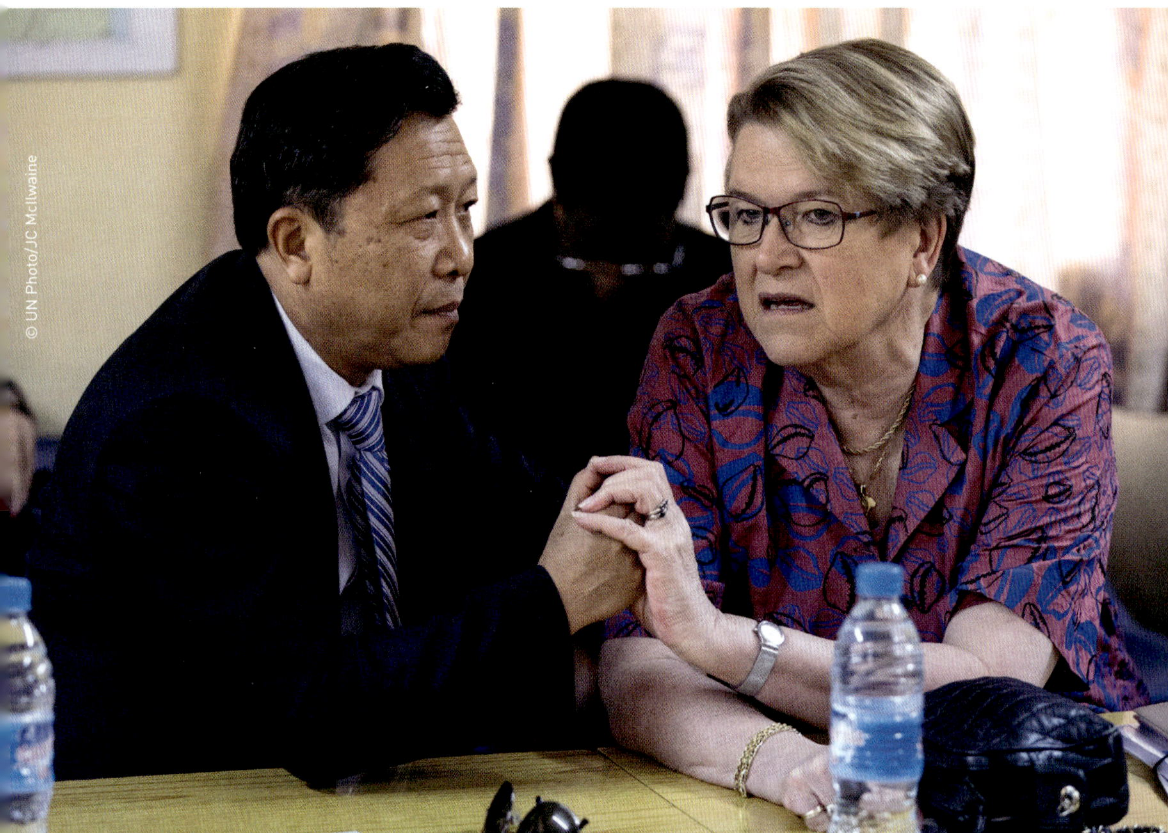

3.3 When should the situation analysis take place?

A health sector situation analysis should be done as a key initial step in the development of a NHPSP. Ideally, it should be undertaken at least once during the health policy and planning cycle, and updated every few years, because an updated, in-depth technical analysis that includes stakeholder viewpoints is an invaluable resource for the whole health sector.

That being said, taking stock of the situation, especially for particular thematic areas that may not be covered in complete depth in an overarching health sector situation analysis, is an activity which may be necessary during any stage in the policy cycle. It is an activity which is worth investing in, as it forms a basis and is a part of good programming and monitoring.

A health sector situation analysis need not always be undertaken on a large scale – it depends solely on the scale of the objective. If, for example, a malaria programme is considering reprogramming small funds, without interfering with the overall health sector strategy and targets, a quick technical analysis on malaria can potentially fulfil this objective. On the other hand, if, for example, a reorientation of the national health plan objectives is foreseen as a consequence of the development of a new national health financing strategy, a more substantial and in-depth situation analysis of the health financing situation and its linkage and potential impact on the health sector as a whole would need to take place.

Thus, the timing is linked to the specific objectives of the situation analysis, the topic in question, and the scope of the situation analysis (full health sector, a sub-sector, a programme).

3.4 Who should be involved in the situation analysis?

There are three main functions taken on by stakeholders for a successful situation analysis: active and inclusive multi-stakeholder participation, decision-making, and organization and coordination.

When examining the roles and responsibilities of the various health sector stakeholders (see Box 3.4), it is important to keep in mind the three main functions which are needed for a successful situation analysis: active and inclusive multi-stakeholder participation, decision-making, and organization and coordination. Some health actors will be active on all three fronts, while others will only be involved in one or another function, as described in more detail below.

Box 3.4

A health sector situation analysis typically brings together some or all of the following stakeholders

Population/beneficiaries

- population and community representatives;
- civil society, including nongovernmental and faith-based organizations;
- special interest groups.

Government and government-affiliated entities

- various central-level MoH departments;
- other ministries whose work is pertinent to health;
- regional MoH departments;
- other institutions and agencies linked to the MoH (e.g. parastatals);
- development partners.

Health providers

- public services providers and in particular local health systems authorities;
- professional associations;
- private for- and not-for-profit health services providers.

Other

- research institutions;
- think tanks.

3.4.1 Ministry of health

In an overall health sector situation analysis, the leader should be the MoH, especially if the objective is the formulation of a new national health plan. The MoH leads the coordination, organization and decision-making of the situation analysis exercise, and besides participating itself, ensures meaningful participation of others. There may be cases where certain preparatory steps, such as the population consultation, or the analysis of health data, are better conferred to outside parties in order to be independent and unbiased in their recommendations. Nevertheless, the MoH is the entity that takes the final decision on how to use the recommendations and results of various analyses and consultations and translates them into a national plan.

A situation analysis needs to be as impartial and objective as possible – ensuring this is a crucial role of the MoH, whether the analysis is actually conducted externally or not. One way to do this is to ensure that no single stakeholder or stakeholder group dominates the discussions and the process. A range and variety of stakeholders should be represented adequately and everyone given a voice and role. Of course this is easier said than done because often, in reality, the interest levels, funding and availability of different participants are not equal – this is where the MoH must make an extra effort to pique participants' interests, to incentivize participation if necessary, and ensure a fair balance in the voices.

3.4.2 Sub-national health systems authorities[IV]

Sub-national health authorities and services providers have an important role in providing data and information as well as in synthesizing this information in a format that is understandable to the vast majority of stakeholders. Their main role thus lies in "active participation"; however, it is advisable to have at least one regional or district health authority in the core team, as much of the knowledge that will be synthesized and analysed for the situation analysis comes from the field. The core team member will certainly contribute to the organization and decision-making of the situation analysis exercise.

A situation analysis needs to be as impartial and objective as possible – ensuring this is a crucial role of the MoH, whether the analysis is actually conducted externally or not.

District and especially regional authorities have a good overview of the challenges and bottlenecks faced in their local health sectors – their role in a situation analysis is thus to ensure that this message from the ground is brought across with the appropriate supporting evidence, in an understandable and clear way.

IV Often called "regional" or "district" health authorities.

3.4.3 Civil society, including professional associations and special interest groups

The private sector is comprised of both for-profit and non-profit entities. Their role in the situation analysis is to actively participate at the very least. In situations where they make up a substantial proportion of health services, it would be wise to include them in the core team and definitely in relevant technical working groups.

Civil society's role is crucial, as these are the organizations which are most often closest to the populations. A CSO representative can also be in the core team, and if not, should certainly actively participate and be transparent in providing relevant data and information. It is essential for CSOs to ensure that legitimate representatives are engaging in the situation analysis process. Where a plethora of CSOs exists working on similar topics, it may not be possible for all of them to participate in the situation analysis process – in this case, CSOs as a group would have the responsibility to ensure legitimate representation.

3.4.4 Private sector

In most countries, the private sector contributes to providing health services and health system inputs such as pharmaceuticals, health technology and human resources for health. It is thus relevant and necessary to bring the private sector into the situation analysis discussion, even though it is often difficult to do so. A complete and accurate understanding of a country's health sector is really not possible in some settings without the private sector angle.

The private health sector comprises "all providers who exist outside of the public sector, whether their aim is philanthropic or commercial, and whose aim is to treat illness or prevent disease".[10] This comprises for-profit and non-profit entities, including faith-based organizations. It also includes the informal health sector such as traditional healers, traditional birth attendants, indigenous systems of medical providers, and market drug sellers.

Their role in the situation analysis is to actively participate at the very least. In situations where they make up a substantial proportion of health services, it would be wise to include them in the core team and definitely in relevant technical working groups. Their insights into the realities on the ground are unique, and they have knowledge and experience with the same issues but from a different angle – therefore, huge efforts should be undertaken to ensure their meaningful participation in the situation analysis process.

3.4.5 Parliament

Ideally, a parliamentary health committee representative would be a part of the thematic working groups or – at the very least – follow the analyses and discussions by keeping in touch with the core team. Health committee parliamentarians will ultimately be involved in approving the national health budget that will be based on the NHPSP; the NHPSP is based on the situation analysis, so ensuring a link between the legislative focal points for health and the technical situation analysis work is beneficial to both sides. During the budget hearings in parliament, it would be extremely useful for health committee members to have the background knowledge of the situation analysis to better defend the health budget.

3.4.6 Media

The media is a special actor, since it is omnipresent and aims to provide information and reflect population opinion in an objective way. In a situation analysis, its role is chiefly to disseminate and inform the population on the situation analysis exercise, thereby ensuring that the analysis process and results are transparent and understandable. The media's role is thus critical and keeps the national health planning process dynamic.

3.4.7 Development partners

Development partners can be represented in the core team, where they would take on more of an organization/coordination as well as co-decision-making role. Where they are not in the core team, their active participation is important, as they have relevant data and information on the projects and programmes that they are involved in and which could add value to the situation analysis discussions. The information should also be made available in as palatable and understandable a format as possible.

During the budget hearings in parliament, it would be extremely useful for health committee members to have the background knowledge of the situation analysis to better defend the health budget.

In aid-dependent contexts, development partners should be careful not to skew or over-influence the debates. MoH and country health sector needs should always be in the forefront of the discussions, rather than partner priorities.

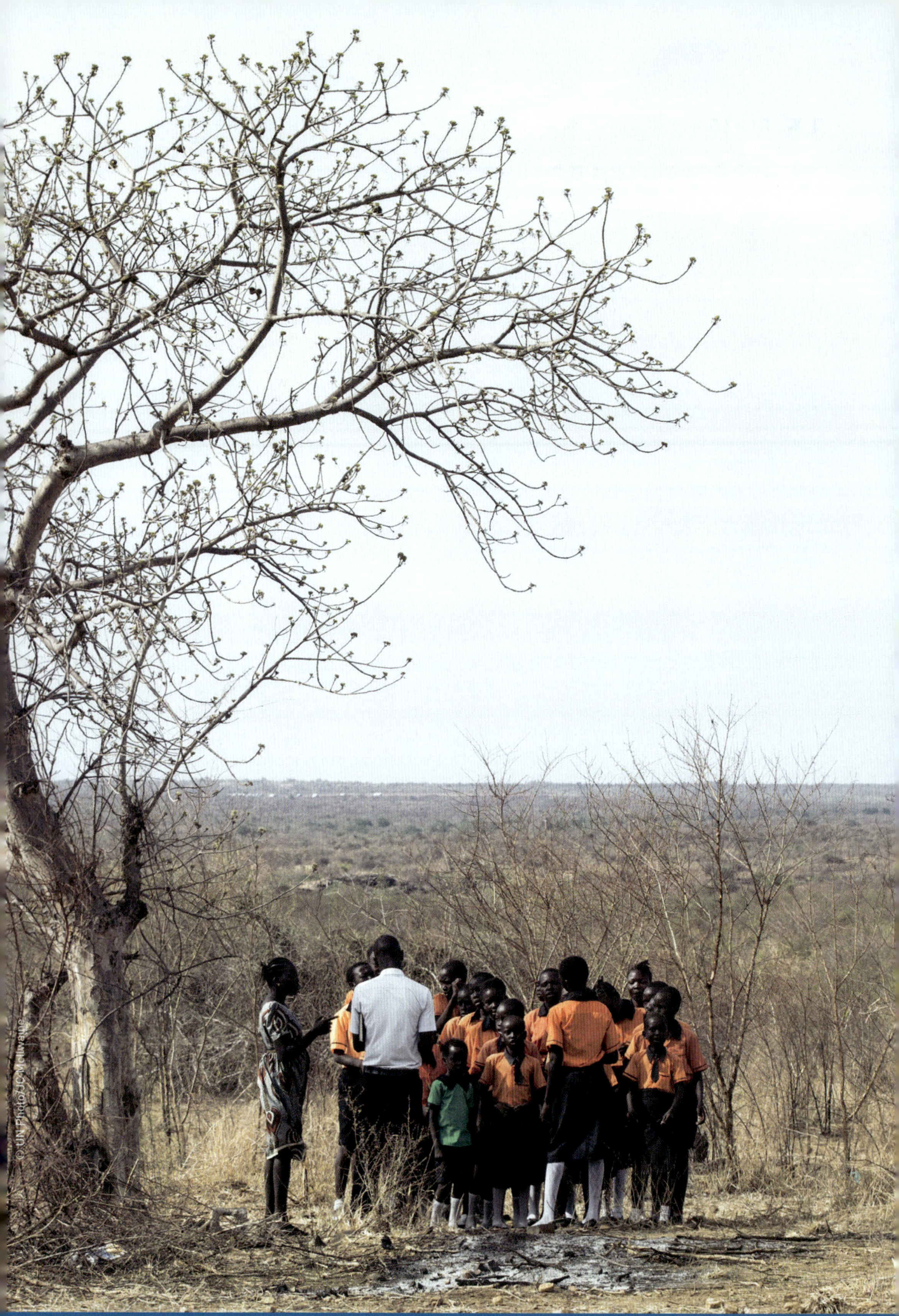

3.5 Methodology: how should a situation analysis be organized and conducted?

A situation analysis must be participatory and inclusive, analytical, relevant, comprehensive, and evidence-based.

A situation analysis can be conducted in different ways but there are key elements which must be in place to ensure that all the chief characteristics (see section 3.1.1) are fulfilled:

- participatory and inclusive;
- analytical;
- relevant;
- comprehensive;
- evidence-based.

In the following sections, organizational aspects of a situation analysis (steering committee, core team, working groups) are detailed, as well as the streams of work which need to be examined by health planning stakeholders.

3.5.1 Organization of the situation analysis

There are two main ways of organizing the situation analysis of the health sector, and it will partly depend on the amount of time and funds at MoH's disposal. The first might be necessary when the analysis must be done quickly; here, international and national expert consultants come and review documents, carry out interviews with key informants, examine existing data and draw conclusions within a few weeks. This will be useful in producing a published analysis rapidly, but it will neither build country capacity nor allow adequate understanding and buy-in from all relevant stakeholders, especially those in the field, such as local NGOs and communities. The second way is through working groups involving relevant experts and health actors with adequate space and time for dialogue. It is true that when the analysis involves a wide array of stakeholders as is advocated in this handbook, it can become heavy and time-consuming. Nevertheless, it is a crucial investment, whose potential to unite those who have a stake in health into a common understanding of health sector challenges and solutions should not be underestimated. The latter methodology is elaborated upon in more detail in this section.

Establishment of a "steering committee"

The creation of a formal "steering committee" (or whatever name chosen by the country), representing the community of stakeholders involved in the exercise, may or may not be necessary; it depends on the scope of the situation analysis and the core team's access to higher-level decision-makers in the government. If it is decided to form one, it would be important to have MoH department heads as well as heads of CSOs or other line ministry directors who are closely linked to health sector activities. In any case, clarity is needed as to who will finally sign off on the situation analysis and formally accept its contents.

Nomination of a "core team"

The nomination of a "core team" (this can go by any other title, depending on the country context) is essential to ensure effective coordination of the situation analysis exercise. This team should have the skills to organize well, have

A participatory situation analysis is mainly organized through thematic working groups, coordinated by a core team. The working group reports should then be submitted to a policy dialogue which includes a broad range of stakeholders, including community and citizen representatives.

relational skills to be able to reach out to the right people for constitution of working groups, and also possess strong technical capabilities to actively participate in and support the working groups. The team should be led by the MoH but its constitution does not need to be exclusively MoH staff. In fact, representation from key donors, CSOs, professional associations, sub-national health authorities or any other relevant bodies (especially relevant for NHPSP implementation) for the particular country setting is explicitly recommended.

The core team's tasks include (but are not limited to):

- preparing the situation analysis, including obtaining official approvals and a budget;
- constituting working groups;
- making available relevant documentation;
- informing and sensitizing relevant stakeholders;
- organizing workshops and meetings between relevant actors and/or working groups on cross-cutting topics;
- technically supporting working groups;
- ensuring that the three streams of work as described below are done well and accurately, and that they are adequately linked.

WHO health systems taxonomy: a tool

In order to ensure comprehensiveness of the aspects covered under the different working groups that will be conducting the situation analysis, WHO has put together a taxonomy for health systems (see Box 3.5), or exhaustive list of subjects which can be covered on health systems-related matters. The taxonomy is organized in a set of health sector categories based on the health system building blocks; most principal country health programme areas come under the "service delivery" building block. Under each category, a series of sub-headings has been developed with the corresponding experts so that an analysis of each area is comprehensive. An annotated taxonomy explains which information is expected for each sub-heading of the taxonomy. Using a comprehensive taxonomy to describe the way the system and programmes function is a good starting point and can help the working groups ensure that all important aspects of the health system in the country are well covered in the situation analysis.

Examples of other situation analysis tools are described in Table 3.1.

Box 3.5

An example of a taxonomy[11]

Medical products

- organization and management of pharmaceuticals;
- regulation, quality and safety of the pharmaceutical sector;
- drug procurement system;
- rational use of medicines.

Clinical biology

- organization and management of clinical biology;
- procurement system of clinical biology inputs;
- maintenance of clinical biology equipment;
- quality control of clinical biology equipment.

Blood

- organization and management of blood products;
- collection and distribution system of blood products;
- quality and safety of blood products.

Vaccines

- organization and management of vaccines;
- vaccines procurement system;
- cold chain and other quality issues.

Priorities and ways forward

Others

Table 3.1 Examples of situation analysis tools

SITUATION ANALYSIS TOOL	WHAT IS IT?	WHO RUNS IT?	TARGET AUDIENCE	EXAMPLE COUNTRIES WHERE APPLIED
Health systems in transition, health system reviews (HiTs)[12]	"Country-based reports that provide a detailed description of each health care system and of reform and policy initiatives in progress or under development"	WHO Regional Office for Europe	Countries of the WHO European Region; some additional OECD countries	Albania, Australia, Canada, Estonia, Hungary, Portugal, Slovenia, Turkey, United States, Uzbekistan
Health System Assessment Approach (HSAA)[13]	Technical Modules used to "produce a comprehensive assessment of an entire health system or parts of the health system" "Widely used in the developing world to diagnose health systems performance and to capture system-wide information"	United States Agency for International Development (USAID)	Policy-makers and analysts; health system planners, policy-makers, practitioners, and program managers	Angola, Azerbaijan, Benin, Viet Nam
Organizational Assessment for Improving and Strengthening Health Financing (OASIS)[14]	"An analytical approach and framework for undertaking a systematic review of a health financing system including a performance assessment"	WHO	Health financing policy-makers of ministries of health, finance, planning and labour, or other ministries; health insurance organizations; other actors in health financing	Benin, Cambodia, France, Jordan, Mali, Morocco, Nicaragua, Pakistan, Republic of Korea, Rwanda, Sudan, Tunisia, Uganda, Viet Nam
Human Resources for Health Toolkit [15]	"Toolkit brings together a set of existing tools that are in use for various aspects of country-level HRH [human resources for health] development, including situation analysis, planning, implementation, monitoring and evaluation"	Global Health Workforce Alliance	Various levels stakeholders and policy-makers involved in health planning	....

Establishment of "working groups"

Ideally, the stakeholders can be organized into working groups, with the aim of balancing out technical input from different levels of the health system, different institutions involved in the topic, and simply, different viewpoints which need discussion and debate. For example, a working group on human resources for health can include representatives from: MoH, from the department dealing with health workforce; a researcher from an academic institution working in this area; health professional association (health worker representative); donor agency if they are interested in or fund this area; and a CSO that may be providing health services and must manage staff. In addition, this group would call upon a wider group of actors to consult them ad hoc on specific issues (sometimes termed a "community of practice") – this could be ministry of labour; district health authorities; community leaders, etc.

Working groups should not only be mixed teams, with experts and experienced actors from various stakeholder groups, but also cover all main aspects of expertise on the topic attributed to them. The WHO taxonomy already gives an idea of the various aspects to be analysed, but as it is very comprehensive, it would not be practical to nominate a member for each section.

Table 3.2 can be used as a checklist for expertise that needs to be covered in working groups on common situation analysis topics. It allows the core team, which is responsible for establishing the working groups, to verify that, together, each group has sufficient expertise and experience to ensure a comprehensive analysis of their topical area.

Table 3.2 Expertise needed for common situation analysis topics

WORKING GROUP	PRIORITY FOR DEVELOPMENT OF AN IMPROVED EVIDENCE BASE
Service delivery	▸ Health service levels, service packages, referral system ▸ Quality of care: continuity, care, drugs ▸ (Universal) coverage, primary health care, outreach, health-seeking behaviour, health service demand ▸ Role of various private sector providers ▸ Traditional medicine
Pharmaceutical and medical supplies	▸ Needs projection, procurement, supply ▸ Drugs, material, blood bank, contraceptives
Equipment and infrastructure, logistics	▸ Asset planning and management, norms and standards ▸ Health facility mapping (existing and projected) ▸ Maintenance
Human resources	▸ Needs projection, production, distribution, registration, supervision, training ▸ Technical assistance
Financing	▸ Costing, medium-term expenditure framework, resource allocation (criteria) ▸ Cost-sharing policy/practices, financial accessibility ▸ Resource projection/budgeting process, mobilisation (National Health Accounts) ▸ Financial management, expenditure tracking, internal control ▸ Auditing arrangements
Governance/ management	▸ Administrative legislation and regulation ▸ Implementation and administrative arrangements ▸ Planning processes and procedures ▸ Procurement
Coordination and leadership and reforms	▸ International Health Partnership (IHP+) compact development ▸ Institutional development ▸ Multisectoral cooperation ▸ International cooperation ▸ Health sector decentralization ▸ Public/private partnership
Information systems	▸ Monitoring and review mechanism ▸ Knowledge management ▸ Research
Sector policies and context	▸ Process of strategy and policy development, validation and review ▸ Gender, equity, human rights ▸ Alignment with overall government directives/processes ▸ International commitments, initiatives
Health outcomes (health status)	▸ Trends of main health indicators (compare with region) ▸ Epidemiological profile ▸ Results of priority health programmes ▸ Results regarding international commitments (Millennium Development Goals, etc.) ▸ Analysis of factors and causes

The working group's principal tasks are to collect, examine and interpret relevant data, knowledge and information around the topic at hand, and through preliminary internal expert discussions, come to joint conclusions which would be the object of policy dialogue. The group's analysis and conclusions should be drafted into a thematic report which can be disseminated to all stakeholders for review and comment, and discussion and debate.

Working groups can be organized along the health systems building blocks,[16] along strategic directions of the current NHPSP, or along cross-cutting topics such as universal health coverage (see Tables 3.3 and 3.4). In practice, the topics of the working groups will depend also on the way the health sector, and the MoH, is organized.

Table 3.3 Situation analysis working groups by health system building block

EXAMPLES OF WORKING GROUP TOPICS BY BUILDING BLOCK	ISSUES TO CONSIDER
▸ Human resources for health ▸ Pharmaceuticals and medical products ▸ Health technologies and infrastructure ▸ Service delivery ▸ Health governance and leadership ▸ Health financing ▸ Health information system	This grouping might reinforce silo thinking. Service delivery working group ends up taking on all programme-related information which can make this group's workload very high compared to other groups. Overlaps must be thought through to ensure joint meetings between overlapping topics. Labelling one group to look only at governance and leadership may be politically sensitive in some settings - it must thus be easier to integrate governance issues into other topics.

Table 3.4 Situation analysis working group by cross-cutting health sector topics

EXAMPLES OF WORKING GROUPS BY CROSS-CUTTING TOPICS	ISSUES TO CONSIDER
▸ Universal health coverage ▸ Social determinants of health ▸ People-centred service delivery ▸ Governance for health	Can support thinking out of the box. Can foster collaboration across existing departments, institutions and sectors. If the sector is not organized in this cross-cutting way, it can be difficult to incentivize full participation during the situation analysis. Understanding of cross-cutting topics may be from the point of view of the expertise of each working group member -- an initial investment in explaining and clarifying the definition and content of cross-cutting topics may be necessary.

Meetings, workshops and communication

Individual working groups can organize their reading, debate and writing work for the analysis in ways that suits them. If team members are doing this work on top of their routine duties, most of the exchanges can take place by email or online. These channels are also useful when some members are based at a decentralized level, or elsewhere.

It is useful to adopt a clear schedule of meetings and workshops that all working group members have agreed upon, for both individual working groups as well as meetings between different working groups on overlapping or cross-cutting topics. These meetings can be the forum where working groups report on the progress in their work, give and receive feedback, receive advice from other experts and a community of practice (who may not necessarily be in the working group) and harmonize content with other groups, especially on cross-cutting topics. They also serve to link the different streams of work together and ensure data and knowledge sharing.

The working groups should agree on text formatting, management of feedback and comments and on procedures for communication. Some groups may decide to organize formally, with a chair and formal roles for members. Others may be more loosely formed, especially if the group is small and the members know each other well.

Box 3.6

Working groups: proposed sequencing of work

1. Review the taxonomy: subheadings and possible key words.
2. Identify main issues and aspects for the working group report.
3. Formulate the identified issues in strength-weakness-opportunity-threat (SWOT; see Box 3.11) bullet points and discuss root causes and effects.
4. Identify key sources of information and assure their availability.
5. Verify if each of the identified aspects is evidence-based, and can be referenced.
6. Identify information and analysis gaps and search for complementary documentation.
7. Based on feedback, especially from other working groups and the Streams 1 and 2 focal points, revise the first SWOT version.
8. Start writing a concise working group report, with quotes and references.

Situation analysis report

Each working group must submit their individual thematic reports, which must then be consolidated into a final report. Writing the first draft of the report may be done jointly in a workshop format, but finalization of it will usually end up being the responsibility of a small group of people or an individual from the core team, or a hired (consultant) by the core team.

Each working group's report, as well as the final report, should summarize key issues and recent developments, relating them to the objectives and plans of the NHPSP. The most important strengths and weaknesses and their underlying causes – as well as determining factors – should be highlighted. The report should be well referenced, especially on issues which are contentious or heated in stakeholder debates. The working group thematic reports, which will go more in-depth onto the topic at hand, may be lengthier, but the final report should focus on a concise analysis and summarize the working group reports and address cross-cutting issues. For a sample outline of the situation analysis report, please see Box 3.7.

Box 3.7

Sample outline of a situation analysis report

Table of Contents
Executive summary
Introduction/Background
Objectives
Methodology/Approach
Limitations
Team members/Coordination
Findings (this can be divided by working group topics, strategic directions of the current NHPSP, cross-cutting topics, or any mix of the above; it can also potentially follow the WHO taxonomy)
Discussion
Conclusion
Annex (list of documents reviewed, field visit reports, list of people interviewed, etc.)

3.5.2 Three streams of analysis

Three distinct streams should be examined by the situation analysis working groups: analysis of health data and measuring health sector performance; analysis of the implementation of sector activities and finances; and policy dialogue on the effectiveness of NHPSP activity areas.

To ensure solid results, three distinct streams should be examined by the situation analysis working groups (see Fig. 3.3):

(i) analysis of health data and measuring the performance of the health sector as per its indicators;
(ii) analysis of the implementation of health sector activities, budgets and finances;
(iii) analysis of the effectiveness of NHPSP activity areas: policy dialogue with a wider stakeholder group on the strengths and weaknesses of the health system (health workforce, pharmaceuticals, health financing, service delivery, etc.) and health programmes (HIV, noncommunicable diseases, nutrition, maternal health, immunization, etc.), their causes and effects, and cross-cutting issues.

Ideally, a focal point or several people acting as a focal point group would be responsible for streams 1 and 2 respectively, liaising with all the working groups as needed.

Fig. 3.3 Three streams of work in a health sector situation analysis

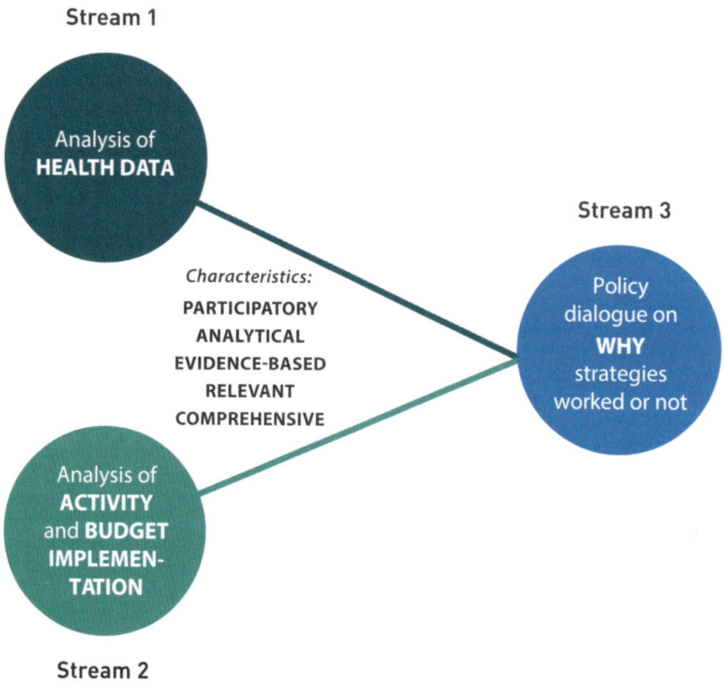

(a) Stream 1: analysis of health data

An in-depth analysis and synthesis of all relevant health data is crucial to assess performance and better comprehend priority problems, main challenges, and urgent needs to be covered in the health sector. Beyond data sets that capture a snapshot of the health sector at a given time point, this step should try to elicit trends and developments over time, especially with regard to the major causes of morbidity and mortality in the country.

The health data analysis should be focused on the priority areas of the NHPSP if that is the objective of the situation analysis. In many countries, health sector indicators tend to focus on service delivery performance (output) and outcome, whereas very important, sometimes more qualitative, reform aspects are ignored (and not captured in a routine monitoring and evaluation system). Even if attainment of reform phases are used as a milestone indicator, the actual effects and impact of the reforms can be easily missed.

Similarly, the effects of unforeseen environmental changes (external to the health care system) sometimes need special attention. For example, unexpected large migrations due to civil unrest can overburden a health system and merit a specific evaluation; decentralization efforts can lead to an increase in the number of administrative districts, which often leads to an increase in the number of health districts. Targeted studies or targeted data/information gathered to evaluate these types of circumstances may be necessary.

Ensuring a wide variety of data types and data sets allows for critical triangulation between the different data and information to get a more complete and realistic picture of the health sector.

Box 3.8

What can a good data analysis report include?

It includes:

- assessment of progress against targets for key indicators (core NHPSP indicators, as well as additional programme specific indicators);
- equity analysis by key stratifiers;
- comparative analyses with peer countries;
- customer satisfaction surveys/health facility exit surveys;
- performance and efficiency analysis comparing inputs and outputs at the sub-national level;
- computation of lives saved through interventions;
- data quality assessment.

First and foremost, existing data sets should be collected, analysed and synthesized, including primary data sets, reports of data collection efforts, existing reviews as well as published and grey literature. Here follows a (non-exhaustive) selection of key questions to ask and issues to appraise. Is data coverage complete, geographically and time-wise? Do existing indicators allow for a comprehensive analysis? Do the existing thematic reports and evaluations allow for a comprehensive analysis? Is there likelihood of contradicting information/data? If so, how can one clarify this? How reliable is the routine data? Should facility-based data be complemented with other sources, like exit surveys?

If a data gap has been identified, a country may choose to do additional surveys or research studies to close that gap (if time permits).

It is to be highlighted that a wealth of data and information may exist which have not been validated, or disseminated, or stored. The task of identifying and centralizing this documentation should not be underestimated: it takes considerable time and effort, but is of course a useful investment.

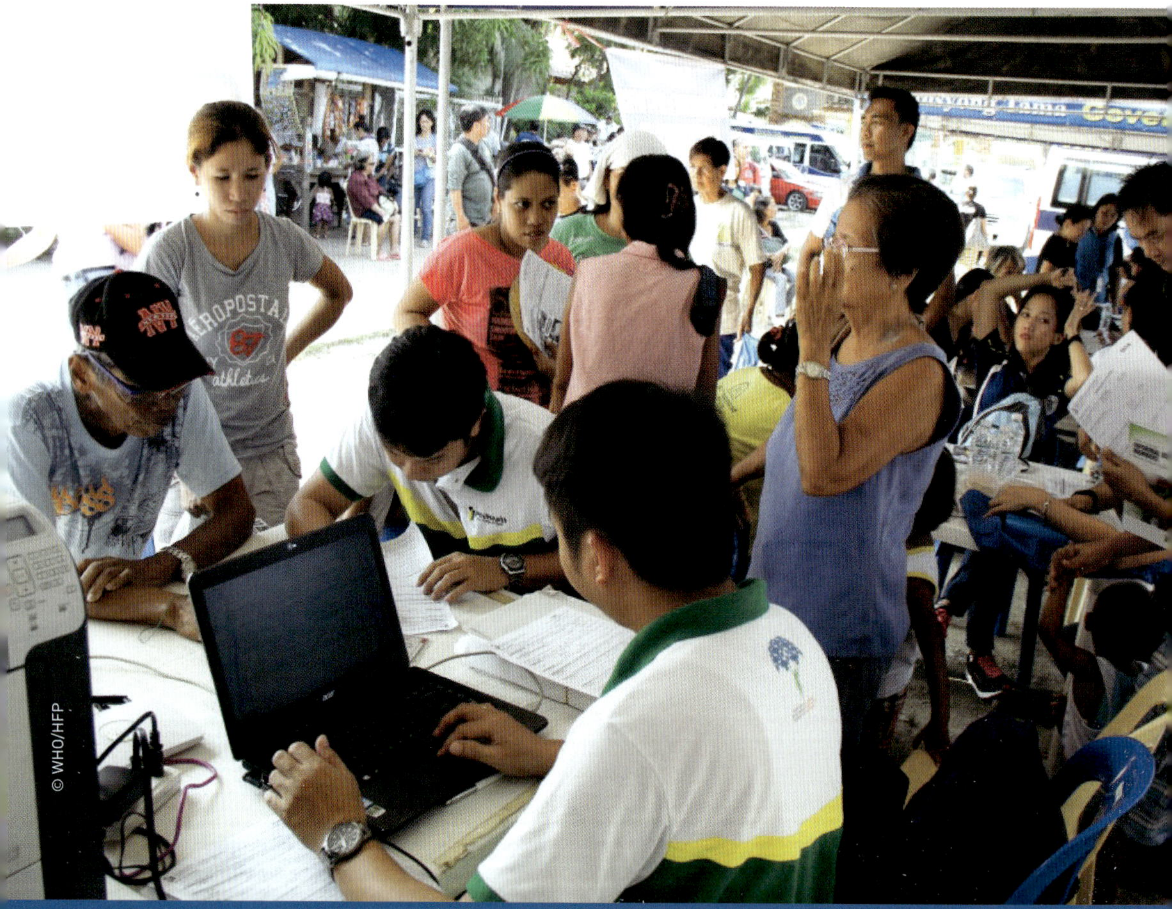

Examples of data sources for health data analysis

1. National health plan
2. Population health surveys
   - reproductive, maternal, neonatal, child health and other issues: Demographic Health Surveys;
   - HIV/AIDS: AIDS indicator surveys, sero-behavioural survey;
   - malaria indicator survey;
   - national household survey;
   - national service delivery surveys;
   - sub-national surveys.
3. National health information system data, including trend data
4. Performance reports
   - annual health statistics report;
   - annual health sector performance reports;
   - HIV/AIDS epidemiological surveillance reports.
5. Facility assessments
   - Service Availability Readiness Assessment (SARA);
   - client satisfaction surveys.
6. Administrative data
   - financing: National Health Accounts, progress reports on public sector management/finance reforms;
   - human resources: Human Resources Information System, professional council databases, training institutions records, progress reports on civil service reforms;
   - infrastructure: Health facility inventory, vehicle inventory, equipment inventory of health facilities (public).
7. Mortality and causes of death
   - hospital reports, Health Management Information System (HMIS);
   - maternal perinatal health review reports.
8. Research/Evaluation studies
   - health systems assessment;
   - programme evaluations – e.g. Malaria Programme review report.
9. Data sets/documents from other ministries (planning, education, local government, finance, etc.)
10. Data sets/documents from civil society – reviews, analyses, evaluations, case studies, etc.

Often, due to time and resource constraints, health sector situation analyses draw heavily from internal, or government, documentation. These are usually data sets and documents which the MoH is familiar with and can easily access. It takes a concerted extra effort to go and find out about the existence of, and obtain, other non-sectoral, non-government material. A solid situation analysis, however, depends on this, since changes in health status are sometimes better explained by other "external" health determinants and activities in which the government may not be directly involved.

Normally, health data analysis is done largely by technical experts who are familiar with the data sets and/or who are trained to analyse data sets. For the interpretation of the data, it is important to collaborate with those who are familiar with health sector activities as well as non-technical experts (see below section 3.5.5).

The technical experts will most likely be the focal points for Stream 1 of the situation analysis. Since health data analysis is relevant and cross-cutting across all working groups, these focal points will be liaising and working closely with all working groups (see Fig. 3.4) – this is the crucial link needed for understanding the numbers and making sense of the data. For the working groups, the input from the health data analysis will be indispensable for understanding if and how health status and indicators have evolved over the medium term and how it potentially correlates with activity implementation on the ground.

Fig. 3.4 Interaction between situation analysis working groups and streams

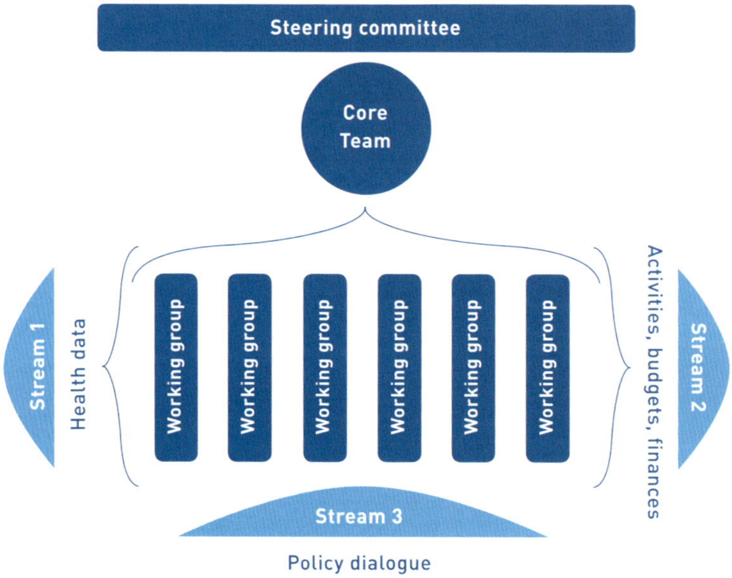

(b) Stream 2: Analysis of the implementation of health sector activities, budgets and finances

The analysis of the implementation of NHPSP activities should be organized around the budget and planning cycle: beginning with the costed NHPSP, the links to the actual health sector budget and health sector expenditures should be assessed. A study of the national health budget and sector finances should be undertaken to better understand whether budget formulation and implementation have adequately reflected the NHPSP objectives. In addition, an assessment of whether the NHPSP has been adequately funded, and if activities have been implemented as per plan, must take place. To this end, a review of public expenditure over the previous years will be necessary, along with an in-depth look at activity reports from districts. The analysis of the implementation of the health sector budget is a necessary link between performance and activity progress. It will be essential to link in with the health data analysis when reviewing clinical activities in health facilities and progress made on performance indicators – this linkage should happen at the level of the working groups, depending on the specific topic at hand.

Box 3.10

Examples of data sources for the analysis of activity, budget, and financial implementation

Activities

- national HMIS data;
- periodic activity reports from the different levels of various ministries involved in health sector activities;
- social audits;
- district and regional sector review reports;
- donor mapping exercises.

Finances

- NHPSP costing;
- ministry of finance reports
  national health insurance or private insurance reports;
- MoH administration and finance reports (including sub-national entities financial reports);
- private sector reports;
- National Health Accounts;
- public expenditure review;
- external donors financial reports if relevant;
- all other relevant reports, data, papers and grey materials from other ministries, partners, nongovernmental organizations, private sector, etc.

Usually, this type of analysis is done with a large range of mainly technical stakeholders, principally from the health sector but also, where necessary, with input from other sectors. The working groups will be responsible for a more in-depth interpretation of the data beyond the technical analysis, as will the work done in Stream 3.

(c) Stream 3: Analysis of the effectiveness of NHPSP activity areas through policy dialogue

Stream 3 is based on a policy dialogue on the strengths and weaknesses of the different elements of the health system and health programmes not only by technical experts, but also by service providers, representatives of the population and beneficiaries, national and international partners and CSOs.

This analysis aims at assessing and analyzing what works and what does not work in the health system as well as in programmes, sub-policies and strategies. It is based on a participatory assessment of strengths and weaknesses of the different elements of the health system and health programmes not only by technical experts, but also by service providers, representatives of the population and beneficiaries, national and international partners and CSOs. The key to this analysis is bringing together experts' views with non-technical opinions of community members who are using the health system on a day to day basis. Health strategies and plans should not be solely based on experts' views, but also on populations' perceptions, opinions, preferences and expectations – so as to help demand meet the supply of health services. Also, contextual issues play a key role in the success of NHPSP implementation – people's views and opinions can be decisive in putting the best-laid plans into context.[V]

In principle, this step should take place after the two other streams, when the stakeholders have a better understanding of what works well and less well through the Stream 1 (data and indicators performance assessment), and Stream 2 (has the implementation taken place as per planned activities and budgets?). Stream 3's objective is to collectively assess if the strategic directions and activity areas adopted have indeed led to expected results, to examine strengths and weaknesses, and deliberate on whether a change in strategies should be recommended to reach higher levels of effectiveness.

Moreover, policy-making is clearly a highly-political process and decisions are rarely done on the sole basis of objective reasons. Consulting population representatives is a critical means to involve them in the political decision-making process in order to avoid a bias in the situation analysis towards the point of view of policy-makers, or any other minority or elite group, only. A situation analysis should go beyond the descriptive stage to where stakeholders can draw adequate lessons from the past. The identified weaknesses and threats should not be a mere repetition of what had been found already in earlier analyses; instead, a serious effort is necessary to learn why an improvement has not, or insufficiently, taken place in order to be able to rectify the issue at hand.

In practice, the Stream 3, fed by Stream 1 and Stream 2 assessments, is organized following the Strengths-Weakness-Opportunites-Threats (SWOT) approach (see Box 3.11). The exercise requires the organization of working groups that will review the different health topics using the SWOT terminology and ultimately assess the overall health sector strategy. The final product will consist in a set of conclusions and recommendations.

V Please also see Chapter 2 of this handbook, "Population consultation on needs and expectations".

Box 3.11

SWOT analysis

SWOT (strengths, weaknesses, opportunities, threats) analysis is a popular method used to compare internal capabilities, in the form of strengths and weaknesses, to external developments, in the form of opportunities or threats. A SWOT analysis can provide a strong and broad base for NHPSP situation analysis and sets the stage for strategic planning, especially because of its unique ability to illuminate new strategic options via evaluating the balance between internal and external factors.[17]

SWOT analysis in its most basic form can be broken down into four steps. The first step is the collection and evaluation of key data and information, including but not limited to population demographics, sources of health-care funding or the status of medical technology. Step 2 is to sort data into the four key categories, where strengths and weaknesses typically stem from internal organizational factors and opportunities and threats from external factors. The following table demonstrates how these four categories are defined and sorted.

The third step involves development of a SWOT matrix that compares different alternatives for consideration following an in-depth data analysis. The fourth step incorporates SWOT anysis into the broader situation analysis and decision-making process. Ideally, SWOT analysis also includes a comprehensive literature search and qualitative input from stakeholders and sector experts.

Examples of SWOT analysis factors:[18]

	DEFINITION	EXAMPLES
S (strengths)	Factors that have stimulated strong sector performance	State-of-the-art medical equipment, investments in health-care informatics
W (weaknesses)	Factors that increase health-care costs or reduce healthcare quality	Ageing health care facilities, lack of standard clinical practices, duplication of programs
O (opportunities)	New initiatives and areas of growth available to the health sector	New development partners for health-care programmes, introduction of standard clinical protocols, increased sector funding
T (threats)	Factors that negatively affect sector performance	Political or economic instability, funding deficits, growing uninsured population

3.5.3 How long does a truly participatory situation analysis approximately take?

A truly participatory and inclusive situation analysis will take at least 3-5 months, ensuring adequate time for real policy dialogue.

From start to finish, a truly participatory and inclusive situation analysis, with adequate room for real policy dialogue, will take approximately 3–5 months at least. Most working group members will do this work in parallel with their routine duties. If it is possible to free up stakeholders' schedules from their more routine duties, the situation analysis could be considerably faster. On the other hand, if they are overburdened with too many other tasks, it could take longer. In addition, if the participatory approach and methodology are new, time will be needed to explain, clarify and justify it.

Please note that some of the working groups will engage separately with the Stream 1 and 2 focal points. The workload for the three streams will overlap in time so they are not explicitly mentioned in the approximate timeline (see Fig. 3.5).

The proposed timeline also assumes that all data and information is available and needs to be found and brought into one place. If collecting additional data is considered indispensable, the necessary time for integrating the results of such small surveys/studies is additional. Also, if heavy input from sub-national levels is deemed necessary, it may require a longer timeline.

Fig. 3.5 Example of a timeline of situation analysis activities

Activities/time frame	Month 1 / Weeks				Month 2 / Weeks				Month 3 / Weeks				Month 4 / Weeks				Month 5 / Weeks			
	1	2	3	4	1	2	3	4	1	2	3	4	1	2	3	4	1	2	3	4
Inception phase (3 days) -- meeting of all working groups + stream 1 and 2 focal points to discuss content delineation, report structure, modus operandi	■																			
Working group sessions: start content development, discuss specifics of working group organization and work schedule		■																		
Groups meet to examine initial evidence and interview key stakeholders. Streams 1 and 2 focal points liaise with all groups			■	■																
1st version feedback with all groups (1 day)					■															
Groups meet individually, potentially do field visits, continue content development.						■	■	■												
Feedback from core team and concerned department heads								■	■											
Workshop with all groups for peer-review of reports (2 days)										■										
Re-work reports based on workshop feedback										■	■	■								
Each group meets with steering committee for feedback												■								
Groups write pre-final version of reports												■	■							
Core team does compilation and last corrections												■	■	■	■					
MoH approves pre-final version												■	■	■	■					
Stream 3: policy dialogue workshop with wide stakeholder group on pre-final version																■				
Editing final version situation analysis report																	■	■		
MoH endorses the report and disseminates / publishes																			■	■

3.5.4 Link between Streams 2 and 3

In Stream 2, the core team's Stream 2 focal point(s) have the main responsibility for the centralization and validation of all progress and financial reports, audits and evaluations. The main challenge is to:

For the analysis of overall strategic developments and reforms (Stream 3), it is necessary to have a good assessment of how activities and finances were implemented (Stream 2).

- centralize plans, data and reports (financial and implementation) from various levels and actors;
- appraise reliability, identify gaps, contradictions, overlaps;
- assist working groups to synthesize data and capture the essence in concise tables and graphs;
- assist working groups to extract key issues from reports (progress, evaluations, surveys);
- assist working groups to comment on features, trends, unexpected developments.

It is vital that the Stream 2 focal point(s) work with and across all working groups, as activity implementation and activity expenditure needs to be adequately examined and analysed on all health sector topics.

Stream 3 is a collective effort of the core team, working groups, the wider community of experts and the wider community of resource persons (the latter two are sometimes deemed "community of practice"). It involves engaging in real dialogue with all stakeholders, including those with diverging or different views, including non-technicians and non-experts, to discuss, exchange, interpret and nuance the results coming out of the situation analysis working groups. Stream 3 draws from the results of the other streams, and takes place sequentially afterwards. In the analysis of overall strategic developments and reforms (Stream 3), it is necessary to have a good assessment of how activities and finances were implemented (Stream 2) (see Box 3.12).

Box 3.12

Interconnection between the three streams: a hypothetical example from the area of medical equipment maintenance

Stream 1: An assessment of health service readiness revealed that in hospitals, 40% of the medical equipment was not operational and that in dispensaries, 50% of the latrines were out of order. Stream 1 focal points' discussions with the health technology working group revealed that many of the after-sales equipment needs as well as the preventive maintenance needs had not been addressed. Common reasons were: no universal reporting system, responsibilities not clearly attributed, non-availability of technicians and/or a functional workshop and budget insufficiency.

Stream 2: Of the planned activities and investments for strengthening the area of maintenance, only a limited number were implemented. While several regional workshops for maintenance of medical equipment were renovated or constructed, an insufficient number of new technicians and engineers were trained. Moreover, several of them left for jobs in the private sector. The supply of spare parts remained erratic due to procedural and budgetary insufficiencies. Only few of the planned new public-private partnerships (for outsourced maintenance) were actually established.

Stream 3: Policy dialogue with the full range of health stakeholders, including facility-level managers and health workers, showed that, on the plus side, the new database for asset management facilitated the strategic shift to a more centralized system of maintenance for medical equipment. However, on the negative side, the lack of a health technology policy, medical equipment norms and standards and clear technical specifications for equipment standardization were all strong limiting factors for more efficient and needs-based procurement, supply and repair management.

3.5.5 Link between situation analysis and priority-setting

Priority-setting processes the recommendations and insights coming from the situation analysis and accords them a specific priority level.

As elaborated upon above, the health sector situation analysis process is where the health system's strengths, weaknesses, opportunities, and threats, including their root causes and effects, are analysed and debated upon among all relevant stakeholders. Of course, a discussion on what has worked well and less well is not completely disconnected from potential solutions and recommendations to overcome health sector challenges; thus those very suggestions, which have already been debated upon, discussed, and sorted through by a broad stakeholder base during the situation analysis, form the starting point for the priority-setting exercise. Priority-setting is where the recommendations and insights coming from the situation analysis are "processed" and examined in view of according them a specific priority level.

The analysis of the sector thus provides the foundation for priority-setting, and greatly determines the quality of priority-setting results. The challenges identified during the situation analysis process, and the debate around potential strategies to overcome those challenges, help make the best possible choices regarding the focus and distribution of means, in order to improve the performance and impact of the health system in an efficient and fair way. The choices made during the priority-setting process will profit from the quality of evidence and the quality of dialogue during the situation analysis process – if one is sound, the likelihood is that the other will be, as well.

Those choices, or priorities, drive the decisions on the key goals and objectives of the health sector for a given period, and will be expressed in the NHPSP. So, in the context of strategizing for health, it is the identified important need from the situation analysis, and reflections on how this need can be addressed, which paves the way for the priority-setting process.

Normally, future challenges – such as an ageing population, climate change, or increasing health inequalities – are issues which will have emerged both during population consultations and a health sector situation analysis. During the priority-setting phase, the consequences of these expected eventualities will be contemplated. The process of setting priorities is the opportunity for policy-makers and health sector stakeholders to pre-empt foreseeable health problems raised during the situation analysis and ensure that their negative impact on health outcomes is mitigated.

Since priority-setting is a trade-off, and trade-offs are difficult, a robust reasoning and justification must be offered. The situation analysis, by examining challenges and possible solutions, is the knowledge base which provides this to health sector stakeholders and the population.

3.6 Some issues to consider

3.6.1 Factors of success

Success of a situation analysis is judged against its stated objectives. As mentioned previously, the objectives of a health sector situation analysis are:

(a) to realistically assess the current health sector situation, with all its strengths, weaknesses, opportunities, and threats;

(b) to provide an evidence-informed basis for formulating future strategic directions for the health sector;

(c) to provide an evidence-informed basis for responding to real health sector needs of the population.

Accordingly, the main factors of success would be achieving each of the above objectives.

- The situation analysis adequately captures a broad range of the stakeholders' views and opinions in a balanced way. It would be especially useful if these views and opinions were formulated such that they could be easily converted into operational steps for future (or adjusting existing plans).
- More importantly, those very stakeholders have accepted, or "bought into", the situation analysis conclusions, even on controversial issues. It is important to note here that accepting conclusions is not equal to being in agreement with them. If the situation analysis presents all major viewpoints in an unbiased way, throwing light on the pros and cons of the different perspectives, it can be seen as "balanced", which can then be accepted by all.
- In addition, the situation analysis can be seen as successfully undertaken if results are the drivers behind health sector priority-setting as well as embodied in the strategic directions of the health sector.

A successful situation analysis realistically assesses the current health sector situation, provides an evidence-informed basis for formulating future strategic directions for the health sector and for responding to a population's real health sector needs.

3.6.2 Dissemination of situation analysis results

Containing a wealth of information, the full situation analysis should be published, promoted, and distributed widely to guide stakeholders during the rest of the strategic planning process.

A situation analysis is in essence a very technical piece of work whose results and conclusions are relevant for the whole population. Therefore, a significant effort to translate the technical into simple population-friendly language is imperative. For that purpose a concise summary of the situation analysis can be written, with illustrations and graphs where necessary, which can be distributed in communities and at districts and regions. The concise summary should clearly highlight the principal challenges and trends, major issues of debate, possible solutions and reasoning. Using various forms of traditional and social media can be an effective way of communicating the key findings of the situation analysis. For example, partnering with the media and collaborating on disseminating and simplifying messages has been used as a successful strategy in many countries.

The full situation analysis report is a wealth of information which should be published, promoted and distributed widely to guide the contributions of all stakeholders during the rest of the strategic planning process. Dissemination includes not just distribution of a hard-copy document; instead, it implies explaining the document to relevant communities and stakeholders, holding special meetings and presentations, making it available online, etc. In effect, it involves a whole communication strategy linked to the NHPSP as a whole, which might require additional resources to be budgeted.

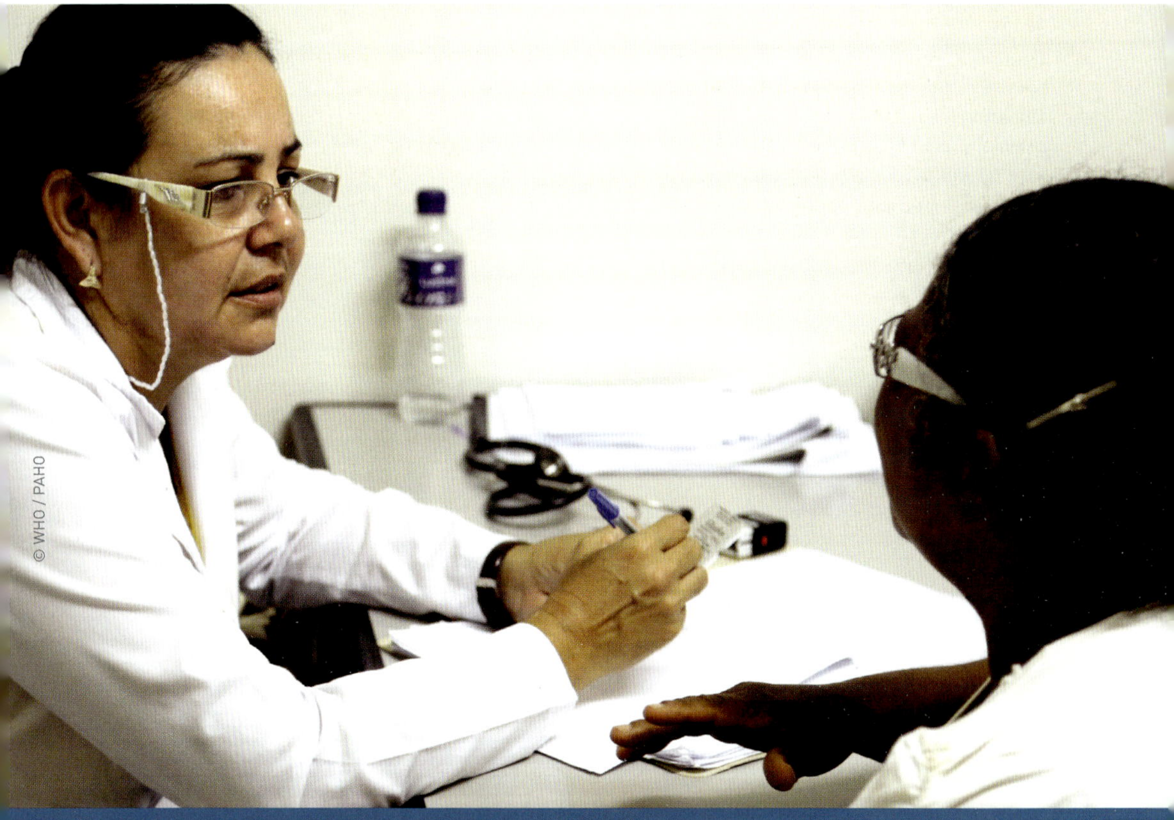

3.7 What if...?

3.7.1 What if your country is decentralized?

A decentralized[VI] setting requires looking more closely at a country's constitutional background and legal framework. If health is a mandate for a sub-national entity, the full health policy and planning cycle, from situation analysis to monitoring and evaluation will fall under that authority. In this case, close cooperation with other decentralized entities and/or a central authority may be necessary on topics that are not confined to one area or region.

A situation analysis at a regional/sub-national level has the distinct advantage of being closer to the reality of health services. This means that a bottom-up approach does not have very far to go to become translated into policy. This is to be taken advantage of, and efforts to disseminate and feedback results of a situation analysis to the population should be easier to undertake. Also, a decentralized system means that those spearheading the health sector situation analysis may have a better knowledge of local realities such as language and customs that can help tailor the situation analysis for maximum results and use in policy-making.

A sub-national health sector situation analysis will also be useful for central-level policy- and decision-making, especially since national policies and plans need to include concerns and be adaptable to sub-national levels. More detailed information, data, and views from specific population groups or remote areas is extremely valuable when designing policies, setting priorities, and allocating resources. It can even merit national-level involvement in the sub-national process – and in some cases, other regional/sub-national levels whose concerns may overlap. A caveat for the national level is to ensure coherence and comparability among sub-national entities – without which it will be extremely difficult to draw more generalized conclusions for the rest of the country.

The table below gives an indication on issues to consider when undertaking a health sector situation analysis in a decentralized context, following the "factors of success" for a situation analysis in 3.6.1.

A situation analysis in a decentralized setting requires looking more closely at a country's constitutional background and legal framework to understand the authority of certain stakeholders and ensure cooperation between entities at various levels.

VI This includes including political decentralization (federal system) as well as geographical decentralization (e.g. islands).

Table 3.5 Factors of success: situation analysis in a decentralized system

DID WE DO A GOOD JOB ...	... IN A DECENTRALIZED SYSTEM?
1. The situation analysis adequately captures a broad range of the stakeholders' views and opinions in a balanced way	▶ Inclusiveness of national as well as sub-national levels in the design of the methodology is ensured even if the actual situation analysis may only be conducted at sub-national level. Both levels can benefit greatly from the situation analysis results and the cross-linkage between the two. ▶ Stakeholders which only exist at sub-national (e.g. state MoH, grass-root organizations, professional associations), or only at national level (e.g. federal MoH, parliamentary groups, ministries of finance and planning, professional associations) are informed and adequately included where useful and necessary. For example, the central/federal MoH should especially be included (potentially in large numbers) in a sub-national situation analysis if a new national health plan is being drafted – input from sub-national level is crucial for this. ▶ All types of stakeholders, even those with diametrically opposing views, have been included and involved and a balanced outlook is presented in the situation analysis report. Please note that this is not specific to a decentralized system; however, it may be even more difficult to present a balanced viewpoint in a localized system where the actors know and interact with each other more closely.
2. And more importantly, if those very stakeholders have accepted, or "bought into", the situation analysis conclusions, even on controversial issues.	▶ Stakeholders who were less present or engaged before have an increasingly active role in policy formulation and implementation. ▶ Roles and responsibilities for NHPSP implementation between national and sub-national levels, and between stakeholders, have been clarified. ▶ National and sub-national levels are adequately represented during the preparation and follow-up of the situation analysis. ▶ Especially more marginalized stakeholder groups have a clear role in and accept the conclusions of the health sector situation analysis.
3. In addition, if the situation analysis results are the drivers behind health sector priority-setting as well as embodied in the strategic directions of the health sector, it can be seen as successfully undertaken.	▶ The results of the situation analysis were made available to all concerned levels. ▶ Priorities which were raised in sub-national situation analyses can be found in local district/regional operational plans as well as the strategic and/or operational plans at national level. ▶ Follow-up to the results should be demonstrated by national as well as sub-national levels – with a clear understanding of which level will be responsible for implementation of the follow-up plan.

3.7.2 What if fragmentation and/or fragility is an issue in your country?

Fragility refers to a country that includes certain areas of limited statehood, "where the state does not have the administrative capacity (either material or institutional) to exercise effective control over activities within its own borders".[19]

When the state does not have effective administrative capacity, its governance and steering capacities are also severely hampered. This can lead to various stakeholders in the health sector working in an uncoordinated way with duplications in procedures, funding streams, and parallel institutions. In this context, a stronger emphasis must be placed on strengthening coordination for planning, funding, and implementation. A joint situation analysis with a comprehensive and solid stakeholder input, bought into by all, can be a very good start.

Especially in post-crisis settings, there is often a tension between those desiring to do a rapid situation assessment with a humanitarian aid focus and those wanting to ensure an overarching policy framework based on a more comprehensive situation analysis to prevent further fragmentation and verticalization. It is key here to enter into dialogue with actors on both sides to come to a common understanding; without it, any situation analysis work, where all stakeholders' input is necessary, will be difficult. In reality, much of the situation analysis itself will be conducted by these very stakeholders anyway, which renders the dialogue beforehand even more critical.

Logistical issues can pose a particularly difficult challenge in a fragile setting and can put into question the feasibility of the exercise in the first place. These issues must be carefully considered with all relevant stakeholders before coming to a decision.

Despite the myriad problems associated with conducting a situation analysis in a fragile setting, this exercise can actually be a huge opportunity to gauge what the new status quo of the health sector is after a difficult conflict/struggle/natural disaster/revolution. It can be the start of gathering relevant information to introduce reforms that may have been necessary before the fragile situation began but were unlikely to go through. It can be seen as the beginning of a clean slate to rebuild the health sector to a state that will be better than it was before.

1. *The situation analysis adequately captures a broad range of the stakeholders' views and opinions in a balanced way*

In a fragile or fragmented context, where steering capacity is diffused and held by those with the most money or power, getting a balanced view on the health sector situation is a challenge. It is all the more important to spend time and effort to build MoH governance capacity in targeted areas as quickly as possible so that it can adequately take on its lead role in ensuring a balanced situation analysis. Development partners can play their part by participating and giving input into a situation analysis exercise, and aligning with the MoH agenda.

2. And more importantly, *if those very stakeholders have accepted, or "bought into", the situation analysis conclusions,* even on controversial issues.

In fragile, post-conflict, or post-emergency settings, a situation analysis will be largely conducted by those involved in emergency relief as well as health sector development professionals. Often, there is a tension between the two groups due to differing views on the objectives and scope of a situation analysis – short-term data and information to feed into humanitarian aid planning, or more in-depth longer-term trends, taking into account the recent or current emergency, for longer-term health system development? Managing this tension will not be easy but the measure of success will be if both sides have truly accepted the situation analysis conclusions.

In an aid-dependent context, a situation analysis should be used as an opportunity to rally donors and aid agencies around the same priorities.

It is important to note here that accepting conclusions is not equal to being in agreement with them. If the situation analysis presents all major viewpoints in an unbiased way, throwing light on the pros and cons of the different perspectives, it can be seen as "balanced" which can then be accepted by all. A good way of assuring a balanced view of a subject in a fragile setting is to actively ensure the meaningful participation and representation of both types of stakeholders into the analysis, even if it might mean that debates and discussions are particularly heated or even conflictual. The conclusions may present the majority view but should take into account other views as well.

3. In addition, if the *situation analysis results are the drivers behind health sector priority setting as well as embodied in the strategic directions of the health sector*, it can be seen as successfully undertaken.

As mentioned in previous chapters, the disconnect between existing policies and plans and realities on the ground is particularly high in fragile settings. A well-done and well-balanced situation analysis can help address this deficiency and support the priority-setting process in a constructive yet realistic way. A direct link between the situation analysis results and the core set priorities in any health sector reform/ health sector plan is particularly imperative here.

3.7.3 What if your country is highly dependent on aid?

A country that heavily depends on external aid might also be dependent on external funding and expertise to conduct the situation analysis in the first place. This could imply undue influence of those who are funding or providing expertise. Unless government stewardship is strong, the situation analysis might end up reflecting external – rather than domestic – priorities or vision. External priorities might imply that certain programmes or project topics receive more prominence than necessary in the situation analysis. It can be a vicious cycle where the situation analysis results find themselves in the national health plan with the same priorities, which are not really the ones the government would like to focus on.

A situation analysis in an aid-dependent context should rather be seen and used as an opportunity to rally donors and aid agencies around the same priorities. If the situation analysis is done correctly with a balanced vision of the strengths and weaknesses of the health system, key problems can be collectively addressed and priorities given funding by donors. A well-done situation analysis could raise the credibility of the MoH and government and give donors confidence to support activities that have been deemed important by the situation analysis.

Table 3.6 Factors of success: situation analysis in an aid-dependent context

WHEN UNDERTAKING A SITUATION ANALYSIS...	... THIS IS WHAT WE NEED TO CONSIDER ADDITIONALLY IF OUR COUNTRY IS HEAVILY DEPENDING ON EXTERNAL AID
1. The situation analysis adequately captures a broad range of the stakeholders' views and opinions in a balanced way	▸ When setting up the methods and deciding on who to be involved (stakeholders), it is important to explicitly recognize and ensure that every stakeholder is considered equally; a categorical effort should be made to create a sense of joint commitment and collective benefit to all. Keep in mind that often, those stakeholders who provide funding (donors) may be perceived as more important than others. The big risk here is the tacit establishment of a certain hierarchy of stakeholders which can create tension, resentment and frustration. The consequences can include the withdrawal of some stakeholders, from the process altogether – with its accompanying loss of "champions" (and the evident possibility of negative propaganda) as well as a group of stakeholders (often donors) taking over the situation analysis to influence it in their own interests. ▸ Linked to the above, it is crucial to clarify in no uncertain terms the roles and responsibilities of each stakeholder, taking into account their respective added value.
2. And more importantly, if those very stakeholders have accepted, or "bought into", the situation analysis conclusions, even on contro-versial issues.	▸ Donor engagement in consultation processes might change the dynamics and reception, and the subsequent results, of the situation analysis. ▸ The technical team coordinating the situation analysis should make a specific effort to ensure that all stakeholders in a sensitive aid-dependent environment feel as if their matters have been adequately considered and its pros and cons weighed up. The aim of any situation analysis result is for it to be balanced and fair.
3. In addition, if the situation analysis results are the drivers behind health sector priority-setting as well as embodied in the strategic directions of the health sector, it can be seen as successfully undertaken.	▸ In an aid-dependent context, it is especially vital to ensure that the results of the situation analysis are immediately translated into either an operational plan or a strategic plan while the momentum and dynamic is still in place. A long gap between the situation analysis and plan development will allow various actors to potentially intervene and influence the plan to their interests, thus creating a disparity between the situation analysis and the plan. ▸ Linked to the above, an adequate follow-up and monitoring body must be set up to see through the implementation of the situation analysis results. A fine balance must be found in enabling the right monitoring body, as it should be a high enough level for decision-making purposes but operational enough for day-to-day follow-up. ▸ Inadequate follow-up can lead to different interpretations of review results by different stakeholders – these varying interpretations may manifest themselves again in the country's health sector vision and priorities.

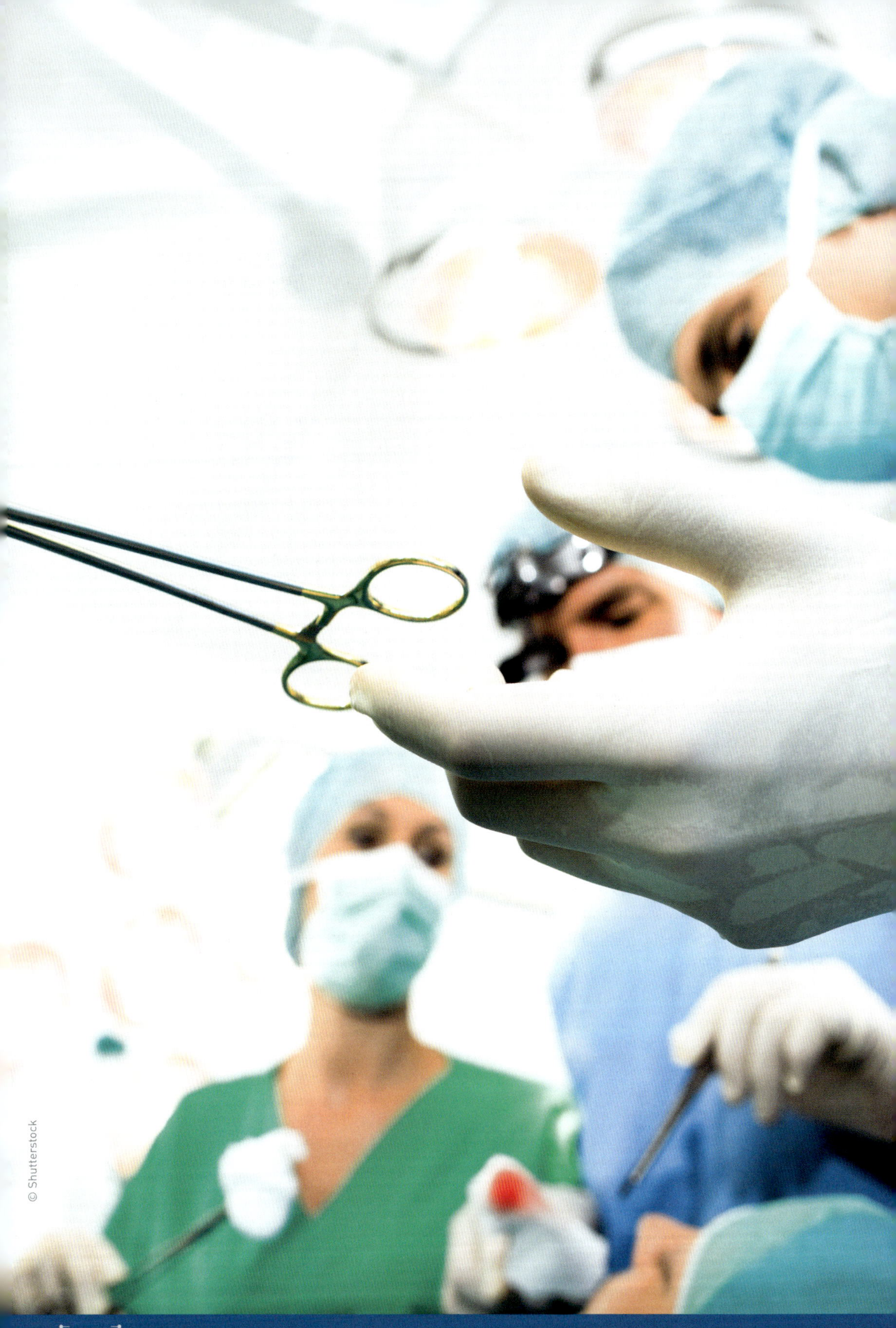

3.8 Conclusion

The strategic directions and the principal orientation of a NHPSP must be firmly grounded in an analysis of the current state of the health sector. A situation analysis helps to provide an evidence-informed basis for the NHPSP strategic directions to respond to real health sector needs of the population. In this chapter, the situation analysis methodology proposed is one that adequately captures not only expert analysis but also stakeholder input that actively includes citizens' voices and population demand.

A situation analysis of the health sector should ideally feed directly into the priority-setting process, as it is the knowledge base for health challenges, potential solutions, what has worked well in the past and what has not. However, regardless of whether it is technically undertaken by external parties or not, the lead and overall coordination should be provided by the MoH.

A health sector situation analysis is a crucial step in the health policy and planning cycle. It is a key platform to give voice to stakeholders in order to obtain their buy-in for better policy design and implementation, and ensure mutual accountability between them.

Methodologically, a situation analysis should include an analysis of health system performance and an analysis of the implementation of health sector activities, budgets and finances. These should then be brought into an overarching policy dialogue on strengths and weaknesses of health system components and health programmes as well as cross-cutting health topics that bring expert views and end user/community opinion together.

A situation analysis should be participatory and inclusive, comprehensive and analytical in nature. This last point is to be emphasized as it is easy to stop at a *description* of the health sector status quo (already useful in and of itself) and not delve adequately enough into the root causes and comprehension of *why* certain activities or programmes worked well or less well. But precisely understanding the root causes and effects will help lead to finding longer-term sustainable solutions or scale-ups.

A situation analysis can be judged as successful if it adequately captures a broad range of the stakeholders' views and opinions in a balanced way; if those very stakeholders have accepted, or "bought into", the situation analysis conclusions; and if the situation analysis results are the drivers behind health sector priority-setting and the strategic directions of the health sector.

Finally, if your country has particular specificities such as a decentralized setting, a distressed health context, or is highly aid-dependent, there may be unique issues to heed when conducting a situation analysis, as has been elaborated upon in this chapter.

References

1 Situation analysis and priority setting. In: National health policies, strategies and plans [website] Geneva: WHO; 2016 (http://www.who.int/nationalpolicies/processes/priorities/en/, accessed 13 October 2016).

2 Berman P, Bitran R. Health systems analysis for better health system strengthening. Washington (DC): World Bank; 2011 (HNP Discussion Paper; http://siteresources.worldbank.org/HEALTHNUTRITIONANDPOPULATION/Resources/281627-1095698140167/HealthSystemsAnalysisForBetterHealthSysStrengthening.pdf, accessed 13 October 2016).

3 Ibid.

4 Jaffré Y, Olivier de Sardan JP. Une médecine inhospitalière. Les difficiles relations entre soignants et soignés dans cinq capitales d'Afrique de l'Ouest. Paris: Apad Karthala; 2003.

5 Brugha R, Varvasovsky Z. Stakeholder analysis: a review. Health Policy Plan. 2000;15(3):239–46 (http://heapol.oxfordjournals.org/content/15/3/239.long, accessed 13 October 2016).

6 Schmeer K. Guidelines for conducting a stakeholder analysis. Bethesda (MD): Partnerships for Health Reform, Abt Associates Inc.; 1999 (Health Reform Tools Series; http://www.phrplus.org/Pubs/hts3.pdf, accessed 13 October 2016).

7 Ibid.

8 Brugha R, Varvasovsky Z. Stakeholder analysis: a review. Health Policy Plan. 2000;15(3):239–46 (http://heapol.oxfordjournals.org/content/15/3/239.long, accessed 13 October 2016).

9 Thow AM. Stakeholder analysis for health policy research. Sydney Health Policy Network and Qualitative Health Research Collaboration Forum; May 2013 (http://sydney.edu.au/health-policy-network//news-events/Thow.pdf, accessed 13 October 2016).

10 Mills A, Brugha R, Hanson K, McPake B. What can be done about the private health sector in low-income countries? Bull World Health Organ. 2002;80(4):325–30 (http://apps.who.int/bulletin/archives/80(4)325.pdf, accessed 13 October 2016).

11 CHPP taxonomy can be found at healthsituation.org [registration required]. See: CHIP annotated table of content. Second draft. October 2, 2009.

12 Health system reviews (HiT series). In: European Observatory on Health Systems and Policies [website] Copenhagen: WHO Regional Office for Europe (http://www.euro.who.int/en/about-us/partners/observatory/publications/health-system-reviews-hits, accessed 7 October 2016).

13 Health system assessment approach: a how-to manual. Bethesda (MD): Abt Associates Inc.; 2008 (Health Systems 20/20 Brief; http://healthsystemassessment.org/wp-content/uploads/2015/03/Health-Systems-Assessment-Approach-How-To-Manual_Brief.pdf, accessed 13 October 2016).

14 Health financing for universal coverage: health systems financing review. Geneva: WHO; 2016 (http://www.who.int/health_financing/tools/systems_review/en/, accessed 13 October 2016).

15 Human Resources for Health Toolkit. Global Health Workforce Alliance. (website] Geneva: WHO; 2016 (http://www.who.int/workforcealliance/knowledge/toolkit/hrhtoolkitpurposepages/en/index3.html, accessed 13 October 2016).

16 World Health Organization: Everybody's business: strengthening health systems to improve health outcomes. WHO's Framework for Action. 2007, Geneva: World Health Organization, (http://www.hoint/healthsystems/strategy/everybodys_businesspdf, accessed 16 October 2016).

17 van Wijngaarden JD, Scholten GR, van Wijk KP. Strategic analysis for health care organizations: the suitability of the SWOT-analysis. Int J Health Plann Manage. 2010;27(1): 34–49 (http://onlinelibrary.wiley.com/doi/10.1002/hpm.1032/full, accessed 13 October 2016).

18 Harrison JP. Chapter 5: Strategic planning and SWOT analysis. In: Harrison JP. Essentials of strategic planning in healthcare. Chicago (IL): Health Administration Press; 2010 (http://www.ache.org/pdf/secure/gifts/Harrison_Chapter5.pdf, accessed 13 October, 2016).

19 Krasner SD, Risse T. External actors, state-building, and service provision in areas of limited statehood: introduction. Governance. 2014;27(4): 545–67.

Further reading

Berman P, Bitran R. Health systems analysis for better health system strengthening. Washington (DC): World Bank; 2011 (HNP Discussion Paper; http://siteresources.worldbank.org/HEALTHNUTRITIONANDPOPULATION/Resources/281627-1095698140167/HealthSystemsAnalysisForBetterHealthSysStrengthening.pdf, accessed 13 October 2016).

Harrison JP. Chapter 5: Strategic planning and SWOT analysis. In: Harrison JP. Essentials of strategic planning in healthcare. Chicago (IL): Health Administration Press; 2010 (http://www.ache.org/pdf/secure/gifts/Harrison_Chapter5.pdf, accessed 13 October, 2016).

Health system assessment approach: a how-to manual. Bethesda (MD): Abt Associates Inc.; 2008 (Health Systems 20/20 Brief; http://healthsystemassessment.org/wp-content/uploads/2015/03/Health-Systems-Assessment-Approach-How-To-Manual_Brief.pdf,accessed 13 October 2016).

Chapter 4

Priority-setting for national health policies, strategies and plans

Frank Terwindt

Dheepa Rajan

Agnes Soucat

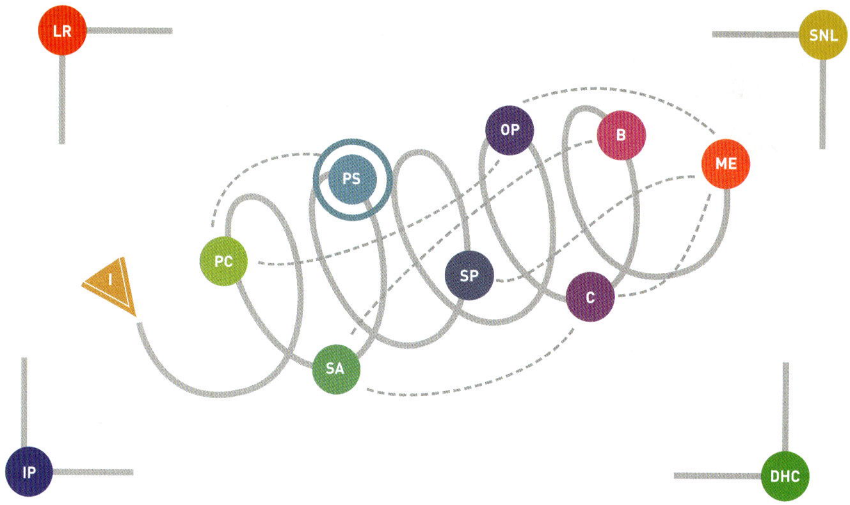

Cross-cutting topics relevant to national health planning

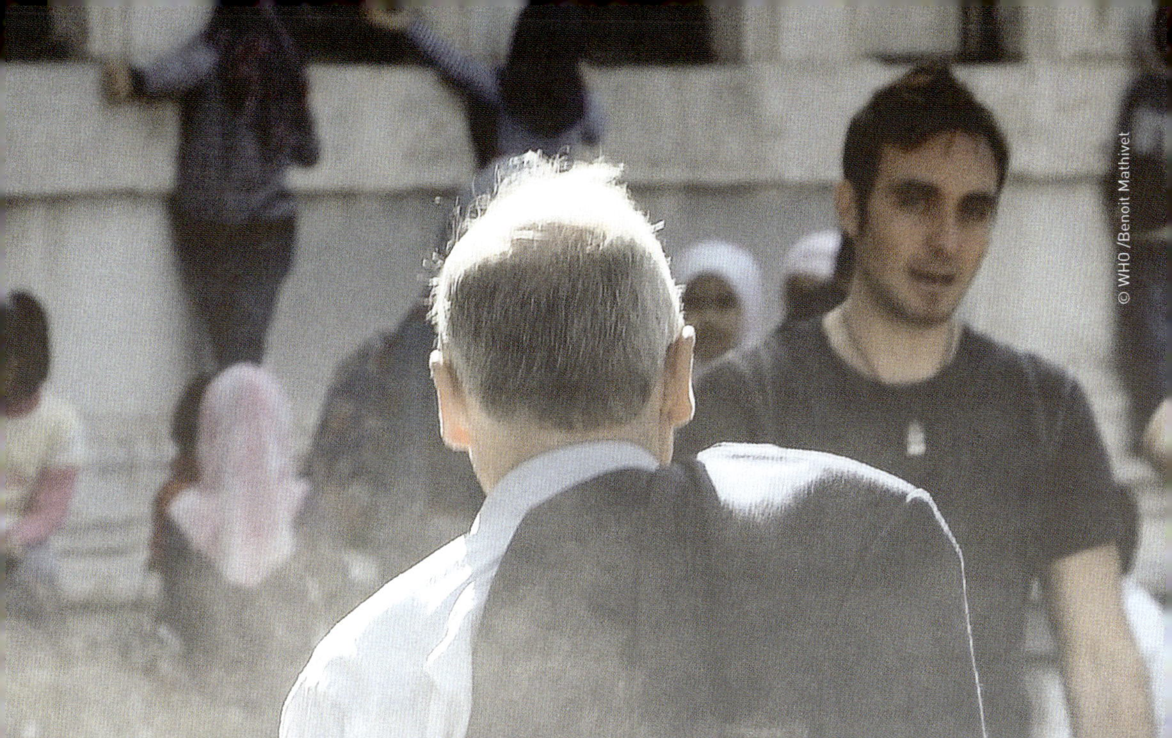

Overview

Priority-setting determines the strategic directions of the national health plan. Led by citizens who are the principals and decision-makers, priority-setting is a shared responsibility between the ministry of health (MoH) and the entire health stakeholder community. This chapter elaborates various criteria and approaches for priority-setting. It closes with some specificities of the priority-setting exercise in particular contexts such as the decentralized and highly centralized setting, fragile states, and an aid-dependent environment.

Summary

What is priority-setting?

The process of priority-setting is inherently political, which means that it is a process where societal values and goals are important, and resulting priorities reflect a compromise among stakeholders. That being said, the aim of the process is to select among different options for addressing the most important health needs, as highlighted in the health sector situation analysis,[I] in the best way ("best" here depends on a number of criteria, explained in the course of this chapter), given limited resources (rationing). In health, priority-setting determines the key objectives for the health sector for a given period, thus directly feeding into the content of the national health plan.

Why is it important?

Priority-setting is necessary everywhere, as resources are never unlimited. Choices must be made that reflect a society's values and vision for the health system, and integrate reflections on explicitly chosen criteria. In addition, a priority-setting exercise is where the principal decisions are made after the situation analysis discussions; these decisions feed directly into national health plan development.

When should priority-setting be done?

The priority-setting exercise generally follows a situation analysis and precedes decisions on resource allocation and planning.

Priority-setting can be done at different intervals in the policy and planning cycle of a sector, a programme or project. For this handbook, it is discussed notably in the context of national health planning in the medium term.

Who should undertake or be engaged in priority-setting?

Actors such as government (ministries) have a formal responsibility for priority-setting. In an inclusive approach, stakeholder groups of various levels are consulted, as are the population.

How can priority-setting be done? What are the criteria and approaches?

Priority-setting is a multifaceted process that is usually informed by the situation analysis. It is based on criteria set by health sector stakeholders. Evidence on the different criteria is then examined jointly. The results of the evidence analysis feed into the formulation of the national health policy, strategy or plan (NHPSP).

Possible criteria and approaches are elaborated upon in this chapter.

Anything else to consider?

- decentralized environment;
- highly-centralized setting;
- fragile environment;
- aid-dependent setting.

I See Chapter 3 "Situation analysis of the health sector" in this handbook.

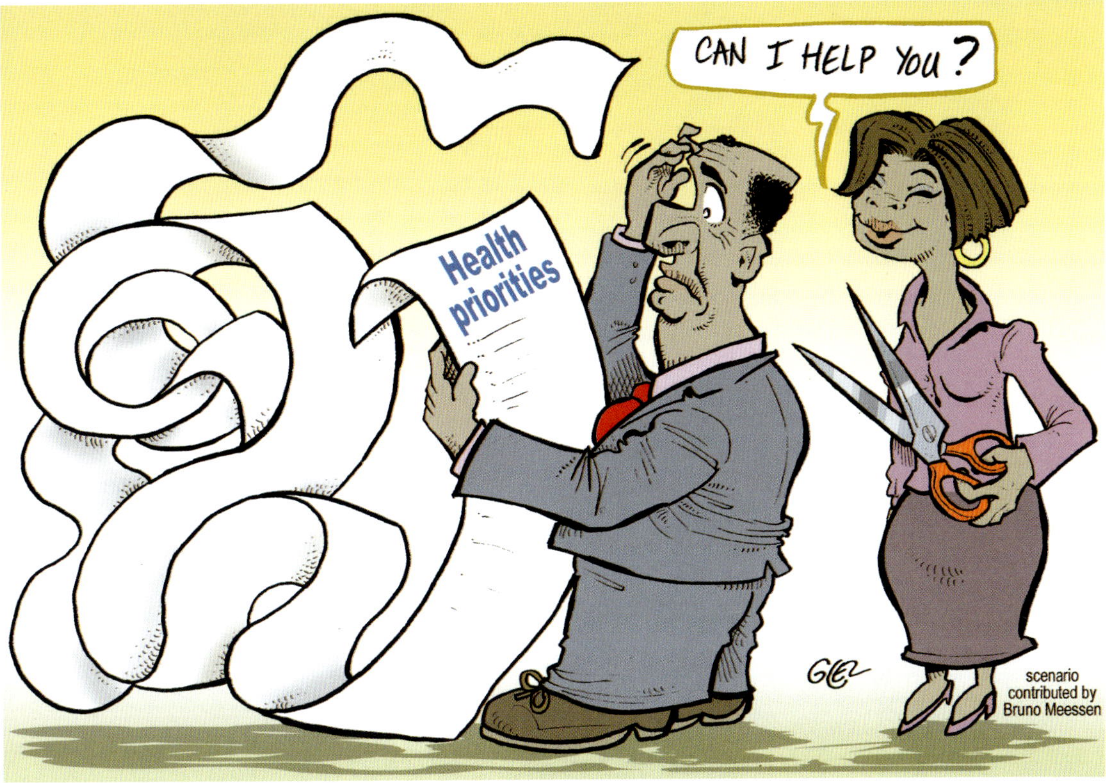
CAN I HELP YOU ?
Health priorities
GLEZ
scenario contributed by Bruno Meessen

Fig. 4.1 Trade-offs are part of priority-setting

Damian Glez; scenario by Bruno Meessen.

4.1 What is priority-setting?

The aim of the priority-setting process is to select among different options for addressing the most important health needs, as highlighted in the health sector situation analysis,[II] given limited resources (rationing). The process of priority-setting is inherently political; it is a process where societal values and goals are important, and resulting priorities reflect a compromise among stakeholders, including the population. Indeed, citizens are the principals and decision-makers of the priority-setting process. In health, priority-setting determines the key objectives for the sector for a given period, thus directly feeding into the content of the national health strategy. The priority-setting exercise generally follows a situation analysis and precedes decisions on resource allocation and planning.

The process of priority-setting is inherently political, which means that it is a process where societal values and goals are important, and resulting priorities reflect a compromise among stakeholders.

II See Chapter 3 "Situation analysis of the health sector" in this handbook.

Priority-setting is closely linked to the challenges identified during the situation analysis process, and the debate around potential strategies to overcome those challenges. It helps to make the best possible choices regarding the distribution of means, since resources are scarce, and trade-offs are thus necessary. The intended consequence is to improve health system performance in an efficient and fair way.

Priority-setting is not only about making the best use of financial resources; it is also about attribution of resources in general in response to population value choices, demand and need.[III] For instance, it may be agreed that certain institutional reforms are a priority. The concerned reforms may necessitate a change in administrative and technical procedures, which in turn may require existing staff to use their time differently – the necessary investment is thus not predominantly monetary in nature.

Priority-setting is often about giving more importance to certain health interventions above others. It must be kept in mind that when importance and resources are attributed to one intervention over another, a reduction of resources or exclusion altogether for the other intervention is the consequence.

In the context of this chapter, the term interventions may cover programmes, sets of activities, policies, strategies, reforms, investments or implementation modalities, undertaken separately or in combination. An intervention is thus any measure whose purpose is to improve health or alter the course of disease, for example, a solution to a health problem or a health promotion activity or a new organigram for the district health management team, etc.

III "Need" in the context of health is something that is necessary for humans to live a healthy life. This can be measured by, for example, self-reporting, health status indicators, biomedical markers, geographic measures, etc. Broadly speaking, "demand" for health-related services is the expression of felt need. Demand is influenced by factors such as illness behaviour, knowledge of services, media, etc.

4.1.1 Priority-setting in the context of universal health coverage (UHC)

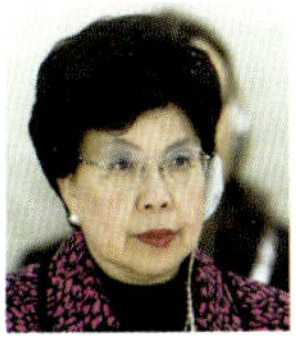

"I regard universal health coverage as the single most powerful concept that public health has to offer," stated the World Health Organization's (WHO's) Director-General Dr Margaret Chan at a ministerial-level meeting on UHC in February 2013.[1]

UHC is a social contract, an overarching goal towards which a health system should steer. WHO Member States committed to this in the World Health Assembly resolution 64.9, with the definition anchored in the 2010 World Health Report: "UHC is defined as ensuring that all people can use the promotive, preventive, curative, rehabilitative and palliative health services they need, of sufficient quality to be effective, while also ensuring that the use of these services does not expose the user to financial hardship."[2] In addition, Sustainable Development Goal 3.8 is to achieve universal health coverage, a goal which all UN Member States subscribed to in September 2015.

There is no blueprint solution for the path towards UHC; instead, it is a process that must be pursued differently in a context-specific way in each individual setting. However, all contexts and all settings will require a health system approach to move closer towards the overarching goal of UHC – an approach that seeks to actively collaborate with other relevant sectors, and bring together all relevant health sector stakeholders to discuss potential interventions to improve the population's health.

The UHC concept takes into account the aspect of financial protection for improving coverage, geographical accessibility and availability of care. To move towards UHC, WHO thus recommends working on three dimensions (Fig. 4.2): extension of health coverage to the population not yet covered, improvement of the health service package provided (in terms of number and quality of services), and a reduction of cost sharing and out-of-pocket payments for health.

Priority-setting exercises can help address these dimensions:

- Reaching vulnerable, marginalized and hard-to-reach populations ("width" of coverage) can be achieved by the extension of services to those segments of the population not yet covered.
- Maximizing service delivery provision ("depth" of coverage) can be achieved by improving efficiency in service package results.
- Improvements in financial risk protection ("height" of coverage) can be achieved for poor and vulnerable populations through targeted reduction of cost sharing and fees.

Moving towards UHC means that priority actions and investments along each axis are needed; for this, trade-offs are constantly necessary. These trade-offs will be influenced by imperatives that change over time as choices of citizens evolve, the economy develops, the population ages, or the disease burden shifts. Hence, moving toward UHC is at the heart of the democratic debate, a political process that involves public information and negotiation between different groups in society over the contribution to and use of the public purse, allocation of health benefits and who should pay for these benefits.

UHC is a process that must be pursued differently in a context-specific way in each individual setting. However, all contexts and all settings will require a health system approach to move closer towards the overarching goal of UHC – an approach that seeks to actively collaborate with other relevant sectors, and bring together all relevant health sector stakeholders to discuss potential priority interventions to improve the population's health.

Fig. 4.2 Three dimensions to consider when moving towards UHC[3]

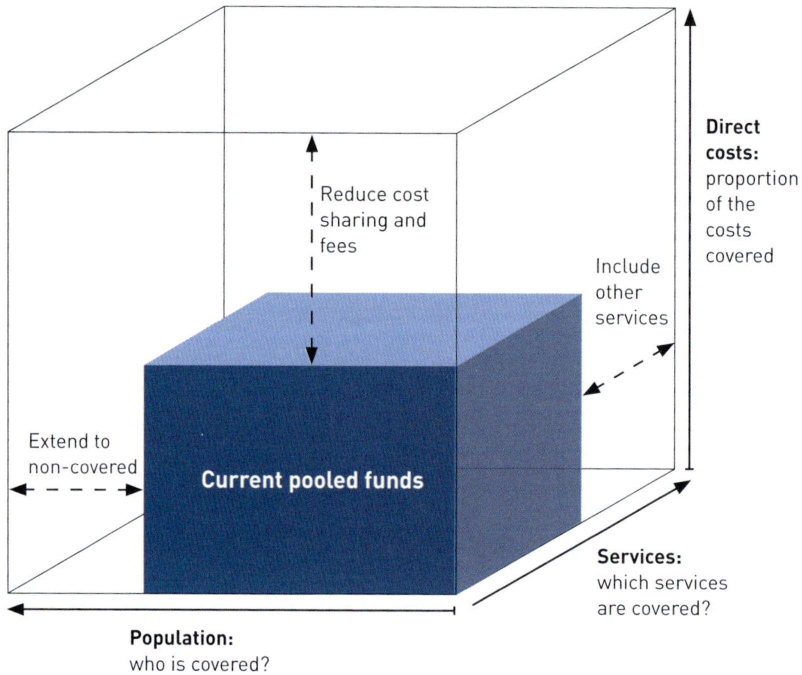

4.1.2 Priority-setting basics

Priority-setting examines the degree to which an identified important need – generally specified in the situation analysis – can be addressed, based on criteria such as, but not limited to, the burden of the health issue at hand, fairness, cost of the intervention, responsiveness, the effectiveness of the intervention and the acceptability of the intervention. A society may also include other criteria that it feels are essential and reflect its culture, history and objectives.

Cost-effectiveness has been an extensively used priority-setting criterion in economic literature and discourse, in this chapter we advance the view that cost-effectiveness analysis is an important and widespread technological approach (and not a criterion), which feeds into the evidence base during the priority-setting process. However, it is only one of several technological approaches, whose results should be deliberated upon carefully during the course of the priority-setting process, along with all other available evidence. More on cost-effective analysis and its place in the priority-setting process is discussed in section 4.5.3.

We distinguish between prioritizing health problems or health sector challenges and prioritizing solutions or interventions to overcome those problems and challenges. Naturally, the two are very closely linked; however, a health problem can have several possible solutions. For example, identifying diabetes as a priority disease in a country is a separate decision from the one that examines the different preventive, promotive and curative interventions available to tackle diabetes.

The priority-setting criteria mentioned in this chapter address both priority-setting for health problems and priority-setting for possible solutions. The criterion of burden looks mainly at the health problem, while effectiveness, cost and acceptability address the proposed health intervention (solution). Fairness can address both.

Resource limitations are taken into account in a priority-setting process. However, the actual resource allocation and budgeting decisions come after the priority-setting, because it is a process of trade-offs. Priority-setting informs the decision-making process. The priority-setting process makes explicit which health problems, challenges and solutions should be given priority based on certain criteria; the decisions then taken are based on the priority-setting process's evidence, giving more or less weight to certain issues based on a (political) debate and discussion. In the end, there might be trade-offs between the various criteria, and the weight of each of them will be a political decision.

In practice, feasibility and implementation issues will be part of the priority-setting dialogue and cannot be artificially extracted from it. Also, feasibility may be included in the priority-setting criteria in some settings. Strictly speaking, the priority-setting process should focus first on what the country's health sector priorities should be for the NHPSP; considerations of feasibility and implementation constraints will be more strongly taken into account in the actual decision-making and NHPSP formulation process.

Because priority-setting is highly coloured by politics, there may be a tendency to focus on shorter-term gains rather than looking at a longer-term strategic vision. Either way, it is useful to keep in mind that a collection of short-term priorities may not necessarily culminate in achieving a longer-term one and that special care might need to be taken to keep the longer-term priorities on the agenda.

In the context of strategizing for health, priority-setting examines the degree to which an identified important need – which is generally specified in the situation analysis – can be addressed, based on criteria such as, but not limited to, the importance of the health issue at hand, the effectiveness of the intervention, the cost of the intervention, the acceptability of the intervention and fairness.

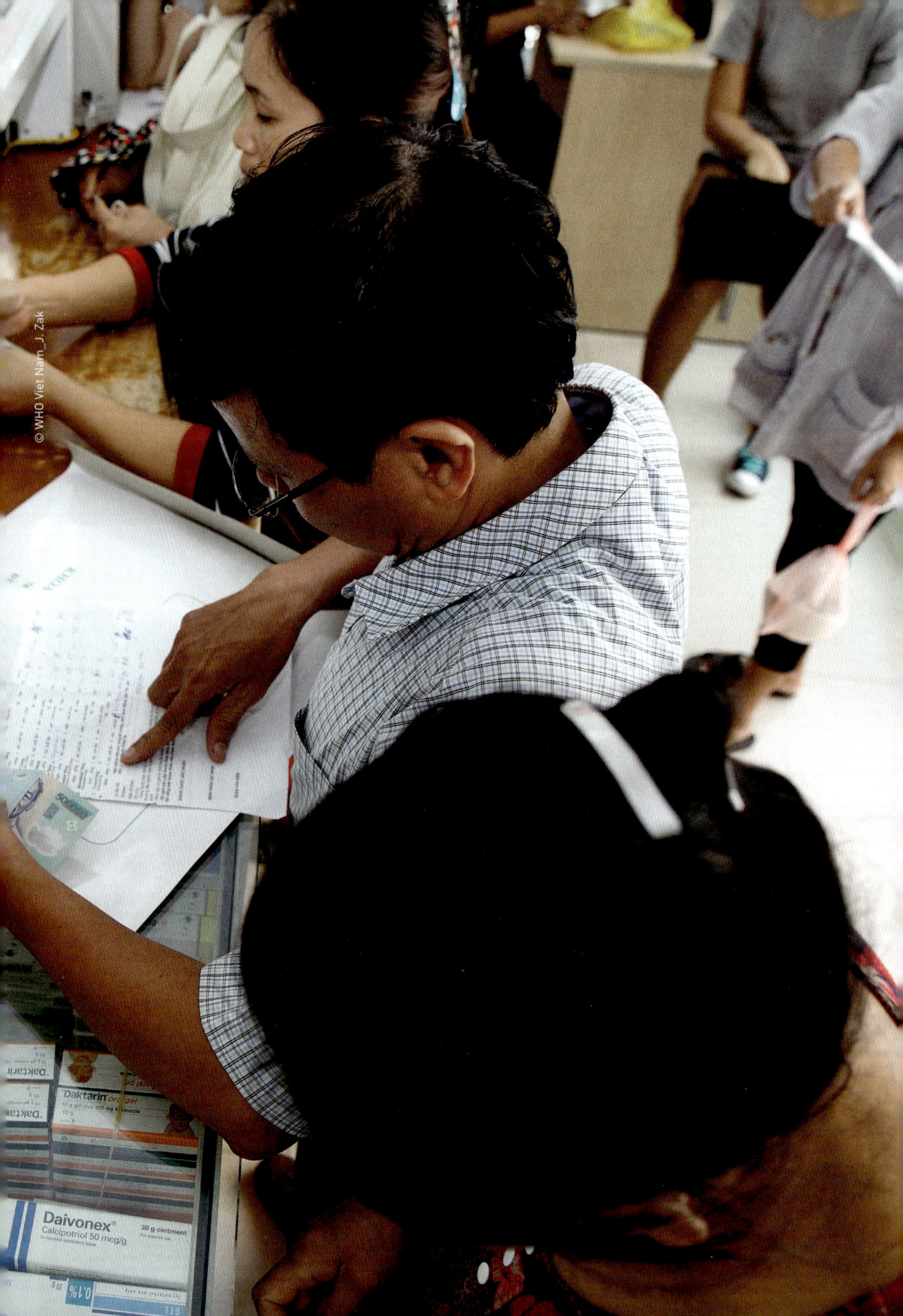
Daktarin
Daktarin oral gel
Daivonex
Calcipotriol 50 mcg/g
30 g ointment

4.2 Why do we want to prioritize?

Priority-setting is necessary, as resources are always limited. A priority-setting exercise is where the principal decisions are made, based on the results of periodic assessments of health needs and solutions.

4.2.1 Priority-setting is necessary to adapt to a changing context

Over time a population's health and its determinants change and a health sector priority-setting exercise can adequately reflect this. For instance, due to the population's increased mobility, new communicable disease threats which, in the past, may have been more geographically contained, may emerge. Or new habits and attitudes, triggered by macroeconomic changes and leading to modifications in lifestyle, may affect the health status of certain population groups (eg. the middle class in emerging economies). Changes in the country's demographic profile (larger percentage of elderly population) may explain the predominance of certain (chronic) disorders. Increased awareness or new technological solutions may cause shifts in mortality and morbidity prevalence and incidence. Fundamental changes in a country's political and or administrative system, such as decentralization, may create new opportunities for a healthier life and more effective health care.

Such trends must be monitored and changes must be detected in a timely fashion for a periodic reassessment of health needs and solutions. This is especially important in the context of public service sectors competing for insufficient government resources.

4.2.2 Priority-setting addresses challenges raised during the situation analysis

The health sector situation analysis process is where the health system's strengths, weaknesses, opportunities, and threats (SWOT) – including their root causes and effects – are analysed and debated upon amongst all relevant stakeholders. A discussion on what has worked well and less well is connected to potential solutions and recommendations to overcome health sector challenges. Thus those very suggestions, already debated upon, discussed, and sorted through by a broad stakeholder base, form the starting point for the priority-setting exercise. Priority-setting is a grand opportunity to take the recommendations and insights coming from the situation analysis work one step further to give them a specific priority level.

Priority-setting is thus a grand opportunity to take the recommendations and insights coming from the situation analysis work one step further and examine them in view of according them a specific priority level.

Box 4.1

Ambitious planning requires prioritization: the case of Sierra Leone

The Sierra Leone IHP+ Compact established a voluntary agreement in 2011 between the government of Sierra Leone and its development partners[4] to reduce inequities in health services and improve the health of vulnerable groups, especially mothers and children. Sierra Leone's National Health Sector Strategic Plan (NHSSP) 2010-2015 was developed around the same time, focusing on the following key pillars: governance and leadership, human resources for health, healthcare financing, medical products and technologies, and health information systems.[5,6] In conjunction, the Basic Package of Essential Health Services (BPEHS) was formulated by MoH with support from stakeholders to ensure a minimum package was offered at different service delivery levels. The Joint Programme of Work and Funding (JPWF) outlined activities and investment decisions by the Government and stakeholders for the 2012–2014 years of NHSSP implementation.[7] These overarching documents' aim was to keep the health sector's focus on reducing mortality rates and improving accessibility of care.[8]

While there was real goodwill to commit to the NHSSP through the IHP+ Compact, it is widely acknowledged that it failed to reach its full potential, as it was poorly implemented. A recent review of the NHSSP concluded that it was overambitious and disconnected with local needs, resulting in minimal improvements in the health sector as evidenced by key indicators. It further established that a lack of priority-setting was the underlying, common misstep made in the development of all of the above documents. The review team concluded that a more participatory process, including more district consultations and input from a broader range of civil society groups, would have easily aided the MoH to identify key health sector priorities. Instead, the NHSSP and the BPEHS were comprehensive in their scope rather than selective in their priorities. Given scarce resources, both ended up being unrealistic, and therefore, poorly implemented.[3,9]

Many of the weaknesses led to a health system which did not demonstrate the necessary resilience to contain the spread of Ebola in 2014. It has been widely documented that the Ebola-affected countries, Sierra Leone included, suffered from low-performing essential health systems functions, hampering the development of a suitable and timely response to the outbreak.[10] Inadequate numbers of qualified health workers, weak basic infrastructure, logistics, health information, surveillance, governance and drug supply systems were the underlying issues which were meant to be addressed through NHSSP implementation.

Though the NHSSP initiatives aimed at strengthening systems, in practice, partners implemented individual initiatives rather than coordinating with district health management teams; more progress could have been made by working within and through existing structures. A gap in ownership was evident in translating the NHSSP and JPWF into action; weak coordination and poor dialogue between stakeholders hindered the harmonization the documents intended to provide. The same review studied the BPEHS and analysed that, although it offered higher quality minimum services and created a more comprehensive set of guidelines for service delivery, operationalization was hindered by a lack of understanding of what the population could afford at district level.

The Sierra Leone example underlines the paramount importance of priority-setting in a situation of massive need, a sector which is struggling and insufficient resources. This illustration also demonstrates the criticality of the conditions which must be created to make it a meaningful and effective exercise: involvement of those who are on the implementing side and input from the population and/or those representing them. The Sierra Leone case also demonstrates the dire consequences of inadequate priority-setting: a weak health system which was unable to successfully face the Ebola threat.

4.2.3 Priority-setting identifies challenges expected to be prominent in the future

When priorities are explicitly set with clear criteria, they can be a subject of dialogue and debate, i.e. they can be challenged. If it can be challenged, there is a potential for improvement.

Future challenges, such as an ageing population, climate change, or increasing health inequalities, may have emerged both during population consultations and the health sector situation analysis. During the priority-setting phase, health stakeholders need to contemplate the consequences of these expected challenges and if available, interpret specific studies for the local context, or commission new ones. The process of setting priorities is the opportunity for policy-makers and health sector stakeholders to pre-empt foreseeable health problems and ensure that their negative impact on health outcomes is mitigated.

With this in mind, priority-setting goals in the health sector are:

- to relate the most important citizens' health needs and demands, as identified in the situation analysis, to the best options for addressing those needs and demands;
- to ensure that programmes and interventions are evidence-based, cost-effective and fairly distributed, addressing health needs of all population groups, particulary the poorest segments of society;
- to inform national strategies and resource allocation of the public purse;
- to provide key reference information and evidence for policy-making, and monitoring and evaluation.

4.2.4 Implicit priority-setting happens if it is not consciously made explicit

A national health planning process always includes priorities. If this is not explicitly done, with a transparent discussion on priority-setting criteria and a joint examination of the evidence, then it will be done in an ad hoc, implicit way. The latter does not encourage accountability, is not transparent and is prone to influences and special interests that may or may not be in the best interest of population health. When priorities are explicitly set with clear criteria, they can be a subject of dialogue and debate, i.e. they can be challenged. If a priority can be challenged, there is a potential for improvement. A recent article by Chalkidou et al.[11] summarizes this as:

"In an explicit process it is clear who made which decisions, the criteria used, whether the criteria used were met, what evidence was considered and whether the evidence was adequately assessed, whether appropriate values were employed, who was consulted, whether those giving advice had significant conflicts of interest and how the various trade-offs were made."

4.3 When should we conduct a priority-setting exercise?

Where does priority-setting start in the planning cycle and where does it end? In principle, priority-setting happens on a continuous basis in some shape or form throughout the policy & planning cycle. Some find that the priority-setting phase is only concerned with the preliminary steps of identifying the most important needs and opportunities, while others include the weighing of resource limitations. Some also include the decision-making process on resource allocation in priority-setting.

Once the health needs/problems and their causes have been identified in the preceding situation analysis phase, the priority-setting should then focus on ranking those identified needs and options, on the basis of a set of criteria, approaches and methods/tools (many of which are described in this chapter). In the planning phases that then follow, decisions will be taken on sequencing priority interventions and on budgeting.

4.3.1 Periodicity and scope of priority-setting

Priority-setting may be done:

- at varying intervals (annually, mid-term, etc.) and for any given timeframe (short-term, medium-term, long-term, or other);
- at any level of the system (national, province/ region, district, or other);
- on varying themes and system components (hospital reform, post-Ebola health system recovery, etc.);
- with any group of actors (authorities, service providers, private sector, communities, etc.).

This chapter focuses particularly on comprehensive, medium-term, health sector priority-setting. Approaching priority-setting from a whole-of-sector perspective is a complex undertaking, encompassing all its levels, types of care, actors, implementation modalities and funding flows. This approach may be at odds with the modus operandi in settings where programmes and projects are vertical in nature since their management timelines may not be in sync with the national governmental planning cycle. Here, there is a risk that the scope of priority-setting for these programmes is limited to the (vertical) programme objectives. In such situations, more integration and alignment with the overall sector planning cycle should be sought and vertical programme priorities should be examined in view of overall sector priorities.

Priority-setting should be a participatory and inclusive process, as part of the health policy and planning cycle. This process itself is transparent and understood by all.

Priority-setting often provides a key milestone for strategic planning. Strategic options are weighed in the priority-setting process. Decisions taken based on criteria such as burden, cost-effectiveness, affordability and fairness will shape the strategic plan, given the resources available for the health sector. Much of the priority-setting process will build on the situation analysis and population consultation phases, closely examining the evidence generated as well as analysed in those processes.

The situation analysis can be seen as the starting point of the priority-setting process.

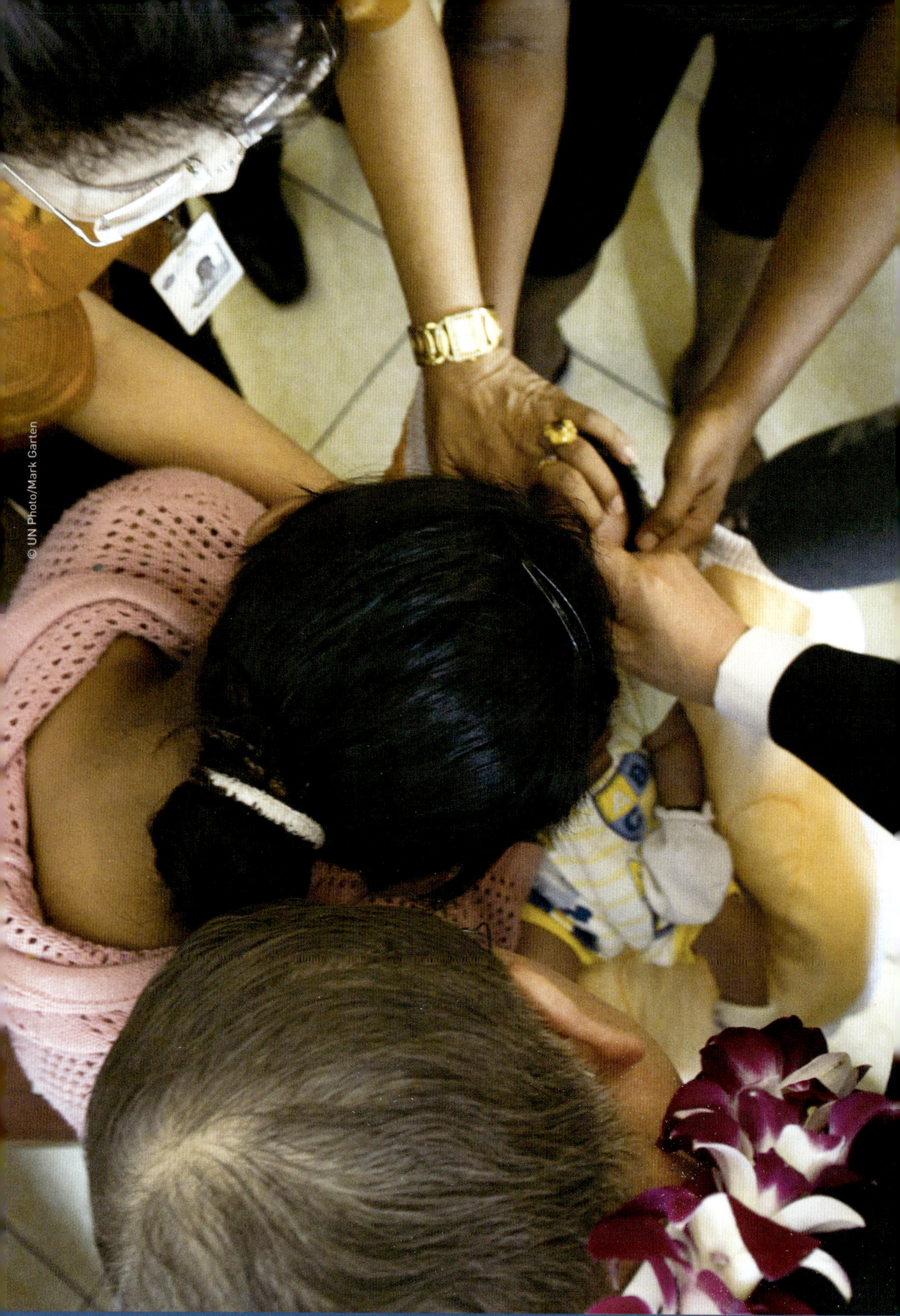

© UN Photo/Mark Garten

Later, the strategic medium-term choices will be translated into annual plans. Priority-setting will also be necessary for guiding this operational planning. It will contribute to budget recommendations on resource allocation for phased implementation of the medium-term strategic directions. This chapter deals with medium-term priorities, while priority-setting to guide operational planning (annual implementation plans and budgets) will be covered in another chapter.[IV]

Priority-setting may or typically come after the situation analysis and before the decision-making and policy debates on key strategic directions for the health sector. Budgeting then follows, after which NHPSP implementation takes place and results are monitored and evaluated.

A comprehensive situation analysis takes an in-depth look at factors that explain success and failure in past implementation. It is retrospective. It can be organized as a mid-term or final health sector review in the case of a medium-term strategic plan. Such a review results in a set of key recommendations (usually for each health system building block[12] and for thematic areas) and sometimes certain priorities are already identified. So the situation analysis can be seen as the starting point of the priority-setting process.

4.3.2 Priority-setting as part of comprehensive health sector development

To ensure adequate priority-setting for the development of national health policies, strategies and plans, it should be assumed that:

- the situation analysis has taken into consideration population needs and demand – through a citizen consultation, by analysing secondary data on patient satisfaction, and by including community leaders meaningfully into the situation analysis process, etc.;
- there is a realistic forecast of the resources likely to become available for the period to be planned;
- criteria and formulae are likely to inform resource allocation;
- budgets will be based on a costing exercise, which in turn is based on an adopted methodology;
- plans and budgets are based on adopted implementation modalities (e.g. horizontal, vertical, decentralized).

A clear distinction is made here between priority-setting and the final decision-making. The priority-setting phase formulates the recommendations for priority areas/interventions/levels, etc., taking into consideration cost implications and assuring fairness, but without going as far as making actual decisions.

IV Please see Chapter 6 "Operational planning: transforming plans into action" in this handbook.

4.4 Who should be involved in priority-setting?

Which actors should be involved in the priority-setting process needs to be considered carefully. An inclusive approach is where different stakeholder groups of various levels are consulted and where the expectations of the population are heard.

Priority-setting rests on judgements informed by evidence, and those responsible for making those judgements need to be held accountable for their decisions. So if priority-setting is to have legitimacy, citizens are to make the final choice through their parliaments.[13]

Some actors have a natural position of participation in the process:

- policy-makers and health planners: MoH, other ministries (such as ministry of finance, ministry of planning);
- administrative and health authorities at decentralized levels;
- health professionals (public and non-public sectors);
- community representatives and/or groups of patients.

Brinkerhoff and Bossert's[14] (see Fig. 4.3) three categories of population groups who have a stake in health governance can be used as a lens to better understand the roles of those stakeholders who have a natural position of participation in the priority-setting process.

Fig. 4.3 Three dimensions to consider when moving towards UHC

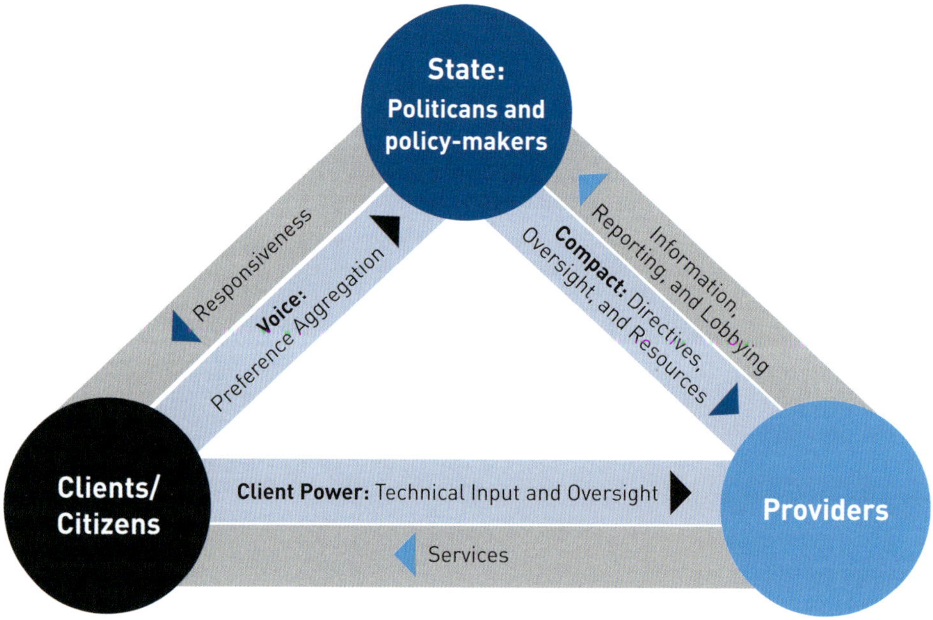

4.4.1 Clients/citizens

Citizens are the final decision-makers on priorities through their parliaments; they thus need to be involved at each step of a priority-setting exercise (see Boxes 4.2 and 4.3).[15] The priorities which are set should ultimately be owned by citizens as part of the democratic process.

Public accountability is one of the principal aims of consulting citizens on their views and needs. As much as possible, the population is to be well informed beforehand about the advantages and disadvantages of various options, and when the methodology is extensive and intensive. The need for and feasibility of an in-depth, large-scale consultation will depend on the national context.[16] Context may also determine to what extent the country chooses a consultation of the population at large or a less complex consultation via appointed population representatives. For this second option, it is assumed that population representation is based on transparent and democratic means.

Consensus-based expert opinion approaches are by definition less inclusive than a large direct citizen consultation because participants are selected based on expertise. However, they are relatively easy to organize and results can be obtained quickly. The main caveat is that external experts may not necessarily be aware of important local developments.[17]

4.4.2 The state: politicians and policy-makers

National leadership (the state: politicians and policy-makers), in particular the MoH, needs to navigate the political complexities of working within and across stakeholders and organizations (both clients/citizens as well as providers) with differing incentives systems and cultures. The role of the MoH is to plan, initiate, coordinate and oversee the priority-setting process, where relevant through health sector coordination mechanisms.

The role of the MoH is to plan, initiate, coordinate and oversee the priority-setting process, where relevant through health sector coordination mechanisms.

The ministry may seek the assistance of independent technical experts for developing and preparing the methodology and tools, as well as for facilitating the process, but the overall coordination and final decision-making is likely to remain with the government side. Policy-makers must thus lead the process, ensure broad and meaningful stakeholder participation, ensure that the priorities that are set reflect stakeholder input in a balanced way, and be held accountable for the results.

In a decentralized environment, the policy-makers are the local government. They must collaborate with service providers (Brinkerhoff and Bossert's "providers"), civil society and the community (clients/citizens) for their insights and input. The process must be transparent, with clear roles and responsibilities, especially when it comes to evaluating and discussing evidence from different angles and viewpoints.

In countries that rely heavily on external funding, the active participation of development partners in the priority-setting process is necessary. In a process lead by the government, it improves their understanding of national considerations, enhances alignment with national priorities and sensitizes for integrated aid contributions.

Box 4.2

Balancing patients' demands with medical needs and cost-effectiveness[18]

A Swedish study in 2012 questioned nurses, general practitioners, and patients on their views on priority health problems in primary health care. The study found that for nurses and general practitioners, the severity of the health condition was the most important priority-setting criterion. Specifically for general practitioners, cost-effectiveness was an additional key criterion. Patients, on the other hand, assigned a relatively higher priority to acute/minor conditions in routine primary care also compared to preventive check-ups for chronic conditions. It was concluded that the challenge for primary care providers is to balance the patients' demands with medical needs and cost-effectiveness. Transparency in applying criteria might contribute to a greater consensus between general practitioners and nurses.

Providers and the population can have differing views regarding health sector priorities – the priority-setting process provides an essential platform for making these different views explicit and discussing them in a spirit of finding a common solution.

4.4.3 Providers

Service providers are the front-line organizations who are at the heart of implementing the priority actions that have been decided upon. Their experience of the health sector comes from the inside, is practical, and offers insights on feasibility. Their input into the priority-setting process is therefore crucial – they essentially translate policy-makers' resolutions into services for citizens.

As the Swedish example demonstrates (Box 4.2), providers and the population can have differing views regarding health sector priorities – the priority-setting process provides an essential platform for making these different views explicit and discussing them in a spirit of finding a common solution. Addressing these differences early on, before the NHPSP is implemented, precludes potential problems and bottlenecks later on during NHPSP implementation.

Box 4.3

More public engagement for health sector decision-making: a meta-study from low- and middle-income countries[19]

Citizen consultations aim to actively engage health system end users in priority-setting. A 2013 meta-study looked at different forms and current trends of such consultations in low- and middle-income countries.

In Uganda, nominated community members were recommended to represent the public on technical committees in health sector decision-making. In Kenya, local health workers developed an annual list of priority activities and targets, informed by the local community. In Indonesia, an annual, bottom-up participatory budgeting process was created specifically to replace Indonesia's former centralized system. In India, the National Rural Health Mission advocates increased stakeholder and public engagement in priority-setting at the village, sub-center, block, district, and state levels. And a recent ordinance in the Philippines requires bottom-up planning for poverty alleviation to incorporate community and grassroots organizations' perspectives at the local government unit level.

The meta-analysis found that affordable, appropriate and effective engagement of the public remains elusive, despite many good initiatives and promising starts. To remedy this situation, it is suggested that, rather than mandating public participation, countries and donors should focus on building a policy environment that is conducive to grassroots initiatives and public involvement in decision-making processes. In addition, a stronger evidence base must be created at local level for what works and what works less well, using small pilot studies.

4.4.4 The media supports all three stakeholder groups

The media can be seen as straddling between the three stakeholder groups, as they bring information to and provide a medium to represent all three groups. The media plays an important role in informing and sensitizing the population about the importance of priority-setting, priority health needs and the consultation process. Media can also function as a forum for public debate on these issues, and act as a key partner in follow-up feedback. Here, the policy-maker and other stakeholders must make a conscious effort to communicate more simply, with less technical jargon, with the media, as well as through the media to the populace. Producing targeted documentation on priority-setting analyses in easy to understand language for the public can be a powerful tool in making choices more transparent.

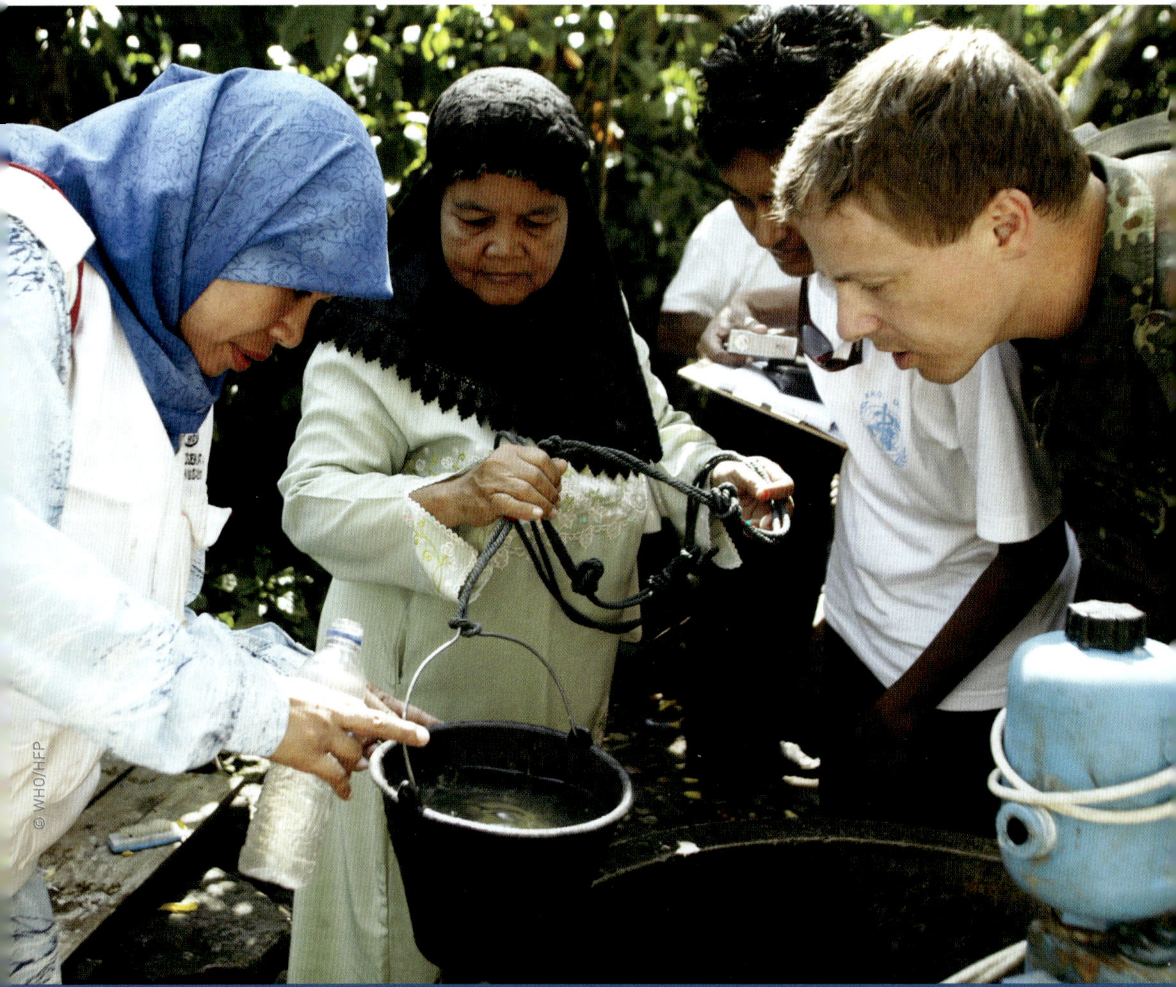

4.5 How should we do priority-setting?

Priority-setting is a trade-off: attributing more attention and resources to a given intervention means to a large extent that less can be done in other areas. That being said, the actual trade-off must be preceded by understanding the health sector challenges (situation analysis), examining possible solutions to overcome the challenges, and then defining the priority-setting criteria explicitly. In this section, five criteria are recommended which underpin the approaches, methods and tools used to set priorities.

Since health status is to a large extent determined by other factors such as cultural, socioeconomic and environmental, it is critical to go beyond the strict remit of the MoH and to consider other sectors when prioritizing solutions for a health problem. Although this might seem obvious, there are few countries which manage to systematically bring intersectoral thinking and action into national health planning processes.[V] An example priority area of focus could be waste management as a solution for lowering the incidence of diarrhoeal diseases – this would imply that the ministry of environment would take the lead, but with key input (and potentially funds) from the MoH. The point here is that some priority options for the health sector may be carried out principally by other sectors and this should be kept in mind.

In the priority-setting process it will usually be possible to identify "quick wins" and "low-hanging fruit" to guide the strategic planning. Some changes to the current set of health sector activities can be relatively easy to achieve and can be addressed first, because they are politically feasible, affordable and technically possible.

4.5.1 Criteria for priority-setting

Five key criteria for setting priorities in the health sector are suggested here, without any pretense that this list is comprehensive; in the end, the choice of and weight given to the criteria themselves will be a product of debate and deliberation by society, stakeholders and policy-makers. They are:

- burden of the health issue;
- effectiveness of the intervention;
- cost of the intervention;
- acceptability of the intervention;
- fairness.

A country may decide to choose different, or additional, criteria according to local needs and norms. The relative weight attributed to each of these criteria may vary as a range of factors influence them. Trade-offs between the various criteria, and the weight of each of them, will be a political decision. Several methods and tools have been developed for measuring and analysing these criteria as far as possible; some are concerned with only one of the five criteria (e.g. health needs assessment), while others combine two criteria (e.g. a method for measuring cost-effectiveness, burden of disease, or several criteria (e.g. health technology assessment)).

Almost all priority-setting is a trade-off: attributing more attention and resources to a given intervention means to a large extent that less can be done in other areas.

(a) Burden of the health issue[20,21]

The burden of the health issue can be viewed from different perspectives. From the MoH or service provider point of view, the ***magnitude severity*** and ***urgency*** of the matter are most pertinent. From the population perspective, it is the ***perception*** of the health burden that is

V For more information, please see Chapter 12 "Intersectoral planning for health and health equity" in this handbook.

most germane. These aspects are not mutually exclusive; for example, a high burden of disease can increase the magnitude of the problem, but can also (but not necessarily) increase the perception of the burden.

From the MoH or health provider perspective, the burden of a health issue can be established by analysing epidemiological trends and data such as prevalence, incidence, and survival rate. For example, in many low- and middle-income countries, the epidemiological profile is rapidly changing, with a growing burden of disease caused by non-infectious, degenerative diseases that are linked to changes in lifestyle and environmental factors. Such a situation (increasing burden of non-communicable diseases (NCDS)) may ask for a review of priorities whereby more focus is given to preventing and treating NCDs. This may result in priority recommendations leading to adjustment of services provided at facility level, etc.

The "burden of disease" is a quantitative, time-based measure combining years of life lost due to premature mortality and years of life lost due to time lived in states of less than full health. The cost of the disease burden permits an understanding that some health issues, if left unresolved, will have more of a cost impact than others on the health system as well as on the society. So the cost of the disease burden itself can influence how it is prioritized.

The ***magnitude*** of a health problem may be indicated, for example, by the proportion of the population at risk or affected in terms of mortality and morbidity. This also means identifying patient subgroups for which treatments have differential benefits and establishing whether or not interventions are effective in all healthcare settings and subpopulations. Projections and trends are essential in ranking health threats, despite the uncertainty of such a judgement. For instance, many countries experience a rapid increase in migrating populations from rural to urban settings. This phenomenon is likely to cause important shifts in the distribution of health risks and health care needs, which may subsequently need prioritizing. Another example of how the magnitude of a health problem can influence priority-setting decisions is sickle-cell disease[VI] in tropical regions and parts of Africa where there are pockets of up to 25% population prevalence of sickle-cell disease gene carriers. In this setting, the magnitude of sickle-cell disease will likely be a deciding factor for allocation of money and resources to programmes to prevent symptomatic sickle-cell disease as well as for disease management. Prioritization of the identified target population (sickle-cell disease gene carriers) with preventive measures and early intervention are likely to have a considerable impact on the burden of this disease.[22]

Severity can be determined by the effects of the health threat: acute or chronic, disabling effects, mortality, measured in quality-adjusted life-years (QALYs) and disability-adjusted life-years (DALYs).

VI Sickle-cell disease is a haemoglobin disorder that affects how oxygen is carried in the body. In this blood disease, misshapen cells lack plasticity and can block small blood vessels, impairing blood flow. The condition leads to shortened red blood cell survival, and subsequent anaemia, often called sickle-cell anaemia. Poor blood oxygen levels and blood vessel blockages in people with sickle-cell disease can lead to chronic acute pain syndromes, severe bacterial infections, and necrosis (tissue death).

Box 4.4

The burden of disease: obstetric fistulas and living in a state of less than full health

Obstetric fistulas remain a major maternal health issue, especially in resource-poor regions, such as some sub-Saharan African and South-East Asian countries, where maternal mortality rates are high and access to emergency obstetric care is limited.[23] The majority of obstetric fistulas result from cases of obstructed labour, one of the top five causes of maternal death and an issue linked closely with young not fully formed girls experiencing pregnancy, the developmental effects of malnutrition, delay in seeking care and poor accessibility to health services.[24] Most women living with the disorder experience urinary or fecal incontinence due to fluid leaking into the vaginal canal through a hole resulting from complications in delivery. The result is not only physical discomfort and constant attempts to mitigate the issue — coping strategies include wearing protective cloths to absorb leaking fluid, linked to an ongoing preoccupation with managing and cleaning the cloth, or applying scented perfumes to mask the smell, both strategies that rarely make a difference—but also shame over ensuing smells, physical isolation from families and communities, and potential divorce or abandonment which further isolates affected women.[25]

Women living with an obstetric fistula can be considered a "state of less than full health" in which their capacities are not necessarily completely debilitated because of the health problem yet they still experience a life of less care, equality, opportunity, and treatment compared to unaffected counterparts. There are vivid descriptions of coping with the disorder that illustrate living in a state of less than full health.

- "In this condition producing odours is inevitable... No perfume is capable of covering up these odours. I give off a bad smell."
- "The sores bother me terribly; I feel as though I am in prison all the time."
- "My life is ruined; I have become like a crazy woman who must live alone cut off from the world. I live far from my parents, my village, and my husband, in order to escape the noise (insults and questions) of others and to look for a cure."

Such recollections exhibit not only the physical consequences of the disorder but the social and cultural ramifications of fistulas. Almost 90% of obstetric fistula cases can be cured by a simple vaginal repair surgery, but transportation limitations because of the disorder, poor accessibility to care, and lack of financial resources can impede on seeking treatment.[26]

According a priority to obstetric fistula treatment and prevention at a national level may be necessary in some settings to minimize the damaging long-term effects of such a condition. The criteria underlying such a decision could be importance (responsiveness – it responds to a demand from a specific population group), effectiveness (vaginal repair surgery is relative simple and effective), and fairness (a vulnerable group in society – women – are suffering and being marginalized due to this health problem).

The *urgency* of a problem may also be a reason for declaring it a priority. The justification would in that case be, for example, the threat of an epidemic outbreak (rate of spread, infectiousness). The recent Ebola epidemic required urgent priority interventions, not only in the three most affected countries (Guinea, Liberia and Sierra Leone), but also at a global scale. Containment of the outbreak in a region with poorly-functioning health and communication systems and porous national borders required large-scale emergency measures and health system recovery investments.

Perception looks at the burden of the health problem from the patient and population perspective, giving more weight to the demand side of the health system in the priority-setting process. Essentially, this criterion seeks to answer the question "what are the most pressing health problems from the citizens' perspective?" (see Box 4.4). People's sense and implicit knowledge are accorded attention here, such that health sector stakeholders, in applying this criterion, examine the demand and preferences of the public.[VII]

(b) Effectiveness of the intervention[27,28]

This criterion considers how well, clinically or practically, the health issue can be solved, not only in terms of output, but also in outcome and impact. In other words: what is the likelihood that the selected strategy or priority will lead to expected results? What are the risks of the identified problem in terms of available technological and organizational solutions? What are feasibility considerations under the given conditions? Other terms often used in this context are: applicability, deliverability, sustainability. What are trends and developments? Examples include emerging technologies, human resource specialization and skill-mix issues.[29]

When determining effectiveness, the "innovation" factor needs to be taken into account: has the strategy or intervention not yet been researched and tested (evidence-based), or is there an existing knowledge base that has already established effectiveness? One must keep in mind that a new solution may have proven technological effectiveness at a global level, but its effectiveness at country level needs to be assessed as well. For instance, is telemedicine adapted to the local context? Can telemedicine be made operational within the planned period? The same applies for organizational effectiveness. Example: Is decentralized governance sufficiently robust in terms of skills, systems and practices for introducing performance-based financing? What are potential limitations and barriers in implementing healthcare strategies? This means assessing the major forces shaping the service, including technological developments, manpower trends and health policy.

VII See Chapter 2 "Population consultation on needs and expectations" in this handbook.

When the effectiveness of certain solutions is to be analysed, it is useful to distinguish between two types of situations.

(i) The evidence base has not yet been established at the global level and will have to be created through scientifically-sound testing.
(ii) The evidence base exists at global or international level, but the applicability and (cost) effectiveness needs to be verified for the local context. Eventually, the solution/intervention may need to be adapted. Also other issues of effectiveness, indirectly related to the problem, may need to be determined, such as communication capacity and geographical accessibility. For example, while the effectiveness of schistosomiasis prevention through pest control by the application of pesticides has been established at the global level, the effectiveness of this solution needs to be verified for each environment. Also the "strategic fit" for the proposed priority solution has to be verified. For instance, while the arguments for a progressive privatization of a certain type of hospital may be convincing, it will still be necessary to verify that this option is in line with other sector strategies. Questions which need to be answered include: do consequences of an ongoing administrative decentralization have to be taken into account? Are the existing price policies for service delivery in line with such a move? Establishing the evidence base at country level may require a study, pilot project or expert appraisal. Ultimately, the decision is often based on the judgement of a mixed group, composed by experts and non-experts alike, including those who are knowledgeable of and closely linked to the policy process.

The potential of new, innovative solutions must be weighed against the effectiveness of current interventions. Hence, an evaluation of the latter is necessary. In certain cases, an in-depth health technology assessment may be necessary.

The effectiveness and applicability of a solution is also determined by the acceptability of the intervention by the target population. Moreover, the availability of resources to execute the intervention will have to be evaluated. This will allow decision-makers to prioritize health issues that have evidence-based, viable and efficient solutions.

The effectiveness criterion considers how well, clinically or practically, the health issue can be solved, not only in terms of output, but also in outcome and impact.

(c) Cost of the intervention[30,31,32]

This criterion is about cost in the sense of affordability (How much does the NHPSP cost? Is it affordable?) as well as efficiency (a value-for-money assessment, which should cover both cost minimization and cost-effectiveness). Both the affordability and efficiency of the solution to address a health problem need to be carefully considered. In other words, this criterion encompasses the issue of whether the health intervention is affordable in absolute terms as well as the relative cost to the health sector, to the community and to individuals for tackling the health problem. The cost of the intervention must be economically feasible and economically sustainable.

The cost criterion is about cost in the sense of affordability (How much does the NHPSP cost? Is it affordable?) as well as efficiency (a value-for-money assessment, which should cover both cost minimization and cost-effectiveness).

An example is the proposal to establish a national health insurance. While for the health sector this may seem an obvious solution for solving the problem of catastrophic health expenditure, the feasibility and sustainability of a comprehensive insurance scheme will to a large extent depend on political commitment and the country's macroeconomic perspective.

Just as for the criteria burden and effectiveness, the quality of the cost analysis depends on the quality of the data and information available. Here, we not only mean cost-related data but also information on planned implementation insofar as it has cost implications. For instance, the strength of support systems in the health sector need to be taken into consideration, as it has implications on the cost of a health intervention, in addition to more classical clinical dimensions.

(d) Acceptability of the intervention

The acceptability of a priority health intervention refers to whether a community or target population accepts the chosen health intervention that addresses a priority problem.[33] It also refers to the willingness by those who will be carrying out the intervention to do so – for example, health service providers, MoH, and subnational health authorities. Acceptability can be further declined as social acceptability or cultural acceptability; to address this criterion, context-specific priority-setting is required.[34] Acceptability is strongly related to the applicability or feasibility of providing a certain intervention in a local setting.[35] On the service provider side, risk aversion and resistance to change can effectively hinder any policy or intervention – reasons cited are often a reduction of revenues or an increased workload. From the government side, a new priority may create resistance from civil servants and administrators if it represents an additional workload with perceived little added value. It is therefore all the more essential to ensure solid policy dialogue with all stakeholder groups from the outset to raise, discuss and clarify concerns.

Acceptability can be further declined as social acceptability or cultural acceptability.

If a priority health intervention naturally goes against social and cultural norms, it has a low chance of success, unless specific interventions addressing the issue of social or cultural acceptance are undertaken. Priority-setting thus requires evidence on the nuances of social and cultural acceptability, and underlying factors which may affect the success or failure of the health intervention.[36] In the national health planning process, community perceptions of acceptability need to be considered at every stage, and especially so during the priority-setting stage.[37] A district health management team member from Kenya explains exemplarily:[38]

"We also look at specific health problems in a given area. For example, if there is a lack of pit latrines in a specific area due to cultural beliefs that a daughter and a father cannot share the same toilet, we design programmes together with the people to ensure that the programmes are relevant and acceptable to them. So we rely on data and reports from the people."

Another eye-opening example of the influence of cultural and societal factors on the success or failure of priority health interventions is female genital mutilation (FGM) and interventions aimed at reducing or eliminating the practice. FGM, the act of partial or total removal of a female's external genitalia, is a deeply rooted societal, cultural, and religious tradition. In order for FGM to be successfully eliminated, communities themselves must decide to abandon it and adopt behavioural change.[39] Health education programmes must be sensitive to cultural and religious concerns of the community or run the risk that information will be taken as offensive and more deeply entrench the practice that workers are trying to dismiss. For instance, a health programme that immediately lists the reasons why FGM has no health benefits in a community that has religious leaders supporting it as an act of faith may view the health programme as a threat to their religion. The most successful interventions are those that are participatory, allowing communities to create their own solutions and involving many families in the community so that collective change is made. No matter what intervention is used, programmes that maintain a mindset of cultural and social awareness will be more successful for long-term elimination efforts of FGM.

(e) Fairness[40,41]

The notion of fairness is defined by the quality of treating people equally or in a way that is right or reasonable.[42] Put in other words, it is "the state, condition, or quality of being free from bias or injustice". It is based on principles such as equality and equity. Fairness must be brought into a priority-setting discussion, as it is closely linked to the judgment and trade-off on the importance of a health need and the effectiveness of an intervention. It also influences the decision regarding how much weight to give to the cost of its solution. For instance, a health problem may mainly affect people with an income level that is too low to assure healthy living conditions and financial access to health care. A health problem may also be particularly prevalent amongst populations living in a hazardous environment. In other circumstances, a particular segment of the population may be at risk because of their unhealthy lifestyle (dietary habits, drug abuse, etc.). In all of these cases, the fairness criteria might lead to a decision to give priority to the health problems of these population subgroups, even though their health need represents a minority of the population, and even though the treatment of this health problem is not the most cost-effective (see Box 4.5).

Fairness is based on principles such as equality and equity. Fairness must be brought into a priority-setting discussion, as it is closely linked to the judgment and trade-off on the importance of a health need and the effectiveness of an intervention. It also influences the decision regarding how much weight to give to the cost of its solution.

Another subjective element linked to fairness which has risen in prominence recently is the "rule of rescue" (RoR) concept, especially when examining the cost effectiveness evidence for intervening early in life. The RoR is a commonly and strictly felt duty to "rescue the doomed", i.e. those with a life-threatening condition. The imperative to rescue is, undoubtedly, of great moral significance, making RoR a predominantly ethical issue linked to the sentiment that those who are "doomed" need special attention and must be "rescued" on grounds of fairness. RoR in health care is commonly invoked as a constraint on cost benefit evaluation, but quite often it may prove the opposite: for example, rescuing patients from a fatal disease prevents patients' premature death. Restoring them to good or full health will "produce" a large number of QALYs.[48]

The RoR concept highlights the ethical dilemma between the two principles "sickest-first" and "maximizing aggregate benefit" (cost benefit). Examples of RoR-principled therapies are renal dialysis and second-chance transplants. Examples of interventions that receive lower priority according to the RoR logic are prevention programmes such as diagnostic screenings.

Box 4.5

The fairness criteria applied to priority-setting: health investments to the marginalized and vulnerable Australian indigenous population

Discernment of what is considered "fair" in priority-setting is sometimes a challenge to perceive. It is a value judgment that a government and society makes collectively. In Australia, it was recently decided to focus public health efforts and resources on the indigenous populations, for objective reasons such as their poorer health status, but also for reasons of fairness (based on principles of equality and equity) linked to decades of having less opportunities and being marginalized.

Indigenous people make up approximately 2.5% of the entire Australian population (with 90% of that group identifying as Aboriginal), in other terms over 710,000 individuals, one third of them under the age of 15.[43] Obvious health disparities exist between indigenous and non-indigenous populations.[44] 13% of indigenous people report some form of cardiovascular disease, 33% are affected by respiratory disease, and communicable diseases are more prevalent in indigenous groups than non-indigenous groups. Smoking rates are twice as high for indigenous people than for non-indigenous people.[32] Furthermore, a large number of indigenous groups have poor accessibility to health services, and are often not treated with welcome and quality care in centres even when they do have access.[33,32]

Through the national health planning process, the Australian government decided to establish a separate fund for indigenous healthcare in efforts to close the gap and ensure equity, thus clearly giving indigenous health an unequivocal priority. The health sector spends 18% more per capita for indigenous than for non-indigenous people, accounting for 3% of the national expenditure on health, and the funding levels for indigenous health continue to grow.[45,46] From 2014–2018 the Australian government plans to spend $A 3.1 billion on indigenous-specific health care and programmes, a 16% increase from the 2009–2013 expenditure.[47] As part of the Indigenous Australians' Health Programme, an updated funding allocation methodology was established to assure investments were directed to the areas of most need, focusing on four different areas: primary health care, child and maternal health, chronic diseases, and a stronger future in health.

4.5.2 Contextual factors

Priority-setting will depend on a number of contextual factors, including political processes and influences, at both national and international levels.

(a) A comprehensive whole-of-government approach

When strategizing for health, including when priority-setting, a sector-wide comprehensive approach has many advantages. First of all, it assures comprehensive and integrated planning for the whole health sector. This means that priority-setting is done for all sector aspects, levels and interventions together. In this way, comparative importance and opportunities are taken into account. Secondly, various stakeholder groups are involved in the priority-setting. This ensures that those who are directly concerned (programme and facility managers, supporting organizations and health system users) contribute in the selection of priorities. Thirdly, a comprehensive sector-wide approach reinforces national (MoH) leadership which, in the context of a priority-setting exercise, enhances country ownership of the priority-setting results. In short, priority-setting in a comprehensive sector-wide approach can lead to improved effectiveness, efficiency, broad commitment and acceptability, and therefore sustainability.

Many countries have stated their adherence to the principles of a comprehensive planning approach and of the Paris Declaration. Many also signed the IHP+ Global Compact and have developed a national Compact.[49] Still, even if concrete commitments in a country's health policy and strategic framework reflect adherence, this does not guarantee that the scope, approach and methodology of medium-term priority-setting for the health sector will be genuinely sector-wide and based on broad stakeholder inclusiveness. For this to become reality, effective stakeholder consultation and coordination mechanisms must be in place with clear principles and procedures for joint decision-making. Secondly, comprehensive sector information, analysed and synthesized, must be shared. This demands clear and strong MoH communication. Last but not least, strong national leadership is required to lead the priority-setting, with MoH proactively managing the process. Here, challenges may include avoiding a politicized environment in priority-setting and withstanding undue pressure from powerful and potentially generous external partners.

(b) Politics and political climate at national level

Priority-setting is inherently a political process. The need to invest in getting all relevant stakeholders on board and ensuring political buy-in cannot be emphasized enough. In addition, the general political climate and political party programmes are an important underlying aspect which needs to be taken into consideration.

The time and resources necessary to invest in getting all relevant stakeholders on board and ensuring political buy-in cannot be emphasized enough.

In the end, citizens, through their governments will determine which health issues are addressed in policy and the allocation of resources within the health system. Political opportunities such as elections or a change in government can greatly impact the nature and methods used on setting priorities within the health sector. Also, the influence of various types of lobbies (including pharmaceuticals, donors, and civil society) is not to be underestimated. In countries where national level governance has been weakened due to political turmoil, special care must be taken to ensure that the population's health

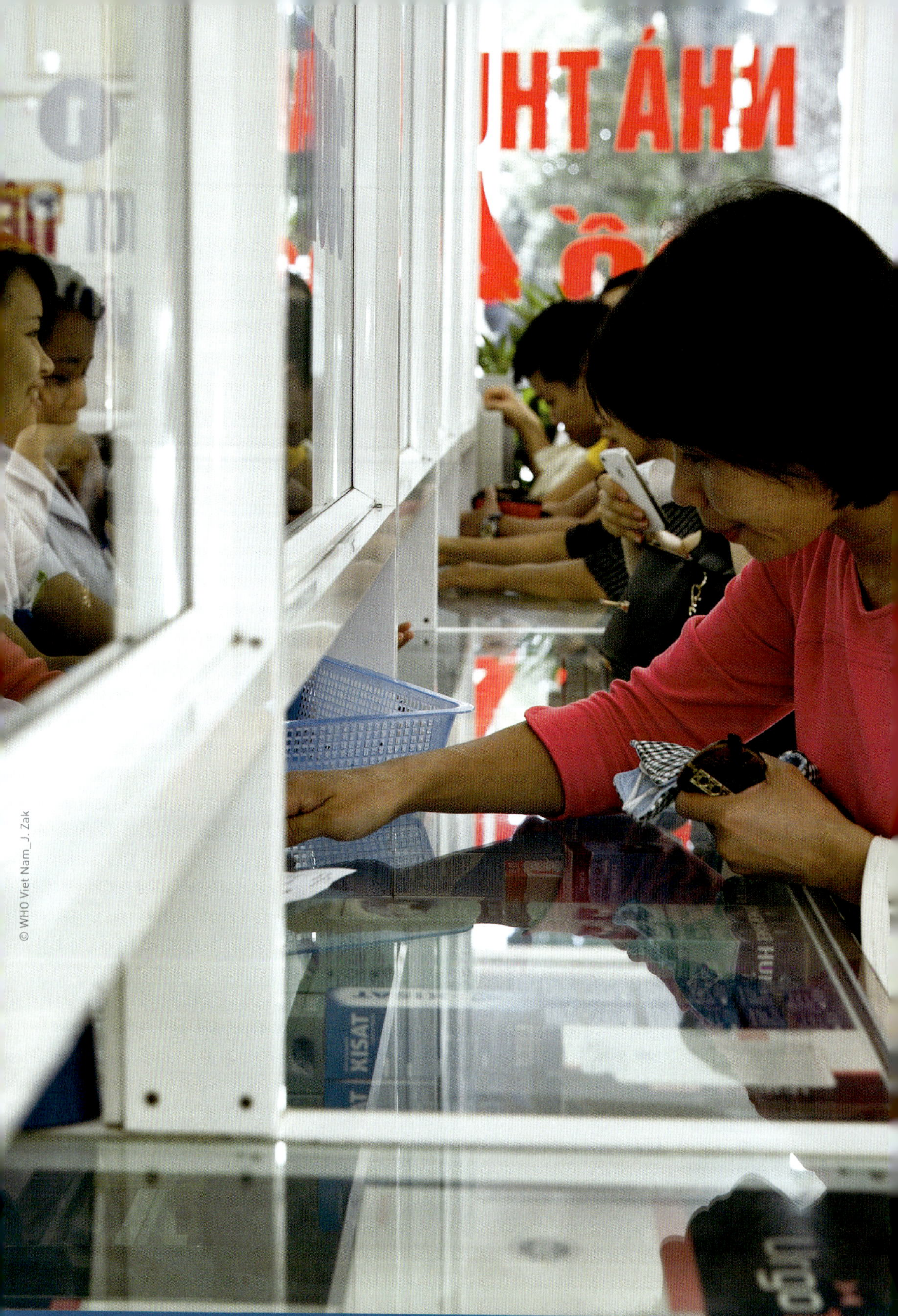

© WHO Viet Nam_J. Zak

remains the strong focus. Even though politics will certainly be omnipresent in priority-setting, health sector stakeholders should ensure that evidence and hard facts are at the centre of the political debate.

(c) International policy relevance

Issues of international policy relevance – whether as a debate, an agenda or a firm national commitment – need to be considered. For example, environmental protection is a key theme in the global debate. The consequences of air/water/soil pollution and of climate change include threats for the health of the concerned populations. Ideally, this would mean that an environmental goal such as the reduction of carbon monoxide levels should also be reflected in priority-setting for health. Similarly, international commitments with regard to the protection of human rights could be reflected in the explicit protection of marginalized groups against discrimination and further marginalization with regard to the accessibility of health care. Regional disturbances and warfare may lead to a sudden massive migration/exodus which would unexpectedly affect health care in neighbouring countries. Another aspect that needs to be taken into account is the pressure of industrial and trade policies on global health policy-making.

4.5.3 Approaches, methods and tools

The literature describes a variety of approaches and hybrids of approaches and models, all of which assist in technical analyses (see Fig. 4.4). That being said, values will underpin the technical approaches and value judgments are never absent from the interpretation of evidence. The technical element of any approach attempts to analyse the available data and evidence to provide a rational basis for a priority-setting decision. The value-based element of an approach will contribute to the priority-setting decision based on a judgment of the rightness or wrongness of a certain principle (examples of such principles are "equity", or "health as a human right"). Most priority-setting methods have both a technical and a value-based element.

A recent comprehensive literature review discusses a long list of existing approaches: Accountability for Reasonableness, multi-criteria, decision analysis, public budgeting and marginal analysis, multidisciplinary approach, business case approach, saved lives, investment case approach, balance sheet combined normative-empirical approach, public participation approach, mixes of qualitative and quantitative approaches, the local level diamond model. The review concluded that no particular approach could be confidently recommended, suggesting that the advantages and limitations of each of these approaches should be weighed in relation to the local situation and context.[50]

Technical approaches such as burden of disease and mortality analyses are methodologies which have been tried and tested, and have less of a subjective element compared to other approaches (see Annex 4.1 for more information on all of the mentioned tools and approaches). The future projections approach or risk factor approaches already bring in certain assumptions, and thus,

Fig. 4.4 Evidence, Transparency, Voice: Three steps of priority-setting

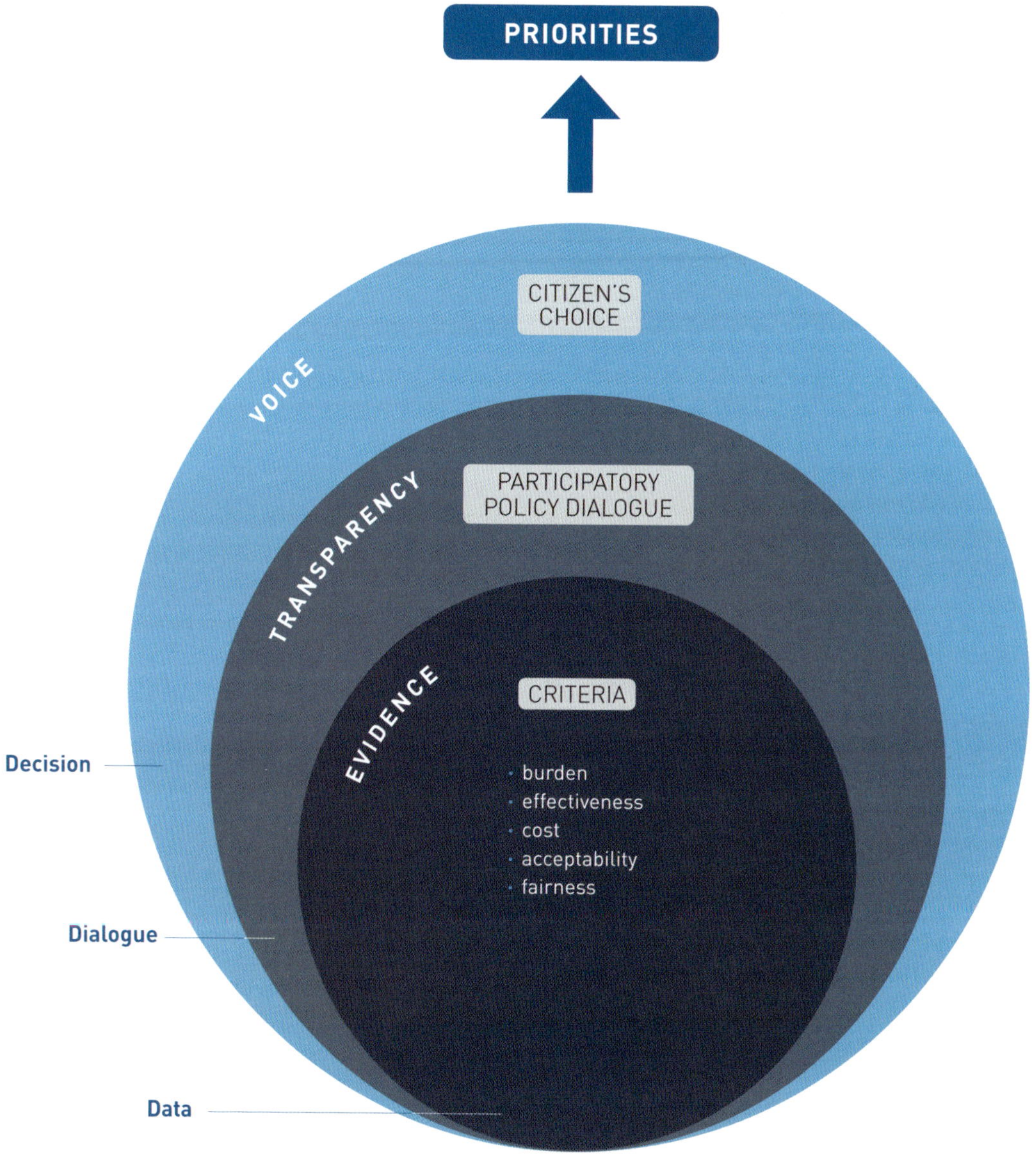

a subjective element. The social solidarity approach has a strong value base, because priority-setting is based on ethical and moral aspects, judged by the society or country that is setting priorities.

That being said, ethics and moral values are never completely absent from a priority-setting process. They are often invoked to mobilize support for various health initiatives, and theories of social justice are often applied to assure fair and equitable treatment of people.[51]

In this chapter, at several places, the argument is made for choosing a combination of several approaches and tools. The reason is clear: used in isolation, none of the approaches is able to examine priority options from different angles, while parallel analyses, with different methods, used by different actors, provide a more comprehensive perspective on questions of the relative importance of a health need, on the potential of a particular solution and on the fairness of a strategy. Also, since the priorities in this context are being ultimately set by the public sector (even if input from private sector and others is actively solicited), it is important to note that the principles, objectives and issues are multiple from the public sector perspective. This calls for putting different arguments and views in balance with one another, which is best done when evidence from a combination of approaches and tools are examined.

In the literature, the distinction between approaches, models, methods and tools used in priority-setting is not always uniform. We use "approach" to mean a particular way of thinking about or dealing with something or someone in space, time, quality or amount, or, more simply: direction and ways of getting to a common goal.

In this handbook, the term "method" stands for a procedure, technique, or way of doing something, especially in accordance with a definite plan. A "tool" is defined as an item or implement used for a specific purpose. The criteria for priority-setting put forth in this handbook should be part of and feed into the decision of which approach(es) is/are chosen.

Used in isolation, no single approach is able to examine priority options from different angles, while parallel analyses, with different methods, used by different actors, provide a more comprehensive perspective.

Box 4.6

Examples of policy priorities in line with the three UHC dimensions

- ***Maximizing service delivery:*** strengthening the gate-keeper function in hospitals.
- ***Reaching vulnerable, marginalized and hard-to-reach populations:*** establishing mobile primary health care (PHC) services for hard-to-reach communities.
- ***Improvements in financial risk protection:*** adopting a pro-poor price policy and preference for generic drugs.

In the following sections, various priority-setting approaches are discussed. All of them help assess the potential for solutions to health problems and health sector bottlenecks against the key criteria for prioritization, mentioned earlier. More detailed information on each of the methods is in Annex 4.1.

Health needs

Identification and ranking of health needs (problems and threats) should be based on an approach that analyses both the burden of diseases and their determinants. This is notably important because the combined approach gives more insight into the vulnerability of a health problem/threat, and subsequently guides the weighing of options to address it. For example, if under-five children frequently suffer from diarrhoea, an assessment of socioeconomic health determinants may link this problem to poverty and to poor water and sanitation infrastructure. The solutions for these determinants exist but are not the mandate of the health sector. Nevertheless, priority-setting should include strategies and interventions to collaborate with other sectors to address the diarrhoea issue.

Three analyses often used to look more carefully at health needs are burden of disease analysis, health needs assessment, and the 2x2 grid.

(a) Burden of disease analysis (BoD)

The burden of disease analysis encompasses a broad range of assessments from multiple data sources to determine health loss from diseases, and its attribution to specific risk factors. Even though this analysis is specific to disease-related health issues, it can also help inform priority-setting in health system related issues. The advantages of using BoD are that, with consistent methods, it critically analyses available information on each health condition, makes this information comparable and systematic, and produces results using standardized metrics.

(b) Health Needs Assessments (HNA)

A HNA involves epidemiological, qualitative, and comparative methods to describe health problems of a population. It may be undertaken as part of the situation analysis phase when routine data and existing information are insufficient for purposes of ranking health needs. HNA provides the opportunity for describing the patterns of disease in the local population, differences between districts, regions and national disease patterns, while highlighting the areas of unmet need. It also allows for learning more about the needs and priorities of the local population. It provides a clear set of objectives to work towards to meet these needs and helps to decide rationally how to use resources to improve their local population's health in the most effective and efficient way.

(c) 2x2 grid

The 2x2 or strategy grid uses need and feasibility criteria to determine which health priorities yield the greatest results. The grid organizes health problems using two dimensions, need and feasibility, to form a quadrant. The combination of a health problem and its solution can be classified either as of

(i) low need/high feasibility,
(ii) high need/high feasibility,
(iii) high need/low feasibility, or
(iv) low need/low feasibility.

An example can be found in Annex 4.1. This grid helps to refocus efforts by shifting emphasis towards addressing problems in a manner that will yield the greatest results. This simple tool may assist in transitioning from brainstorming with a large number of options to a more focused plan of action and can be used also by stakeholder groups with limited capacity.

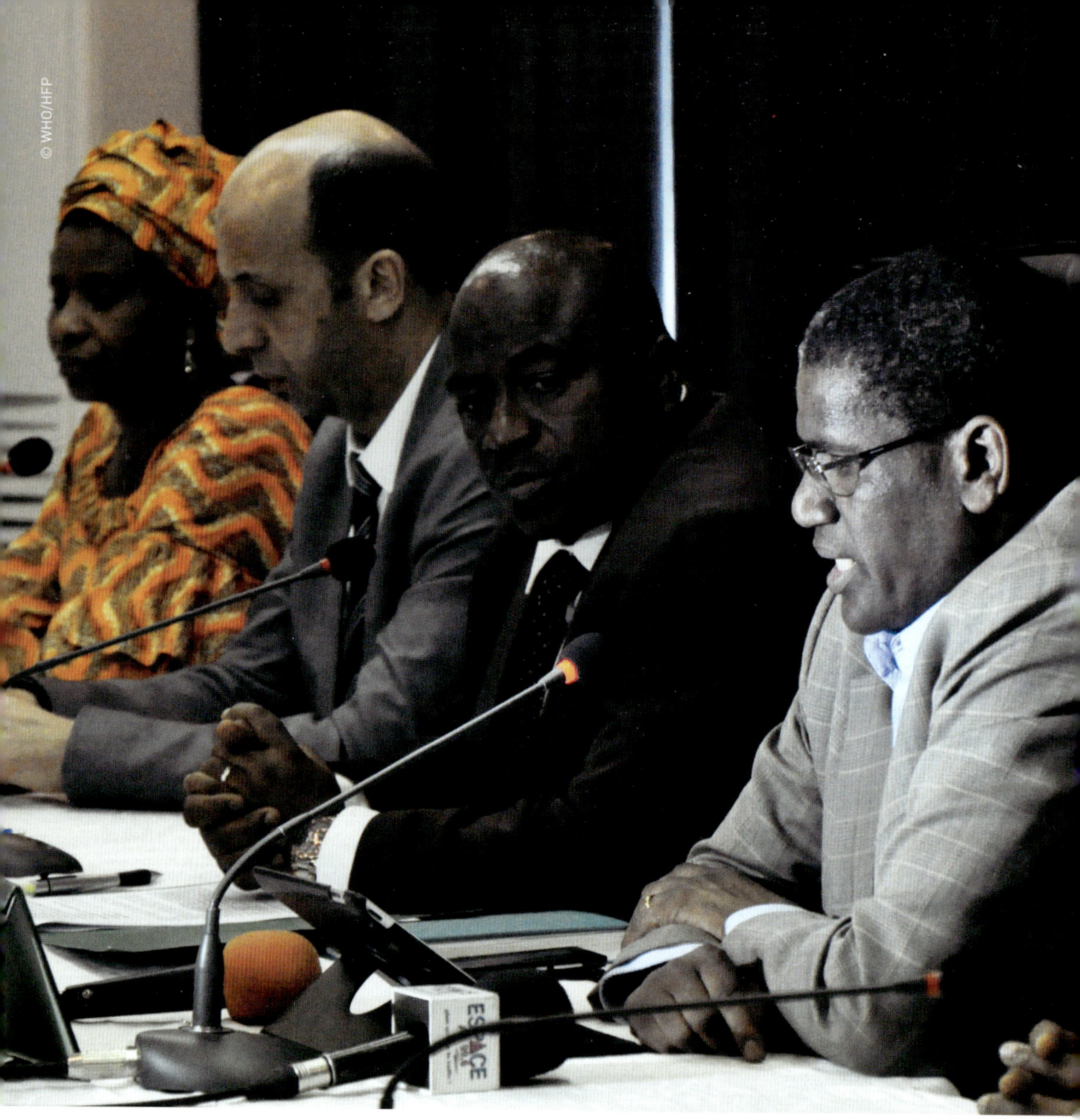

Health technology assessment (HTA)

HTA is a multidisciplinary form of research used to generate evidence about the performance of health technologies. HTA not only includes cost-effectiveness analysis but also identifies new technologies for health problems. HTA works under an explicit legal and institutional framework, aiming to channel and manage political, commercial, advocacy and donor interests fairly and ethically.

More recently, HTAs have focused more attention to the assessment of weaknesses and inefficiencies in existing interventions. In the same way, HTAs increasingly take into account the country's broader development context, visions, and goals; for instance, the quest to move towards UHC. A comprehensive HTA thus may be the technical approach which provides the most comprehensive set of evidence for priority-setting.

When doing a comprehensive HTA of a programme, one may be tempted to expect that all the technologies of that programme have a high score on cost-effectiveness. This is not always the case. For example, while the strategy for screening may be cost-effective, certain palliative technologies may not be. Therefore, when prioritizing between programmes, it is recommended to do a HTA separately for each individual health technology. Within a programme HTA may be done, for example, for devices, drugs, procedures and/or systems. Similarly, a cancer-control programme usually includes a variety of technologies, for prevention interventions, screening, early-detection, diagnostics, therapies and palliative treatment, evaluated in appropriate combinations.

Cost-effectiveness and affordability

Maximizing health is usually the goal of health policy-makers. Economic considerations in priority-setting are important for furthering such goals. Economic models and their measurements offer the decision-maker a rational approach to making policy choices to maximize health.

Cost-effectiveness analysis

The main type of economic evaluation is the CEA, which compares the cost of a potential health intervention with the expected (or in some cases, known) health gain. CEA is a powerful tool for priority-setting; from an economic perspective, it looks at the problem of choosing the optimal portfolio of programmes that can be afforded from a limited national healthcare budget. It forces the decision-maker to define explicitly the objectives of the priority-setting process, even if these cannot be easily measured. CEA promotes value for money in health in order to allocate available resources. CEA can be a central factor for decision-makers when choosing health issues to prioritize. An economic perspective recognizes that the priority-setting process will often involve a series of conflicts, but instead of obscuring such conflicts, it provides a framework for their exploration, and trade-offs can be made explicit.

Cost-effectiveness analysis is a powerful tool for priority-setting; from an economic perspective, it looks at the problem of choosing the optimal portfolio of programmes that can be afforded from a limited national healthcare budget.

CEAs are popular with the public health community because the method offers a coherent measure of benefit while avoiding the difficulties involved with the valuation of health. The value of health can be seen as the "price" of health multiplied by its quantity. However, this "price tag" is based on the most obvious health benefit, i.e. those that can be easily expressed in mortality, disability avoided, etc. The caveat here is that it may lead to a narrow focus on benefits related to health care only, rather than broader health-related development goals. It is more difficult to attach a value to some of the broad development goals which influence health.

It is important to keep in mind that despite many decades of advancement in addressing the technical and methodological issues, it is widely recognized that economic models such as this one should be put in context and combined with other approaches in order to paint a more complete picture of health sector priorities.

The traditional economic approach proposes maximizing health gain (however measured) subject to a budget constraint, which implies ranking programmes according to their cost-effectiveness ratio. The traditional approach generally ignores the numerous practical constraints arising from the political, institutional, and environmental context in which priority-setting takes place. A few such limitations to keep in mind when undertaking CEA are listed below.[52]

Methodological concerns include identifying whose perspective to adopt, the generalizability of results to multiple settings, the treatment of uncertainty and timing, and the treatment of interactions between programmes.

Equity considerations are either related to some concept of need or related to access to services. However, it has been reported that many contributions to the debate on equity concepts are theoretical and remote from practical implementation issues.

Practical constraints arise from the political, institutional, and environmental context in which priority-setting takes place. These include the influence of interest groups, the transaction costs associated with policy changes, and the interactions between the provision and financing of health services.

The following tools look at either cost or effectiveness or cost-effectiveness; they do not explicitly put effectiveness/feasibility in relation to the local context. Especially in settings of weak, poorly-managed institutions and insufficient capacities, context should be taken into account in other ways within the priority-setting process.

(a) Lives Saved Tool (LiST)

LiST is a software tool used to model the impact of scaling-up health interventions aimed to reduce mortality and morbidity in mothers, newborns, and children under five years of age. It allows users to set up and run multiple scenarios, called projections, in order to estimate the impact of different health intervention packages based upon coverage at the national or subnational (e.g. region, state, or district) level.

(b) Basic Priority Rating System (BPRS)

The BPRS, also known as the Hanlon method, helps to quantify public health problems. It proposes a priority rating, based on attributing scores from 1 to 10 for three sets of variables on

(i) weight;
(ii) severity, urgency, economic consequences, and willingness/involvement of others;
(iii) the effectiveness of the intervention. The tool is used by health administrators and decision-makers and uses various data in order to quantify public health problems and set reasonable priorities[53] Though a complex method, the Hanlon method is advantageous when the desired outcome is an objective list of health priorities based on baseline data and numerical values.

(c) Propriety, Economics, Acceptability, Resources and Legality component (PEARL)

The PEARL[54] rates preselected priorities on five factors of feasibility. These factors are not directly related to the health problems; however, they contribute greatly to deciding which priorities should be addressed. PEARL can be used in combination with BPRS. The PEARL component requires sufficient data about both the characteristics of the health problem and the target population.

(d) Programme budgeting and marginal analysis (PBMA)

This economic framework can be used to set priorities in health by examining how resources are currently spent and subsequently linking those expenditures to possible marginal health gains. PBMA relies on an advisory panel, which is charged with identifying areas of health service growth (for a given budget cycle) and resource distribution (to fund proposed growth). It is usually carried out within or across interventions for comparison.

Values which may underpin assumptions and interpretation

Value-based approaches are used for the assessment and ranking of the fairness criterion. Fairness is the principle that all members of society should have guaranteed access to adequate health care.

Social value judgements are an important element in any public justification of how priorities are set. Some key ethical values underpinning priority-setting exercises are listed below.

Equity through solidarity: solidarity is both a shared moral sentiment and norm, arising from the sense of belonging. It is expressed in the union or fellowship of a community that shares feelings, purposes, or responsibilities and interest. Solidarity implies that, on a voluntary basis, the community helps the disadvantaged (equity).

Rights, societal obligation, and self-interest: this argument asserts that basic human needs (such as food, shelter, education, justice) create an obligation on society to provide some level of common access to these fundamental goods. The obligation is acceptable because of the self-interest of the society members. Access to health care is an element of the common good.[55]

Social wisdom: directs us to shape our systems of health care so that we accomplish what we value. Social wisdom is the society's implicit recognition of how it perceives health and what it values in health care. Such a foundation of common understanding and consensus guides national policy-making and planning. In its absence, a narrow focus, for example, on medical care access, would prevent society from focusing on social and economic factors that lead to major public health problems.

Social value judgements are an important element in any public justification of how priorities are set.

In addition to the above, the following can also be seen as formal values which play a role in priority-setting in specific contexts: legality, faithfulness to constitutional provisions and respect for international obligations.[56] Expressed in trust and accountability, these can be easily formalized.[57]

Furthermore, there exist some classical ideologies coming from the economics field that are essentially linked to the above-mentioned values of equity through solidarity and fairness. Priority-setting exercises in some countries may be rooted in one of these ideologies, albeit not necessarily explicitly.[58]

While the research and analysis for technical/ rational approaches can be left to professionals, value-based approaches subjectively weigh formally adopted as well as perceived values.

Libertarianism considers personal responsibility for achievement as very important and that this is weakened when others are offered unearned rewards.[59] This would be the case for instance, when certain risk groups are entitled to specific privileges in health care in terms of access or price.

Utilitarianism claims that pleasure promotion and pain avoidance could be measured and that interpersonal comparisons of utility could be made. Utilitarians are often criticized for ignoring individual freedom. Indeed, when only consequences matter, methods used can be questionable.[60] The utilitarian approach is not considered fair, because it is solely based on the framework that "greatest good is for the greatest number". Critics argue that preferences used for valuing health outcomes should be representative of the entire at-risk population, with due regard for the sentiments of minority disadvantaged groups such as the disabled. Therefore, valid scientific evidence on differential outcomes must exist.

Egalitarianism calls for the most equal distribution of available goods. Economic failure is not equated with moral depravity or social worthlessness. The destitute are not to be punished for alleged economic failure by limiting their access to goods. A "difference principle" calls for every arrangement to be evaluated in terms of the interest of the least advantaged. Alternative arrangements are compared first from the interest of the least advantaged only. If the least advantaged are equally badly off in two different health intervention options, then it is the situation for the second least advantaged that matters, etc.

While the research and analysis for technical/ rational approaches can be left to professionals, a society, through participatory policy dialogue, must subjectively weigh formally adopted as well as perceived values. Policy dialogue platforms will therefore seek representative working groups and/or public engagement. The latter is captured in the literature under the term "deliberative approaches".

Deliberative approaches in weighing ethical values for priority-setting is about public involvement. It can be defined as an approach that seeks to actively involve citizens in the process of formulation, passage, and implementation of public policies through action aimed at influencing decisions. It is acknowledged that, in most cases, policy decisions are ultimately taken by public representatives and officials so the focus is on the interaction between citizens and those making health care decisions.[61]

A literature review on public participation in health care priority-setting found that there is a growing interest in deliberative approaches. However, formal evaluation efforts of deliberative approaches are rare. Also, it is unclear how public views might be integrated with other decision inputs when allocating social resources.[62]

A process for deliberative priority-setting should ideally meet four necessary conditions:[63]

- it must be relevant to the local context as determined by accepted criteria;
- its eventual decisions – and the reasons behind them – must be publicized;
- it must include appeal mechanisms for challenging, revising, and reversing decisions
- its leaders must be able to enforce the above three conditions.

Examples of deliberative approaches are:

(a) Citizen consultation processes

Citizen consultation can capture a population's demands, opinion and expectation on health-related matters in order to improve the transparency and relevance of the priority-setting process. Please refer to Chapter 2 on population consultation for more detail.

(b) Accountability for Reasonableness (AFR)

Accountability for Reasonableness (AFR) is an ethics-based approach to a legitimate and fair priority-setting process that builds upon key conditions that must be fulfilled to gain support for their implementation.

Multi-stakeholder finalization and validation

Validation means the formal adoption of the priority agenda and this is the final stage of priority-setting. Decision-making on how to translate priority choices into planning and resource allocation will be discussed in the following chapters.

(a) Multivoting technique (MVT)

The multivoting technique (MVT, also known as nominal group technique, NGT), is notably used to make collaborative decisions when the list of propositions is long and team members have differing opinions. Based on a more or less exhaustive list of options (ideas, problems, issues or solutions) produced in a brainstorming session, it seeks to ensure a good and common understanding of the items in the list. Each idea is then jointly defined by the team members in clear terms, so as to ensure that all participants have a fair idea of what each item means. Ideas are grouped or merged and a few new, related ideas may be added. The team then reduces the total number of items that can be voted for to about one third of the initial number. The last step of voting should result in a consensus. This method is also useful in the early stages of priority-setting and works best for smaller group processes.[64]

(b) The Delphi technique

Just as the MVT, the Delphi method is a type of consensus method. Through questionnaires, a panel of independent experts is consulted over two or more rounds. Whereas focus groups purposely use group dynamics to generate debate on a topic, Delphi methods maintain anonymity of the participants, even after the study. The most important advantages of this technique are:

(i) a rapid consensus can be achieved,
(ii) participants do not have to be in the same room together to reach agreement,
(iii) individuals are able to express their own opinions as opposed to "group think",
(iv) consultation can include a wide range of expertise, and
(v) relatively low cost to administer and analyse.[65]

(c) Multi-criteria decision-making (MCDM)

MCDM is a quantitative decision analysis model that captures preferences of decision-makers and discovers the most desired solution to the problem (see Box 4.7). It is a hybrid method in that it incorporates both technical and value-based approaches.[66] It is based on a performance matrix where each row describes an option and each column describes the performance of the options against each criterion. To do so, five criteria are applied: maximization of general population health, the distribution of health in the population, specific societal preferences, budgetary and practical constraints, and political considerations.

All the above tools, and others not mentioned here, have a variety of purposes and objectives. They can be used at various stages of the priority-setting process in health. Each of them has advantages and disadvantages. The majority can be used as a stand-alone tool, but they can also be used in conjunction with one another. Traditional methods, such as evidence-based medicine, burden of disease analyses, cost-effectiveness analyses (classical method) and equity analyses concentrate on a single criterion, whereas in reality, policy-makers need to make choices taking into account multiple criteria simultaneously. Advantages and disadvantages of various methods and tools are summarized in a table in Annex 4.2 together with a list of limitations of traditional single criteria methods.

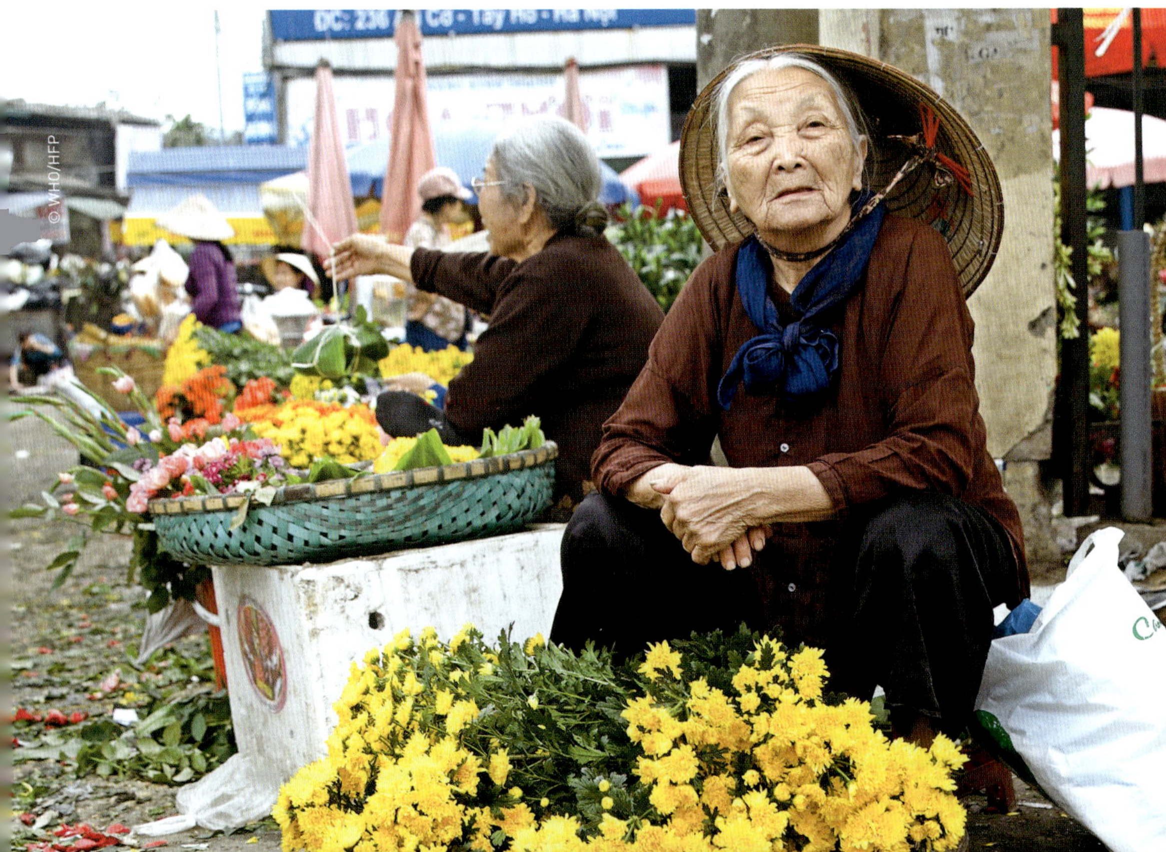

Box 4.7

Economic justification for public funding targeted at the whole population or the poor only[67]

Governments often attempt to provide free services to the whole population, and often spend resources on low-impact services. A study proposed a rational approach to targeting and prioritization of public spending in Ghana in order to better balance equity and efficiency in the country. It employed the priority-setting approach MCDM analysis on the following criteria: number of potential beneficiaries, severity of disease, cost-effectiveness, poverty reduction and vulnerable population. The study considered a selection of interventions related to childhood diseases, communicable diseases, noncommunicable diseases, reproductive health and injuries.

First, interventions were tested against the economic justification for public funding to define to whom spending should be targeted. Second, resulting interventions were prioritized on the basis of medical and non-medical criteria. A rank ordering emerged of interventions with a specification on whether public spending should be targeted at the whole population or the poor only. For example, whereas improved complementary feeding in childhood would be given low priority on the basis of cost-effectiveness alone, it would receive much higher priority when severity of disease, its number of potential beneficiaries, the vulnerability of children, and its potential for poverty reduction would be taken into account as well.

The MCDA resulted in the following disease control priorities: prevention of mother-to-child HIV/AIDS transmission, and oral rehydration therapy to treat diarrhoea in childhood. Therefore, public funding of these interventions was warranted for the whole population. However, case-management of pneumonia in childhood was also considered a priority, but public funding was to be targeted at the poor only.

The study concluded that the application of MCDA in the priority-setting process of health interventions can help health systems to move towards a more equitable and efficient use of resources and that, in Ghana, it was a step forward to transparency and accountability in policy-making. However, it was recommended that policy-makers should not only use such a formulaic approach to prioritize interventions, because here only criteria that were amenable to quantification were analysed. It was stressed that addressing also non-quantitative concerns through a deliberative process to reach consensus (when possible) by different stakeholders was also warranted.

4.5.4 Process

The success of the priority-setting process depends on an honest debate to forge a common understanding of the criteria and approaches to use for priority-setting.

Priority-setting is one of the crucial stages of the national health planning process because it links the results of a health sector situation analysis with the strategic orientations of a national health strategy. Its success depends on an honest debate to forge a common understanding of the criteria and approaches to use for priority-setting. Decision-makers must agree on the interpretation of key values, assumptions and concepts and make those interpretations transparent. Diverging views and conflicts of interests should be explicitly acknowledged and managed. It is important to ensure that all stakeholder groups understand what they will gain through their active participation in a medium-term sector priority-setting exercise for it to be successful.

Different interpretations of key notions like health, health risk, disease, quality of life or necessary care can lead to different decisions regarding the health sector interventions to prioritize (see Box 4.8). Decision-makers must agree on the interpretation of key concepts and reference standards used. A choice must be taken whether a narrow (biological) or a broad (bio-psychosocial) interpretation of health and disease is to be applied, and which standards of normality and abnormality (minimum, average or optimum) will be applied with regard to the (expected) quality of life.

"All views are entitled to be aired. It is through vigorous and constructive debate that together we will chart the path ahead."
-- Nelson Mandela speaking at the Opening of the 48th National Conference of the ANC, University of Durban-Westville, Durban, South Africa, 2 July 1991

Box 4.8

Differences in attitudes between national health workers and donors in weighing cost-effectiveness and severity of disease in Uganda?[68]

In Uganda, the relative preference of key players in priority-setting was studied with regard to two criteria: cost-effectiveness of interventions and severity of disease. Respondents of the questionnaires were health actors at national, district, and health subdistrict and facility levels: health workers, development partners or donors and politicians. Above 90% of the respondents recognized the importance of both severity of disease and cost-effectiveness of intervention. In the three scenarios where they were to choose between the two, a majority of the survey respondents assigned highest weight to treating the most severely ill patient with a less cost-effective intervention. However, in in-depth interviews, international development partners preferred the consideration of cost-effectiveness of intervention. The study recommends that discrepancies in attitudes between national health workers and representatives from the donors should be openly debated to ensure legitimate decisions.

Steps

The following steps are suggested for the priority-setting process.[69]

1. Adopt a clear mandate for the priority-setting exercise.
2. Define the scope of the priority-setting and who will play what role.
3. Establish a steering body and a process management group.
4. Decide on approach, methods and tools.
5. Develop a work plan/roadmap and assure availability of the necessary resources.
6. Develop an effective communication strategy.
7. Inform the public about the priority-setting and engage internal/external stakeholders.
8. Organize the data collection, analysis and consultation/deliberation processes.
9. Develop or adopt a scoring system.
10. Adopt a plan for monitoring and evaluating the priority-setting exercise.
11. Collate and analyse the scores.
12. Present the provisional results for discussion; adjust if necessary.
13. Distribute the priority list to stakeholders.
14. Assure the formal validation of recommendations of the priority-setting outcome.
15. Plan and organize the follow-up of the priority-setting, i.e. the decision-making steps.
16. Evaluate the priority-setting exercise.

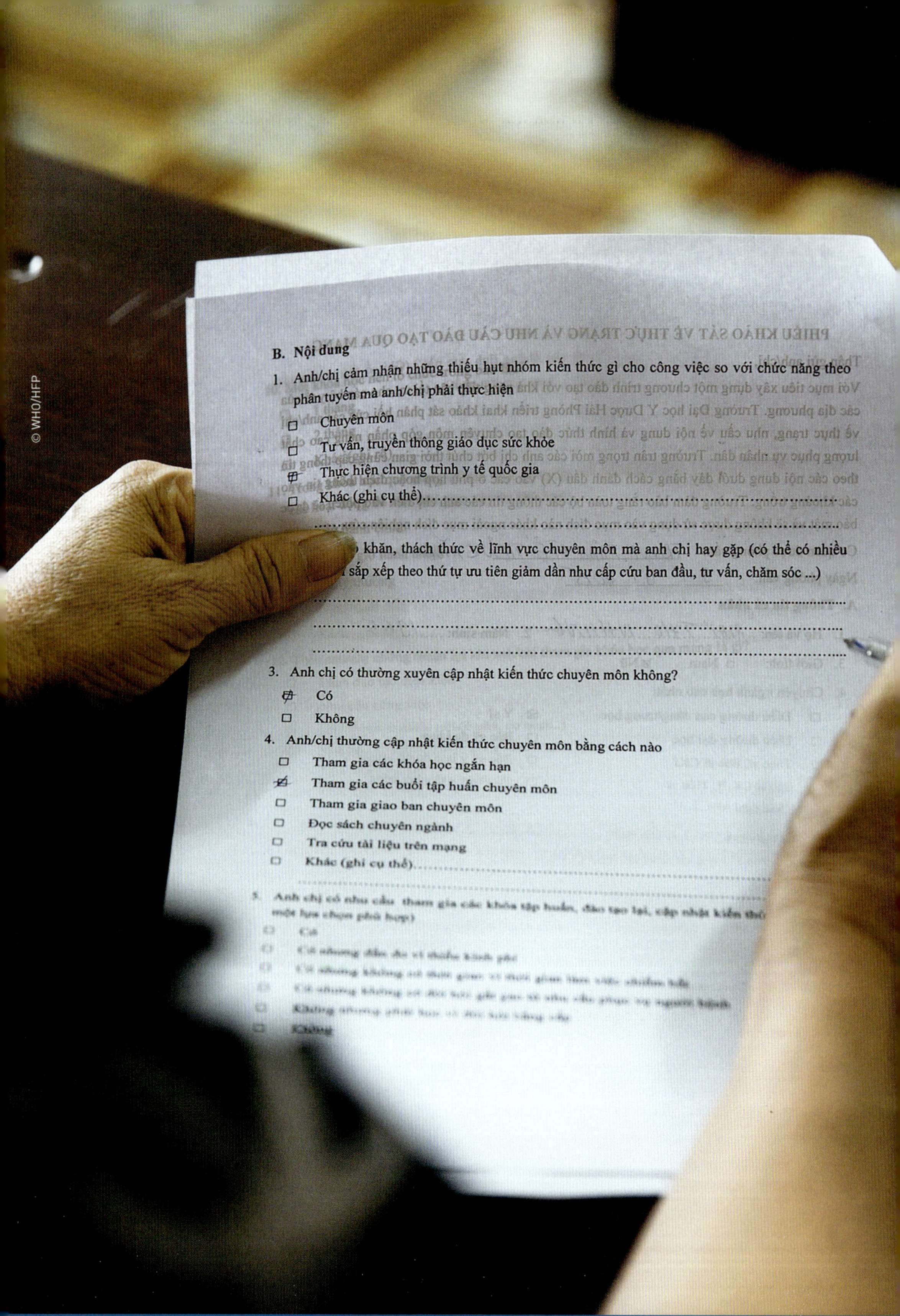
B. Nội dung
1. Anh/chị cảm nhận những thiếu hụt nhóm kiến thức gì cho công việc so với chức năng theo phân tuyến mà anh/chị phải thực hiện
Chuyên môn
Tư vấn, truyền thông giáo dục sức khỏe
Thực hiện chương trình y tế quốc gia
Khác (ghi cụ thể)
khăn, thách thức về lĩnh vực chuyên môn mà anh chị hay gặp (có thể có nhiều
sắp xếp theo thứ tự ưu tiên giảm dần như cấp cứu ban đầu, tư vấn, chăm sóc ...)
3. Anh chị có thường xuyên cập nhật kiến thức chuyên môn không?
Có
Không
4. Anh/chị thường cập nhật kiến thức chuyên môn bằng cách nào
Tham gia các khóa học ngắn hạn
Tham gia các buổi tập huấn chuyên môn
Tham gia giao ban chuyên môn
Đọc sách chuyên ngành
Tra cứu tài liệu trên mạng
Khác (ghi cụ thể)

4.6 Common challenges and factors of success

4.6.1 Constraints and challenges

Several constraints have been observed in priority-setting. Some of these are rooted in a given country's overall political, institutional or legal context, while others are health system related. There are also process-related constraints.[70]

Context constraints

- Weaknesses in the country's legal frameworks may hamper implementation and monitoring and evaluation (M&E) of national policies, as well as adequate leadership and governance, notably in terms of transparency and accountability.
- Insufficient intersectoral coordination and collaboration, due to weak institutional frameworks, may cause inadequate priority-setting and may result in incompatible decision-making on public and donor budgets.

Health system constraints

- A poorly functioning health sector information system, marked by incomplete and flawed data, may lead to erroneous conclusions regarding the relative importance of health problems and the effectiveness of strategies. If the health system lacks the necessary entrepreneurial spirit and learning culture, the priority-setting exercise may become a formality that will not effectively provide guidance for further sector development.
- Incomplete legal frameworks for the health sector and unclear decision-making procedures may hamper programme evaluation. As a result, the evidence base for priority-setting may become biased.
- In a strongly centralized health system there is a risk that representatives of service providers and civil society are not sufficiently on board.
- If the panel for advising on health sector priorities lacks health economic knowledge and/or allocation experience, there may be insufficient capacity to translate analysis results into revised and updated plans.

Process constraints

- In a health system that is facing too many administrative demands, priority-setting and/or its follow-up may end up as an activity of low priority.
- Absence of strong MoH leadership and of effective two-way communication between the various stakeholders may lead to a poorly accepted outcome of the priority-setting and, ultimately, to uncertainty about the availability of the necessary future resources (national and external).
- Another challenge is the natural inclination of those who are involved in priority-setting to focus on the continuation of existing strategies and modalities, with slight modifications. However, ongoing interventions and programmes are usually the product of a multitude of driving forces, motivations and compromises. Understanding those driving forces can help prevent undue influences from playing a role in reviewing sector priorities, thereby better customizing existing strategies and modalities.

4.6.2 Factors of success

One major success factor is having, prior to priority-setting, an in-depth sector review or situation analysis that has examined aspects such as effectiveness, efficiency, and cost-effectiveness on the basis of not only a quantitative data analysis but also on qualitative information on cross-cutting factors that influence health system performance and potential.

One major success factor is having, prior to priority-setting, an in-depth sector review or situation analysis that has examined aspects such as effectiveness, efficiency, and cost-effectiveness on the basis of not only a quantitative data analysis but also on qualitative information on cross-cutting factors that influence health system performance and potential. For this, it is not enough to only identify SWOT of the past. We must know what worked and what did not work in the past, but above all we must find out why interventions of the past period were effective or not. A classic example is health information, an area that in many countries was diagnosed again and again as suffering from serious systemic weaknesses, in spite of repeated strategic (medium-term) decisions to strengthen it. In many cases this was to no avail, because the root causes were not addressed in subsequent new plans. In other words, the "why" question was not adequately addressed. If, once again, the insufficiencies of the health information system are seen as a key problem to be addressed in the coming years, it is only useful to select this area as a priority when the proposed renewed efforts and investments are based on a clear understanding of the root causes of dysfunction.

The priority-setting can be considered successful when a number of criteria have been met.[71]

- The priority-setting process is based on a clearly defined scope, approach and methodology.
- The process of priority-setting has evolved in a transparent manner, with adequate information management, whereby communication and feedback were ensured, the organizers were accountable and opportunity existed for a decision review (appeals mechanism).
- The analysis has taken into consideration values and local context.
- If undue driving forces have co-determined the previous priority agenda, there is space for "alternative agenda setting".
- The next (stage of the) plan and budget show a more balanced and rational resource distribution, based on needs, cost-effective interventions and values.
- It transpires clearly from the next (stage of the) plan and budget that the most important health threats are adequately addressed.
- Resources are allocated for interventions that benefit the population groups and regions most affected and at risk.
- The implementation of the plan/budget shows better cost-effectiveness because strategies and implementation modalities have been adapted to evidence-based technologies, whereby the local context was taken into account.
- The next (stage of the) plan and budget show that priority needs of disadvantaged population groups are explicitly addressed.
- The adopted priorities and following resource allocation and plans have taken into account the views of various stakeholder groups through an explicit process that has resulted in their engagement (buy-in) and the priority-setting outcomes are socio-culturally acceptable to the population. As a result, stakeholders have shifted priorities and/or reallocated resources changes in strategic directions.

Factors that facilitate the priority setting:[72]

- senior-level managerial and clinical championship;
- strong leadership in coordination and oversight;
- culture to learn and change integrated management of budgets;
- resources earmarked for the process itself and for follow-up on recommendations.

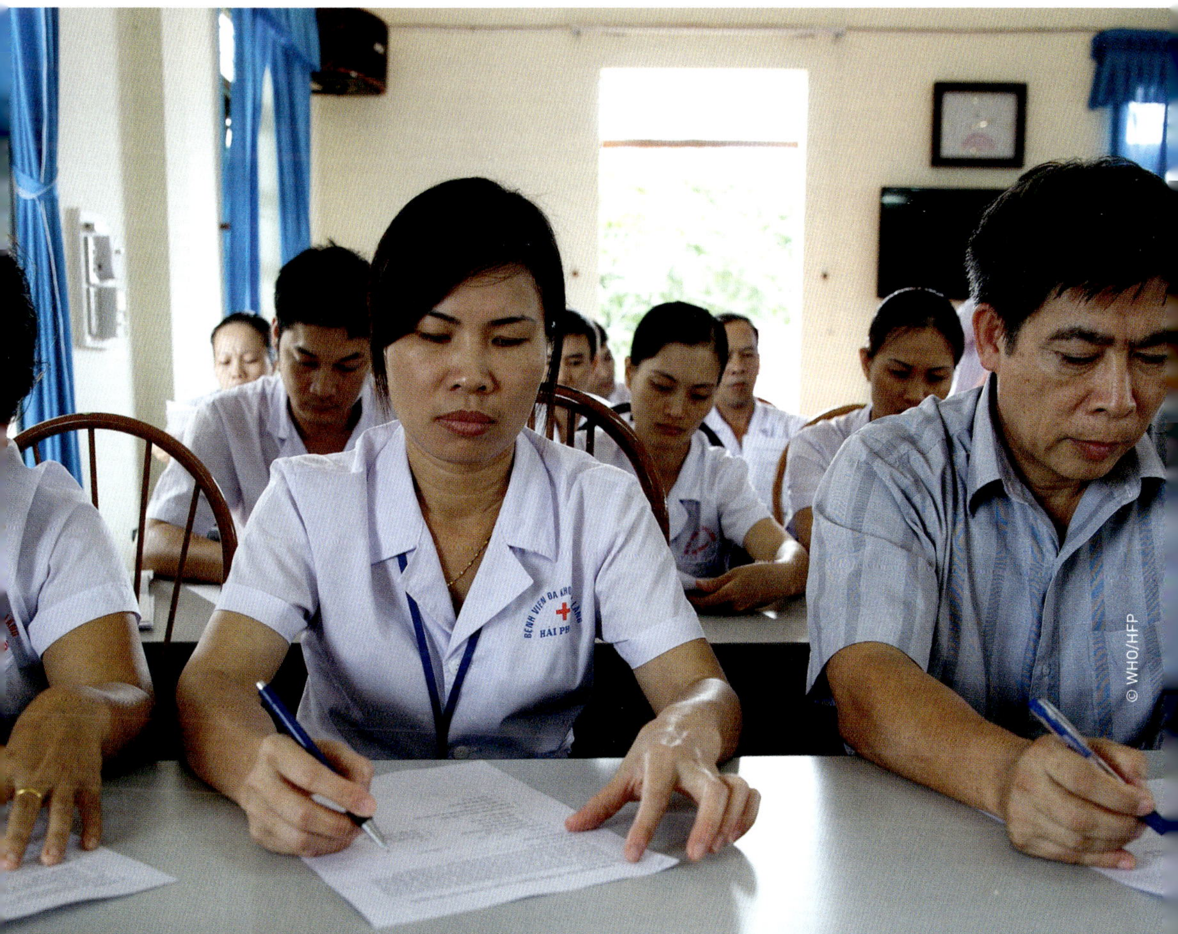

4.7 What if ...?

4.7.1 What if your country is highly centralized?

In a highly centralized setting, those who are responsible for the priority-setting exercise must be aware of four risks.

- If communication (two-way) between central level and intermediate and operational levels is insufficient, the MoH may not have all the necessary information about the situation "in the field", for identifying and adopting priorities. For instance, the ministry may not have a complete picture of different situations and needs between regions and may not have full insight in the perceptions, opinions and demands of local stakeholders.
- If MoH's communication strategies, mechanisms and means are insufficient, there is a risk that various groups of actors and beneficiaries of the health system are not adequately informed and sensitized for the priority-setting exercise in a timely manner.
- The existing institutional and organizational framework may not provide the necessary platform function for consulting various stakeholder groups and for facilitating their participation in the priority-setting process (including repeal mechanism).
- If decision-making in the health sector is highly centralized, the translation of the results of the priority-setting (i.e. the recommendations for prioritizing specific needs, interventions and for resource allocation) in planning and budgeting may be unduly influenced by political issues, thereby weakening its legitimacy.

The following case (Box 4.9) describes some of the potential threats experienced in a highly-centralized system:

Box 4.9

Influences in priority-setting at the meso and micro levels in a highly-centralized system[73]

A study in Kerman province in Iran sought to understand how the national priority-setting programme worked. What factors influenced the implementation process, at the meso and micro levels, in this centralized health system? The analysis showed that the process of priority-setting was non-systematic, that there was little transparency, and the priority decisions were made independently from their implementation. This was found to be due to the highly centralized system: priorities are set at the macro level without involving meso or micro local levels or any representative of the public. The two main benefit packages are under the responsibility of different ministries and there was no coordination between them. The process was also heavily influenced by political pressure exerted by various groups, mostly medical professionals. The weaknesses were exacerbated by a growing gap between rural and urban areas in terms of access to health services.

In order to avoid the above-mentioned risks, it is useful for central-level authorities to think about its existing health sector policy cycle to ensure improved communication and participation. This is only of benefit to the central authorities as more input from and better communication with the sub-national levels will lead to better adherence and more meaningful contribution to new plans and budgets.

4.7.2 What if your country is decentralized?

In many countries, decentralization of the health sector involves decision-making and resource management being delegated to regional and district health managers. In a situation of comprehensive political/administrative decentralization, there is even devolution of powers and responsibilities to local government. Consultation in health sector priority-setting will take place in line with the type and degree of decentralizing. The main challenges will be to:

- organize, coordinate and guide the consultation at all levels, and to adequately synthesize the results of all phases;
- allow for sufficient flexibility in setting priorities, respectful of mandates at decentralized levels, while also keeping in mind national guidelines, targets and norms for the whole country.

Especially in a situation where health sector responsibilities and powers have been devolved to local government, it is important that local administrators are well prepared for the task at hand. This means that

(i) they must have a good understanding of public health issues;
(ii) their mandate is clear and that coordination and collaboration with local health authorities is adequate;
(iii) they receive clear guidelines and instructions regarding any norms, priority areas, resource allocation decisions etc, that have been defined at national level. Hence, central-level MoH and the ministry of local government jointly have a key role to play in preparing local government for priority-setting in the local health system (see Box 4.10).

Box 4.10

Challenges in participatory planning and priority-setting in Uganda's decentralized health system[74]

In Uganda, participatory planning is fairly established; many decentralized district leaders involve the public in local health priority-setting processes. In an attempt to draw lessons from Uganda's experience, one study conducted in-depth interviews with health planners at the national, district and community levels, and organized five group discussions at community level. Participants revealed a number of challenges.

District-level respondents reported to have gained decision-making powers, but were concerned about the degree of financial independence they had to implement decisions. The national-level respondents were concerned about the capacity of the districts to absorb their new roles. Meaningful involvement of the public in priority-setting, and poor communication between the different levels of the decentralization system, despite the existing structures, were additional concerns.

To address these challenges, the authors proposed several potential solutions. Regarding district health planning capacity, the authors suggested providing stronger technical assistance and supporting districts to hire qualified technical personnel. In addition, they recommended that the national level ensure true financial decentralization so that districts actually have more control over the decisions and plans they make. The authors also encouraged mapping of resources allocated to districts so that resource distribution can be better visualized and understood at the national level. This would have positive spillover effects on the level of financial independence granted to districts. Finally, to address the issue of poor public participation, the authors advocate for more resources to facilitate continuous discussion and dialogue between the public and leaders.

4.7.3 What if fragmentation and/or fragility is an issue in your country?

Determinants of fragility include conflicts, weak institutions, external shocks, poverty, disease and regional instability. It is the interplay of these determinants that determines the outcome. Drivers of dysfunctional governance are often self- and mutually-reinforcing. In this environment, short-term gains may outweigh an uncertain long-term vision, and any priority-setting exercise will certainly reflect this.

In a fragmented and/or fragile environment, health needs are likely to be very diverse and extreme, varying from rampant infectious diseases to malnourishment, injuries caused by violence and chronic effects from failed primary-level care. On the other hand, effectiveness and efficiency of available solutions/interventions may be very low, due to local implementation constraints such as insufficient service providers, poor maintenance, interrupted access due to insecurity and corruption. Meanwhile, the situation on the ground may evolve rapidly and in an unplanned way. In combination with poor communication lines, it makes it difficult for central government to keep a good overview of the situation and trends for the whole country. The problem is often compounded by incomplete and possibly flawed data/information, which is to provide the basis for the sector analysis. This makes the assessment of health needs, feasibility of solutions and cost implications difficult.

A weak public sector is one of the common characteristics of a fragmented and/or fragile environment. The MoH may have insufficient human resource capacity (in numbers and in expertise). The institutional framework may be suboptimal as well as the internal organization, leading to ineffective communication and coordination. Weak leadership by the MoH and insufficiencies in the coordination of stakeholders and actors make it difficult to organize a comprehensive and inclusive approach for the priority-setting.

Before formulating recovery strategies as per sector priorities, stakeholders should consider what the main characteristics of the crisis are, and what the future country context might look like. Important questions to be answered are, for instance: Is the present turmoil structural or transient? What are the chances that a legitimate government will eventually emerge from the protracted crisis? What are the economic prospects (recovery of livelihoods, resettlement of displaced people and refugees)?

The supranational landscape needs to be understood as well. Will external actors remain involved in domestic affairs, and if so for how long? Will donors support transition and health system development? What will be the role of neighbouring countries?

In addition, priority-setting must take into account the role of the national government and the MoH in a situation of fragmentation and/or fragility. Is the national government politically legitimate and technically capable? Is the MoH willing to lead healthcare developments, disinterested or resource-less? Are health authorities able to play a leading role in the healthcare field? Are there no contested regions? Is there no opposition by powerful donors on political or human-rights grounds?

A medium-term priority-setting exercise for the health sector in such an environment will probably need an adapted and simplified approach in various areas.

In a fragile state context, a "quick and dirty" assessment could be organized that would provide a "good enough" understanding of the essential issues.

1. **Data/information collection and analysis**
   If the health information system is poorly organized, turning out incomplete and unreliable data, the usefulness of (the analysis of) certain data for priority-setting may be doubtful. One might be tempted then to immediately invest in repairing/completing the entire database and to start strengthening the health information system. However, this is a comprehensive, complex and sizeable undertaking, even under more favourable circumstances. Therefore, instead, some "quick and dirty" assessments could be organized that would provide a "good enough" understanding of the essential issues

2. **Consultative approach, scope and time horizon**
   When communication with certain parts of the country is disturbed due to insecurity or failing logistics, or when partner organizations from the non-public sector have started operating more or less independently due to failing coordination mechanisms, a comprehensive consultation process will be difficult to organize and is likely to become a costly exercise. Moreover, due to the disturbed environment, those to be consulted may not have been adequately informed in advance on the health sector issues at stake. In such circumstances, the concessions may be necessary with regard to the scope of the consultation, the methods to be used and the degree of representativeness of various stakeholder groups.

3. **Flexibility of the resulting recommendations**
   While the recommendations that result from the consultation may be relevant and fair, their feasibility may become questionable due to rapidly changing circumstances in a volatile environment. Therefore, it may be useful to formulate these recommendations in such a way that they can be used in different situations. A few scenarios may be considered, for example, with regard to the likelihood of achieving in the near future a planned government reform and implementation of measures towards governance strengthening. Because of this need to allow for flexibility in the recommendations, it is preferable that their total number be limited.

If there are indications of serious health threats, specific for a certain population group or region, or of paralysed service provision in certain service areas (types, levels or geographical), efforts must be made to establish a clear picture of the current situation and trends. Such problems need to be quantified and their likely consequences are to be documented. This will allow for situation- or area-specific priority-setting recommendations.

4.7.4 What if your country is highly dependent on aid?

As we move from Millennium Development Goals (MDGs) to the Sustainable Development Goals (SDGs), the fragmented priorities seen in global health for decades are being counterbalanced with more sustainable, system-focused solutions. The SDGs are applicable to all countries, and go well beyond the MDGs.[75]

Accordingly, the role of donors and global health initiatives is evolving greatly over the last decade. The Millennium Development Goals (MDGs) adopted by the United Nations in 2000 had set the tone for much of the international agenda for health and directed the nature of health as priorities at national level. Looking back 15 years at the trends and positive forces during the MDG era, several limitations have also become apparent. These are, a limited focus, resulting in verticalization of health and disease programmes, a lack of attention to strengthening health systems, the emphasis on a "one-size-fits-all" development planning approach, and a focus on aggregate targets rather than equity. The MDGs is perceived by some as a typical case of bypassing the will of developming countries' citizens.

The MDGs spurred large global health initiatives to donate millions to national governments for very specific health issues; this has shifted the perspective of national governments when deciding on resource allocation for health. It may be the case, as is seen with HIV in Malawi (see Box 4.11), that certain diseases take prominence because of the available financial resources from large donors and not initially because of the prevalence or burden of disease.

The importance of high aid dependency for the priority-setting process depends on several factors.

(a) The extent to which the external aid and donors are integrated in the overall health sector development, in terms of coordination, alignment, etc.

In aid-dependent settings, it is especially crucial to keep striving for better collaboration and coordination in planning, especially for joint sector analysis, comprehensive needs assessment, resource allocation, budgeting, predictability of resource flows, resource utilization and management. Stronger national leadership and formal arrangements for harmonized sector development by the entire stakeholder community are important goals to work towards and keep working towards.

While structural high dependency on external aid itself is a barrier for establishing a sustainable national health system, the consequences of scattered and poorly coordinated aid probably have an even more negative impact on the planning process, especially on priority-setting. Medium-term and comprehensive health sector priority-setting in an environment of poorly integrated and coordinated aid is undermined by parallel steering and decision-making, which is often guided by different agendas and based on different criteria and decision-making processes. Even when in such a situation, development partners express support for national leadership and adhere to the adopted sector plan and priorities, this does not guarantee that their financial and technical resources can be harnessed towards the implementation of the adopted sector priorities. These constraints have been extensively documented and have led to initiatives such as the Paris Declaration, the Accra Agenda and IHP+. Experience to date with countries where a National IHP+ Compact was signed indicates that important gains could

Fig. 4.5 Inexistent lines of accountability between donor agencies, their citizens and recipient citizens

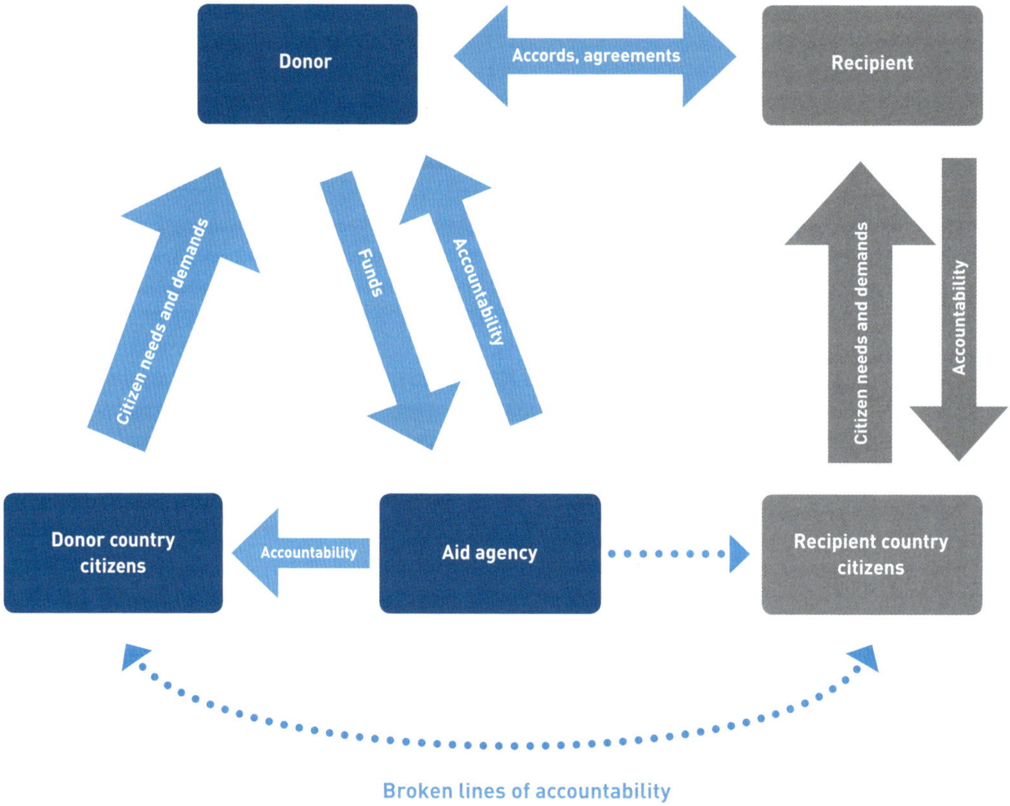

Adapted from the World Development Report 2004:
Making services work for poor people, World Bank, 2004

be made in assuring that external aid is used adequately.

(b) The opportunities and prospects for reducing aid dependency

The options may be limited, when

(i) solutions for solving the country's health problems are costly;
(ii) the country's economic basis is weak;
(iii) extensive efforts have already been made to reduce costs through efficiency gains by introducing reforms, adapted strategies and implementation modalities.

In such a case, national government and development partners should jointly develop ideas and plans for efficiency gains and review resource redistribution. This may require institutional reforms or adaptation of standard strategies and care systems for improving efficiency. New strategies and implementation modalities will have to be tested in a pilot before they are implemented. In addition, it may be necessary to review the economic sustainability of certain care solutions. Such a review may lead to a decision to disinvest in a certain area/service in order to increase resource availability for more crucial health needs.

Integration of priority (disease-based) programmes in comprehensive health system development is often an uphill battle. The vertical nature of some of these programmes in terms of planning, implementation modalities, funding flows, allocation criteria and M&E is usually seen as a condition for obtaining rapid and significant results, especially in an environment of weak public-sector leadership and governance. The risks that come with well-funded vertical programmes are also well documented.[76] They are related to the multiplication of implementation systems, norms and standards, misbalanced sector funding, conflicting interests and ownership issues. It is, therefore, important to carefully manage the role of such vertical programmes and their funders in a sector-wide priority-setting process. National IHP+ Compacts should help to avoid that pressure from powerful, sometimes semi-autonomous disease programmes and the temptation of their lavish funding that can distort the processes of ranking priorities and subsequent decision-making in resource allocation and planning.

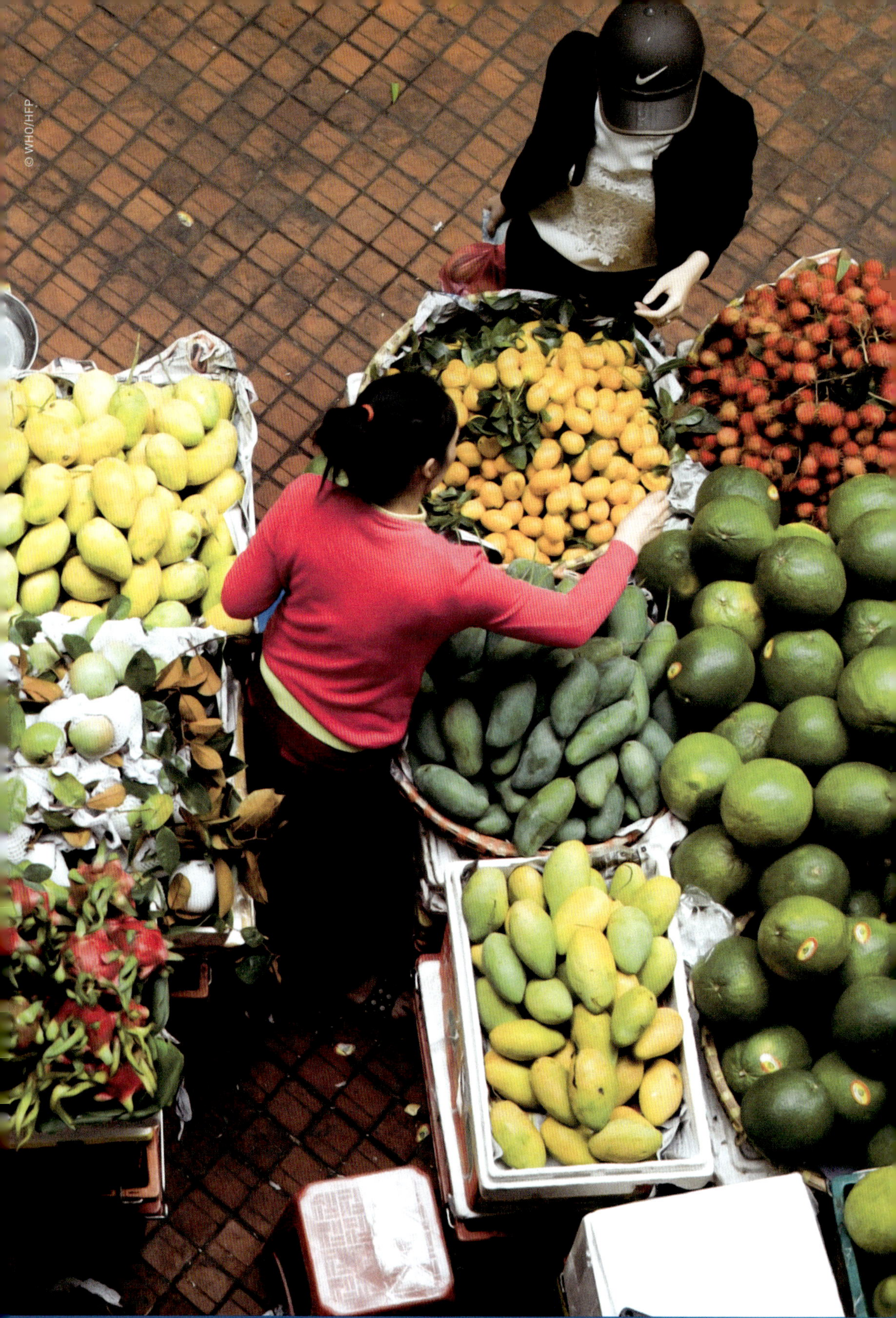
© WHO/HFP

Box 4.11

The impact of earmarked aid contributions on national health priority-setting mechanisms in Malawi[77]

This case study in Malawi on external influence in priority-setting looked at the involvement of the international community in the campaign to tackle the HIV/AIDS epidemic, and found that it had an unprecedented impact on national health priority-setting mechanisms in Malawi. The example shows how, despite the country's commitment to comprehensive sector development based on national leadership and strengthened coordination, massive earmarked external funding interfered with rational and just priority-setting.

Malawi has a high prevalence of HIV (12%). In response to the MDG goal No. 6 several Global Health Initiatives (GHIs) provided increased financial assistance to Malawi for addressing HIV/AIDS within the health sector. Among them were the Global Fund to Fight AIDS, Tuberculosis and Malaria (GFATM), United States Agency for International Development (USAID), UN Development Programme (UNDP), the World Bank, UK Department for International Development and the African Development Bank, among others. In 2002, donor contribution to the total HIV/AIDS resource envelope held by the National AIDS Commission was 46%, but rose to 73% by 2005. In addition, the majority of the aid contributions for health were also earmarked for HIV/AIDS. Due to this shift in the overall sector budget, attention was diverted away from other important health priorities. GFATM became the largest donor, with US$ 300 million in aid since 2002, of which around 80% was earmarked for HIV/AIDS programmes. Not surprisingly, GFATM's role in national priority-setting and planning grew and complications arose. Concerns were reported about the poor integration of its activities into the Malawi's health sector SWAp (Sector-Wide Approach). For instance, there were parallel planning structures for the Malawi National AIDS Committee Integrated National Working Plan. These developments were not in line with Malawi's earlier efforts to better coordinate the different GHIs and development agencies even before the SWAp. Vertical funding towards HIV/AIDS has compromised the distribution of human resources for health. There has been a noticeable task-shifting impact on the health system as health workers leave other services, such as antenatal care and reproductive health, to work for HIV/AIDS programmes funded by international donors. Although there have been improvements in HIV/AIDS incidence rates in Malawi, it is important to consider the gravity of the impact of these external influences on priority-setting in the wider health sector.

4.8 Conclusion

Priority-setting is an indispensable step in the health sector development process because it guides medium-term sector development. It is important to choose approach, methods and tools carefully, taking into account the national setting with regard to important contextual developments and overall development trends, availability of key data and evaluations on performance, the role of citizens and various stakeholder groups, the organizational and leadership capacity of the public sector, and – last but not least – the resources that are available.

Priority-setting requires detailed and timely preparation as well as a formal follow-up of the results especially with regard to enabling and empowering citizens to make an informed choice through their parliaments. A crucial aspect of the process is ensuring that criteria and values are made explicit so that they can be openly discussed.

Priority-setting starts with a reflection on the criteria to be used to set priorities, followed by a series of analyses where value-based and technical approaches may be used. Technical considerations are then weighed against value considerations. This means that an analysis on the basis of explicit criteria is done with contributions from experts as well as from population representatives.

Priority-setting starts with a reflection on the criteria to be used to set priorities, followed by a series of analyses where values and technical approaches may be used. This chapter argues in favour of a combination of approaches in priority-setting, in which technical considerations are weighed against value considerations. This means that analysis on the basis of explicit criteria (such as, but not limited to: burden of the health issue, effectiveness of the intervention, cost of the intervention, acceptability of the intervention, and fairness) is done with contributions from experts (for technical aspects) as well as from population representatives (deliberation, notably on weighing values). The latter is crucial as, in the end, citizens should have the final say in decision-making through democratic processes.

There is not one single set of methods and tools that is considered appropriate in all settings. All those presented in this chapter have advantages and disadvantages or limitations (see Annex 4.2). For this reason, approaches which combine different criteria are recommended. At the moment, a comprehensive HTA process comes the closest to bringing together analyses of different criteria, although it still needs to be complemented by further analyses.

From priority-setting to planning

In priority-setting, the ranking exercise will result in a set of recommended interventions that are considered most important, most effective and least costly. The ranking must take into account preliminary cost implications in order to determine cost-effectiveness, but does not go into detailed operational costing.

The decision-making about how to apply the ranked priorities with regard to the existing resource allocation criteria and formulae is done in a following phase. This decision-making will require compromises and trade-offs. The national criteria and formulae will be applied by the ministry of finance and the MoH, taking into account the expected total volume of resources (fiscal space), after which the planning, detailed costing and budgeting will follow.

Predictability of all types of external financial resources is paramount, since these may determine to a large extent how realistic the scenarios of a Medium-Term Expenditure Framework (MTEF) are.

The sector policy and planning cycle then proceeds with the strategic planning, costing and budgeting, after which follow the implementation stage and M&E.

References

1 The place of health in the post-2015 development agenda: opening remarks at at an informal Member State consultation on health in the post-2015 development agenda. Geneva, 14 September 2012 (http://www.who.int/dg/speeches/2012/mdgs_post2015/en/, accessed 20 September 2016).

2 Health systems financing: the path to universal coverage. world health report 2010. Geneva: World Health Organization: 2010 (http://www.who.int/whr/2010/en/, accessed 20 September 2016).
Green A. An introduction to health planning for developing health systems, 3rd edition. Oxford: Oxford University Press; 2007, 18–20.

3 Ibid.

4 Government of Sierra Leone. Health compact. 2011 (http://www.internationalhealthpartnership.net/fileadmin/uploads/ihp/Documents/Country_Pages/Sierra_Leone/Government%20of%20S.%20Leone%20Health%20Compact.pdf, accessed 12 September 2016).

5 Government of Sierra Leone. National health sector strategic plan 2010-2015. [Freetown]: Ministry of Health and Sanitation; 2009 (http://www.internationalhealthpartnership.net/fileadmin/uploads/ihp/Documents/Country_Pages/Sierra_Leone/NationalHealthSectorStrategicPlan_2010-15.pdf, accessed 12 September 2016).

6 The Government of Sierra Leone. Review of the implementation of the national health sector strategic plan (2010–2015). [Freetown]: Ministry of Health and Sanitation; 2015 (http://uhcpartnership.net/wp-content/uploads/2014/03/Sierra-Leone-NHSSP-Final-Report_FINAL.pdf, accessed 12 September 2016).

7 Government of Sierra Leone. National health sector strategic plan 2010-2015: joint programme of work and funding (JPWF) 2012-2014. [Freetown]: Ministry of Health and Sanitation; 2012 (http://www.nationalplanningcycles.org/sites/default/files/country_docs/Sierra%20Leone/jpwf_final.pdf, accessed 12 September 2016).

8 Government of Sierra Leone. Basic package of essential health services for Sierra Leone. [Freetown]: Ministry of Health and Sanitation; 2010 (http://www.unicef.org/wcaro/wcaro_SL_basic_package_health2010.pdf, accessed 12 September 2016).

9 The Government of Sierra Leone. Review of the implementation of the national health sector strategic plan (2010–2015). [Freetown]: Ministry of Health and Sanitation; 2015 (http://uhcpartnership.net/wp-content/uploads/2014/03/Sierra-Leone-NHSSP-Final-Report_FINAL.pdf, accessed 12 September 2016).

10 Kieny MP, Evans DB, Schmets G, and Kadandale S. Health-system resilience: reflections on the Ebola crisis in western Africa. Bull World Health Organ. 2014; 92: 850.

11 Chalkidou K, Glassman A, Marten R, Vega J, Teerawattananon Y, Tritasavit N, et al. Priority-setting for achieving universal health coverage. Bull World Health Organ. 2016;94(6):462–75 (https://www.ncbi.nlm.nih.gov/pmc/articles/PMC4890204/, accessed 13 September 2016).

12 Everybody's business: strengthening health systems to improve health outcomes: WHO's framework for action. Geneva: World Health Organization; 2007 (http://www.who.int/healthsystems/strategy/everybodys_business.pdf, accessed 13 September 2016).

13 Ham C. Priority-setting in health care: learning from international experience. Health Policy. 1997;42: 49-66. pmid:10173493.

14 Brinkerhoff DW, Bossert TJ. Health governance: concepts, experience, and programming options. Washington (DC): U.S. Agency for International Development; 2008 (Health Systems 20/20, Policy Brief; https://www.hfgproject.org/health-governance-concepts-experience-programming-options/, accessed 13 September 2016).

15 Mitton C, Smith N, Peacock S, Evoy B, Abelson J. Public participation in health care priority setting: a scoping review. Health Policy. 2009;91(3):219–28. doi:10.1016/j.healthpol.2009.01.005.

16 Mitton C, Donaldson C. Health care priority setting: principles, practice and challenges. Cost Eff Resour Alloc. 2004;2(3) (http://www.resource-allocation.com/content/2/1/3, accessed 13 September 2016).

17 Robinson S, Williams I, Dickinson H, Freeman T, Rumbold B. Priority-setting and rationing in healthcare: evidence from the English experience. Soc Sci Med. 2012;75(12):2386–93. doi:10.1016/j.socscimed.2012.09.014.

18 Arvidsson E, André M, Borgquist L, Andersson D, Carlsson P. Setting priorities in primary health care – on whose conditions? A questionnaire study. BMC Fam Pract. 2012;13:114 (http://bmcfampract.biomedcentral.com/articles/10.1186/1471-2296-13-114, accessed 13 September 2016).

19 Bolsewicz Alderman K, Hipgrave D, Jimenez-Soto E. Public engagement in health priority-setting in low- and middle-income countries: current trends and considerations for policy. (PLoS Med. 2013; 10(8) (http://journals.plos.org/plosmedicine/article?id=10.1371/journal.pmed.1001495, accessed 13 September 2016).

20 Mitton C, Donaldson C. Health care priority setting: principles, practice and challenges. Cost Eff Resour Alloc. 2004;2(3) (http://www.resource-allocation.com/content/2/1/3, accessed 13 September 2016).

21 Arvidsson E, André M, Borgquist L, Andersson D, Carlsson P. Setting priorities in primary health care – on whose conditions? A questionnaire study. BMC Fam Pract. 2012;13:114 (http://bmcfampract.biomedcentral.com/articles/10.1186/1471-2296-13-114, accessed 13 September 2016).

22 Sickle-cell disease and other haemoglobin disorders. Geneva: World Health Organization; 2011 (Fact sheet N308; http://www.who.int/mediacentre/factsheets/fs308/en/, accessed 13 September 2016).

23 Living with obstetric fistula: qualitative research findings from Bangladesh and the Democratic Republic of Congo. USAID. (https://www.engenderhealth.org/files/pubs/fistula-care-digital-archive/1/1.2/living-with-obstetric-qualitative-brief-english.pdf, accessed 13 September 2016).

24 Wall LL, Arrowsmith SD, Briggs ND, Lassey A. Urinary incontinence in the developing world: the obstetric fistula. In: Abrams P, Cardozo L, Khoury S, Wein A, editors. Incontinence. 2nd international consultation on incontinence, Paris, July 1–3, 2001. 2nd edition. London: Health Publications Ltd.; 2002: 893–935 (http://www.ics.org/publications/ici_2/chapters/chap12.pdf, accessed 14 September 2016).

25 Luwam Semere L, Nour NM. Obstetric fistula: living with incontinence and shame. Rev Obstet Gynecol. 2008 1(4):193–7 (http://www.ncbi.nlm.nih.gov/pmc/articles/PMC2621054/, accessed 14 September 2016).

26 Goh JTW, Krause H, Tessema AB, Abraha G. Urinary symptoms and urodynamics following obstetric genitourinary fistula repair. Int Urogynecol J. 2012;24(6):947–51 (http://worldwidefistulafund.org/wp-content/uploads/2011/06/Goh-Urodynamics-after-VVF-repair-2013.pdf, accessed 14 September 2016).

27 Robinson S, Williams I, Dickinson H, Freeman T, Rumbold B. Priority-setting and rationing in healthcare: evidence from the English experience.

Soc Sci Med. 2012;75(12):2386–93. doi:10.1016/j.socscimed.2012.09.014.

28 Tromp N, Baltussen R. Mapping of multiple criteria for priority setting of health interventions: an aid for decision makers. BMC Health Serv Res. 2012;12:454 (http://www.ncbi.nlm.nih.gov/pmc/articles/PMC3565954/, accessed 14 September 2016).

29 Primary Care Trust Network. Priority-setting: strategic planning. London: The NHS Confederation; 2008 (http://www.nhsconfed.org/~/media/Confederation/Files/Publications/Documents/Priority%20setting%20strategic%20planning, accessed 14 September 2016).

30 Mitton C, Smith N, Peacock S, Evoy B, Abelson J. Public participation in health care priority setting: a scoping review. Health Policy. 2009;91(3):219–28. doi:10.1016/j.healthpol.2009.01.005.

31 Tromp N, Baltussen R. Mapping of multiple criteria for priority setting of health interventions: an aid for decision makers. BMC Health Serv Res. 2012;12:454 (http://www.ncbi.nlm.nih.gov/pmc/articles/PMC3565954/, accessed 14 September 2016).

32 Baltussen R, Niessen L. Priority setting of health interventions: the need for multi-criteria decision analysis. Cost Eff Resour Alloc. 2006;4:14 (https://www.ncbi.nlm.nih.gov/pmc/articles/PMC1560167/,accessed 15 September 2016).

33 Guide for establishing public health priorities. Course notes, modified from CDC case study: Translating science into practice. 2004.

34 Tromp N, Baltussen R. Mapping of multiple criteria for priority setting of health interventions: an aid for decision makers. BMC Health Serv Res. 2012;12:454 (http://www.ncbi.nlm.nih.gov/pmc/articles/PMC3565954/, accessed 14 September 2016).

35 Buffett C, Ciliska D, Thomas H. Can I use this evidence in my program decision? Assessing applicability and transferability of evidence. Hamilton (ON): National Collaborating Centre for Methods and Tools; 2007 (http://www.nccmt.ca/uploads/media/media/0001/01/110008a2754f35048bb7e8ff446117133b81ab13.pdf, accessed 14 September 2016).

36 Public Health Science Team. Priority-setting in public health. Los Angeles: County of Los Angeles Public Health; 2010. (Quality Improvement Brief; http://publichealth.lacounty.gov/qi/docs/qibrief-prioritysettinginpublichealth.pdf, accessed 14 September 2016).

37 Mendenhall E, De Silva MJ, Hanlon C, Petersen I, Shidhaye R, Jordans M, et al. Acceptability and feasibility of using non-specialist health workers to deliver mental health care: stakeholder perceptions from the PRIME district sites in Ethiopia, India, Nepal, South Africa, and Uganda. Soc Sci & Med. 2014;118:33–42 (http://www.sciencedirect.com/science/article/pii/S0277953614004973, accessed 14 September 2016).

38 Bukachi SA, Onyango-Ouma W, Siso JM, Nyamongo IK, Mutai JK, Hurtig AK, et al. Healthcare priority setting in Kenya: a gap analysis applying the accountability for reasonableness framework. Int J Health Plann Mgmt. 2013. (https://profiles.uonbi.ac.ke/onyangoouma/files/publication_2013.pdf, accessed 14 September 2016).

39 Eliminating female genital mutilation: an interagency statement: UNAIDS, UNDP, UNECA, UNESCO, UNFPA, UNHCHR, UNHCR, UNICEF, UNIFEM, WHO. Geneva: World Health Organization; 2008. (http://apps.who.int/iris/bitstream/10665/43839/1/9789241596442_eng.pdf, accessed 14 September 2016).

40 Mitton C, Donaldson C. Health care priority setting: principles, practice and challenges. Cost Eff Resour Alloc. 2004;2(3) (http://www.resource-allocation.com/content/2/1/3, accessed 13 September 2016).

41 40 Tromp N, Baltussen R. Mapping of multiple criteria for priority setting of health interventions: an aid for decision makers. BMC Health Serv Res. 2012;12:454 (http://www.ncbi.nlm.nih.gov/pmc/articles/PMC3565954/, accessed 14 September 2016).

42 Cambridge Dictionary. Fairness. (http://dictionary.cambridge.org/dictionary/english/fairness, acccessed 14 September 2016).

43 Australian Indigenous HealthInfoNet (2016) Summary of Aboriginal and Torres Strait Islander health status, 2015 Perth (WA): (http://www.healthinfonet.ecu.edu.au/health-facts/summary, accessed 14 September 2016).

44 Why does the health gap exist? Melbourne: Oxfam Australia. (https://www.oxfam.org.au/what-we-do/indigenous-australia/close-the-gap/australias-indigenous-health-crisis-in-depth/, accessed 14 September 2016).

45 Australia's disturbing health disparities set Aboriginals apart. Bull World Health Organ. 2008;86(4):241–320 (http://www.who.int/bulletin/volumes/86/4/08-020408/en/, accessed 15 September 2016).

46 The health and welfare of Australia's Aboriginal and Torres Strait Islander people 2011. The Australian Institute of Health and Welfare. (http://www.aihw.gov.au/indigenous-observatory/health-and-welfare/, accessed 15 September 2016).

47 Indigenous health: 2014–2015 budget outcomes. Canberra: Australian Government Department of Health. 2016. (https://www.health.gov.au/Indigenous, accessed 15 September 2016).

48 Schöne-Seifert B. The 'rule of rescue' in medical priority-setting: ethical plausibilities and implausibilities. In: Baurmann M, Lahno, editors. Perspectives in Moral Science. Rationality, Markets and Morals. 2009:0;421–30 (http://www.rmm-journal.de/downloads/030_schoene_seifert.pdf, accessed 15 September 2016).

49 The International Health Partnership. (http://www.internationalhealthpartnership.net/, accessed 15 September 2016).

50 Hipgrave DB, Alderman KB, Anderson I, Soto EJ. Health sector priority-setting at meso-level in lower and middle income countries: lessons learned, available options and suggested steps. Soc Sci & Med. 2014;102:190–200.

51 Kaplan W. Approaches to priority setting. Geneva: World Health Organization; update of 2004 version of article (Priority Medicines for Europe and the World, Background Paper 3; http://www.who.int/medicines/areas/priority_medicines/BP3_Approaches.pdf, accessed 15 September 2016).

52 Hauck K, Smith PC, Goddard M. The economics of priority setting for health care: a literature review. Washington (DC): World Bank, Human Development Network; 2004 (Health, Nutrition and Population Discussion Paper; http://siteresources.worldbank.org/HEALTHNUTRITIONANDPOPULATION/

Resources/281627-1095698140167/Chapter3Final. pdf, accessed 15 September 2016).

53 Issel LM. Health program planning and evaluation: a practical, systematic approach for community health. Sudbury (MA): Jones & Bartlett Learning; 2004.

54 Guide for establishing public health priorities. Course notes, modi ed from CDC case study: Translating science into practice. 2004.

55 Garland M, Stull J. Public health and health system reform: access, priority-setting, and allocation of resources. In Jennings B, Kahn J, Mastroianni A, Parker L, editors. Ethics and public health: model curriculum. Washington (DC): Association of Schools of Public Health; 2003.

56 Clark S, Weale A. Social values in health priority setting: a conceptual framework. J Health Organ Manag. 2012;26(3):293–316 (http://www.ucl.ac.uk/socialvalues/downloads/files/Social_Values_and_Priority_Setting_in_Health_-_Background__paper.pdf, accessed 16 September 2016).

57 Daniels N. Four unsolved rationing problems: a challenge. Hastings Cent Rep. 1994;24(4):27–9. pmid:7960702.

58 Olsen JA. Theories of justice and their implications for priority setting in health care. J Health Econ. 1997;16(6): 625–39. pmid:10176776.

59 Williams A. Priority setting in public and private health care: a guide through the ideological jungle. University of York Centre for Health Economics, 1988 (Health Economics Consortium Discussion paper 36; http://www.york.ac.uk/che/pdf/dp36.pdf, accessed 15 September 2016).

60 Hadorn DC. The problem of discrimination in health care priority setting. JAMA. 1992;268(11):1454–9. pmid:1387422.

61 Williams I, Phillips D, Nicholson C, Shearer H. Evaluation of a deliberative approach to citizen involvement in health care priority setting. Leadership in Health Services. 2014;27(1):5–19. doi: 10.1108/LHS-01-2013-0002..

62 Mitton C, Smith N, Peacock S, Evoy B, Abelson J. Public participation in health care priority setting: a scoping review. Health Policy. 2009;91(3):219–28. doi:10.1016/j.healthpol.2009.01.005.

63 Campbell S. Deliberative priority-setting. CIHR KT module. Ottawa: Canadian Institutes of Health Research; 2010 (http://www.cihr-irsc.gc.ca/e/43533.html, accessed 15 September 2016).

64 National Association of County and City Health Officials (NACCHO). Guide to prioritization techniques. (http://www.naccho.org/topics/infrastructure/accreditation/upload/Prioritization-Summaries-and-Examples-2.pdf, accessed 15 September 2014).

65 Blackwood R. The use of Delphi methods. 2009. (http://www.healthknowledge.org.uk/public-health-textbook/research-methods/1c-health-care-evaluation-health-care-assessment/use-delphi-methods, accessed 15 September 2016).

66 Baltussen R, Niessen L. Priority setting of health interventions: the need for multi-criteria decision analysis. Cost Eff Resour Alloc. 2006;4:14 (https://www.ncbi.nlm.nih.gov/pmc/articles/PMC1560167/,accessed 15 September 2016).

67 Baltussen R. Priority-setting of public spending in developing countries: do not try to do everything for everybody. Health Policy. 2006;78:149–56 (http://www.who.int/choice/publications/p_2006_priority_setting.pdf, accessed 20 September 2016).

68 Kapiriri L, Arnesen T, Norheim OF. Is cost-effectiveness analysis preferred to severity of disease as the main guiding principle in priority setting in resource poor settings? The case of Uganda. Cost Eff Resour Alloc. 2004;2:1 (https://resource-allocation.biomedcentral.com/articles/10.1186/1478-7547-2-1, accessed 15 September 2016).

69 Baltussen R, Niessen L. Priority setting of health interventions: the need for multi-criteria decision analysis. Cost Eff Resour Alloc. 2006;4:14 (https://www.ncbi.nlm.nih.gov/pmc/articles/PMC1560167/,accessed 15 September 2016).

70 Glassman A, Chalkidou K. Priority-setting in health: building institutions for smarter public spending. Washington (DC): Center for Global Development; 2012 (http://apps.who.int/medicinedocs/documents/s19985en/s19985en.pdf, accessed 16 September 2016).

71 Hipgrave DB, Alderman KB, Anderson I, Soto EJ. Health sector priority-setting at meso-level in lower and middle income countries: lessons learned, available options and suggested steps. Soc Sci & Med. 2014;102:190–200.

72 Health System Intelligence Project. The Health Planner's Toolkit. Health System Intelligence Project. Ontario: 2008. (http://www.hclinkontario.ca/resources/14-hclink/resources/45-resources-planning.html, accessed 16 September 2016).

73 Khayatzadeh-Mahani A, Fotaki M, Harvey G. Priority setting and implementation in a centralized health system: a case study of Kerman province in Iran. Health Policy Plan. 2013;28:480–94 (http://heapol.oxfordjournals.org/content/28/5/480.full.pdf, accessed 16 September 20.16).

74 Kapiriri L, Norheim OF, Heggenhougen K. Public participation in health planning and priority setting at the district level in Uganda. Health Policy Plan. 2003;18(2);205–13 (http://heapol.oxfordjournals.org/content/18/2/205.long, accessed 16 September 2016).)

75 Health in 2015: from MDGs, Millennium Development Goals to SDGs, Sustainable Development Goals. Geneva: World Health Organization; 2015 (http://www.who.int/gho/publications/mdgs-sdgs/en/, accessed 16 September 2016).

76 De Maeseneer J, Willems S, De Sutter A, Van de Geuchte I, Billings M. Primary health care as a strategy for achieving equitable care: a literature review commissioned by the Health Systems Knowledge Network. Witwatersrand: Health Systems Knowledge Network; 2007. http://www.who.int/social_determinants/resources/csdh_media/primary_health_care_2007_en.pdf, accessed 16 September 2016).

77 Adjei S, Nazzar A, Seddoh A, Blok L, Plummer D. The impact of HIV and AIDS funding and programming on health system strengthening in Malawi. KIT, University of Malawi; 2011 (Health System Research Series No. 4; https://www.kit.nl/health/wp-content/uploads/publications/1919_111114_KIT_Ghana.pdf, accessed 16 September 2016).

Annex 4.1

Methods and tools for technical approaches

Health Technology Assessment

The health technology assessment system defines the following 7 steps.

1. **Registration** assures safety and efficacy of new products and provides a gateway for considering a technology for public or donor funding.

2. **Scoping** identifies and selects technologies (broadly defined as policies, interventions, drugs, diagnostics, and other products) for evaluation depending on country or donor priority-setting goals.

3. **Cost-effectiveness** analysis uses widely-accepted economic evaluation methods, tools, and systematic evidence reviews, building on defined priority-setting criteria, such as health impact, equity, and financial protection, as relevant.

4. **Budget impact analysis** examines and projects the potential financial and fiscal impact of adopting and diffusing a technology.

5. **Deliberative process** considers the results of cost-effectiveness analysis and budget impact analysis as well as more subjective decision-making criteria dependent on national values and context to recommend public or donor funding.

6. **Decision** assesses recommendations and makes decisions to include a technology in public or donor budgets.

7. **Appeals, tracking, and evaluation** allows for the appeal of recommendations and associated analysis, as well as the tracking and evaluation of the impact of decisions.

Cost-effectiveness analysis (CEA) compares the relative costs and effects (outcomes) of two or more courses of action.

(a) Marginal cost-effectiveness analysis (MCEA), also called incremental cost-effectiveness analysis, is only concerned with spending the marginal (i.e. the "next") dollar on the most cost-effective option. It is exclusively based on an assessment of existing interventions, regardless of any explicit constraints. MCEA relies on a threshold as a simple decision rule for choosing whether or not to do something: if the cost-effectiveness of that activity is under the threshold, the activity should be implemented, but not otherwise. The threshold can represent some notion of social benefit but in practice it is usually defined by precedent. Such marginal decision-making on new priorities is likely to allow only for marginal improvements. The difference between the optimal position and the current position will tend to grow if marginal decision-making with respect to such criteria is repeated over many periods.

(b) Generalized cost-effectiveness analysis (GCEA) does not assume that current practice is economically worthwhile. It estimates the cost-effectiveness of both the new and existing technology compared with a hypothetical "null" comparator. In GCEA, this null position is estimated by simulating the effects of "stopping" activities relevant to the domain of analysis. It does not mean removing all the effects that may persist after such activities are stopped -- the effects will usually wane as the population ages. In the WHO GCEA toolbox, known as CHOICE (http://www.who.int/choice/en/), the null reference scenario does not demand that they be artificially removed. Instead, the WHO CHOICE approach assumes that priority-setting seeks to maximize benefit in a real-world setting. Therefore, CHOICE takes into account an explicit budget constraint (e.g. the current health expenditure) and realizable health gains are analysed with respect to this constraint. WHO CHOICE produces a set of interventions (activities, policies or projects) which, for a given budget, yields the highest achievable health gain. GCEA may identify opportunities for disinvestment or for increased investment in existing activities. In MCEA, such opportunities will be systematically missed.

(c) Extended cost-effectiveness analysis (ECEA) "extends" GCEA by estimating, in addition to the health gains of an intervention, the benefits in financial risk protection and fairness (i.e. equity). These benefits can be assessed independently and reported in a "benefits dashboard".

Program Budgeting and Marginal Analysis (PBMA) is used to determine the optimal mix of a particular set of services for a given amount of resources. While programme budgeting was originally conceived as a tool for tabulating expenditure of different programmes within an organization, marginal analysis was required as an evaluative technique to examine the reallocation of resources in order to improve benefit to the defined population. Based on the underlying economic principle of opportunity cost, use of marginal analysis can aid decision-makers in identifying potential changes in the mix of services provided which may lead to maximizing the health gains.

Limitations of PBMA mentioned in literature are:

(i) the method is exclusively based on current programmes/priority areas and allocation criteria, and
(ii) it is both time and data-intensive.

Burden of disease analysis (BoD)

Burden of disease analysis aims to quantify the gap between the ideal of living to old age in good health, and the current situation where healthy life is shortened by illness, injury, disability and premature death. BoD analysis can include epidemiological measures such as incidence, prevalence and mortality rates. The impact of a health problem is measured by financial cost, mortality, morbidity, or other indicators. Morbidity can be quantified in terms of quality-adjusted life-years (QALYs) or disability-adjusted life-years (DALYs), both of which quantify the number of years lost due to disease. Since DALYs/QALYs measure for loss of quality and productivity in life, these indicators are notably interesting in a setting where chronic conditions due to non-communicable diseases (such as diabetes type 2) are gaining importance over life-threatening communicable diseases (e.g. malaria).

The following examples illustrate models for BoD analysis that can also be considered in addition to the traditional BoD means of analysis.

- The Patient Generated Index (PGI) is self-administered, and aims to quantify (via questionnaire) the effect of a medical condition on a patient's quality of life in a way that has meaning and relevance in the context of the individual's daily life.

- The Lives Saved Tool (LiST) is a decision-making computer software that enables the estimation of intervention impact on mortality at national, regional and global levels. It contains an expansive evidence base of context-specific intervention effectiveness. A possible disadvantage of the tool is that it could encourage a vertical approach in health care strengthening, and does not take into account contextual factors that influence feasibility and effectiveness.

Health Needs Assessments (HNA)

Health Needs Assessments can include various epidemiological measurements on patterns of disease within a community or population. Examining these patterns can help to identify inequalities in health. The assessment outcome may, however, not be entirely in line with economic evaluations that focus on health problems with cost-effective soltions, because the emphasis with HNA is on high-mortality health problems (which may not be cost-effective). Despite this, HNAs provide a foundational basis for evaluating fundamental health problems.

2x2 grid

The 2x2 grid helps to evaluate priorities according to certain criteria. The grid consists of four quadrants; one broad criterion is assigned to each axis (e.g. "importance/urgency", "cost/impact", "need/feasibility", etc.). Arrows on the axes indicate "high" or "low". Each quadrant is labelled as either "high need/high feasibility", "high need/low feasibility", "low need/high feasibility", "low need/low feasibility". Competing activities, projects, or programmes are evaluated against how well this set of criteria is met. They are then categorized and prioritized.

- **High need/high feasibility** – With high demand and high return on investment, these are the highest priority items and should be given sufficient resources to maintain and continuously improve.
- **Low need/high feasibility** – Often politically important and difficult to eliminate, these items may need to be redesigned to reduce investment while maintaining impact.
- **High need/low feasibility** – These are long-term projects which have a great deal of potential but will require significant investment. Focusing on too many of these items can overwhelm an agency.
- **Low need/low feasibility** – With minimal return on investment, these are the lowest priority items and should be phased out, allowing for resources to be reallocated to higher priority items.

Box A.4.1 shows a hypothetical 2x2 grid assessment of priorities in an Ebola outbreak situation. The need and feasibility parameters evolve over time, demonstrating that this sort of exercise can be done at regular intervals.

Box A.4.1

Priority-setting at national level after an Ebola outbreak

Emergency phase:
should stopping the outbreak be a priority?
High need/low feasibility
Need: Risk of outbreak further spreading, possibly becoming a pandemic.
Feasibility: No cure readily available; isolation of cases and prevention difficult.

Health system recovery:
should short-term investments be a priority?
High need/high feasibility
Need: Due to system breakdown (e.g. shortage of human and other resources), care in the affected areas is increasingly insufficient.
Feasibility: Emergency funding allows for rapid investments (e.g. by recruitment of new staff and by adding laboratory services) and for strengthening of key services (e.g. improvement of surveillance practices).

Resilient health system building:
medium-term strategies
Low need/high feasibility
Need: Parallel to the system recovery investments, an in-depth analysis of structural health system flaws (including those related to socioeconomic health determinants, and therefore multisectoral) can be thoroughly planned and implemented. Based on the results of this analysis, medium-term strategies can be developed for tackling deeply-rooted system weaknesses.
Feasibility: Firm political commitment at national and international level allows for strengthening the overall health system so that it can better prevent similar outbreaks and their spreading, as well as improve service readiness for the care of affected populations.

Basic Priority Rating System (BPRS)

The BPRS (Hanlon method) prioritizes health problems based on the nature of the problem and the effectiveness of the solution. The nature of the problem is defined by key variables, including the weight, severity, urgency, economic consequences, willingness and involvement of others and the effectiveness of the intervention. Each variable is given a rating on a scale of 1–10 (low to high). The method uses the steps outlined below.

Step 1: Rating against specified criteria – Once a list of health problems has been identified, on a scale from one through ten, each health problem is rated on the following criteria: size of health problem, magnitude of health problem, and effectiveness of potential interventions.

Step 2: The PEARL test is applied (see below).

Step 3: Priority scores are calculated, based on the three criteria.

Step 4: The health problems are ranked, based on the priority scores calculated in Step 3 of the Hanlon method, the highest priority score receiving a rank of "1", the next highest priority score receiving a rank of "2", and so on.

Propriety, Economics, Acceptability, Resources and Legality component (PEARL)

Once health problems have been rated by criteria, PEARL is used to eliminate any health problems which receive an answer of "No" to any of the questions below on aspects of feasibility. Alternatively, corrective action is planned to ensure that potential health priorities meet all five feasibility factors.

- Propriety – Is a programme for the health problem suitable?
- Economics – Does it make economic sense to address the problem? Are there economic consequences if a problem is not addressed?
- Acceptability – Will a community accept the programme? Is it wanted?
- Resources – Is funding available or potentially available for a programme?
- Legality – Do current laws allow programme activities to be implemented?

Annex 4.2

Methods and tools for value-based approaches

Accountability for Reasonableness (AFR)

AFR is a decision-making approach that builds upon four conditions:

(i) relevance to the local setting, decided by agreed criteria;
(ii) publicizing priority-setting decisions and the reasons behind them;
(iii) the establishment of revisions/appeal mechanisms for challenging and revising decisions;
(iv) the provision of leadership to ensure that the first three conditions are met.

Citizen consultation processes

Citizen consultations can capture a population's demands, opinion and expectation on health-related matters in order to improve the transparency and relevance of the priority-setting process. Please refer to Chapter 2 "Population consultation on needs and expectations" in this handbook for more detail.

Multivoting technique (MVT)

1. Round-one vote: on a note card, all participants anonymously vote for as many priority focus areas as desired.

2. Update list: all votes are tallied and a small number of focus areas receiving most votes are posted for the group to view.

3. Round-two vote: all participants vote up to three times for the remaining focus areas.

4. Update list: all votes are re-tallied and the three focus areas receiving three or more votes are posted for the group to view.

5. Round-three vote: all participants vote up to two times and the only item with three or more votes is the chosen focus area.

Nominal group technique (NGT)

The technique involves a facilitator to direct a round-robin series of voting whereby an issue or problem is brought forward by each participant in the group. This is done "silently" with no group discussion and produces a lengthy list of areas that are recommended by the group for prioritization; this is also known as silent brainstorming. The items are then grouped together and categorized by nature of the issue and a discussion is facilitated to determine if the items measure up to the criteria decided upon prior to the NGT process. Participants are then asked to individually rank the various health problems identified on a scale of 1–10 (or most appropriate scaling measure). Responses are then collected, and calculated by the facilitator, who reports the scores back to the group. This process is then repeated, either by group consensus or individual ranking until the results are narrowed down further.

Delphi technique

The Delphi technique facilitates decision-making based on the results of questionnaires sent to a group of experts. Several rounds of questionnaires are sent out, and the anonymous responses are aggregated and shared with the group after each round. The experts are allowed to adjust their answers in subsequent rounds. Since multiple rounds of questions are asked and the panel is told what the group thinks as a whole, the Delphi technique seeks to reach the correct response through consensus.

Table A.4.1 Example Delphi questionnaire

In your view, which of the following clinical areas should be high priority for development of an improved evidence base on minority ethnic groups and their health needs?

CLINICAL AREA	PRIORITY LEVEL FOR DEVELOPMENT OF AN IMPROVED EVIDENCE BASE	COMMENTS – INCLUDING ANY PARTICULARLY IMPORTANT TOPICS FOR ACTION
Mental Health	Low 1 2 3 4 5 High 0 (don't know)	
Cancer	Low 1 2 3 4 5 High 0 (don't know)	
Immunization	Low 1 2 3 4 5 High 0 (don't know)	

The questionnaire provides space for respondents to raise any other issues relating to the topic. The first round of the questionnaire aims to categorize opinions under common headings. Based on an analysis of round 1 responses, a second questionnaire is then prepared.

Table A.4.2 Example Delphi questionnaire

Cancer has been identified as a high priority for developing an evidence base relating to minority ethnic groups. Within this clinical area, what aspects should research focus on?

RESEARCH AREA	PRIORITY FOR DEVELOPMENT OF AN IMPROVED EVIDENCE BASE	COMMENTS, IMPORTANT TOPICS FOR ACTION
Identifying risk factors of disease	Low 1 2 3 4 5 High 0 (don't know)	
Identifying barriers to access to services	Low 1 2 3 4 5 High 0 (don't know)	
Improving the patient experience for minority ethnic groups	Low 1 2 3 4 5 High 0 (don't know)	

After analysis of the round 2 responses, a third round questionnaire may be designed. Here, the second round questionnaire is repeated but incorporates scores from the second questionnaire results. This gives participants a chance to see how the rest of the group prioritized the areas. If the participant then wants to change his/her opinion on the basis of the group consensus, he/she has the opportunity to do so.

Finally, the results of the third round questionnaire are analysed for agreement and degree of consensus and the findings are reported.

Multi-criteria decision-making (MCDM)

MCDM is a quantitative decision analysis model that captures preferences of decision-makers and discovers the most desired solution to the problem. It is a hybrid method in that it incorporates both technical and value-based approaches. It is based on a performance matrix where each row describes an option and each column describes the performance of the options against each criterion. To do so, five criteria are applied: maximization of general population health, the distribution of health in the population, specific societal preferences, budgetary and practical constraints, and political considerations.

Chapter 5

Strategic planning: transforming priorities into plans

Frank Terwindt

Dheepa Rajan

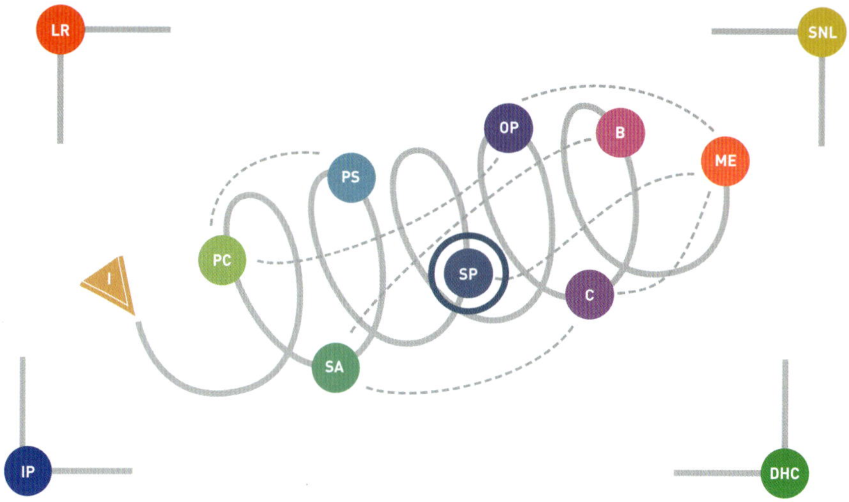

- I — CHAPTER 1 Introduction
- PC — CHAPTER 2 Population consultation on needs and expectations
- SA — CHAPTER 3 Situation analysis of the health sector
- PS — CHAPTER 4 Priority-setting for national health policies, strategies and plans
- SP — CHAPTER 5 Strategic planning: transforming priorities into plans
- OP — CHAPTER 6 Operational planning: transforming plans into action
- C — CHAPTER 7 Estimating cost implications of a national health policy, strategy or plan
- B — CHAPTER 8 Budgeting for health
- ME — CHAPTER 9 Monitoring, evaluation and review of national health policies, strategies and plans

Cross-cutting topics relevant to national health planning

- LR — CHAPTER 10 Law, regulation and strategizing for health
- SNL — CHAPTER 11 Strategizing for health at sub-national level
- IP — CHAPTER 12 Intersectoral planning for health and health equity
- DHC — CHAPTER 13 Strategizing in distressed health contexts

Overview

In health, strategic planning aims at identifying, sequencing and timing medium-term interventions for the health sector in a comprehensive way. The end product is the sector strategic plan which guides the activities and investments that are necessary for achieving medium-term outcomes and impact.

In line with this definition, the purpose of strategic planning in health is to define a medium-term orientation and focus for the development of the health system. Decision-making should be based on a thorough analysis of the current situation, lessons learned from previous plans, expected available resources and chosen priorities.

In this chapter, guidance is provided on developing a relevant NHPSP that is referred to, consulted and used. Steps are proposed to manage the NHPSP development process and common challenges and mistakes are pointed out with suggested solutions.

Summary

What is strategic planning?

In health, strategic planning aims at identifying, sequencing and timing medium-term interventions for the health sector in a comprehensive way. The end product is the medium-term sector strategic plan that guides activities and investments necessary for achieving medium-term outcomes and impact.

Why is it important to transform priorities into a plan?

Key reasons for transforming priorities into plans are:

- to concretize priorities;
- to keep focus on the medium to long term without deviating from the optimal path;
- to avoid fragmentation of the health sector;
- to help focus the policy dialogue on health sector priorities;
- to guide operational planning, resource allocation, and sector monitoring and evaluation.

When should operational planning take place?

In the context of ongoing comprehensive health sector development, strategic planning is an iterative process that should be conducted every 3–5 years (medium-term). The strategic planning exercise generally comes after the phase of priority-setting and precedes operational planning.

Who should be a part of strategic planning?

Strategizing for health will be more effective if a wide range of stakeholders are involved in it, and both the process and the product are truly owned by the country. To make the process effective, health sector stakeholders will need to come to a common understanding of the key issues and share institutional goals and expectations. Such an inclusive approach is likely to be more potent, not only in terms of planning the right vision and activities, but also in ensuring that implementation of the strategic plan is jointly undertaken by all actor groups.

How do we transform priorities into plans?

In this chapter, guidance is give on:

- preparation of NHPSP development;
- setting goals (or strategic directions) in line with commonly agreed priorities;
- setting objectives in the form of targets (and their baselines);
- formulating broad activity areas;
- providing orientation on NHPSP implementation;
- approval and dissemination of the NHPSP;
- NHPSP document structure.

Anything else to consider?

- decentralized environment;
- fragile environment;
- highly aid-dependent context.

5.1 What is strategic planning?

5.1.1 Definitions

Planning is a method of trying to ensure that the resources available now and in the future are used in the most efficient way to achieve explicit objectives.[1] Planning also includes organizing and preparing the necessary interventions for meeting those objectives.

In terms of timing, three types of planning can be distinguished in health sector development:

1. long-/medium-term planning, which is mostly used for strategic orientation;
2. short-term planning, which guides operational aspects of implementation;
3. ad-hoc plans/disaster preparedness plans, which are necessary in a situation of important unforeseen developments.

Three characteristics of strategic planning, different from those of operational planning, taken from entrepreneurial business theories, are:

1. a long-term, rather than a short-term, focus;
2. a comprehensive, "whole-of-business" perspective, rather than a collection of divisional business plans;
3. a concern to "fit" the business within the external environment expected to affect the business in the longer term.

In health, strategic planning aims at identifying, sequencing and timing medium-term interventions for the health sector in a comprehensive way. The end product is the NHPSP, which guides activities and investments necessary for achieving medium-term outcomes and impact. The details on implementation of the NHPSP, i.e. the most appropriate course of action to fulfil the goals or strategic directions of a NHPSP, are reflected in operational plans (see Fig. 5.2).

Strategic planning aims at identifying, sequencing and timing medium-term interventions for the health sector in a comprehensive way.

In line with this definition, the purpose of strategic planning in health is to define a medium-term orientation and focus for the development of the health system, based on a sector vision, policies, strategies and priorities. In essence, it is the development of the NHPSP.

In strategic planning, decision-making is based on a thorough analysis of the current situation, lessons learned from previous plans, expected available resources and chosen priorities.

Health sector strategic planning covers:

- delivery of comprehensive health services, including personal and non-personal, clinical and non-clinical services;
- support functions for health service delivery;
- health systems governance;
- health research;
- overall health systems development;
- reforms (institutional, organizational and administrative, including for decentralization);
- collaboration/coordination with other sectors.

5.1.2 Strategic planning in relation to other phases in the policy and planning cycle

Health sector strategic planning includes:

- sequencing and timing;
- attributing general responsibilities;
- linking interventions (activities and investments) with resource attribution;
- establishing a sector monitoring and evaluation system that allows for measuring implementation (inputs and outputs), effectiveness and result (outcomes and impact), as well as adjustments of the plan in the course of its implementation, as per need.

In any case, NHPSP development is in a sense an ongoing process. While the overarching NHPSP document is developed jointly by health sector stakeholders once every 3–5 years, an adjustment for an area-specific strategy such as, for instance, community health or malaria, may be slightly earlier or later but impacts on the core substance of the NHPSP. In the same vein, specific activities may require a separate strategy, such as performance-based financing, which will affect the NHPSP content. In practice, only very major changes and events elicit a completely new NHPSP. Smaller changes can be taken into account through modifications to the operational plans, which are more flexible and closer to the actual tasks undertaken on the ground.

A strategic plan defines above all the direction in which the health sector should go, while an operational plan describes in detail how to get there.

(a) Strategic planning vis-à-vis operational planning

The processes for strategic and operational planning can be viewed as a continuum made up of a series of "whats" and "hows".[2] A strategic plan defines above all the direction in which the health sector should go, while an operational plan describes more in detail how to get there.[I] For example, "strengthen primary health care services" can be an objective of a strategic plan. The strategic plan may then lay out proposed broad activity areas for strengthening primary health care services, such as "ensure implementation of the essential health services package". An operational plan would detail the activities to be undertaken to provide the services mentioned in the essential health services package, such as "training programme on nutrition for district hospital staff" or "support and supervision visits by district health management team".

Operational plans specify the different activities which are suitable to implement the strategies. The strategic plan takes a longer-term view (generally 3–5 years or more), while operational plans focus on shorter time segments (annually, semester, quarterly, monthly) (see Table 5.1).

I See Chapter 6 "Operational planning: transforming plans into action" in this handbook

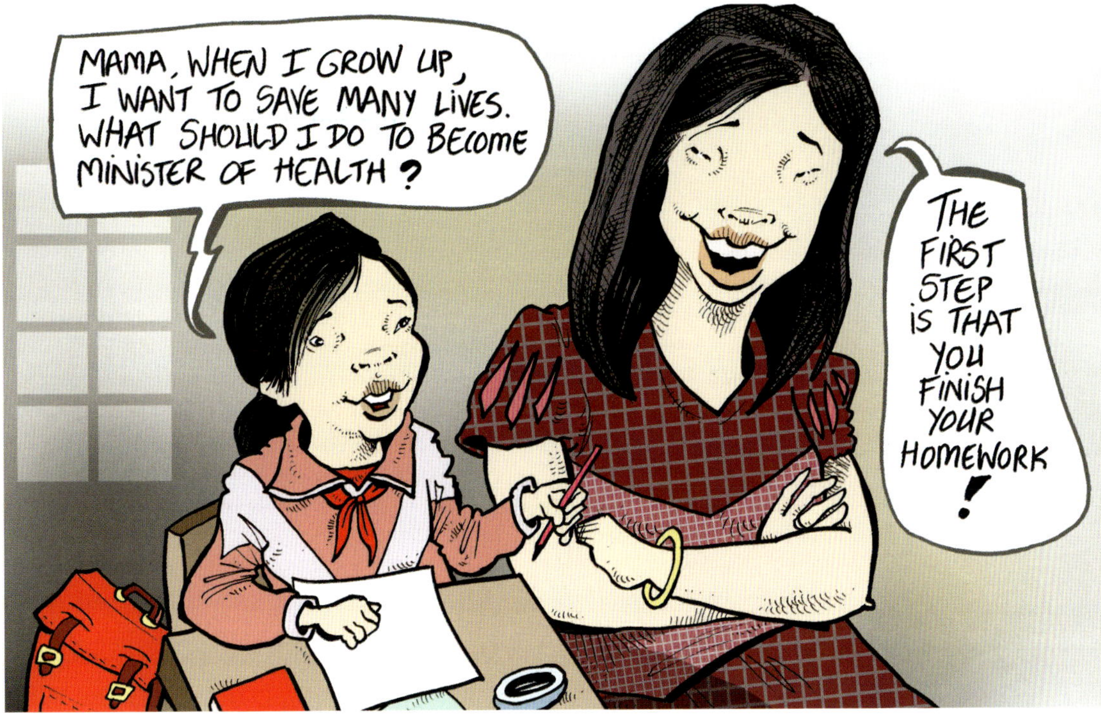
MAMA, WHEN I GROW UP, I WANT TO SAVE MANY LIVES. WHAT SHOULD I DO TO BECOME MINISTER OF HEALTH?
THE FIRST STEP IS THAT YOU FINISH YOUR HOMEWORK!

Damian Glez; scenario by Bruno Meessen.

Fig. 5.1 Strategic planning: sequencing actions to reach a long-term vision

Table 5.1 Key characteristics of strategic and operational planning

	STRATEGIC PLANNING	OPERATIONAL PLANNING
PERSPECTIVE	Medium- to long-term development	Short(er)-term interventions
FOCUS	Strategic direction for the health sector	Concrete activity implementation
TIME FRAME	3- to 5-year document	1 year, sometimes shorter time frame
FLEXIBILITY	Less likely to change during its term	Can more easily be adapted and modified according to changing circumstances

Operational plans are sometimes also called implementation plans. This can lead to confusion because strategic plans are also implemented. Also, operational plans are sometimes considered to be plans specifically for middle- and lower-management levels. This is incorrect, as high-level staff at the central ministry of health (MoH) work on the basis of both the sector strategic plan as well as on their unit's operational plan.

Operational plans must be linked to the strategic plan (see Fig 5.3) by defining the actions that are to be taken to produce outputs in a specified period of time as defined by the strategic plan.

The operational plan should identify the resources required, activities to be carried out and those involved in and responsible for carrying them out. For the strategic plan, there will always be a certain degree of uncertainty about the feasibility to achieve outcomes and impact, as it will depend on the details of implementation during a medium term (approximately five years) period which one cannot always foresee. By contrast, the feasibility to fully implement the operational plan must be assured as much as possible. For a time horizon of one year or less, this is possible because targets, responsibilities and resources are quantified and the operational plan is usually linked to an approved sector budget.

Fig. 5.2 Link between the strategic (NHPSP) and operational plan

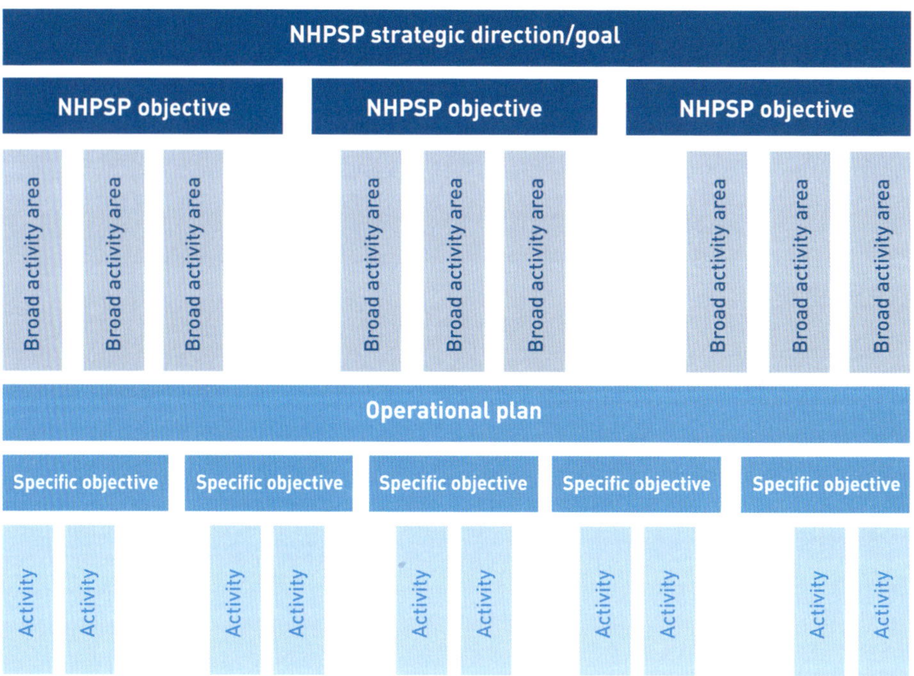

Box 5.1

Linking strategic and operational planning in the United Republic of Tanzania[3]

The United Republic of Tanzania's health sector is guided by its national health sector strategic plan, which is implemented through operational plans at different levels of the health system, including in districts. The MoH provides overall strategic directions, guidance, supervision and training for districts in operational planning, with the aim of bridging the strategic plan at a national level with operational plans on the ground. In 2007, the MoH developed training manuals for this purpose, in the recognition that district operational plans in the past had very little linkage to broad NHPSP objectives and activity areas, thus rendering the tracking of long-term objectives difficult.

The training module encourages districts to study the NHPSP objectives and discuss with MoH planners how those objectives can be realistically operationalized at district level, given the donor landscape, local epidemiology and public health needs.

(b) Strategic planning vis-à-vis costing and budgeting

Strategic planning and costing go hand in hand.[II] The initial, more approximate, cost estimation should be considered as a reference point to inform the strategic planning process, while further fine-tuning of cost calculations should reflect a back-and-forth dialogue with health planning stakeholders. Understanding the costs and resource implications is imperative to the policy dialogue on the affordability of the stated aims of the NHPSP, and more importantly, whether they are feasible and realistic, given the existing state of the health system.

In order to ensure realism of the exercise, it is imperative that the link between planning and costing is very strong from the beginning – any NHPSP discussion on planned reforms and targets should take into consideration the resource requirements. The process is highly iterative because planning decisions must take into consideration operational and financial feasibility, while the cost projections need to adjust between planned activities and available fiscal space.

A cost estimation of a NHPSP can thus help anchor the planning process in reality. The costing process often serves to demonstrate that a NHPSP may be too aspirational, in that it does not consider the constraints of limited financial resources available. The costing needs to be combined with realistic projections of available

II See Chapter 7 "Estimating cost implications of a national health policy, strategy, or plan" in this handbook.

financing (all sources included), in order for the analysis to be credible. Countries may use frameworks such as the Medium Term Expenditure Framework (MTEF) or other approaches to organize and present the information.[III]

If a MTEF is being developed simultaneously with the NHPSP, it is possible to go back and forth between the drafts of both documents before finalizing them, in order to ensure that they are compatible.

III See Chapter 8 "Budgeting for health" in this handbook.

5.1.3 A brief overview of strategic planning approaches

(a) Health sector planning may be more top-down or more bottom-up

In top-down planning cycle stages, terminology and orientation are predetermined by the central level for the whole planning process, starting with overall design, goal and objective-setting, up to implementation modalities, possibly even targets. The lower levels of the health system are mainly seen as implementation arms of the central level. In bottom-up planning, the central level acts to support managers and directors of different budget centres (where the operational planning will take place) in the identification of issues that are important and relevant to them, which helps feed into the strategic planning process. The input from the various operational units is then used as the principal starting point for central-level planning.

In the context of this chapter, we categorically advocate for the latter approach, with a process as participatory as possible, bringing in a wide range of expert and non-expert stakeholders at various points during the health policy and planning cycle.

In reality, many countries may practice a mix of top-down and bottom-up planning. Bottom-up planning does not mean a disengagement of the central level – instead, the central-level health authority has a pivotal role to play in providing guidance and collaborating with the different health sector institutions and sub-national entities to ensure alignment with the strategic directions given by the NHPSP.

(b) Strategic planning may be done in a more normative or a more flexible way

If the approach is normative, it is a rational, orderly progression of predefined steps in a policy cycle, usually set by the central health authority. In such a situation, the central-level decision-making capability tends to be located at the top, concentrated at the level of a limited number of actors from senior management.

Strategic planning can be approached in different ways: top-down or bottom-up; normative or flexible.

If the approach is more flexible, it allows for a certain degree of autonomy of the various interest groups, population groups and government agencies involved in the planning process. The emphasis here is on discussion and negotiation where a pragmatic path helps to sift through the often divergent values and views.

Again, in reality, many countries practice a mix of both. One can also have a normative bottom-up as well as a flexible top-down approach. A certain level of normative central-level guidance and authority is necessary to ensure coherence across the different topics discussed as well as consistency across geographical regions. The central level should approach its collaboration with other stakeholders in the spirit of a partnership, where all views are taken into consideration in a balanced way and feed into the final decisions made collectively. Flexibility is necessary here in order to accommodate and/or challenge the diverging views.

5.2 Why is it important to transform priorities into a plan?

Priorities must be translated and articulated into a written strategy and orientation for action. The rationale for this is elaborated upon in this section.

5.2.1 To concretize priorities

A good strategic plan translates long-term sector vision and priorities into concrete implementation phases and incremental steps, thereby providing a medium-term horizon for overall sector development. This ensures continuity and direction of the longer-term priorities, considering that many problems are complex and cannot be solved within a short time frame.

A good strategic plan translates long-term sector vision and priorities into concreate implementation phases and steps, providing a medium-term horizon for sector development.

Strategic planning is a function that – if well done – translates leadership vision, objectives and priorities into a robust document that will ensure not only effective and smooth implementation of activities but also efficiency and sustainability. If one views all of the health planning stakeholders as co-managers of the health sector, a strategic plan is necessary to define roles and responsibilities, giving each of them direction, clarifying what they can expect and what is expected from them. This clarity on involved institutions' and individuals' roles and responsibilities is essential for broad adherence and commitment of health stakeholders, and thus, better implementation.

5.2.2 To keep focus on the medium to long term

A plan can help keep the country on the chosen, optimal path towards health sector development underpinned by universal health coverage, given outside influences and events.

As mentioned previously, a written vision is important for orientation of the health sector. The strength of it is the fact that it has been debated and discussed, and carefully pinned down with a solid evidence base. This can help keep the country's health sector on this optimal path as far as possible, despite political or other changes. Robust strategic planning can thus be a means of minimizing the effects of outside influences that may cause unwanted deviation. It helps avoid priorities being set in an ad hoc way by reacting to external pulls and pushes, rather than following a discussed, debated and agreed upon plan. A solid NHPSP can also be seen as a way to minimize the level of uncertainty or risk faced from the outside environment.

5.2.3 To avoid fragmentation of the health sector

Because of its comprehensiveness, a sector strategic plan involves and includes all programmes and services, including support functions. This facilitates coordination and can help avoid fragmentation due to parallel planning and implementation.

A big part of avoiding fragmentation is ensuring that the baseline data as collected for and presented in the NHPSP is agreed upon by the full range of health sector stakeholders, including programmes, services and support functions. These numbers set the tone for all future activities in the health sector as progress will be assessed and measured against them.

5.2.4 To help focus the policy dialogue on health sector priorities

The strategic plan provides a focus towards priority areas and interventions, as it is directly linked to the situation analysis, costing and budgeting. The NHPSP is the reference document against which all subsequent health sector activities will be assessed, oriented and revised. The topics which will be at the centre of policy dialogue during all of the planning cycle steps will be those highlighted in the NHPSP.

The topics and goals highlighted in the NHPSP serves as a reference against which subsequent health sector activities are assessed, oriented and revised.

Box 5.2

The role of strategic planning in progressing health sector development in five country studies[4]

In a study done by the Overseas Development Institute, an analysis of health sector development in five countries— Cambodia, Mozambique, Nepal, Rwanda and Sierra Leone — highlights various strategic planning pathways that were used to improve governance and result in positive gains for maternal and child health (MCH) and neglected tropical diseases (NTDs). The key disease areas of MCH and NTDs were selected as indicators due to their centrality to the Millennium Development Goals and as such their ability to act as proxy for general health services. Countries were chosen based on quantitative indicators denoting health improvements, both in terms of key disease areas studied and compared with other countries in their respective regions.

Case studies from 2013 to early 2014 and extensive literature reviews served as the basis to analyse concerted efforts made in different country contexts to improve strategic policy-making and their consequences in the health sector. In Mozambique, improvements in strategic health plans, with targeted objectives and broad activity areas linked to MCH and NTDs, resulted in increased sector investment by donors through sector budget support. In Cambodia, national commitment to the strategic health plan which included an emphasis on NTDs, facilitated a key partnership between the MoH and the Ministry of Education, Youth and Sport; this was critical for scaling up the NTD response. In Rwanda, the MoH placed a strong focus in the health sector strategy on decentralized health planning, with reforms allowing for more community and local-level participation in planning. This has led to more community ownership of the strategy, and a greater willingness to take part in implementation.

The study suggests that, despite the various economic and political constraints, multilevel efforts to improve health sector governance and strategic policy-making can lead to more successful policy implementation and thus bring about positive results in health.

5.3 When should strategic planning be done?

In the context of ongoing comprehensive health sector development, strategic planning is an iterative process that should be conducted every 3–5 years (medium-term). Most health sectors work with long- and/or medium-term strategic plans, as well as with annual and quarterly operational plans. The strategic planning exercise generally comes after the phase of priority-setting and precedes operational planning.

It may be useful to ensure adequate bridging of the strategic plan with the annual operational plans through a rolling implementation plan or programme of work and forward budgets. Such a bridging planning document is necessary when the strategic plan is too broad in orientation for guiding implementation, often because it does not provide enough detail on phases/steps, targets, implementation modalities and/or responsibilities.[5]

The term prospective planning is used in the case of long-term strategies, i.e. one that covers at least a 10-year period. Increasingly such a long-term view is used in combination with short-term rolling plans which have shorter cycles. Such a combination is seen as a flexible response to the need for short-term detailed plans within the context of a longer-term view.[6]

A strategic planning exercise with a narrower scope can be necessary whenever there is a broad and open question to be answered, for example, in the case of the emergence of a new health problem or when a new vision or strategic direction emerges. In such cases, it is not necessary to review the entire existing sector strategic plan. The area-specific newly developed medium-term strategic orientation can be considered as an addendum to the sector strategic plan.

When (donor funded) programmes and projects are vertical in nature, their management cycle may be different from the national governmental planning cycle. Fig. 5.3 illustrates a recent analysis of vertical programme plans and their synchronicity with the national health plan – it is clear that many vertical programme plans are not synchronized with the national health plan. This lack of synchronicity means that probably different specific programmatic stakeholder groups met in different places at different times and may have developed sub-plans in isolation from each other, and from the overall health sector strategic group of stakeholders. This situation may lead to duplication and overlap. To overcome this, it is important not to settle for a sequenced planning exercise for individual programmes, but rather to integrate their planning elements into the sector-wide NHPSP exercise. Efforts should be made to progressively adapt the planning cycles of programmes that are still vertical in nature to the government/ sector NHPSP cycle.

Strategic planning is an iterative process that should be conducted every 3-5 years (medium-term); operational plans are more often annual or quarterly.

Fig. 5.3 Programme-specific plans and national health plans: to what extent are they synchronized?[7]

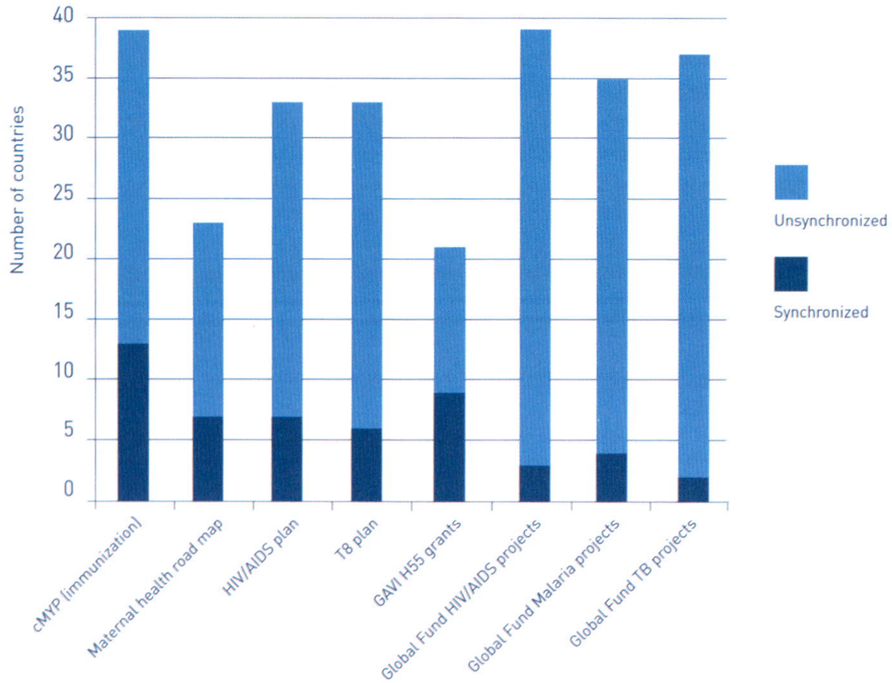

At some point in the course of 3–5 years, the need may be felt to revise the strategic plan. The temptation may arise, for instance, when a new government defines new development priorities that affect the health sector considerably, or when a particular health problem is labelled as a particular priority by the global (health) community. The risk of a complete revision of the entire strategic plan in such a case is that it will cause confusion in the health sector stakeholder community. It may cause interference with ongoing implementation of operational plans, stall sector coordination and even disrupt continuity in service delivery. Usually, it is better to maintain the existing sector strategic framework and only adjust, as per need, the sector priority agenda and directives for annual operational planning. These unforeseen important developments can then be integrated into the following strategic plan.

The above recommendation does not hold in countries where the NHPSP covers a whole decade; in that case, the NHPSP is not really a medium-term plan but a long-term one. Since important sector-specific and contextual changes can be expected over such a long period, it may be necessary to revise or update such a 10-year plan halfway, i.e. after five years.

5.4 Who should be part of strategic planning?

All levels of the health system have their own unique role to play in strategic planning. Strategizing for health will be more effective if a wide range of stakeholders is involved in it, and both the process and the product are truly owned by the country. Health sector stakeholders will need to come to a common understanding of the key issues and share institutional goals and expectations. Such an inclusive approach is likely to be more potent, not only in terms of planning the right vision and activities, but also in ensuring that implementation of the strategic plan is jointly undertaken by all actor groups.

Another angle to take when considering whom to involve in the strategic planning process is to examine stakeholders' contribution to planning based on their function. Categories could be for instance: idea generators, entrepreneurs, managers, networkers and champions. The aim would be to include not only those who will write the plan but also those who will implement it and those who will benefit from it.[8]

Brinkerhoff and Bossert's three categories of population groups who have a stake in health governance (see Fig. 5.4) can be used as a lens to better understand the specific roles of the different stakeholders in the NHPSP development process.[9]

Fig. 5.4 Population groups with a stake in health governance

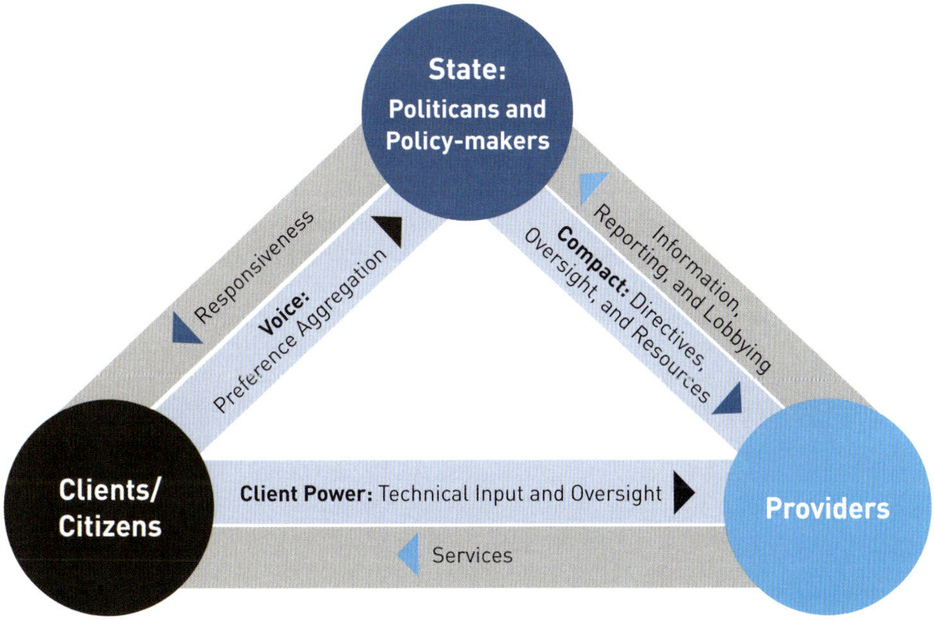

5.4.1 The state: politicians and policy-makers

The central-level MoH coordinates and leads NHPSP development and is responsible for informing, instructing and guiding the concerned stakeholders at all levels through the development exercise.

This group includes:

- policy actors within the government (policy-makers, health managers);
- parastatal institutions;
- representatives of other sectors (e.g. finance, gender, education);
- representatives of local government global, multilateral and bilateral development partners.

We include development partners here because those acting at global level, through multilateral or bilateral channels, usually engage directly with policy-makers, most commonly at the national level or at least through the national level to lower levels of the health system.

The central-level MoH initiates, coordinates and leads NHPSP development according to a chosen approach, methodology and process. In some settings, a uniform planning framework and calendar may be provided by national government for all sectors. The MoH is responsible for informing, instructing and guiding the concerned stakeholders at all levels through the NHPSP development exercise.

The perspective of relevant citizen groups and institutions is important for providing feedback and evidence on the most pressing health priorities being discussed in the NHPSP planning process.

All these tasks cannot be simply delegated to MoH departments as part of their routine work. It is a considerable extra workload. In addition, in the spirit of participation, it can be extremely useful to involve a few representatives of main stakeholder groups in the organization itself of the NHPSP development process. Establishing a core team of not more than 10 people is one way to do this. This group could include 2–3 senior MoH staff – usually from the planning and/or monitoring and evaluation department – as well as representatives of key health sector stakeholders groups and other sectors.

The MoH may seek the assistance of international, (sub)regional or national independent experts for developing and preparing methodology and tools, as well as for facilitating the process.

5.4.2 Clients/citizens

This group includes:

- civil society/ NGOs;
- for-profit private sector;
- community representatives;
- academic/research institutions.

The core team established with MoH coordination should ideally include the most relevant citizen groups and institutions that can provide the necessary feedback and evidence for the most pressing health priorities.

Obviously, not all levels of all stakeholder groups can be intensively involved in all the stages of the strategic planning process, so it is important to determine the best role for each of them at each stage, depending on the aspect(s) in which they can contribute: defining the scope, preparation, write-up of the plan, validation, etc. For instance, through their membership in thematic (or technical) groups, research institutes can play an important role in defining medium-term roadmaps for implementing specific activities, while regional health offices and district health management teams can ensure that the strategic planning takes into account district-specific needs for increasing health service coverage or for strengthening a particular intervention. In some countries, non-profit or faith-based institutions provide the bulk of local health services; their input into defining the scope and preparation of the NHPSP would then be vital, given their insights and stakes in the health sector.

In some settings, bringing on board the for-profit private sector has proven difficult, as interests and viewpoints diverge considerably with the public sector. Nevertheless, a concerted effort must be invested in making the case for an added value for both sides to be involved in the NHPSP development process. This should be an ongoing effort as there may be issues to resolve, concerns to look into and a common ground to be found – all of which can take time.

5.4.3 Providers

Health providers are at the crux of implementing the NHPSP. Their experience of the health sector comes from the inside, is practical, and offers insights on feasibility. Their input into the NHPSP development process is therefore crucial, as it is a complementary perspective to those of patients and the population. In addition, any hesitance or outright opposition will become a major hindrance to NHPSP implementation; health providers' reservations need to be addressed openly and dialogue channels actively sought to find a joint solution. This investment is key to the credibility of the NHPSP as well as to the implementability of the plan.

Health care providers are at the crux of implementing a NHPSP; their input is crucial as a complementary perspective to those of patients and the population.

Box 5.3

The health policy formulation process in Thailand: who are the different stakeholders?

Policy formulation in Thailand underwent a change in 1997 following enactment of the People's Constitution, effectively increasing public participation in policy decision-making.[10, 11] While policy in the past was mostly characterized by a power struggle between military rule and elected bureaucrats, the 1990s political reform has led to improvements in other stakeholders' involvement in the policy process.[12, 13] Today, formulation of national health plans and policies involves an array of policy actors, each with their own perspective and agenda for action and each influencing policy at various stages of the process.[14] The prime minister serves as the agenda setter, influenced by a large support system made up of research institutions and nongovernmental organizations. State bureaucrats and health professionals are closely linked, demonstrating the long tradition and mindset of a centralized hierarchical health system structure which may be changing, but only slowly. Civil society also holds a large stake in the process as representatives of people's voice. NGOs provide a large number of specific health services, often with funds from different donor groups, and hence are interested in better collaboration with public services. Additionally, private hospitals are mainly concerned with access to funding and resources. Understanding the different vantage points of each stakeholder is critical and facilitates the development of strong policy reforms.

For example, the Thai Universal Coverage (UC) policy was borne out of a series of communications between different policy actors, starting among a small number of civil servants and elected officials. The explicit objective of the UC policy was to expand health insurance coverage to all citizens through the means of two main features: a single standard for all in terms of benefits and care, and a decentralized sustainable insurance system. Policy elites and members of government, such as the prime minister, minister of health, minister of finance etc., held mostly pro-market economic viewpoints and had reservations regarding the creation of a welfare system; however, this was overridden by the Party's commitment to ensuring citizens' entitlement to health care. Results from focus group discussions with villagers and commentary from civil society representatives revealed concerns that the rich might have more opportunities to use public resources than the poor. Health providers and hospitals, especially in the private sector, were eager to join the scheme as soon as possible, hoping that the insurance system could be a major source of income. In the end, no single stakeholder had absolute power to dominate every decision in the policy; the space for interplay between multiple policy actors was key for the decision-making process.[15]

5.5 How do we transform priorities into plans?

Medium-term sector strategic planning is a complex undertaking that can be done in different ways. Its complexity comes from the sheer comprehensiveness of the exercise, involving all aspects of the full health sector, as well as other sectors with a stake in health. A wide variety of actors must be an active part of the process for it to be successful – thus adding to the complexity of the task. However, if done well, the NHPSP process will pave the way for operational planning as well as activity implementation for all aspects of the health system (health care, support systems, other determinants), for all actors and for all levels. Depending on how the government and the health sector and the services are organized, the type of planning process may vary (result-based, programme-based, etc.) and the role of the different actors may differ (stronger bottom-up planning in decentralized settings, influence of donors in a setting of strong dependence on external financing, etc.). The national context will determine how the NHPSP process will be organized and phased.

The NHPSP process will pave the way for operational planning and activity implementation for all aspects of the health system, for all actors and for all levels.

Of course, policy-making does not take place in a vacuum. The process is set within the constitutional and legal framework – as well as the history and culture – of each country. The NHPSP process will take into account demographic, economic and fiscal trends, as well as international and regional commitments. Health sector stakeholders leading the NHPSP process should keep the general policy environment in mind at all times and work within its confines.

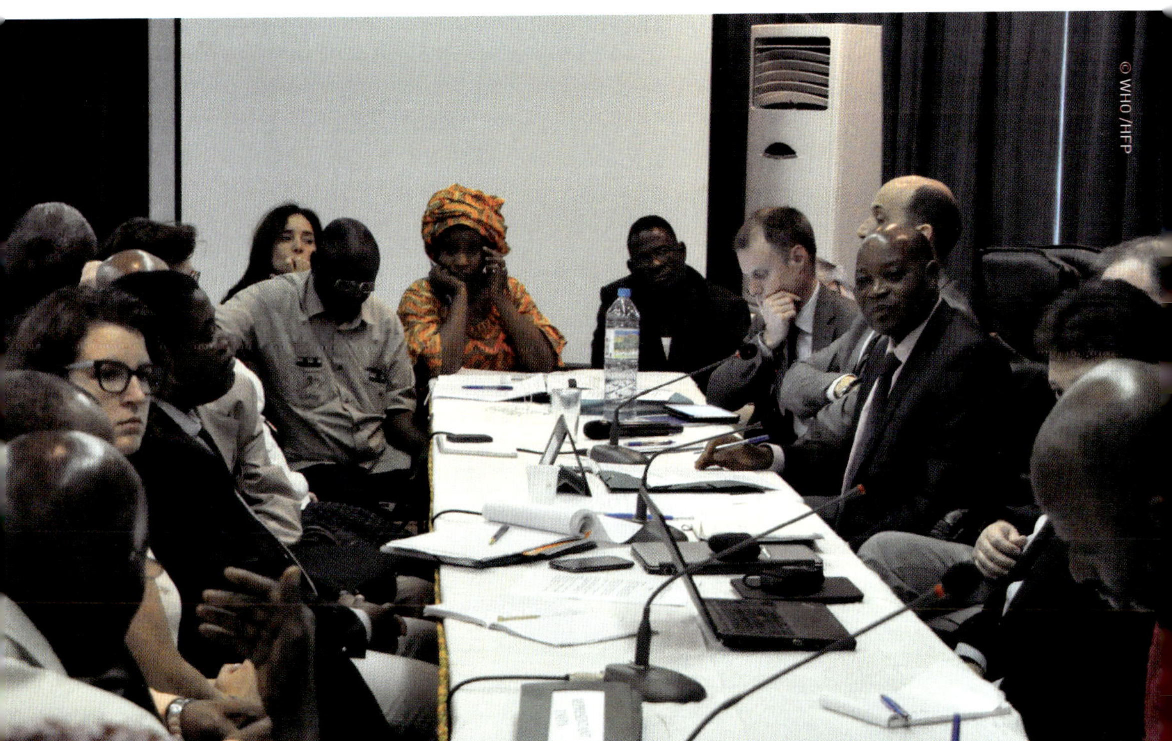

Ensuring buy-in from all stakeholders and keeping it realistic and feasible is the key to ensuring the NHPSP is a dynamic document.

Box 5.4

National planning cycle database: a WHO resource[16]

The Country Planning Cycle Database is an open, online resource that provides information on all 195 WHO Member States and their national health policies, strategies and plans. Initiated in 2009, the goal of the database is to provide countries with the necessary information to improve the coordination and synchronization of health sector planning efforts. The database provides a country-by-country overview of different planning, programme and project cycles in the health sector, and generates country profiles with a snapshot of important milestones and graphical representations of donor commitments. It also offers access to an online repository of NHPSPs.

Information in the database is continuously updated through the efforts of WHO and collaborating partners to maintain the accuracy and comprehensiveness of the resource. The database can be accessed through the WHO national planning cycles website (www.nationalplanningcycles.org).

5.5.1 How can we ensure that the NHPSP is actually used as a key orienting text?

In some countries, the NHPSP process has become a periodic, bureaucratic formality, a mere obligation met behind closed doors in government offices. In such cases, there is a considerable risk that, in the implementation phase, the plan will not be considered a fundamental reference document; it will just gather dust on the shelves. Without this important steering function, sector development efforts are likely to become fragmented, inefficient, with poor final outcomes and impact as a consequence.

The key to ensuring that the NHPSP is truly a living, breathing document, which is used dynamically to achive buy-in from all stakeholders and keeping it realistic and feasible, while still expressing ambition for the future. Ensuring buy-in from all stakeholders is only possible when all stakeholders are adequately represented in the national health planning process, and are able to meaningfully participate. This requires a skilled MoH to convene all relevant actors and broker a decision among potentially divergent views. The final result should be a balanced and evidence-informed decision on the strategic directions for the health sector.

5.5.2 Some strategic planning basics

Comprehensive, balanced and coherent NHPSP content

National health policies, strategies and plans must articulate a country's goals, objectives and broad activity areas for the health sector in a comprehensive, balanced and coherent fashion.[17]

Comprehensive

This includes all aspects impacting on the health sector, such as human resources for health, health sector governance, pharmaceuticals, health information systems, health financing arrangements, personal and non-personal health services, all specific programmes (disease-specific and others) and all actors and budget centres, public or private.

Balanced

The content of the NHPSP must be well-balanced in terms of finances and inputs, as well as depth of analysis on the principal health issues of the country. In other words, each strategic direction needs to be developed with the same level of detail as the others, and with a level of resources that corresponds to its extent and scope.

Coherent

(a) Coherence with other sectors and the national development plan

Strategic planning for health should ideally be based on a government-wide policy framework laid out for all sectors. Success in implementation will be influenced by whether health strategies and planned reforms are coherent with overall government policies. It is crucial for health planning stakeholders to examine the national development plan, or any other relevant overarching vision statement for advancing the country as a whole.

(b) Coherence with programme-specific or subsector plans

Ideally, programme-specific or subsector plans have already been established before the comprehensive sector NHPSP process starts. It is then principally a matter of integrating these elements into the NHPSP. Even without finalized subplans, the active and meaningful participation of programmes and subsectors in the overall national health planning process is important for ensuring harmonization and alignment, and for shaping the strategic directions for the health sector.

Coherence with other plans can also imply coherence with a large injection of funding which may arrive during an emergency situation. A case in point is the recent Ebola crisis in West Africa, which was accompanied by a proliferation of plans that were developed separately from the NHPSP: Ebola emergency plans and health system recovery plans. Ideally, these plans would fall under the umbrella of the existing NHPSP, if the course for the health sector as outlined in the plan remains relevant; if not, it might make most sense to prepare a new NHPSP, or write an amendment to the existing one. A plethora of plans overlapping with each other does not give clarity for the health sector in any way. It is thus desirable in most country settings to have one overarching document giving orienting

A NHPSP must be comprehensive, balanced, and coherent to effectively articulate a country's health sector's goals, objectives and activity areas.

guidance overall, with all other plans linking with and aligning with that strategic orientation.

(c) Coherence with the epidemiological and socioeconomic context

A strategic plan will only be valid if it addresses the principal concerns of the health sector in its broadest definition – this includes not only the epidemiological but also the socioeconomic context. This implies working with the health sector across all levels and actors, but also beyond the health sector with other ministries and stakeholder groups. The NHPSP must include input from all of those institutions, interests and actors in order for it to be relevant and valid for implementation on the ground.

(d) Coherence with the available current and estimated future resources

The resources and costs necessary to implement the NHPSP must be reasonable and within the fiscal space for health estimated for the period.

Baseline data

The strategic plan will define the intended sector development and will indicate the expected results in terms of outcomes and impact. In order to measure progress during the course of plan implementation, and evaluate the end result based on NHPSP targets, it is necessary to know exactly where the starting point is. For this reason, baseline indicators on service availability, workforce distribution, vaccination coverage, prevalence and incidence of major health conditions, performance of support functions, and progress on institutional and organizational reforms, among many others, are crucial. This baseline information will be used in the monitoring and evaluation of the NHPSP.

Demographic trends are decisive: information on population trends, with gender and geographical disaggregation, is basic to strategizing for health. For example, the population by age cohorts is often the starting point for the allocation of health services. Outward migration (and internal migration within the national territory) is obviously another key element in health service investment. The same holds true for mortality and morbidity data, which may come from the national government or may be the responsibility of an independent health agency. The point here is: the quality of the NHPSP will be largely influenced by the quality of the (baseline) data available for review.

Working within a given budget ceiling

The MoH is expected to translate government policy goals (as described in the NHPSP) into cost estimates to fit into the suggested budget ceiling for health. The budget ceiling is given by the ministry of finance (MoF) based on its revenue forecast outlining the country's macroeconomic prospects in the medium term.

In many settings, the full quantity of resources available might be known with considerable accuracy, and the NHPSP guides the maximum possible progress toward a goal, using these available resources (see Box 5.5). In some cases, the availability of resources is only approximate (for example, where large donor monies are not on-budget, but fund many health sector activities), and the plan may be produced to justify a request for resources to reach a stated goal. Whether the NHPSP is developed before or after the allocation of resources, it is intended to ensure the best return on investment, that is, the greatest possible achievement of results given the available resources.[18]

Macroeconomic projections and fiscal space analysis will provide the information on opportunities and constraints within which the health sector will operate.[IV] Equally important are the population's income levels — which are themselves influenced by employment — and their distribution, as they will impact on the nature of their health problems and health-seeking behaviour. Regarding fiscal trends, three aspects will be salient in the NHPSP process, and should thus be kept in mind during NHPSP development:

(a) the budget for the current year;

(b) the forecast for the medium term, for example, three years ahead;

(c) any unforeseen circumstances that force immediate and short-term adjustments to spending plans.

Box 5.5

Developing a NHPSP within a fixed budget ceiling in Uganda[19, 20]

Uganda's Ministry of Finance gives the health sector fixed budget ceilings. For the fiscal year 2014–2015, the health budget ceiling in Uganda was USD 385 million, about 9% of the GDP.[21] With this number in mind, the MoH must guide NHPSP cost estimation to ensure maximum progress towards NHPSP goals.

Budget Framework Papers, or medium-term budgets, are then prepared by sector working groups, based on the given budget ceilings, to reflect the sector's priorities and expenditure plans as outlined in the NHPSP. The cabinet and parliament subsequently decide on sector budget allocations. Once the Budget Framework Papers are finalized, there is room for renegotiating sector budget allocations within the given sector ceiling.[22]

IV See Chapter 8 "Budgeting for health" in this handbook.

5.5.3 Multisectorality

It is necessary to involve, and if necessary guide, other sectors from the outset in the NHPSP process to ensure that, in the end, much-needed cross-sector interventions happen.

Since health is to a very large extent determined by other factors than those which can be influenced by health service delivery, the NHPSP process should consider elements which can and should become part of the agenda for other sectors. Governments usually acknowledge the need for this broader approach; in a general way, intentions for a multisectoral modus operandi are often reflected in overall national development plans. Mechanisms may exist for coordination between sectors. However, when it comes to assuring joint planning for the implementation of multisectoral interventions, there is often hardly any content in NHPSPs, with defined targets that can guide resource allocation and operational planning. The risk is then that the synergy between efforts of and with other sectors is insufficient, or worse, that intended health-related interventions which require multisectoral collaboration do not end up in operational plans and budgets. It is therefore necessary to involve, and if necessary guide, other sectors from the outset in the NHPSP process and to ensure that, in the end, much-needed cross-sector interventions actually happen.[V]

5.5.4 Mitigating risks

To the extent possible, the strategic planning process should include dialogue on possible and probable risks and the means to mitigate them.

Any strategic planning process will have to deal with uncertainties related to developments that are beyond the control of the health sector. Under normal circumstances, there should be no uncertainty about the availability of national and donor resources for the implementation of the NHPSP; however, an important downturn in the country's macroeconomic situation or an unforeseen epidemic outbreak (e.g. Ebola) may hamper complete NHPSP implementation. In a similar way, important political reshuffles can also negatively influence strategic plan implementation. Therefore, to the extent possible, the strategic planning process should include a dialogue on such possible and probable influences in terms of risks and conditions, and think through means to mitigate them.

V For more information, please see Chapter 12 "Intersectoral planning for health and health equity" in this handbook.

5.5.5 Approaches to policy development

The rationalist model developed by Howlett and Ramesh[23] is characterized by an orderly progression of well-defined steps:

1. identification of objectives — agenda-setting;
2. evidence-gathering — formulation of options;
3. decision-making — weighing the options in terms of cost and benefit;
4. implementation — putting the chosen solution into effect;
5. evaluation — monitoring results; and
6. termination/adaptation/confirmation.

The systematic approach of this model clearly has appeal, but in reality policy-making rarely proceeds in a rational and orderly manner. Objectives often cannot be agreed upon. The evidence is often incomplete or ambiguous, and political considerations often intrude at all points, disrupting the orderly sequence. Busy policy advisers will rarely have the opportunity to approach their daily work in terms of such a model. The model implies that the steps identified follow each other in a linear sequential fashion. In practice, the process tends to take place in a more haphazard manner, driven by circumstances. Nevertheless, the labelling of the stages draws attention to the logic of a rational policy process. It underlines the point that policy-making is more than isolated decisions; it is a process in which more than one party is involved and in which the issues may be revisited in an iterative process.

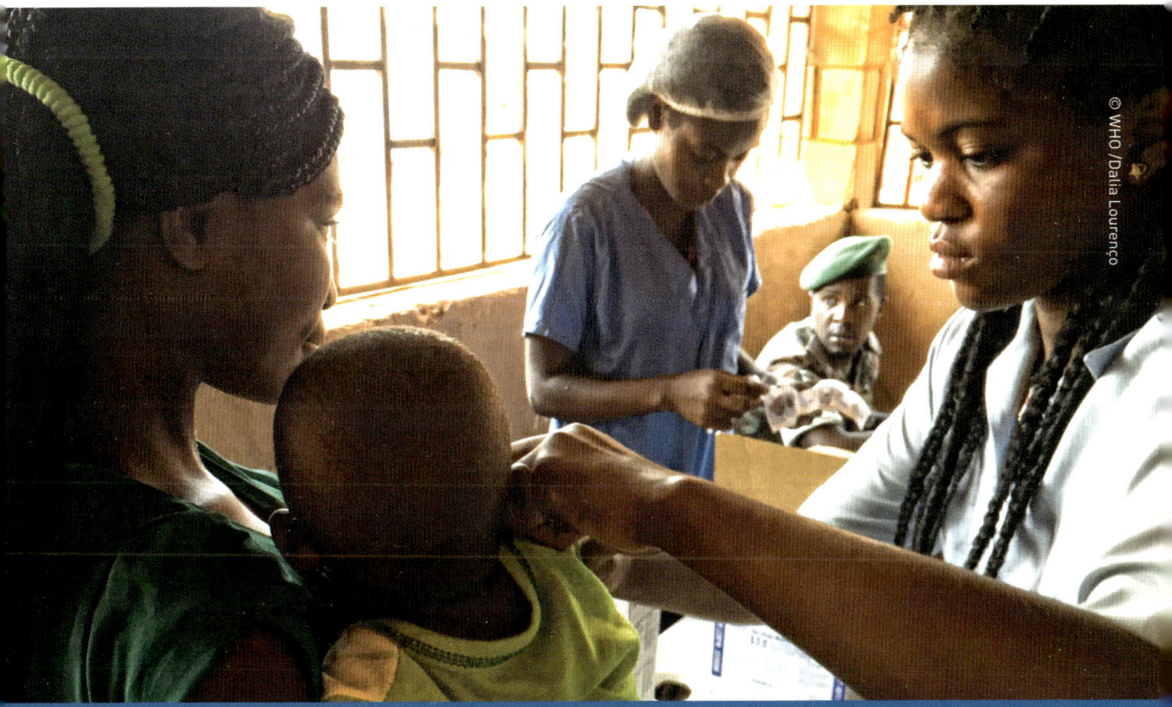

The **stakeholder model** focuses more on the interaction between principal policy actors, and tries to negotiate a pragmatic path through the often divergent values and views of the various interest groups and government agencies. In reality, stakeholder bargaining can be undemocratic and exclusive, and is often captured by the most powerful players. It requires very skilled and diplomatic leaders to ensure that a balanced viewpoint emerges from the policy-making process.

At different times, and in various ways, any subset of stakeholders can exert power and influence over the health system. Ways must be found to ensure that all legitimate interests are assessed and weighed in the policy-making process. The success of NHPSP development may well depend upon the extent to which the key stakeholders have been involved and are committed to supporting its implementation.

Some important preparatory activities for NHPSP development are defining the schedule, putting together a core team, determining budgetary requirements, assigning tasks, informing the health stakeholder community of the chosen methodology and process, and collecting reference documentation for review.

The **participatory model** can be considered a particular form of the above-mentioned stakeholder model. It takes more of a socially democratic and inclusive approach, and is the model that is explicitly endorsed here. It is the most recent arrival in policy studies literature, but it is by no means new. The participatory process requires that the resulting policy or strategy is "democratically legitimate". In practice, this implies an open, inclusive, interactive and highly politicized approach. The contention is that multiple criteria should guide policy-making processes. Such criteria could include relative dependence on expertise, the availability of an evidence base, the analytical policy support available, resource and time pressures, the political sensitivity of the issues, and the relative power of the principal stakeholders involved.

This model has also been described as incrementalism, or a deliberative process, which recognizes the political nature of planning in a far more overt manner than in the rational approaches.

In practice, an evidence-based, flexible and pragmatic approach to policy-making will most likely move things forward.

5.5.6 Process and steps for developing the NHPSP

Preparation of NHPSP development

NHPSP development requires considerable time and resources. It should therefore be planned and budgeted for, and funds made available. Health planning stakeholders in the core team are expected to set aside adequate time for preparation, which may take two weeks or more. The important preparatory activities to be considered are:

- defining the schedule for NHPSP development;
- putting together the core team for NHPSP development;
- determining the budgetary requirements for NHPSP development and matching them with available funds in the current annual work plan;
- assigning specific tasks and responsibilities to each member of the core team;
- developing a methodology and selecting indicators for evaluating the NHPSP development process;

- securing funds for NHPSP development;
- informing citizens and the broader health stakeholder community of the methodology and process;
- collecting reference documentation for review.

The steering, organization, implementation and monitoring of the NHPSP development process are functions that should be attributed to the appropriate stakeholder groups and structures. Steering can be done by a mixed group of health sector stakeholders under the leadership of MoH, while the responsibility for the actual organization of NHPSP development activities may be given to the core team. The whole process should be coordinated and led by the MoH (usually its department of planning).

Mixed thematic groups of area-specific experts from a broad range of stakeholder groups are needed to provide targeted technical expertise. The thematic groups should include ministries (health and other sectors), service providers, private sector (for-profit and not-for-profit), research institutions, sub-national health authorities, etc.

The core team should prepare a roadmap for NHPSP development, inform all sector stakeholders about the work at hand, develop terms of reference on the exact role to be played by various actors, provide instructions on methodology, coordinate and provide technical and organizational support. This core team should also ensure mobilization of the resources which were budgeted for the NHPSP exercise.

Setting goals (or strategic directions)

A goal, sometimes called a "strategic direction" in NHPSP documents, is a broad statement of the overall outcome(s) which the health system is expected to achieve. For instance, the United Nations' eight Millennium Development Goals, valid from 2000–2015, included goals such as "improve maternal health" as an expected outcome of the health system. Usually only a few goals, or perhaps only one, are mentioned in strategy documents, as they are general and all-encompassing in nature. Setting a goal will be the result of policy dialogue during the population consultation, situation analysis and priority-setting phases of the policy and planning cycle. Mostly, these goals will not change drastically over time and will not entail huge surprises.

NHPSP development requires setting goals, setting objectives, formulating broad activity areas, creating medium-term implementation guidance, and approving and disseminating the NHPSP.

Setting objectives

According to the WHO *Health Systems Strengthening Glossary*,[24] an objective is a statement of a desired future state, condition or purpose, which an institution, a project, a service or a programme seeks to achieve. It is thus a broad approach to be followed to achieve a health system goal. Taking "improve maternal health" as an example, an objective could be "reduce the maternal mortality ratio by two thirds within the next 20 years".

A NHPSP objective can lay out the path to reach a goal or fulfill a strategic direction. Like goals, objectives describe planned outcomes resulting from implemented activities – they are not activities themselves. Setting objectives is essential for three main reasons.

First, they define in a clear and precise way what the plan is designed to achieve.

Second, the objectives largely determine which key activities should take place during NHPSP implementation.

Third, objectives provide the required guidance for health planning stakeholders and implementers to apply appropriate monitoring and evaluation tools.

The SMART approach describes a set of key criteria to ensure in an objective.[25] Adapted to the medium-term NHPSP context, they are:

(a) measurable: quantifies the change to be achieved (in the above example, the quantification is "reduce by two thirds");

(b) appropriate: logically relates to the overall goal/strategic direction ("reduce maternal mortality ratio" is directly linked to "improve maternal health");

(c) realistic: provides a realistic dimension which is achievable with available resources and implementation capability (this evidence-informed discussion begins during the priority-setting debates and is specific to each country);

(d) time-limited: specifies an expected time for the objective to be achieved ("within the next 20 years").

Measurable, appropriate, realistic and time-limited objectives are those that can be achieved with hard work. Objectives that are too ambitious will discourage implementers or will be bypassed. Objectives that are too easy to achieve will foster complacency.[26] It is an art to agree upon objectives that are truly attainable for an entire health sector, but an art which health planning stakeholders must master if achievements and progress are to be made.

Formulating broad activity areas

After setting goals and objectives, health planning stakeholders must address the means of reaching their goals, at least in a general way. The operational plans will address it in a more specific and concrete way; however, even the operational plan will take guidance from the NHPSP, so broad activity areas should be explicitly mentioned. These activities can address expansion, testing, reform or strengthening of sector areas. The activities should be feasible, given the strengths and weaknesses of health sector stakeholders.

In formulating broad activity areas, it is necessary to identify:

- the levels, organizations and sectors to be targeted;
- which population(s) or geographic areas are targeted;
- the personal and environmental factors to be addressed;
- those who can most benefit and contribute.

Broad activity areas, when formulated well and thought through adequately by the health sector stakeholder group, should fulfill the following characteristics:[27]

- they point out the overall path, in line with goals/strategic directions, and sometimes a specific approach;
- they match resources;
- they take advantage of opportunities, current skills and strengths, and public opinion;
- they minimize resistance and barriers;
- they reach those who are most affected;
- they involve communities.

Box 5.6 describes an example of how broad activity areas can evolve, starting from a goal/ strategic direction and objectives, and how they provide a starting point for operational planning.

Box 5.6

Example of a goal, objectives and broad activity areas in a NHPSP

Goal

- decrease under-five mortality rate by strengthening and expanding primary health care services.

Objective

- increase the focus on health promotion and prevention services as an integrated part of the maternal and child health programme;
- strengthen staff skills at primary and secondary care level;
- intensify collaboration with other sectors on health prevention issues (education sector, water and sanitation, etc.).

Broad activity areas included in the medium-term NHPSP

- expand the community health worker (CHW) network;
- training in "Integrated Management of Childhood Illnesses" (IMCI) for all health facility staff;
- link district health plans with local water and sanitation development plans.

Activities as they might appear in annual operational plans

- recruit and train additional CHWs; provide refresher training for existing CHWs.
- develop an IMCI training module adapted to the local context and organize training courses locally;
- develop a guide for district councils to better link health and water and sanitation plans.

Ideally, the relevance and feasibility of the proposed broad activity areas will have been verified during the priority-setting exercise, and if necessary tested, with a team of experts and advisers with different capabilities. Since the broad activity areas will require the active involvement of a range of actors, often at several levels, and possibly co-financing by development partners in some countries, it is imperative that various stakeholder groups are part of, understand and agree to the broad activity areas. This cannot be overemphasized. Apart from the useful input they can provide to this process, it will enhance their willingness to contribute and cooperate in later implementation. Stakeholder buy-in can make or break the success of implementation.

NHPSP implementation guidance

A medium-term NHPSP will not go into detail on implementation issues. However, some key aspects related to implementation can be extremely useful, depending on the activity area. Those key aspects include synergy with other sector development strategies, assumptions, preconditions to be fulfilled, resource requirements, attribution of responsibilities, establishment of a monitoring and evaluation (M&E) mechanism, sequencing and timing. Many of these aspects enable the practicability of the broad activity areas. In the NHPSP, these activity areas will be linked to milestones and targets.[VI]

A number of other plans or strategy documents might be developed to expand on specific areas covered in the NHPSP, and to support NHPSP implementation. These could include:

- specific intervention plans (e.g. HIV voluntary testing and counselling, prevention of mother-to-child HIV transmission, antiretroviral therapy, etc.);
- M&E plan;
- health financing strategy;
- donor technical assistance plan;
- procurement and supply management plan;
- health workforce strategy.

In some settings, a NHPSP can provide enough guidance for direct annual operational planning in terms of:

- reforms and programme interventions;
- key activities per level;
- sequencing with milestones and targets;
- levels of responsibility and tasks;
- implementation and management modalities for the M&E system.

If the NHPSP is less specific about these issues, one possibility is to bridge the NHPSP and the operational plans with a rolling programme of work or MTEF for two or three years.[VII]

VI See Chapter 9 "Monitoring and evaluation of national health policies, strategies and plans" in this handbook.

VII See Chapter 6 "Operational planning: transforming plans into action" and Chapter 8 "Budgeting for health" in this handbook.

Approval and dissemination of the NHPSP

Once the core team agrees on the pre-final version of the NHPSP, it can be presented to the wider stakeholder community for final comments. For that purpose a concise, two-page summary of the plan can be written in simple language, with the purpose of:

- informing the population about the proposed plan;
- informing other services and sectors;
- championing the cause of improved services among local authorities, development partners and the government.

This summary should highlight salient points of the NHPSP and should include:

- major health problems and system development needs;
- goals, objectives, broad activity areas, and expected outcomes;
- major reforms to be implemented for the planning period;
- roles and responsibilities;
- total resource needs estimate, potential sources of funding and, if applicable, financial gaps;
- relationship/synergies of the plan with other ongoing programmes.

A broad range of health sector stakeholders must reach consensus on the content and presentation of the NHPSP. One way to arrive at consensus is through an intense and ongoing involvement of major stakeholders in the NHPSP development process. This may not always be possible due to the heavy time and resource commitments involved; however, it is the ideal option as it enables stakeholders to provide their perspectives and assent at each step of the process. The second approach is by circulating a draft of the NHPSP as widely as possible, to all stakeholders and interested parties, allowing sufficient time for review and feedback. This provides an opportunity to assess the big picture, raise any additional concerns, and correct factual errors. A consensus meeting could provide a forum to openly express views and for making compromises.

It may be decided to undertake an assessment of the quality of the NHPSP. The purpose of the assessment or peer review is to verify that the NHPSP demonstrates the attributes of a good plan that allows for feasible implementation and provides a sound basis for domestic and international investment. An assessment is usually undertaken jointly by all parties directly involved in developing the NHPSP; other interested external parties may also be invited when it is a larger exercise. One NHPSP quality assessment tool which is widely used is the Joint Assessment of National Strategies (JANS);[VIII] it was developed to assess NHPSP and their constituent plans, such as programme plans and subsector (human resource, financing, procurement, etc.) plans (see Box 5.7).

VIII http://www.internationalhealthpartnership.net/en/tools/jans-tool-and-guidelines/

Box 5.7

Joint Assessment of National Health Strategies (JANS)

The JANS[28] approach is a tool and set of guidelines that can be used to check the quality of a national health plan. The approach emphasizes the "joint" inclusive process, meaning that the assessment is conducted by a wide stakeholder group, based on dialogue and consensus on the final conclusions.

The three main goals of JANS are: to improve the quality of the national health strategy; to increase confidence and help inform funding decisions; and to reduce costs and eliminate the existence of multiple assessments. The idea is that through a systematic assessment of an existing NHPSP, insights can be realized to improve future NHPSPs.

The assessment itself includes a review of the NHPSP as well as the national development framework. In addition, numerous other documents, including multisectoral and subsectoral strategies and budgets, are studied in detail. The JANS focuses the analysis on five main areas: situation analysis and programming; process; costs and budgetary frameworks; implementation and management; and monitoring, evaluation and review. For each area, a series of desirable attributes and criteria gives the evaluator a lens through which to assess the NHPSP.

A number of countries have applied the JANS as part of their NHPSP development process. Feedback has shown that, besides the actual assessment results, the process of assessing jointly, with external and internal parties, brought unexpected insights and forged a sense of ownership around the NHPSP.

"The JANS process significantly improved the quality of the 5-year health plan. Outcomes: more trust and confidence from development partners; more streamlined support to the sector."
--Dr Long, Ministry of Health, Viet Nam[29]

For example, in Viet Nam, to ensure the "joint" aspect of the assessment, government, development partners and NGOs were all involved in the core team, preparing and conducting the evaluation. In Ethiopia, separate assessments were carried out in the form of workshops at various health system levels to ensure that civil society organizations and other local stakeholder groups could participate in the JANS process.

Regardless of the approach taken, the output from JANS is a structured judgement on the NHPSP's strengths and weaknesses, as well as concrete recommendations for improvement that can feed policy dialogue and debate.

Once broad consensus on the NHPSP has been reached and it has perhaps been assessed for quality, the NHPSP must be formally endorsed by the relevant national authorities. The NHPSP final draft will usually be submitted for approval to the minister of health or an interdepartmental committee. Sometimes an official validation workshop or ceremony might be planned.

A NHPSP without formal endorsement will be perceived as lacking legitimacy. Here, two issues are relevant:

(a) internal legitimacy within the health sector: endorsement must be provided by authorities within the health sector, including the minister of health, to demonstrate that it is a formal element within the overall direction the MoH wishes the health sector to go;
(b) external legitimacy beyond the health sector.

Once the plan has received official endorsement, the document must be promoted and distributed widely to guide the contributions of all stakeholders. Dissemination includes not just distribution of a hard copy document; instead, it implies explaining the document to relevant communities and stakeholders, holding special meetings and presentations, making it available online, etc. In effect, it involves a whole communication strategy around the NHPSP that might require additional resources to be budgeted. This issue is pivotal to ensuring that the document is actually used and becomes the point of reference for all activities, tasks and initiatives within the health sector in the medium term.

NHPSP document structure (see Box 5.8)

Usually, a NHPSP begins with an executive summary, after which the overall context of the health sector is introduced, together with the NHPSP goal(s). Before describing the actual plan contents, a summary can be given of the results of the situation analysis, since this analysis has provided the justification for the priority-setting and beyond. The NHPSP objectives should then be presented clearly, with an explanation provided for each, linking with the broad goals/strategic directions.

Next, the various broad activity areas for sector development can be presented, indicating phases and relevant orientation for implementation modalities. In an annex the NHPSP contents can be presented for quick review by readers in a table format, highlighting vital elements such as goals, objectives, expected outcomes (targets), description of all proposed broad activity areas, estimated required resource inputs (financial, human and other), timeline and responsible structures/institutions.

A NHPSP should mention assumptions as well as risks and how these will be managed. Last but not least, the NHPSP must indicate when and through which system its progress and achievements will be monitored and evaluated. The NHPSP can refer to a MTEF.

The M&E section of a NHPSP should be well prepared, allowing space for periodic assessments of inputs, processes, outputs, outcome and, eventually, impact. It requires a well-defined set of key indicators, quantitative and qualitative, often used in combination with a scorecard. To the extent possible, baseline data should be gathered and mentioned in the M&E plan. More details on monitoring and evaluation of NHPSPs can be found in Chapter 9 of this handbook.

Box 5.8

NHPSP sample outline

Foreword/Preface
Acknowledgements
Acronyms and abbreviations
Executive summary
Introduction
NHPSP development process
Community of stakeholders involved in the process
Roles and responsibilities (mapping)
Section I: Background and situation analysis
- Country profile
- Socioeconomic status
- Health status of population
- Health system/sector profile

Section II: NHPSP strategic directions/goals
- Link to long-term vision for the health sector or for country's development as a whole
- Mission
- Guiding principles
- Priority areas
- Main objectives and broad activity areas

Section III: Implementation of NHPSP
- Policy and regulatory framework
- Implementation framework
- Mitigating risks

Section IV: Financing the NHPSP
- Available funds and costing
- Financing gap
- Strategic investment plan

Section V: Monitoring and evaluation strategy
- Monitoring and evaluation systems – indicators, baselines, targets
- Approaches for data collection
- Results strategy

Section VI: Conclusion
References
Annexes

Estimating cost implications of a NHPSP and ensuring necessary resources

Examining the costing implications of a NHPSP must be part of the NHPSP development process from the beginning.[IX] This leverages the costing process to enable fine-tuning and adjustments to the contents and targets of the NHPSP, and prevents the NHPSP from becoming an unrealistic plan which is quickly shelved and not actively used. Scenarios can be modelled by costing experts, especially if resources appear to not match NHPSP ambitions.

Costing a plan requires planners to project the financial expenditures that will be required to achieve the results set out in the plan. Cost estimations provide invaluable input into the NHPSP development process and can inform priority-setting by highlighting resource constraints. Cost estimations provide guidance to decision-makers on the feasibility of a plan. Perhaps most importantly, cost estimates can be matched to available funds to identify funding gaps and mobilize additional resources from the national budget or international sources.

Scenario-building will be a useful tool within the NHPSP development and costing process, with several rounds of iterations between those who primarily perform cost analyses and those who are more involved with NHPSP development. For example, a scenario can be projected for different possible budget ceilings or different health coverage targets to understand and think through the resource implications in order to make strategic decisions.

IX For a more detailed discourse on this topic, please see Chapter 7 "Estimating cost implications of a national health policy, strategy or plan" in this handbook.

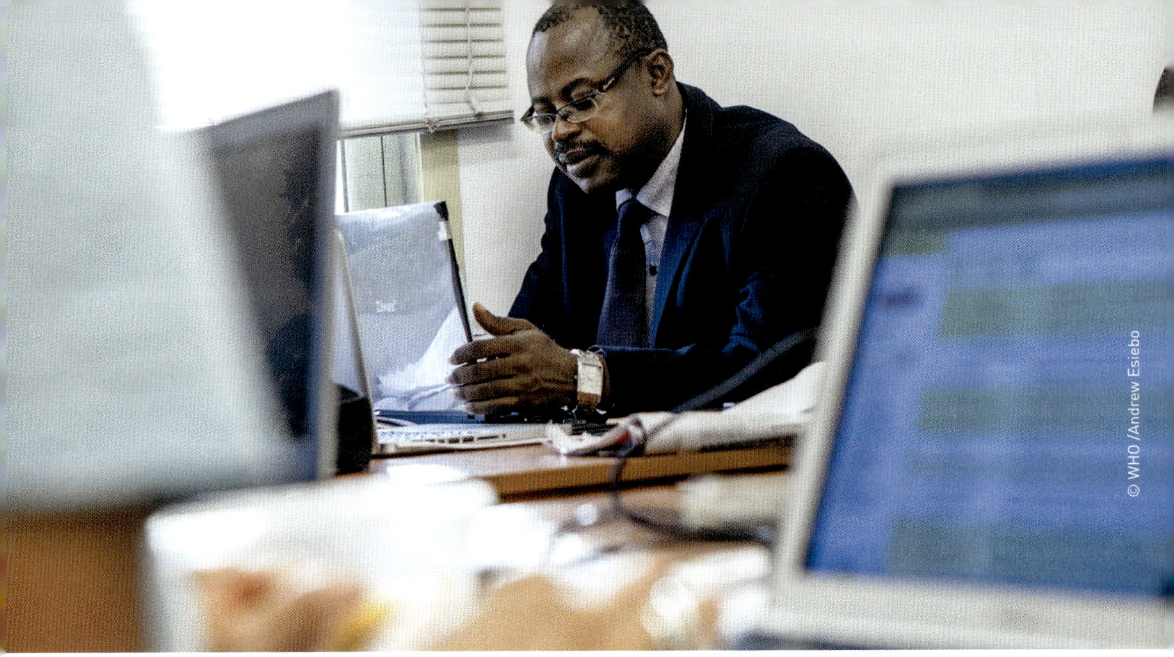

© WHO /Andrew Esiebo

5.6 Common NHPSP development challenges, mistakes and possible solutions

5.6.1 Common challenges to the NHPSP development process and possible solutions

Tight timelines, not allowing for a thorough review of evidence

In a comprehensive planning process in a time-limited context, decisions may have to be made to reduce the planning process by some steps or parts of steps. For example, if strategic directions are required in three months' time, it may not be possible to engage comprehensively with the community or collect new data on targeted health sector issues. An effective way to address the lack of time is to establish parallel activity processes through working groups. The working groups should be in close communication with the core groups; what seems to work best is ensuring that core group members are part of the working groups as well, ensuring information exchange and a relationship of trust.

Some common challenges to the NHPSP development process are tight timelines with not enough time to review evidence thoroughly, a rapidly changing environment, insufficient stakeholder involvement, a weak link to planning, costing and budgeting, and weak coordination between programme plans and the overarching NHPSP.

A rapidly changing environment which can render any medium-term planning uncertain

In a rapidly changing environment, medium-term planning can be done for shorter time frames, for example 2–3 years, rather than five years. In addition, flexibility will be crucial to keeping the plan relevant, which may mean keeping the wording general on issues whose details should rather be worked out in the operational planning phase. In any case, in an environment where the future is not predictable, operational plans can fill in the gaps. It is important to ensure that operational plans, linked to the strategic plans, fill the gap, instead of parallel plans overlapping with the NHPSP.

The operational plan takes on a more significant meaning in the context of a constantly changing environment, as it is here that activities can be flexibility adapted and changed. The flexibility of operational plans is absolutely central to the implementability of the NHPSP. The NHPSP gives the strategic orientation for the sector which serves as a basis for the content of operational plans. The operational plans should "operationalize" the strategic plan, allow modifications where necessary (such as in a volatile context), as and when situations change.

Insufficient stakeholder involvement at all levels (not only top leaders)

Stakeholders will be interested in participating meaningfully in the NHPSP development process when they can see an added value for them and when the criticality of the NHPSP for steering the health sector is made clear. Much of the lethargy around partaking in NHPSP development often centres around the place the NHPSP is given in the health sector and its actual feasibility and role as an orienting document. In many countries, especially non-state (private) actors do not see the point in being a part of the process when they see a one-way contribution with no return for them.

The level of stakeholder involvement points back to the steering capacity of MoH and the core team (i.e. not just MoH, but key planning stakeholders as well) to effectively lead, coordinate and motivate the right people to give their input on the one hand, and assist implementation on the other. Investment in and reflection on NHPSP preparation will be crucial in settings where the NHPSP has traditionally been written for a donor audience or to tick off a planning to-do list, and then subsequently shelved.

A weak link between planning, costing and budgeting

In many countries, a lack of understanding of budget-related issues results in delinked processes such that health policy-making, planning, costing and budgeting take place independently of each other, leading to a misalignment between the health sector priorities outlined in overall strategic plans and policies, and the funds that are ultimately allocated to the health sector through the budgeting process. This misalignment has negative consequences: resources are not used as intended, and accountability is weakened. On the contrary, a good understanding of the budget process and solid engagement by the MoH and other health sector stakeholders at the right time during the budget cycle will increase the chances that the final resource allocation matches planned health sector needs.

Early engagement on the part of the MoH with the Ministry of Finance (MoF) can provide a better understanding of the financial management rules and the system within which expenditures must happen. Closer cooperation and inclusion of MoF representatives in key MoH consultations (such as those related to the estimation of NHPSP costs) can help both sides better understand each other's needs and challenges.

Weak coordination between programme plans and the overarching NHPSP

As shown in Fig. 5.3, many countries evince vertical programme plans that are not synchronized with the national health plan, and vice versa. Fig. 5.3 is based on an analysis that simply examined the timing and the years covered by programme plans vis-à-vis the NHPSP, without looking at the content of those plans and how they were harmonized and aligned – this would probably reveal even more inconsistencies. Especially in settings where large programmes are fully externally funded, they are perceived as "independent" from the rest of the health sector, yet are, in practice, influential when it comes to ad-hoc priority-setting for health. The risks are therefore great if a bridge is not adequately built between the NHPSP and programmes: the vertical programme will continue programme activities in a vertical, unsustainable way, with activities ceasing if funds cease. There may be duplications, overlap and wastage of resources, especially with the health workforce if the vertical programme is better funded and organized than the government.

On the other hand, a well-funded programme may be an opportunity to address goals that are in the NHPSP anyway – instead of overlaps and duplications, it would be more beneficial to join forces and ensure that priorities for a programme as well as priorities for the health sector are adequately reflected in both documents. This might entail a good amount of groundwork during the NHPSP preparation if the two sides are not used to engaging with each other. At the very least, during the NHPSP development process, existing programme plans should be studied, programme representatives brought in to contribute on their expert area, and M&E executed for both programme and NHPSP purposes concomitantly.

5.6.2 Common mistakes observed in NHPSPs

Insufficient connection between available inputs and intended outputs and outcomes

It is not uncommon to find NHPSPs in which inputs (resources used, such as personnel and equipment) are inadequate or inappropriate, and show no obvious connection to the achievement of the NHPSP outputs and outcomes. In order to avoid this trap, it helps to always remind oneself of the final result and the ultimate aim of the exercise. Keeping in mind the overarching health sector vision and NHPSP goals and objectives, steps can be plotted and actions thought through that would be required to arrive at the final end point of the NHPSP.

Proposed broad activity areas and implementation modalities are too vague

There may be contexts where NHPSP activity areas and guidance on implementation are deliberately vague – for example, in fragile or rapidly changing situations, or in very decentralized countries. However, in such cases, the MoH and health planning stakeholders should make explicit provisions for strong technical support when operational plans are being drafted and/or disseminate additional guidance documents at a later point in time in order to ensure that the health sector is moving in the intended direction. The risk of not doing so is a potentially fragmented health sector and a NHPSP that is inconsequential.

In situations where it is not really necessary to keep wording vague, there is no reason to not make the requisite effort to provide more detail and orientation. Reasons for not doing so often lie in an insufficiently participatory process, too short a time frame and simple lack of information on the needed details. Investing in the process and having the right people on board can fill in information gaps, for example, based on implicit knowledge and experience.

The plan is static, therefore discouraging a flexible response to change

Sometimes the NHPSP process can end up becoming much too routine. A lot of zeal and enthusiasm might have characterized the beginning stages, but when and if the process stagnates or drags on, it can be perceived as an added burden, with the principal aim being simply to finish the document and move on. This can happen when the national health planning process has not set aside adequate resources for any extra work involved, which the core team is unable to do. In addition, if the NHPSP in and of itself is seen as a separate "project", apart from the key tasks at hand, it is understandable that once it is finished, normal activities resume and the plan becomes a static document, with little chance of being implemented.

In some countries, an overemphasis on formalities and formal procedures built into the NHPSP development process has made it into a largely bureaucratic function. This can weigh down the process unnecessarily and its principle objective gets lost in paperwork and signatures.

The key to ensuring that the NHPSP is a real point of reference is ensuring that the document is realistic and feasible, provides a sector orientation broadly enough without being vague, and giving some detail without getting too operational. In addition, it is imperative that it is truly driven by meaningful input by a wide array of stakeholders – this quality of process aspect is key and should not be mired in bureaucracy.

It is crucial to ensure close links to operational planning by providing enough operational guidance to enable follow-up operational plans. Milestones can be useful here, as they give in-between targets without laying out the operational details. At the same time, the NHPSP should not go into too much unnecessary detail that can better be taken care of at the operational level, where a flexible response is possible.

If evidence analysis is superficial, there may be no convincing options for doing better in the future

Some NHPSPs are based on an analysis of the evidence that remains superficial. A solid, in-depth analysis of evidence is necessary to project what the health sector environment might look like in the future. It goes without saying that the whole policy and planning cycle must be anchored in reliable data – this means not only ensuring the generation and preservation of this data but also putting effort and resources into adequately understanding and interpreting it for purposes of strategizing for health. Otherwise, even if the NHPSP is implemented, the chances are it will not be as effective as expected.

Goals, objectives and broad activity areas reflect departmentalism, silos culture, the tendency to protect own territory and individual interests

A common criticism of national health plans is that they are unrealistic and simply reflect a wish list of desirable actions in the health sector, with little feasibility. This can happen when the NHPSP development process is not a real collaborative effort where stakeholders come together and engage in evidence-informed debate and dialogue and touch upon the contentious issue of setting priorities. Prioritization means that some groups' or institutions' activities may not be selected, and others will. When stakeholder input is piecemeal and individual – i.e. on a one-on-one basis with the MoH or other central planning authority – and not dialogue-based and joint in nature, NHPSP goals, objectives and broad activity areas become a simple collection of each actor's own separate workplan.

The solution to this problem lies in the convening and brokering role of the MoH and its capacity to bring together stakeholders – those who agree and do not agree with each other – and coordinate policy dialogue such that the result is a balanced, realistic and feasible NHPSP. In settings where MoH capacity acknowledged as weak, improving health sector governance should be prominent in the NHPSP.

5.6.3 Health sector governance

Good health sector governance involves stakeholders, leaders, and managers being aligned around the same vision, with the planning process being comprehensible to all.

Most of the above-mentioned challenges and mistakes can be linked to the absence of sound health sector governance. For example, leadership might not motivate their staff and managers at all levels of the health system, i.e. those who are at the frontline for NHPSP implementation. Leaders may not prioritize dissemination efforts with the NHPSP communicated in an understandable way to service delivery personnel and managers. If the intended results and value added for local levels are not clear to implementers, the necessary will and drive to execute will be lacking.

In essence, good leadership ensures that leaders and managers are aligned around the same vision. The point of the planning process must be comprehensible to everyone. Much of the trust in the intended NHPSP results is linked to the level of openness and transparency of the NHPSP process itself. Astute leaders will ensure that all relevant health sector stakeholders have access to the data, information, process and decision-making logic.

5.6.4 Intersectoral action and NHPSPs

Health equity and social determinants of health (SDH) are acknowledged as critical components of the post-2015 sustainable development agenda, and are essential elements of any country's path towards universal health coverage (UHC). Governments and other stakeholders should proactively address social determinants and health inequities by identifying and promoting intersectoral action as an integral and vital component of the national health planning process. Without intersectoral action as a fully-integrated component – and indeed, mindset – embedded in the national health planning process, health inequities will likely persist, and as a result, the population's health will suffer.

As mentioned in Chapter 12 of this handbook "Intersectoral planning for health and health equity", intersectoral planning, as part of the national health planning process, is not a linear process and thus several entry points exist. In particular, the situation analysis phase is an immense opportunity to ensure that the right questions regarding equity and the determinants of health are raised, and that those key issues are adequately assessed. Actions may be undertaken all along the planning cycle; however, without the principal matters coming to the forefront during the situation analysis phase, these actions will not be slated in.

Intersectoral action should be kept in mind when formulating goals, objectives and broad activity areas.

For purposes of NHPSP development, once the situation analysis and priority-setting have been undertaken, intersectoral action should be kept in mind when formulating goals, objectives and broad activity areas. In settings where intersectoral action has long been neglected, this might entail a separate objective specifically on intersectoral action. Otherwise, if it is to be embedded into other objectives and/or broad activity areas, operational guidance can be given specifically on intersectoral action to ensure that it is not forgotten during the operational planning stage.

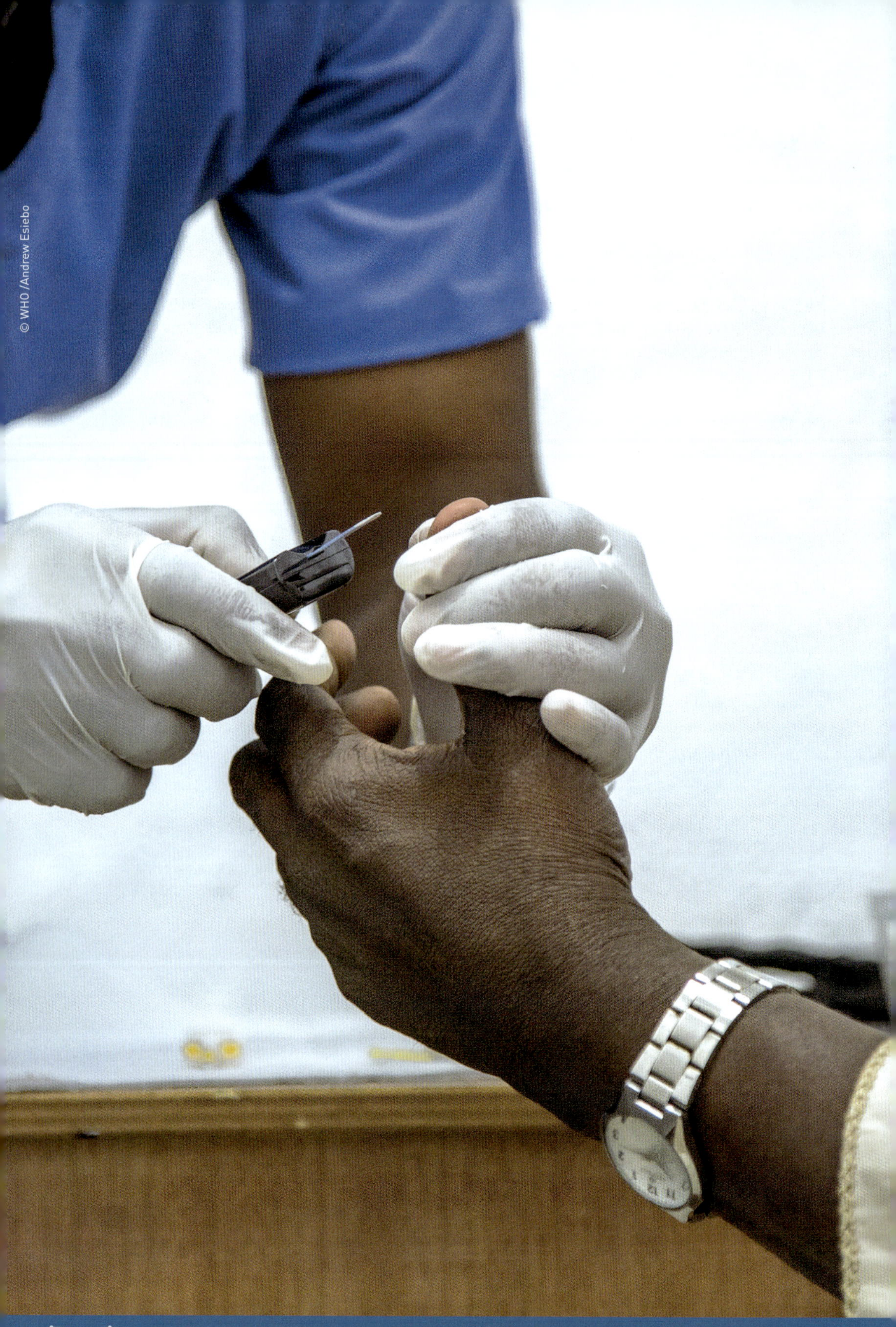

5.7 What if ...?

5.7.1 What if your country is decentralized?

A distinction should be made between strategic planning at sub-national level, which is usually only done in highly devolved settings, and national-level strategic planning in a decentralized context. Here, we address the latter.[X]

National-level strategic planning in any context, but especially in a decentralized one, is dependent on data, information, and active input from districts and regions. Central-level guidance, templates and capacity-building initiatives are key here, as sub-national levels will put together their own medium-term and operational plans anyway. Consistent and clear guidance from central level not only assists the national level to better aggregate and understand the information coming from districts and regions, but also supports the strengthening of local health systems to the benefit of all levels.

A decentralized setting may help to achieve more effective planning and decision-making in the health sector, but it can also create new challenges, especially in finding the right balance between national- and local-level planning, as the systems at each level need to be developed appropriately and consistently with each other. Especially in a decentralized setting with bottom-up planning, the dynamics of back-and-forth between levels are of importance. Districts will communicate their most important medium-term needs to central level, while the central MoH will communicate new or adjusted sector strategies and priorities to the districts. Districts may then react with proposals for strengthening certain system components or for adapting national strategies and programme roadmaps to their particular local circumstances. In turn, the central MoH will then have to verify the financial feasibility of such proposals and, if found acceptable, harmonize and coordinate the local adaptations.

Although the principles and broad processes will be similar at each level, as one moves down to the lower levels, plans will be more specific with national-level guidance providing the broad strategic envelope into which they are placed. Each level therefore needs to take into account the other plans, i.e. those being developed both in other organizations working at the same horizontal level, and also plans of both higher and lower levels in the system (the vertical dimension).

Ultimately, district plans should be validated and integrated into the NHPSP; it should then be clear which contribution the peripheral units will play in its achievement and what key results are to be achieved at their level.

X More information on both aspects can be found in Chapter 11 of this handbook "Strategizing for health at sub-national level".

5.7.2 What if fragmentation and/or fragility is an issue in your country?

In a fragile setting, decision-makers must be opportunistic in strategic planning and focus on the feasible.

NHPSP development in a rapidly changing environment sometimes renders a comprehensive health plan difficult, especially when the plan is not tailored enough to the specific environment. Complex situations require considerable flexibility in planning and a greater focus on learning and adaptation.

As a result of the uncertainty, the temporal horizon of NHPSPs in fragile settings should make room for potential revisions and changes; it should still stay concrete, with proximate objectives and mechanisms for revising objectives and broad activity areas in place. In particularly unstable situations, the absence of a prescriptive strategy can be an advantage, allowing for more flexibility and easier learning and adaptation.[XI]

Decision-makers must be opportunistic, focusing on the feasible, which is usually distant from the desirable. The challenge is to give a sector-wide purpose to assorted measures taken because they are considered feasible (see Box 5.9). Even modest success may attract other players, and generate the willingness to tackle more difficult issues. Partners should seek concrete responses to real problems, which bring benefits to the whole system and stand a chance of working even in a possible worst-case scenario.

Bottom-up planning focuses on strengthening structures already in place, integrating them into a functional system, and establishing new ones as the case permits. This is usually more valuable than an ambitious NHPSP with a distant time horizon. In many contexts under stress, the most promising level for pursuing the rationalization of health service delivery seems the provincial or local one.

Adapting to the evolving context and learning from experience are key: "The more complex and elusive our problems are, the more effective trial and error becomes... Yet it is an approach that runs counter to our instincts, and to the way in which traditional organisations work".[30]

XI For more information, see Chapter 13 "Strategizing for health in distressed contexts" in this handbook.

Box 5.9

Strengthening strategic planning in Liberia after the end of the civil war in 2003[31]

Following two civil wars, Liberia is on the road to recovery. Since its 2003 Comprehensive Peace Agreement, the country has experienced relative peace and stability through democratic elections and support from the international community. Due to the fragile nature of the post-conflict state, characterized by years of uneven political, economic and social development, strategic policy-making was vital to ensure the development of a solid policy framework void of gaps. The first Liberian National Health Policy (NHP) created in 2007 came at a crucial time for health system development.

Health planning stakeholders were aware of the importance of being opportunistic and flexible in planning, thus the NHPSP consisted of two broad but feasible goals to start rebuilding the health system. The first goal was to establish a basic package of health services that would be free to the entire population, focusing on the most urgent health priorities (communicable disease control, emergency care, maternal and newborn health, mental health care), following a long period of minimal investment in health. The war had had a devastating effect on health and development indicators; ensuring that basic services could be delivered to Liberia's citizens would hopefully set a policy foundation for broadening the services provided by the Ministry of Health and Social Welfare. The second goal placed an emphasis on building strong, sustainable and capable health institutions, particularly through a process of decentralization and integrating health system plans with other development sectors' plans. This goal was deliberately kept broad in order to enable sub-national levels to more easily adapt in their plans to the overarching NHPSP.

The challenges in rebuilding health system infrastructure are far from over. The Ebola crisis in 2014 exacerbated these challenges, especially issues linked to poor monitoring and evaluation systems, continued reliance on donor support, large out-of-pocket payments, low quality of basic and essential services, and health worker shortages. The 2015 Investment Plan for Building a Resilient Health System in Liberia has attempted to build on feasible objectives, with lessons learned from the past, to make progress in Liberia's health sector.

5.7.3 What if your country is highly dependent on aid?

In an aid-dependent context, a robust and inclusive NHPSP development process is likely to increase the ability of the government to set its own agenda and rally external partners around it.

The capacity of multilateral and bilateral agencies to exert leverage over national policy-making processes can increase in proportion to the dependency of the country's government on donor support for financing recurrent costs of the health system. Especially in such cases, a robust and inclusive NHPSP development process is likely to increase the ability of the government to set its own agenda and rally external partners around it.

In an aid-dependent context, a transparent and open consultation is crucial, in order to both ensure relevance of the NHPSP vis-à-vis donor interests and to come to a consensus on any contentious issues. In addition, health planning stakeholders must recognize the need to put effort into developing cohesive support by a broad range of interest groups. Even groups who may have shown little interest should be actively brought into the NHPSP process where possible.

High aid-dependency often goes hand-in-hand with the vertical nature of national disease programmes. This entails the risk of a disconnect between planning for disease-specific programmes and the NHPSP, leading to fragmentation and increased transaction costs. Well-funded programmes may be reluctant or unwilling to participate in the full-sector strategic planning process. Targeted partnership arrangements with these programmes and external partners under national leadership along the lines of national IHP+ compacts,[XII] memoranda of understanding, and bilateral agreements can help to avoid these problems.

XII For more information please the visit IHP+ website: http://www.internationalhealthpartnership.net/en/key-issues/compacts/

5.8 Conclusion

A strategic plan is the overarching guidance document which should steer the health sector towards its stated goals for a medium-term period (generally 3–5 years). The decision on where the health sector should go, as captured in the NHPSP, should be a joint one involving a variety of health stakeholders, with the MoH coordinating and leading the process. A strategic plan is necessary because it has the potential, if done well, to help concretize priorities; to keep the focus on the medium- to long-run, thereby avoiding deviation in vision and optimal strategies; to avoid fragmentation of the health sector; and to help focus the policy dialogue on health sector priorities.

Much has been said on the limited usefulness of strategic plans – but the problem here is not the strategic plan itself; rather it is a lack of coherence in the way it is developed, disseminated and used. For a NHPSP to take on its rightful role as the health sector reference document, it must have adequate buy-in and relevance, be solidly evidence-based and include and involve all programmes, regions, districts, population groups and viewpoints. In the 21st century, the multi-stakeholder process is key, with the aim being a consensus-based strategic document that reflects the priorities of its intended beneficiaries, its providers and the government.

Nevertheless, there are definitely limitations to a NHPSP. It is just a document in the end. In and of itself, it will not ensure success in implementation. It does not replace the need for sector steering capacity and leadership, energetic and innovative management and constant evidence-based policy dialogue on pertinent issues.

In this chapter, guidance is provided on developing a relevant NHPSP which is referred to, consulted and used. Steps are proposed to manage the NHPSP development process and common challenges and mistakes are pointed out with suggested solutions.

References

1 Green, A. An introduction to health planning in developing countries. Oxford: Oxford University Press; 1992.

2 Vriesendorp S, de la Peza L, Perry CP, Seltzer JB, O'Neil M, Reimann S, et al. Health systems in action: an ehandbook for leaders and managers. Cambridge (MA): Management Sciences for Health; 2010 (http://www.msh.org/sites/msh.org/files/msh_ehandbook_complete.pdf, accessed 2 October 2016).

3 Ministry of Health and Social Welfare Tanzania. Module course in district health management. core module 4: planning of district health services. Dar-es-Salaam; 2007 (https://www.pdffiller.com/en/project/78987100.htm, accessed 2 October 2016).

4 Samuels F, Amaya AB, Rodríguez Pose R, Balabanova D. Pathways to progress: a multi-level approach to strengthening health systems: findings on maternal and child health in Nepal, Mozambique and Rwanda, and neglected tropical diseases in Cambodia and Sierra Leone. London: Overseas Development Institute; 2014 (Dimension papier 1, http://www.developmentprogress.org/sites/developmentprogress.org/files/case-study-report/pathways_to_progress_-_a_multi-level_approach_to_strengthening_health_systems.pdf, accessed 2 October 2016).

5 Chatora R, Tumusiime P. Planning and implementation of district health services. Brazzaville: WHO Regional Office for Africa; 2004 (District Health Management Team Training Modules ,Module 4); www.afro.who.int/index.php?option=com_docman&task, accessed 2 October 2016).

6 Green A. An introduction to health planning for developing health systems, 3rd edition. New York/Oxford: Oxford University Press; 2007.

7 Country Planning Cycle Database [online database]. Geneva: World Health Organization; 2016 (http://www.nationalplanningcycles.org/ , accessed 3 October 2016).

8 Bower CE. Guide and template for comprehensive health improvement planning, version 2.1. Hartford (CT): Connecticut Department of Public Health, Planning and Workforce Development Section; 2009 (http://www.ct.gov/dph/lib/dph/state_health_planning/planning_guide_v2-1_2009.pdf, accessed 2 October 2016).

9 Brinkerhoff DW, Bossert TJ. Health governance: concepts, experience, and programming options. Washington (DC): United States Agency for International Development; 2008. (Health Systems 20/20, Policy Brief; https://www.hfgproject.org/wp-content/uploads/2015/02/Health-Governance-Concepts-Experience-and-Programming-Options.pdf, accessed 2 October 2016).

10 Green, A. Reforming the health sector in Thailand: the role of policy actors on the policy stage. Int J Health Plann Manage. 2000:15(1);39-59. doi:10.1002/(SICI)1099-1751(200001/03)15:1←39::AID-HP-M567→3.0.CO;2-9.

11 Rasanathan K, Posayanonda T, Birmingham M, Tangcharoensathien V. Innovation and participation for healthy public policy: the first National Health Assembly in Thailand. Health Expectations 2012;15(1): 87–96 (http://onlinelibrary.wiley.com/doi/10.1111/j.1369-7625.2010.00656.x/full , accessed 3 October 2016).

12 Green, A. Reforming the health sector in Thailand: the role of policy actors on the policy stage. Int J Health Plann Manage. 2000:15(1);39-59. doi:10.1002/(SICI)1099-1751(200001/03)15:1←39::AID-HP-M567→3.0.CO;2-9.

13 Pitayarangsarit S. The introduction of the universal coverage of health care policy in Thailand: policy responses. (2004 dissertation, London School of Hygiene and Tropical Medicine). Bangkok: National Health Security Office; 2010 (http://www.coopami.org/en/countries/countries/thailand/social_protection/pdf/social_protection03.pdf, accessed 3 October 2016).

14 Rasanathan K, Posayanonda T, Birmingham M, Tangcharoensathien V. Innovation and participation for healthy public policy: the first National Health Assembly in Thailand. Health Expectations 2012;15(1): 87–96 (http://onlinelibrary.wiley.com/doi/10.1111/j.1369-7625.2010.00656.x/full , accessed 3 October 2016).

15 Rasanathan K, Posayanonda T, Birmingham M, Tangcharoensathien V. Innovation and participation for healthy public policy: the first National Health Assembly in Thailand. Health Expectations 2012;15(1): 87–96 (http://onlinelibrary.wiley.com/doi/10.1111/j.1369-7625.2010.00656.x/full , accessed 3 October 2016).

16 Country Planning Cycle Database [online database]. Geneva: World Health Organization; 2016 (http://www.nationalplanningcycles.org/ , accessed 3 October 2016).

17 WHO. A framework for national health policies, strategies and plans. Geneva; 2010 (http://www.who.int/nationalpolicies/FrameworkNHPSP_final_en.pdf, accessed 3 October 2016).

18 Vriesendorp S, de la Peza L, Perry CP, Seltzer JB, O'Neil M, Reimann S, et al. Health systems in action: an ehandbook for leaders and managers. Cambridge (MA): Management Sciences for Health; 2010 (http://www.msh.org/sites/msh.org/files/msh_ehandbook_complete.pdf, accessed 2 October 2016).

19 WHO Country Cooperation Strategy 2009–2014: Uganda. Brazzaville: WHO Regional Office for Africa; 2009 (http://www.who.int/countryfocus/cooperation_strategy/ccs_uga_en.pdf, accessed 3 October 2016).

20 Health Sector Strategic Plan III 2010/11–2014/15. Kampala: Government of Uganda Ministry of Health: 2010 (http://www.health.go.ug/docs/HSSP_III_2010.pdf, accessed 3 October 2015).

21 Government of Uganda. National budget framework paper: section 3: health sector. 2015 (http://budget.go.ug/budget/sites/default/files/Sector%20Budget%20Docs/Health%20Sector%20BFP.pdf, accessed 3 October 2016).

22 Odaga J, Lochoro P. Budget ceilings and health in Uganda. Kampala: Caritas, Uganda; 2006.

23 Howlett M, Ramesh M. Studying public policy: policy cycles and policy subsystems. Toronto: Oxford University Press; 2003 (http://works.bepress.com/howlett/12/, accessed 4 October 2016).

24 WHO. Health systems strengthening: glossary. Geneva; 2011 (http://www.who.int/healthsystems/Glossary_January2011.pdf, accessed 3 October 2016).

25 SMART goal criteria can be found at: http://hr.tufts.edu/wp-content/uploads/ODT_smart_goal_criteria.pdf, accessed 4 October 2016.

26 Spiegel AD, Hyman HH. Strategic health planning: methods and techniques applied to marketing and management. Nordwood (NJ): Ablex Publishing Corporation; 1991.

27 Bower CE. Guide and template for comprehensive health improvement planning, version 2.1. Hartford (CT): Connecticut Department of Public Health, Planning and Workforce Development Section; 2009 (http://www.ct.gov/dph/lib/dph/state_health_planning/planning_guide_v2-1_2009.pdf, accessed 2 October 2016).

28 International Health Partnership. Joint Assessment of National Health Strategies (JANS) tool and guidelines. (http://www.internationalhealthpartnership.net/en/tools/jans-tool-and-guidelines/, accessed 3 October 2016).

29 JANS lessons. In: International Health Partnership+[website]. 2016 (http://www.internationalhealthpartnership.net/en/results-evidence/jans-lessons/, accessed 3 October 2016

30 Harford T. Adapt: why success always starts with failure. London: Abacus; 2012: 35.

31 Rocha Menocal A., Sirgrist, K. Capacity gaps at centres of government: coordination, implementation monitoring, communications and strategic planning in cost-conflict and fragile situations. Liberia case study. London: Overseas Development Institute; 2011 (https://www.odi.org/sites/odi.org.uk/files/odi-assets/publications-opinion-files/8495.pdf, accessed 3 October 2016).

32 Ibid.

33 Republic of Liberia. National Health Policy: National Health Plan 2007–2011. Monrovia: Ministry of Health & Social Welfare; 2007 (http://apps.who.int/medicinedocs/documents/s18363en/s18363en.pdf, accessed 3 October 2016).

34 Downie R. The road to recovery: rebuilding Liberia's health system. Washington (DC): Center for Strategic and International Studies; 2012 (https://csis-prod.s3.amazonaws.com/s3fs-public/legacy_files/files/publication/120822_Downie_RoadtoRecovery_web.pdf, accessed 3 October 2016).

Further reading

Chatora R, Tumusiime P. Planning and implementation of district health services. Brazzaville: World Health Organization Regional Office for Africa; 2004 (District Health Management Team Training Modules: Module 4; http://www.who.int/management/district/planning_budgeting/PlanningImplementationDHSAFROMd4.pdf, accessed 2 October 2016).

Green A. An introduction to health planning for developing health systems, 3rd edition. New York/Oxford: Oxford University Press; 2007.

Health policy development: a handbook for Pacific Islands practitioners. Manila: WHO Regional Office for the Western Pacific; 2006 (http://www.wpro.who.int/health_services/documents/health_policy_development_pacific_island_practitioners/en/, accessed 3 October 2016).

Joint Assessment of National Strategies and plans: combined joint assessment tool and guidelines. version 3, August 2013 (online) (http://www.internationalhealthpartnership.net/fileadmin/uploads/ihp/Documents/Tools/JANS/JANS_updated_guidelines_August_2013.pdf, accessed 2 October 2016).

Annex 5.1

Review of existing policies and strategies to ensure inclusion in and harmonization with NHPSP

When developing a NHPSP, it is necessary to review other existing policies and strategies with regard to their relevance for the health plan in development. In view of this, the questions listed below can be helpful.

1. Where does the policy/strategy idea come from? Government manifesto, the minister, the agency, chief executive, policy branch, delivery staff, an interest group, a community consultation?

2. Is the policy/strategy defined adequately?

    - Do we have a clear authoritative statement of intent of the desired outcome? Is there agreement on the nature of the problem?
    - Are there feasible solutions?
    - Is it a problem for the government or someone else?
    - Is there adequate "evidence" to justify the proposal?
    - What is the optimal timing of: (a) the decision? (b) implementation?

3. Is the underlying analysis adequate?

    - Are the objectives and goals explicit and unambiguous?
    - Has there been a thorough search for options?
    - Have the appropriate methodologies (mix of policy instruments) been employed?
    - Is there a preferred option?
    - Has implementation been considered?
    - Is legislative action required?
    - Has the proposal's relationship to "the health plan" been considered?
    - Has a consultation process been developed: (a) within government? (b) with other stakeholders? (c) with the community?
    - Have the possibilities of external assistance been explored?

With regard to inclusion and harmonization into the NHPSP, the following questions should be asked.

- What is the time line for presentation to the decision-maker, chief executive, minister, cabinet?
- Are there dissenting views of which the decision-maker should be informed?
- Are the "right" options exposed to the decision-maker?
- Is there a clear expression of the relationship of the proposal to: (a) the budget? (b) the "health plan"? (c) the "national plan"?
- Are the workforce implications clear?
- Are the legal implications (authority and enforcement) identified?
- Has the proposed involvement of donors, including international agencies, been discussed with them? Are there concrete proposals or commitments?
- Who has been consulted; who should be informed before the decision is announced?
- What should be done to "sell" the policy?
- Is the implementation time line sufficiently detailed; are those to be held accountable identified?
- What are the risks for the government and the community?

Annex 5.2

Mind-mapping

Mind-mapping is a way of capturing a combination of information and ideas, and of organizing them. It relies on pictorial representations of the flow and synthesis of ideas. It is used for standard flip chart-based discussions, as well as computer-based exercises.

This tool is particularly useful when a group of planners with different backgrounds is considering the option of introducing or adjusting strategies or reforms. It helps the group to find common ground in weighing options.

Source: www.mindmapping.com, accessed 4 October 2016

Annex 5.3

Formulating strategic objectives on the basis of SMART criteria

Goal # ______ *(write goal number or statement here)*	**Objective Number**					
Test Questions	1	2	3	4	5	6
1. Will attainment of the objective help the goal?						
2. Does the goal have at least one objective?						
3. Is the objective evidence-based (supported by data and theory)?						
4. Does the objective specify a starting (baseline) value or condition and a desired accomplishment (target value or condition)?						
5. Can progress toward achieving the objective be measured?						
6. Is the objective attainable and realistic, given the planning period and available recources?						
7. Does the objective specify a ***realistic result***, rather than an ***activity***?						
8. Is a time frame specified for attainment of the objective or implied in the Plan, itself?						
9. Would someone unfamiliar with the planning group understand what the objective means?						
10. Have you indentified who will be accountable for achieving the objective?						

Source: http://hr.tufts.edu/wp-content/uploads/ODT_smart_goal_criteria.pdf, accessed 4 October 2016.

Annex 5.4

Intervention logic as a tool for strategic planning

Intervention logic attempts to tease out the steps between the activity and final outcome. Within the context of NHPSPs, the technique focuses the planner on each intermediate step necessary to go from a broad activity area to the intended outcome or goal. It helps avoid big leaps in logic from the most easily identified output to a more distant outcome, without thinking through the intermediate steps. Assumptions are explicitly stated and risk scenarios are considered. Intervention (or programme) logic can be employed for policy design, programme planning and policy evaluation.

An important advantage of this technique is that it focuses attention on what the government plans to do with what it hopes to achieve. At the heart of the process is the notion of a "hierarchy" or 'cascade' of outcomes (intermediate results).

Annex 5.5

Gantt chart

A Gantt chart is a simple aid used to develop an action plan and monitor that plan, with tasks and timelines visually linked. In the NHPSP context, a Gantt chart can be used for the NHPSP itself, or to prepare and follow up on the NHPSP process. For example, each activity can be listed with start and end dates, depicted on a linear timeline using a horizontal bar. The advantage of a Gantt chart is that activities are presented visually in logical sequence. The chart makes visually clear which tasks need to be carried out and when. For the NHPSP process, a Gantt chart can depict tasks by semester or quarter, with key phases and steps, as well as the person or institution responsible for steering, coordinating, supporting, oversight reporting and implementation.

Source: www.gantt.com, accessed 4 October 2016.

Chapter 6

Operational planning: transforming plans into action

Dean Shuey

Maryam Bigdeli

Dheepa Rajan

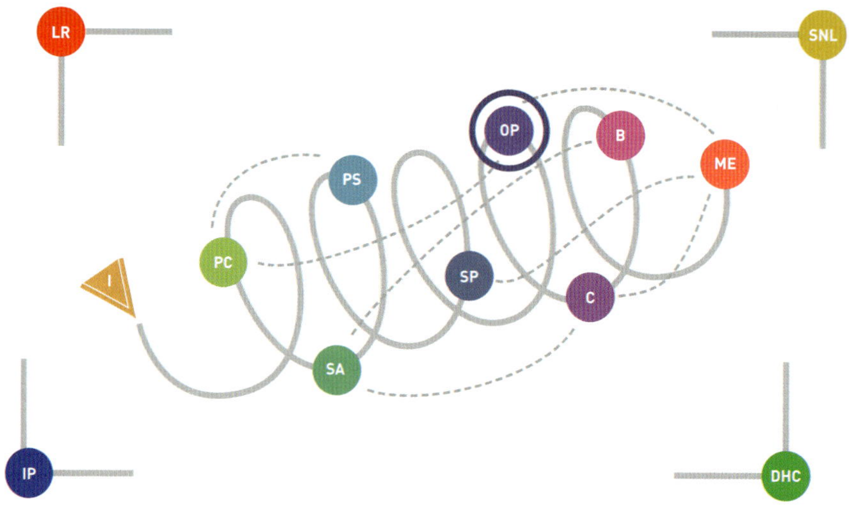

Cross-cutting topics relevant to national health planning

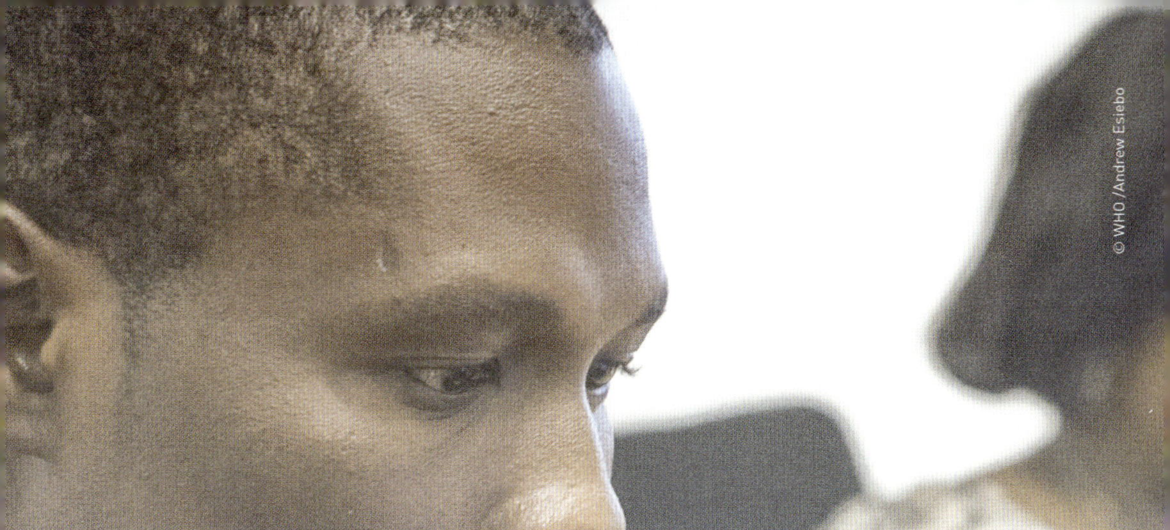

© WHO /Andrew Esiebo

Overview

Operational planning is the link between strategic objectives of the national health policy, strategy or plan (NHPSP) and the implementation of activities. It is about transforming the strategic-level plan into actionable tasks. At this stage, most steps of the NHPSP have been completed and the budgeting has been done. Operational planning is done by budget centre and will identify the activities to be carried out to achieve the objectives of the strategic plan.

Planning is often made into something complicated, a mystery wrapped in jargon, process and politics. Planning is sometimes left to the professional planners or the managers to control and do. That

is a mistake. The best operational plans, and certainly the ones most likely to be implemented, are those that are developed with the people who will carry them out (as well as other stakeholders).

Everyone in the health sector is an operational planner and everyone has a plan, even if they don't recognize it as such. The simplest operational plan is a "to-do" list, which may be written down or carried in a health worker's head. A calendar of activities that defines the what, when and who of tasks is also a plan. The operational plan determines the day-to-day activities of the unit for which it is written.

Summary

What is operational planning?

Operational planning is typically based on a NHPSP that defines the vision, goals and objectives for the health sector. Operational planning is managerial and shorter term, as opposed to strategic planning, which usually has a 5–10 year horizon, sometimes even longer. Operational planning deals with day-to-day implementation and often has a one-year time horizon.

An operational plan is a practical plan of activities to undertake that are in line with the overall NHPSP, but is concrete enough for practitioners at each level of the health system to know what they are responsible for.

Operational planning takes place when most other steps of the planning cycle are completed, at the level of budget centres.

Why is operational planning crucial to strategizing for health?

Operational plans are necessary to concretize NHPSPs. They provide a framework for action based on the strategic vision given by the NHPSP. The operational planning process has the potential to greatly assist stakeholders in gaining a better understanding of the NHPSP target population and its needs, as well as stakeholders' own capabilities and limitations in implementation. Especially when defined jointly, an operational plan is critical for the clarity it offers as to what needs to be done, by whom, how, and with which monies.

When should operational planning take place?

The health operational planning process should be synchronized with the budgeting process of the financing entity. This typically means a complete operational plan with budgets done on a yearly basis. This can be on a two-yearly basis in settings that are very stable from a political or social point of view. Operational planning can be done even more frequently, for example every six months or even three months, in situations where insecurity and instability force decision-makers to adapt activities to a rapidly-evolving context.[I]

I For more information, please see Chapter 13 "Strategizing in distressed health contexts" of this handbook.

How does operational planning work?

An operational plan should typically include:

1. a description of activities and a statement as to which major objective of the NHPSP it falls under;
2. the timing and sequencing of those activities;
3. a quantity of activity;
4. the person(s) responsible for the activity;
5. the resources required, including financial resources, and the origin of those resources;
6. a method of measuring progress (monitoring).

The following steps are necessary for sound operational planning:

1. taking stock of the situation (where are we now?), including identification of stakeholders (who is involved?);
2. setting operational priorities;
3. putting together the operational plan (what are we going to do?), including the operational budget;
4. implementation of planned activities (how are we going to do it?);
5. monitoring and evaluation of the operational plan (what have we accomplished so far?);

Who are the main actors involved in operational planning?

Ideally, all of those who are responsible for an activity in the health sector will be involved in operational planning, either directly or through having their interests represented by someone involved in the formal planning process. Key stakeholders are the national and local health authorities, health service providers and health system end users.

Anything else to consider?

- decentralized environment;
- fragile environment;
- highly aid-dependent context;
- strong vertical programme.

6.1 What is operational planning?

6.1.1 Concepts and definitions

"Planning is a method of trying to ensure that the resources available now and in the future are used in the most efficient way to obtain explicit objectives."[1]

Another way to see operational planning, taken from a business consultancy, is "the process that determines the day to day activities of the business".[2] This point of view is transferable to the public sector. An operational plan is about doing. It defines what actions will be taken. Implementation planning, activity planning, and work planning are alternative terms used for operational planning.

An operational plan is a practical plan of activities to undertake that are in line with the overall NHPSP, but it is concrete enough for practitioners at each level of the health system to know what they are responsible for. In other words, an operational plan will describe the tactics that must be employed as the preferred method for achieving certain objectives, or targets. A simple example of a target might be "90% of pregnant women receive four antenatal care visits". A tactical (or specific) objective would choose whether the preferred method of reaching this target is through outpatient consultations at maternal and child health clinics, during outreach activities, through community health workers, or some combination of these methods or tactics.

Operational planning is undertaken by "budget centres" (or "cost centres"), ideally when the overall health budget is formally known. A "budget centre" is an accounting term used to describe a department, division, or other subunit for accounting purposes; usually, a budget centre has some level of autonomy in activity implementation. With regard to health sector planning, this can refer to a unit within a ministry of health (MoH), a parastatal institution, a sub-national entity, or any other establishment for which the income and expenses are separated out and monitored. It can also be a contracted facility or group of facilities (which could be in the private sector). The level of budget details may vary with private entities, but all facilities working in the health sector – public, private for-profit and private non-profit, need to do operational planning exercises; at the very least, all stakeholders need to be aware of what the others are doing.

That being said, all units that have activities and budgets should have an operational plan. There will be cases where several units (such as health centres) together form a budget centre; the contrary holds true as well – a large well-funded programme may end up being several budget centres. In the former case, it might mean that a "sub-unit", for example a health centre, might still need to do a separate operational plan for its own purposes; in the latter case, the large programme might have to do a separate, unified operational plan for it to work off of. Either way, the principles of operational planning as elucidated in this chapter apply.

The operational plan of units that do not provide direct services, such as units at a central MoH,

An operational plan is a practical plan of activities to undertake, concrete enough for practitioners at each level of the health system to know what they are responsible for.

should include the activities undertaken to technically support those units that are providing direct services. An important decision is whether MoH units include the actual service delivery carried out by health facilities or district teams in their plans. There is a strong inclination to do so, but it can lead to a proliferation of planning exercises, and also lead to double counting of activities. In a well-organized system it is preferable for the operational plan to only include activities actually performed by the unit that is planning. For example, in a malaria control programme, the central malaria unit would not include the distribution of bednets to community members in their operational plan if members of a district health team do that distribution.

Operational plans are sometimes described as something that is needed for lower levels of the health sector, typically sub-national structures such as regions or districts and individual facilities such as hospitals and health centers. That is true, but incomplete. All who carry out activities benefit from having an operational plan. The planning unit of a MoH needs an operational plan to define what it will do on a day-to-day basis to implement the plan. Each department at a central MoH needs an operational plan, not to set strategy, but to determine activity. Even a minister's office needs a plan of the activities it will carry out to provide stewardship for the sector.

If the unit undertaking the operational planning is a sub-national entity, the specificities of planning is linked to the decentralized level and is addressed in the "what if" section 6.1.3.

A formal operational plan at a minimum should include:

1. a description of activities linked to the overarching strategic objectives (normally contained in the strategic plan);
2. the timing and sequencing of those activities;
3. a quantity of activity;
4. the person(s) responsible for the activity;
5. the resources required, including financial resources, and the origin of those resources;
6. a method of measuring progress (monitoring).

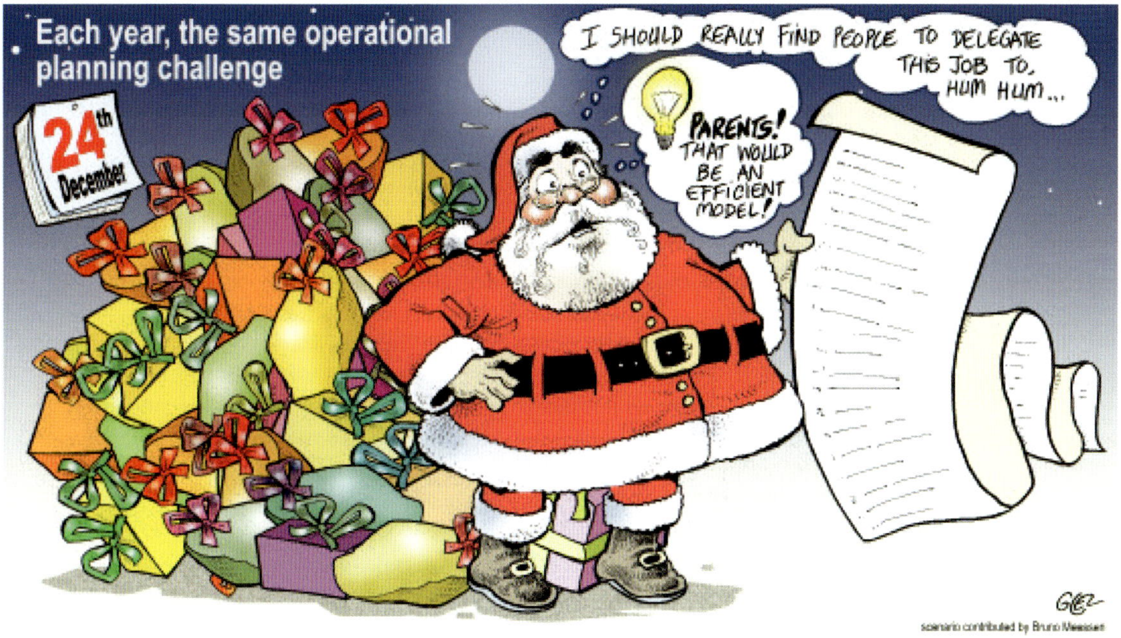
Each year, the same operational planning challenge
24th
December
I SHOULD REALLY FIND PEOPLE TO DELEGATE THIS JOB TO, HUM HUM...
PARENTS! THAT WOULD BE AN EFFICIENT MODEL!
Glez
scenario contributed by Bruno Meessen

Damien Glez; scenario by Bruno Meesen

Fig. 6.1 Operational planning

6.1.2 Strategic planning vs operational planning

Strategic health planning refers to the long-term vision, goals and objectives for the health sector. Operational planning is managerial and shorter term. Strategic planning usually has a 5–10 year horizon, sometimes even longer (see Table 6.1). Operational planning deals with day-to-day implementation and often has a one-year time horizon. The time frame is usually the same as the budgeting cycle of the organization or government. Strategic plans, once completed and agreed, tend to stay relatively constant throughout their agreed term. Operational plans, on the other hand, should be dynamic, open to change if situations change or targets are not being met, and remain open to regular revision as circumstances change. Examples of changing circumstances requiring a change of plan would be an unexpected epidemic or a natural disaster, changes in the resources available, or clear signs that goals are not being met.

The flexibility of operational plans is absolutely central to the implementability of the NHPSP. The NHPSP gives the strategic orientation for

The flexibility of operational plans is absolutely central to the implementability of the NHPSP. The operational plans should "operationalize" the strategic plan and can only adequately do so if they can be modified along the way, as and when situations change and new context-specific learning can be applied.

the sector, which serves as a basis for the content of operational plans. The operational plans should "operationalize" the strategic plan and can only adequately do so if they can be modified along the way, as and when situations change and new context-specific learning can be applied. An example illustrating this point is the interaction between Cambodia's second Health Sector Strategic Plan (HSP) and Annual Operational Plans (AOPs). The AOPs for the health sector, which became mandatory in 1999, are put together through a combination of bottom-up and top-down processes, and are further broken down into quarterly action plans and monthly workplans.[3,4] The last HSP 2008–2015 was not altered during its duration, as its objectives were aligned with the Millennium Development Goals; however, the AOPs were constantly modified when corrective action was necessary, based on regular supervision and monitoring results.

Table 6.1 Key characteristics of strategic and operational planning

	STRATEGIC PLANNING	OPERATIONAL PLANNING
VISION	Long term	Short(er) term
FOCUS	Strategic direction for the health sector	Concrete activity implementation
TIME FRAME	3- to 5-year document	1 year, sometimes shorter time frame
FLEXIBILITY	Less likely to change during its term	Can more easily be adapted and modified according to changing circumstances

6.1.3 Operational planning and budgeting

Ideally, the sector budget ceiling as well as the exact allocations to the budget centres should be clear before putting together an operational plan. If the public budget negotiation process is still not completely concluded at the time of operational planning, the approximate sector budget allocation as well as the NHPSP disaggregated costing can be used as an approximate ceiling within which to plan.[II]

The structure of the operational plan will be heavily dependent on the type of budgeting used in the country. Ideally, it can be developed based on the specific objectives for the operational unit, as this is usually most useful from the point of view of the unit. However, if operational plans and budgets need to be submitted using line-item budgeting, one of the two options below can be used.

(a) The operational plan can still be done by specific objectives but an additional step will be necessary to "translate" the budget lines linked to activities and objectives to line items (sometimes called a "chart of accounts"). Several iterations will be necessary here if the exact amounts of each of the line items are fixed and inflexible, in order to make the objective-driven budget match the line items. If the line item amounts are not fixed and there is flexibility within the budget centre's allocation of funds to change the amounts linked to the line items, then the line-item budget can be more easily molded to the needs of the operational unit's objectives.

(b) The operational plan is created from the beginning according to line items. The risk of not ensuring a link between the country's budgeting system and the structure of the operational plan is that resource allocations may not match the needs nor the capacity of the operational unit. If there is room for flexibility in the line item allocations, at least ensuring that those allocations meet the objectives of the operational plan is possible, but will entail an extra workload for health planning stakeholders in securing allocations by line items that tally up to the necessary resources per objective.

6.1.4 Participation and inclusiveness of operational planning

Operational planning is a method of formally organizing activities through a process that involves key stakeholders, with the results of the process shared with all involved. The process is meaningful in and of itself to encourage and solicit participation and input of major stakeholders of the (local) health system. The absolute criticality of broad and inclusive participation cannot be emphasized enough, all the more so for operational planning (vis-à-vis strategic planning) because the decisions made regarding what to include into the operational plan concretely and directly affect those who will be carrying out the decisions. Success or failure will depend largely on the buy-in, understanding and willingness to implement the plan by health sector stakeholders; hence, those very stakeholders must be consulted and heard. Many countries have well-functioning, recognized participatory bodies (health committees, management committees, etc.) that can be used as a vector to ensure that all interests are represented in the decision-making process.

While operational plans are a guide for day-to-day action, they are not a detailed description of every action taken; the correct amount of detail is vital to ensure the planning process is not burdensome.

II For more information, please see Chapter 7 "Estimating cost implications of a national health policy, strategy or plan" and Chapter 8 "Budgeting for health" in this handbook.

Box 6.1

Inclusive planning in Senegal: regional health sector reviews[5]

"[We have been able to focus] more on the communities in need, in their own environment, by putting in place much-needed regional health sector reviews," said Dr. Farba Lamine Sall, Director of the Minister of Health's Office, Senegal.

In 2014, the Senegalese Ministry of Health was looking to improve coordination among national, regional and local health administrations. It was decided to put in place regional health sector reviews (RHSRs), in addition to the annual health sector review, the idea being to more closely involve the health community, civil society and implementers on the ground, as it was usually not feasible to involve them all at the annual health sector review.

Over a period of two years, the RHSRs have been formally institutionalized as a means to monitor sub-national operational plans. In addition, the RHSR has proven to be a key instrument for allowing greater and more meaningful participation from different players in the local health system, since much of civil society and various population groups are represented at regional, rather than national, level. Also, most of the practitioners on the ground were more motivated to actively participate in the regional – rather than national – reviews, as the issues discussed directly affected their daily lives.

The Senegalese MoH has noted better quality operational plans from the regional level since 2014, and a more profound understanding of national-level stakeholders for challenges in the different regions. All in all, monitoring of operational plans, and the subsequent adjustments made to operational plans in the regions, have proven to be essential means to increase community and population participation and make the participation more useful and meaningful.

6.2 Why is operational planning crucial to strategizing for health?

Operational plans are necessary to concretize NHPSPs. They provide a framework for action based on the strategic vision given by the NHPSP. They are the only instrument that allows for a formulation of implementation modalities, and an identification of financial and other resources needed and of the timelines against which the tasks must be achieved. Without an operational plan to make the NHPSP more tangible, stakeholders will not be clear about their own roles and responsibilities, and implementation will suffer. Especially when defined jointly with all relevant health sector stakeholders, an operational plan is critical for the clarity it offers as to what needs to be done, by whom, how, and with which monies.

The operational planning process has the potential to greatly assist stakeholders in gaining a better understanding of the NHPSP target population and its needs, as well as stakeholders' own capabilities and limitations in implementation. The operational plan provides an opportunity on at least an annual basis to constantly adjust activities and actions according to need and circumstance, also by other actors from other sectors.

The process can help increase transparency and avoid confusion about what is expected, and guide the implementation of activities. It is a useful tool for both the manager and the person being managed. Each worker should know where he or she fits in the overall plan and what is expected.

6.3 When should operational planning take place?

Although an operational plan may have activities described for a year, the exact timing of most activities need to be planned on a shorter time period, often quarterly or even monthly. For example, it may be possible to describe a certain number of primary health care activities per month to cover a district, but fixing the exact dates of the activities needs to be done closer to the time of actual implementation.

Operational plans are necessary to the NHPSP planning process because they provide a framework for action based on the plan's strategic vision.

The operational planning process should be synchronized with the budgeting process of the financing entity. This typically means a complete operational plan with budgets done on a yearly basis. This can be on a two-yearly basis in settings that are very stable from a political or social point of view. Operational planning can be done even more frequently, for example every six months or even three months, in situations where insecurity and instability force decision-makers to adapt activities to a rapidly evolving context.[III] Close cooperation between the finance and health sectors – and indeed other relevant sectors – is ideal.

Typically, operational plans with budgets are done on a yearly basis to ensure that the planning process is synchronized with the budgeting process of the financing entity. They can be done more frequently in situations in insecurity or less frequently in a very stable context.

The central health planning authority should provide operational units clear guidance on dates that planning milestones must be met and the processes for approval of the plans. It is helpful if guidance can be given as to the estimated length of time that is required for preparation of the various steps in the process. A checklist with due dates is extremely useful (see Box 6.2).

III For more information, please see Chapter 13 "Strategizing in distressed health contexts" in this handbook.

Box 6.2

Example: operational planning checklist from a Cambodian Provincial Health Department (PHD) Office[6]

TASK	WHEN	WHO	CHECK
Task 1: Attend the MoH Annual Performance Review Meeting	End of February	PHD Director	
Task 2: Provincial workshop for annual review and setting provincial objectives and targets	March	Provincial Health Technical Advisory Team (PHTAT), PHD staff, referral hospital management team, health centre chiefs, partners	
Task 3: Provide technical support to the referral hospitals and health centres	March and April, during development of annual operational plans	Directors of PHD, key staff of PHD technical bureau, key staff of PHD finance bureau	
Task 4: Appraisal of PHD, referral hospitals, and health centre annual operational plans	May, as soon as operational plans developed	Directors of PHD, key staff of PHD technical bureau, key staff of PHD finance bureau	
Task 5: Preparation of the provincial 3-year rolling plan and the provincial annual operational plan	May, as soon as operational plans developed	Directors of PHD, key staff of PHD technical bureau, key staff of PHD finance bureau	
Task 6: Meeting to review the provincial 3-year rolling plan and the provincial annual operational plan based on feedback from the MoH	Early August, as soon as PHD received feedback from MoH	PHTAT, PHD staff in charge of national programs activities, referral hospital management team, health centre chiefs, partners	
Task 7: Meeting to finalize the provincial annual operational plan	December	PHTAT, PHD staff in charge of national programs activities, referral hospital management team, health centre chiefs, partners	
Task 8: Monthly Meeting of PHTAT with referral hospitals and health centres	Every month of the next year, while operational plan implemented	PHTAT, PHD staff in charge of national programs activities, referral hospital management team, health centre chiefs	
Task 9: Provincial quarterly review meetings	The first week of each quarter	PHTAT, PHD staff in charge of national programs activities, referral hospital management team, health centre chiefs, partners	
Task 10: Attend the MoH Mid-year Performance Review Meeting	August next year	PHD Directors	

One problem encountered in some countries is constant change to the guidance and formats of planning. Typically, central health planning authorities may find that the format of the operational plans are not perfectly adapted for monitoring and evaluation purposes, or for tracking the use of resources for a particular programme or for better access to specific earmarked funding. They may therefore change the format of the operational plan from one cycle to the other (from one year to the other). It must, however, be kept in mind that every change requires time and effort to adapt to it. The change must be a significant improvement to justify the disruption it causes. The pursuit of perfection should not drive out planning processes that are good enough.

It is wise for the unit undertaking operational planning to try to finish work at least a week or two before the deadline, leaving ample time for a leisurely review and fine-tuning, as necessary. Last-minute planning often leads to mistakes.

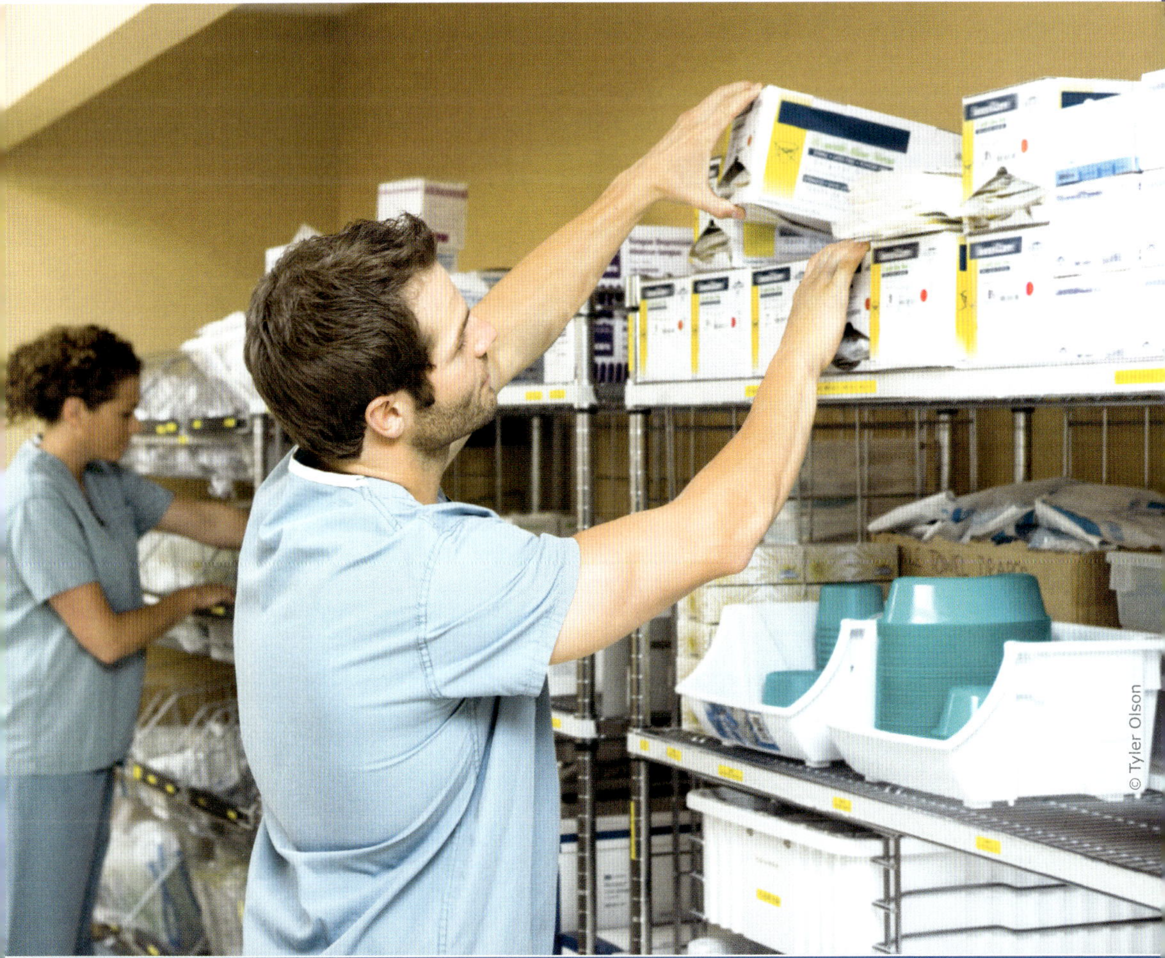

6.4 How does operational planning work?

Central-level guidance to the different budget centres and operational units on operational planning should typically include information on timing for completing the different steps, information on the stakeholders expected to be involved in the planning process, and a guidance framework, often a matrix, that includes at a minimum:

A formal operational plan should include: a description of activities linked to the strategic objectives; the timing, sequencing, and quantity of those activities; the person(s) responsible for and resources required for the plan; and a method of measuring progress.

1. a description of activities and a statement as to which major objective of the NHPSP each falls under;
2. the timing and sequencing of those activities;
3. a quantity of activity;
4. the person(s) responsible for the activity;
5. the resources required (including financial) and the origin of those resources; and
6. a method of measuring progress (monitoring).

The guidance must also include instructions concerning the degree of decision-making authority that lies with the budget centre. Is the operational planner required to follow goals, objectives, budgets, and tactics that are determined by a central authority? Or, can the budget centre set its own goals, objectives, budgets and tactics? In most situations, the reality is somewhere in between these two extremes. The national health planning authority should give guidance as to where the balance lies in that particular system.

In addition, major policy orientations based on the NHPSP should be detailed and explained right at the beginning of the operational planning process, in order to orient the content of the operational plans.

6.4.1 Some operational planning issues to consider

Operational plans are still needed even if there is no useful strategic plan

There are times when the strategic planning process is less effective, and clear and reasonable guidance is not available. In such circumstances, an operational planning exercise is still necessary and useful as a management tool for health managers or health care workers who have responsibilities to fulfil.

Level of detail needed in an operational plan

A word of caution on the amount of detail needed is in order. Operational plans are a guide for day-to-day action. They are not a detailed description of every action taken. When too much detail is required, the planning process becomes burdensome and uses excessive amounts of time. The plan can become so large that it is not useful. A plan for immunization services might include an activity to maintain the cold chain in all of the health centres in a district. It will not include every step taken to maintain a refrigerator. However, a cold-chain technician might have a to-do list that does detail those steps, but it would not be part of the district plan. If maintaining the cold chain has been a problem, however, an operational plan might include developing a to-do list for cold-chain maintenance. Finding the correct amount of detail requires common sense and experience.

Flexibility

Operational plans must be iterative. They are subject to change depending on feedback on results that come from monitoring and ongoing field experience. If something is not working, it is often necessary to change what is being done. Depending on the circumstances, those changes do not always have to wait for the end of the formal planning period (see Box 6.3 on medium-term rolling plans).

Box 6.3

Medium-term rolling plans

In some settings, an intermediate or medium-term plan is also developed, which is usually three years in duration, and can be seen as a bridging plan between the NHPSP and the operational plans. Medium-term plans are commonly associated with a medium-term expenditure framework (MTEF), which is discussed in detail in a separate chapter.[IV]

MTEFs have been popularized by the international financial institutions and ministries of finance. In countries where a medium-term plan is developed, there may be a rolling plan process, where on a yearly basis, the operational plan for the coming year is refined, and an additional year of planning is added so that there is always a three-year plan in place.[7] The idea is to make the operational planning process less heavy and more connected with the budgeting process.[8]

Critique of MTEFs has been mainly focused on planning and reporting requirements from international development partners who have heavily supported the MTEFs. It is true that in settings with large donor monies in the health sector, MTEFs have helped give more clarity to development partners' financial and technical commitments. For example, in Benin, some development partners found it difficult to commit beyond three years. A three-year rolling plan was thus more feasible for many partners to commit to. In recognition of this, Benin's 10-year NHPSP (Plan national de développement sanitaire, 2009–2018) was divided into three-year rolling plans with MTEFs.

On the other hand, it has been acknowledged that MTEF processes have contributed to greater linkages between operational planning and budgeting and have helped countries to adjust their plans to be more realistic and feasible.

IV For more information, please see Chapter 8 "Budgeting for health" in this handbook.

Bottom-up or top-down process

A major decision is whether operational planning will be a bottom-up process, a top-down process, or some combination of the two. In most cases, it ends up being the latter.

A top-down process works best in a highly-structured civil service or business setting with strong central budgetary and supervisory controls. Instructions can be sent and the plans have to be completed, as instructed, before any of the resources flow. It should work like clockwork, but rarely does. Nevertheless, even if the organization is highly centralized, there are advantages in letting units and individuals develop their own plans within the limits of that highly centralized structure. Operational plans that are dictated from above frequently do not reflect on-the-ground reality and therefore lead to poor performance.

The pathway for operational plan approval should be clear, both with regard to who can approve and the deadlines for when decisions are to be made.

However, a bottom-up process can be lengthy, requires much training, and large numbers of human resources, and their time, to prepare and consolidate. Whether it is feasible is a judgement that depends on local capacity and local priorities, but such processes frequently become delayed and bogged down.

An alternative is a local operational planning process based on clear guidance from a national health planning office. Such a process usually works better if there is input from the national level during the planning process, before local plans are far advanced. This input can take the form of written guidance, the physical presence of planners to facilitate the planning process, or workshops to familiarize local planners with the national plans and priorities. It can also include remote support such as emails and teleconferences, something that is becoming more feasible as technology improves. The art of planning involves finding the proper balance between these methods.

Finalization and approval of the operational plan

A particularly important issue is to provide guidance on the process of finalization and approval of the operational plan, including clear criteria for acceptance of plans. A clear pathway for approval should be described, both with regard to who can approve and the deadlines for when decisions are to be made. In the real world, there are often multiple layers of approval, and it can become quite confusing unless it is clearly specified who has the right and responsibility of approval and when that is to occur. An even more difficult issue is what to do with the entities that miss submission and approval deadlines (see Box 6.4). Complexity cannot be avoided, but it is only fair that operational planners be given a clear roadmap of the approval process.

Aggregating plans

Another issue to consider is where the aggregation of operational activities is done. Will activities be aggregated at district level and then passed up to a regional office, if it exists, and then on to the national level? Or will activities be aggregated by programme? The decision will depend on how the budget centres are organized and which entities need a separate budget that will be monitored for expenditures and outputs. For example, the district malaria team's operational plan can be aggregated at the district health plan level; the operational plan can also be sent to the national malaria office and aggregated there. Aggregating by programme, i.e. organizing budget centres by programme, is often felt to be more satisfactory by the individual programmes, but is at risk of leading to a plethora of plans– one for each individual programme – which may not be coherent with each other.

Box 6.4

What happens when local units do not complete or submit their operational plans?

Does failure to submit mean no funds or decreased funds? Does it mean that the plan will be identical to last year? Or does it mean reorienting resources towards those teams that do meet the deadlines? The unfortunate truth is that those district teams that are weakest or least experienced with developing plans are frequently in districts that have the greatest health needs. Indeed, more remote geographical areas with poorer or hard-to-reach populations may potentially be understaffed and under-resourced because of the classical challenges of deploying and retaining health staff in these areas or establishing proper communication channels such as internet connection etc. They may therefore be in a weaker position to develop and submit their plans on time. Rather than a punitive approach towards those who miss planning deadlines, it may be better to allocate resources to assist the weaker teams in developing their plans. It is not particularly fair, or a wise public health decision, to take resources away from high-need areas because their public health teams have less experience or capacity in planning.

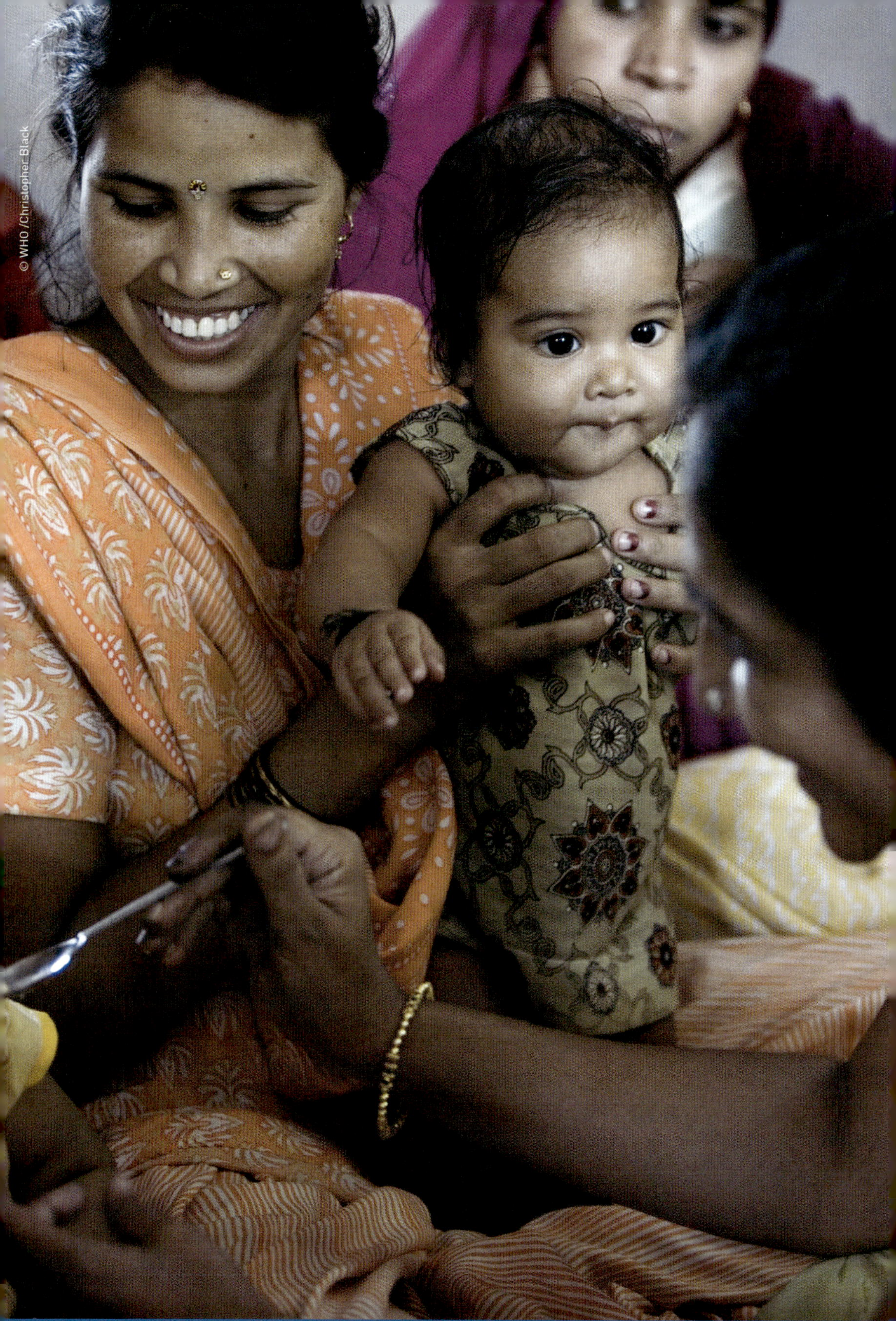
© WHO /Christopher Black

6.4.2 Steps in operational planning

Similar to overall strategic planning, the steps in the operational planning process include:

(a) taking stock of the situation (where are we now?), including identification of stakeholders (who is involved?);

(b) setting operational priorities;

(c) putting together the operational plan (what are we going to do?), including the operational budget;

(d) implementation of planned activities (how are we going to do it?);

(e) monitoring and evaluation of the operational plan (what have we accomplished so far?).

Shorter operational planning cycles that group some of the above-mentioned steps together and longer cycles that split up multiple steps can be considered, but they all contain the same or similar steps. Examples of different cycles can be found in many sources.[9,10]

The operational planning cycle places less emphasis on costing and budgeting compared to the overall national health policy and planning cycle, with more emphasis on the implementation. This is because the overall budget should already have been developed and the budget centre doing the operational planning has its specific budget lines which need to be planned for. Hence, the costing and budgeting is done at a much smaller scale, and is less complex, than in the strategic planning cycle. That being said, if national-level costing is not done well and is based on gross assumptions, a more detailed cost estimation exercise at operational unit level may be useful, also in view of providing valuable feedback to national-level costing and potentially influencing resource allocation decisions. On the other hand, operational planning will of course put more emphasis on the implementation, which is the primary objective of an operational plan.

In the following sections, each operational planning step is described in more detail. As many of the steps mirror the overall national health policy and planning cycle, the possible methodologies for each step are not described in detail, as they are elaborated upon in other chapters of this handbook and can be applied here as well.

Similar to the steps of strategic planning, the operational planning process should take stock of the situation, set operational priorities, put together the operational plan and budget, plan for the implementation of activities, and monitor and evaluate the operational plan once implemented.

(a) Taking stock of the situation (where are we now?), including identification of stakeholders (who is involved?)

Taking stock of the situation from the point of view of a budget centre need not be as extensive as the situation analysis for the NHPSP. It should build upon it, examining more closely the specific issues relevant to the budget centre and its mandate. In addition, it is important to look particularly at any significant differences from the analysis in the national plan. This need not be a problem per se but must be flagged, explained and made clear. Examples of this might be if a certain district has a health problem, such as guinea worm, that is present in that district, but not in the rest of the nation.

What is worth investing in at operational unit level is a tailored stakeholder analysis, examining the local playing field in more detail. The analysis done at central level may be too broad-based to be directly applicable for each operational unit. Local stakes may be very different from central-level stakes and interests.

(b) Setting operational priorities

Based on the national-level situation analysis and any additional context-specific complementary information, a ranking of the different recommendations can be made which then leads to a first draft priority list.

At budget centre level, the prioritization exercise is focused on activities, ideally linked to the overarching priorities already set in the NHPSP. Based on the national-level situation analysis and any additional context-specific complementary information produced by taking stock on the local situation, a ranking of the different recommendations can be made which then leads to a first draft priority list. Through several rounds of dialogue, health sector stakeholders' key operational priorities will crystallize. Part of the discussions on operational priorities will include sequencing of activities, based on level of priority accorded to that activity (even if the final timeline happens in the next stage of actually developing the operational plan).

Any local evidence will be crucial to ensuring that local operational priorities reflect realities on the ground. Other national and international evidence will, of course, also be examined where relevant, but context specificity is so vital here that any data and information from other contexts should be discussed with regard to adaptation to a specific setting.

(c) Putting together the operational plan (what are we going to do?), including budgeting

As explained above, operational planning is usually documented through the use of a predetermined planning matrix or grid provided by the national planning authority. There are many models for this.[11-13] If no template is available, at the very minimum, the elements described in section 6.4 should be included.

Crucial guidance from the central health planning authority to operational planners includes an outline of the operational plan, which should ideally be linked to and follow the headings of the NHPSP. This will allow activities of the operational plan to be clearly identified as contributing to NHPSP objectives. If the NHPSP was developed in a bottom-up manner, then much of the input to the NHPSP will have come from the various operational units anyway, which means that matching NHPSP and operational plan headings should not be particularly difficult. Otherwise, the operation plan headings are often organized around the main local priorities without any distinct link to anything beyond the local. If the operational plan is for a particular programme, reference should be made to the strategic directions of the NHPSP.

Ideally, as mentioned in section 6.1.3, the operational plan headings would also correspond to the budget line items ("chart of accounts") of the financing authority, for example the ministry of finance at the national level and the district treasury office at district level.

Frequently there is poor alignment between the health planning process and the national and sub-national budgeting processes.[14] In actual practice, health planning stakeholders often find the headings from the national chart of accounts to be ill suited to strategizing for health. The temptation to ignore the national chart of accounts should be resisted, even if they do not seem appropriate for an operational plan. A compromise is to do a "translation exercise" by adding another column to the operational plan matrix for the national budget line items so that the operational plan can be sorted to reflect the NHPSP or the national budget line items as appropriate. Another column can also be added for "source of funds", in situations where there are multiple sources of funds that must be accounted for separately, such as funds from different government levels or from external donors.

The pivot table function of a spreadsheet, if that is what is used for the matrix, can be used to provide an operational plan (see Box 6.5) in a format that is suitable for the operational planner or for the planner/accountants from the district treasury, or other development partners. The national health planning staff should help the local planning staff put together the most adequate matrix and technically support the process in areas where it is needed.

Box 6.5

Example of a hypothetical operation plan using the pivot table function of a spreadsheet

Original table of activities for the operational plan

ACTIVITY	COST (IN MILLION USD)	ACQUIRED COSTS (IN MILLION USD)	SOURCES OF FUNDING	MOBILIZATION (IN MILLION USD)	EXECUTION RESPONSIBILITY	T1	T2	T3	T4
Activity 1.1 Create new district health centres in peripheral districts	300	300	World Bank	10	Ministry of Finance	x	x		
Activity 1.2 Acquisition and delivery of enough vaccinations to cover district population	200	200	GAVI	50	Ministry of Health		x		
Activity 1.3 Re-train district and regional health staff in proper immunization techniques	100	80	Foreign donor	20	Regional Health Administration	x			
Activity 1.4 Community engagement by health workers to improve immunization awareness	100	50	Ministry of Finance	40	District Health Administration	x	x	x	x
Activity 1.5 Design and deliver traveling clinics for vaccines to underserviced areas	200	100	Ministry of Finance	20	Ministry of Health			x	
Activity 1.6 Record rates of immunization while performing annual census	100	70	Ministry of Finance	10	Ministry of Housing				x

Pivot table showing the distribution of activity cost by responsible entity

Sum of Cost (in million USD)

ACTIVITY	DISTRICT HEALTH ADMINISTRATION	MINISTRY OF FINANCE	MINISTRY OF HEALTH	MINISTRY OF HOUSING	REGIONAL HEALTH ADMINISTRATION	GRAND TOTAL
Activity 1.1 Create new district health centres in peripheral districts		300				300
Activity 1.2 Acquisition and delivery of enough vaccinations to cover district population			200			200
Activity 1.3 Re-train district and regional health staff in proper immunization techniques					100	100
Activity 1.4 Community engagement by health workers to improve immunization awareness	100					100
Activity 1.5 Design and deliver traveling clinics for vaccines to underserviced areas			200			200
Activity 1.6 Record rates of immunization while performing annual census				100		100
Grand Total	**100**	**300**	**400**	**100**	**100**	**1 000**

Central planners should identify the category of activities and level of detail that they want to see reflected in operational plans, especially in view of bottom-up aggregation of the plans (for example delivery of health services, training activities, management activities, etc. will all need to be coordinated or supported by the central level, sometimes just to ensure that there is no duplication). Clear guidance should also be provided on the methodology and the level of detail needed on the resource calculations for the described activities. The same goes for the selection of resource persons and focal points for activities and the level of details required for the timelines.

The above guidance will ensure that operational plans developed by different units are coherent, comparable and can be aggregated.

The spreadsheets in such situations, particularly if they are long and involve multiple levels of activities and funding sources, can become complicated and difficult to manipulate. Ideally, such complexity is handled within an efficient budgeting and planning database programme. A good database management system can make it easier to enter and extract information, store data over time, make comparisons across activities from different plans and years, etc. In practice, such programmes are often difficult to initiate and expensive to maintain, but if they function well, they are superior to using spreadsheets. But, spreadsheets can be used to manage the planning matrix if proper guidance on their use is given and care is taken in the initial set-up. It is the responsibility of the central health planning authority to provide guidance and capacity building on the issue of proper formats and IT platforms in their setting. It is advisable to avoid each budget centre having their own formats and IT methods.

Another decision to be made is whether the operational planning will be done using an incremental approach, with the new plan based on making changes and adjustments to what activities were carried out in the past, or whether an attempt should be made to plan from a blank slate or matrix. There are theoretical advantages to looking at everything anew, but if it is known that certain services will continue, there is no reason to pretend that you can plan them starting from scratch. Don't waste the precious time of health workers.

Another decision to be made is whether the operational planning will be done using an incremental approach, with the new plan based on making changes and adjustments to what activities were carried out in the past, or whether an attempt should be made to plan from a blank slate or matrix.

In many situations, it can be a recommended approach to start with looking at what has been done in the past. Then look at what is new as far as demographics, epidemiology or the resource base, including human resources, infrastructure and financing, are concerned. Then make adjustments to the operational plans based on what is new in the situation. The rolling 2- to 3- year plan is meant to be particularly well suited to adjust to incremental change. A calendar of deadlines and deliverables can be provided from central health planning authorities to operational planners to allow submission of draft versions of operational plans that can be reviewed and refined. The iterative process will help reconcile an operational plan based on the needs of the implementing units with the resources that are available for implementation.

(d) Implementation of planned activities (how are we going to do it?)

For actual implementation, individual managers should be encouraged by their team leaders to break their planned activities into individual sub-steps that make sense. Operational plans identify the activities that are required to meet the plan's objectives. Managers will then need to identify the concrete to-dos that will allow the team to implement these activities in a given timeline. Not every detailed step needs to be approved and planned by the overall in-charge, but in many respects, each detailed step needs to be thought through by the person who has the direct responsibility for that activity. Operational plan implementation is thus perhaps more about management than about planning.

Operational plan implementation is perhaps more about management than about planning.

For example, a district health plan may list as an activity a fixed number of outreach visits in a fixed number of remote villages per month. The responsible officer will list the steps necessary to actually perform the agreed number of outreach visits – for example, "arrange transport", which involves the tasks "organize car and driver, purchase fuel". Other steps could be:

- identify staff;
- forecast supplies (tests, vaccines, preventive medicines, health education materials, etc.) and ensure they are available at the time of the visits;
- organize coordination meetings;
- etc.

An important aspect of this work is to ensure coordination between different activities: for example, that all staff are not on outreach activities at the same time, that there are not multiple orders of the same kind of supplies but that orders are placed in bulk, and so on.

(e) Monitoring and evaluation of the operational plan (what have we accomplished so far?)

Monitoring and evaluation (M&E) are frequently written together. They are closely related, but they are two different activities.

Monitoring operational plans typically refers to the continuous assessment of whether planned activities are occurring and whether the expected results are being achieved. Monitoring is usually internal, something performed on a continuous or regular schedule by those who are actually doing the activities. It consists of comparing activities actually performed and the outputs actually achieved with what was planned. For example, monitoring will tell you that the planned number of outreach visits to remote villages has not taken place, or that the attendance of the outpatient clinic is declining or, on the contrary, has dramatically increased. Monitoring should be an activity listed in the operational plan in order to ensure it is done and that the resources needed are available. The frequency of monitoring should be defined to allow implementers to correct the course of action. Monitoring will also tell you if something unusual is being reported, such as increased numbers of cases of a certain disease, and therefore action needs to be taken, and perhaps changes made to the operational plan.

If monitoring shows that the implementation of planned activities is behind schedule or that some important outputs are not reached (for example, a decrease in utilization of services), managers need to investigate the reasons for such a situation in order to take adequate corrective measures. For example, they may find that activities are not happening because the funds have not been received on time, because the expected health staff have not been deployed in the area, because medicines or vaccines are out of stock, etc. Other challenges to timely implementation are more complex to understand: the target population may be reluctant to use the services or certain categories of stakeholders may be unhappy and resisting the implementation arrangements. Ideally, managers should try to understand the underlying reasons for such bottlenecks; for example, if the necessary supplies are out of stock, is this because the orders have not been placed on time, or because there were delays in supply? This should be done in collaboration with those who are directly responsible for implementing the activities and in a supportive manner. After examining underlying reasons for slow or delayed implementation, managers can apply corrective measures. Depending on the underlying cause of the problem, these may consist of increasing productivity, reallocating the necessary resources to meet the initial targets, etc. Correcting the course of action may require some amount of dialogue and negotiation; for example, pharmaceutical suppliers may be approached to discuss and solve delays in supply of medicines.

Some implementation bottlenecks may be addressed by managers who are directly responsible for the formulation and implementation of operational plans. Other kinds of bottlenecks are not directly under their control. Typical problems of this kind are delays in disbursement of funds to replenish the budgets of implementing units or perverse incentives created by provider payment methods used by national health insurance organizations. In such cases, the issue should be taken up with central health planning authorities and corrective actions should be taken by them or with their support.

Evaluation seeks to determine the impact of activities, typically after a fixed period of time. It will tell you whether the targets have been met both efficiently and effectively. The implementers themselves can and should evaluate their own performance, usually at the end of the implementation period. And, of course, evaluations are also often done by external evaluators.[V]

Following up on activity implementation should not only be done at local level (including community level); feedback to the national level at least once a year, for example, during the annual health sector review, is just as important.

V For more information, please see Chapter 9 "Monitoring and evaluation of national health policies, strategies, and plans" in this handbook.

Box 6.6

Is a specific operational planning workshop necessary?

Operational planning can be organized through a planning workshop, by operational staff at their worksite, and/or as a topic of discussion at one or a series of meetings with the district health coordinating body.

There are several options with regard to how to organize the operational planning: the common planning workshop, or planning by operational staff at their desks or worksite, or it can be made a topic of discussion at one or a series of meetings of the district health coordinating body. Of course, there is an option for a combination of these possibilities. If the workshop option is chosen, then a decision has to be made whether the workshop is held peripherally, or the involved parties are called to a central location for planning. The latter is often more convenient for the centrally located stakeholders (MoH and external donors). Doing the planning closer to the actual site of implementation, for example in the district, is more consistent with the principle that the best plans are done by those who will implement them.

In many situations, there have been a proliferation of planning processes, often consisting of workshops, involving the same participants. For example, separate workshops for disease control programmes, multilateral and bilateral agencies active in health, and the national planning process have been a common occurrence. This is to the detriment of work on the ground. It is particularly a problem in settings where health worker pay is low and workshops have become a source of income supplementation. Having said that, there are also numerous positive examples of countries where planning exercises were used to strengthen coordination between partners and to strengthen the implication of key actors in decisions related to health system strengthening. In the Democratic Republic of the Congo, for example, when the district model was implemented in the late 1980s, a three-week training package for district management teams was used as an opportunity to jointly develop an operational plan for each district.

A workshop can be useful for team-building and introducing new concepts. There are very few workshops that actually produce a plan, particularly if the planning process is not far advanced before the workshop is held. So, the participants have to take their initial draft back to the office and complete the planning matrix at their desks. Therefore, if a planning workshop is chosen, considerable work should be done on completing a draft before the workshop. Likewise, follow-up activities to support staff in completing their plans should be considered.

Operational planning is probably best done through a mix of on-the-job work, using a clear matrix with clear instructions, with the final product discussed and vetted through a meeting or workshop.

6.5 Who are the main actors involved in operational planning?

6.5.1 Planning is best done best by those who will be carrying out the plans

Operational planning is best done by those who will be carrying out the plans, both by managers and staff and with other stakeholders who are affected in the implementation of the plan.

To some degree, everyone who is responsible for an activity in the operational plan should be involved in the planning for that activity. However, operational planning is often done by managers. That said, the most successful managers will have meaningfully engaged the staff that they supervise in developing the plan. In addition, other partners and stakeholders who are affected by the implementation of the plan should have a say in the operational plan itself.

For example, in the case of an operational planning exercise of a MoH unit, it would mean having consulted partner institutes and state agencies (bureau of statistics, inspector-general's office, etc.) and those working on health in other sectoral ministries of government offices (health advisor in the prime minister's office, health advisor in the ministry of finance, etc.). For a national disease-specific programme, it might mean consulting civil society organizations (CSOs) that have a large stake in how the operational plan is implemented.

In the case of operational planning at a district level, the entire district management team will need to be involved. Furthermore, representatives of community members, representatives from each health unit in the catchment area, and representatives of CSOs that are active in the health sector in the area should participate in the planning exercise. Private practitioners might also be included if they are willing, especially if their services are being included in some of the activities or they are partially financed by public funds.

6.5.2 Multi-stakeholder arena (see Table 6.2)

Negotiating the agreements between the various departments, programmes, donors and non-state actors requires a lot of effort, good will, and political support at the highest level in many cases. Dialogue at all levels is important, but especially with implementing partners, which can be CSOs, community groups or religious organizations. For example, if immunization tactics include mobilization through religious leaders, then discussions with them must take place in order to negotiate their role and responsibilities in the operational plan.

Having a wide variety of stakeholders on board also implies that all parties are transparent about their budgets. This can be immensely helpful to avoid confusion and double reporting. Even though it is strongly discouraged, some stakeholder financial contributions may be separate from the online budget. In this case, a separate column in a table or spreadsheet

Operational planning involves many stakeholders, and thus negotiating between the various government departments, programmes, donors, and non-state actors.

for these contributions can make the overall financial situation clear to everyone.

In the era of the Paris Declaration,[VI] most agencies, and governments, are becoming more willing to share information. They should be encouraged to do so. New developments in information technology can support this effort, for example through shared online planning dashboards that relevant stakeholders can access.

Finally, when drawing up any operational health plan it is also necessary to identify stakeholders outside the government sector and decide to what degree their activities are included in the district operational plan.

VI The Paris Declaration on smart aid: five principles for aid effectiveness (http://www.oecd.org/dac/effectiveness/45827300.pdf, accessed 28 September 2016).

Table 6.2 Key stakeholders and their roles in operational planning

ACTOR	ROLE
MoH	▸ Ensures link between strategic and operational planning ▸ Provides clear guidance on operational planning (templates, tools, modalities, etc.) ▸ Technically supports budget centres in their operational planning processes ▸ Synthesizes and aggregates operational plans to feed into national health planning exercises
State and parastatal agencies (e.g. bureau of statistics, inspector general's office)	▸ Lead operational planning for their respective budget centres ▸ Liaise with MoH for guidance and technical support ▸ Ensure that all stakeholders relevant to the work of the budget centre are adequately involved in the operational planning process
Other sectors (e.g. education, labour, etc.)	▸ Where intersectoral action is needed to reach a specific objective or target, the relevant other sector(s) must be brought into the budget centre's operational planning process
CSOs	▸ Provide data, information and knowledge ▸ Ensure that CSO activities are aligned with and part of the relevant budget centre's operational plan
Regional/district health authorities	▸ Lead and coordinate at local level the operational planning process ▸ Bring all stakeholders on board into the operational planning process, ensure coordination between different activities ▸ Provide supervision and guidance for lower levels of the health system ▸ Implement operational plan ▸ Liaise with national level for guidance and coherence in plans across the country
Community groups	▸ Represent the community in operational planning dialogue ▸ Provide feedback on health services and system ▸ Work with local health authorities to implement operational plan, pointing out any bottlenecks and challenges when necessary
Private sector	▸ Participate meaningfully in district-level operational planning exercise ▸ Strategize with stakeholders how the private sector can contribute and work towards operational planning targets
Development partners	▸ Technically support budget centre where necessary to convene and coordinate operational planning exercise ▸ Actively participate in operational planning evidence examination, dialogue and debate ▸ Provide monies for implementation

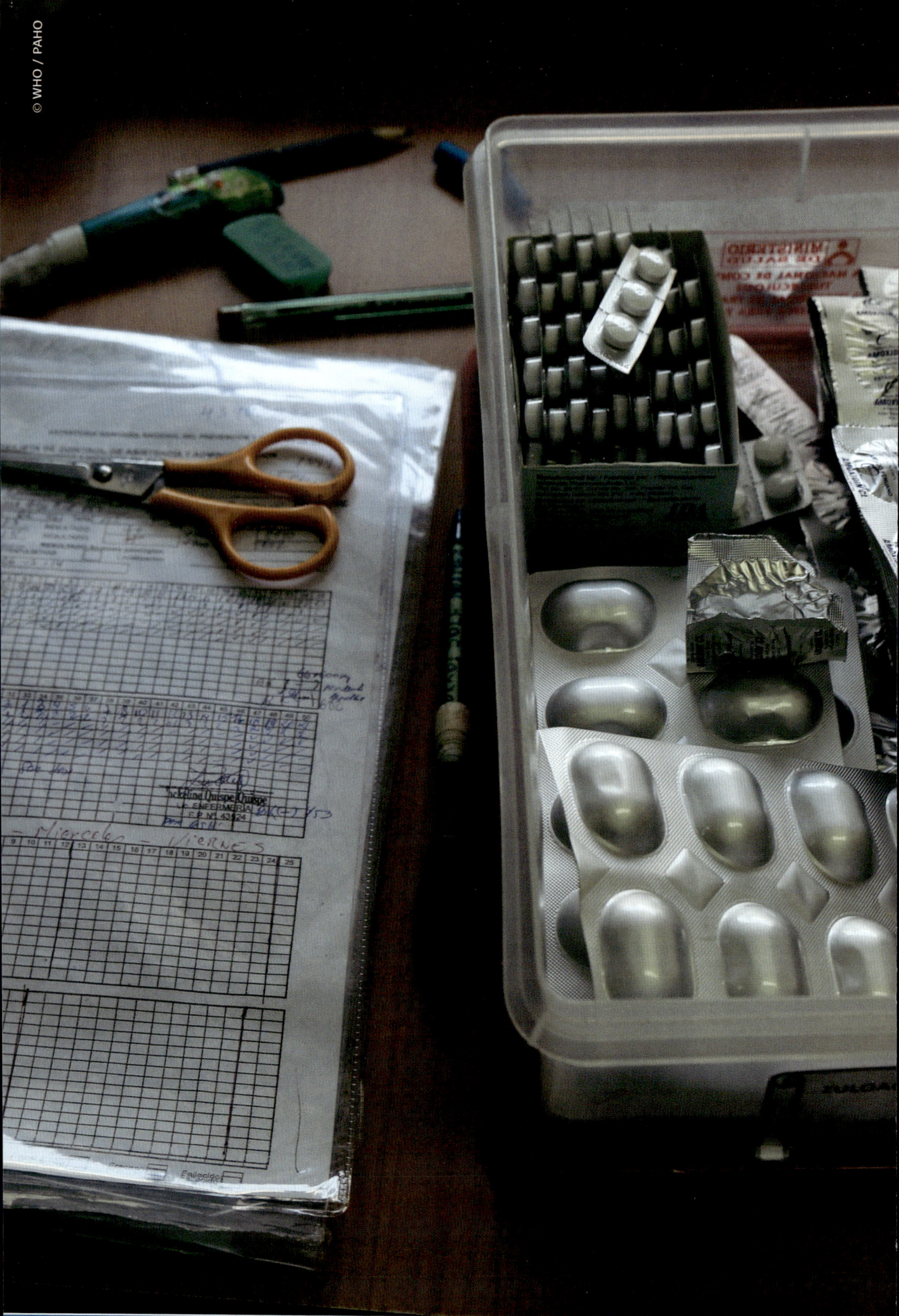

6.6 What if...?

6.6.1 What if your country is decentralized?

Shift in roles and responsibilities

The operational planning process in a decentralized setting must identify who is responsible for governance of the health system at whatever level the plan is being prepared. The operational plan must be developed in a manner that involves and can be understood by and sold to that entity, be it a local government council, a faith-based organization tasked with providing health services, or external funding agencies.

That being said, local government councils may have priorities that do not make sense to public health managers, and may not always reflect population needs. There are examples where public health programmes, such as primary health care, are neglected by local councils, while politically popular projects, such as building new hospitals and health centres, are given undue attention. The operational planners in a decentralized system will need to become educators and negotiators as well as public health professionals if they want to succeed.

It is also important to note that central-level planning authorities may also not have the right answers to a local health system's most pressing needs. Different types of experiences and knowledge will reside with different people and institutions, at different levels of the health system. Bringing those views and realities together in a process of frank dialogue will most likely yield the most pragmatic and effective results.

It is important that national health authorities be involved in the planning process before all the decisions are made and the resources have been committed. In countries that opt for decentralization after having had a long history of highly centralized services, this requires a large shift in attitude on the part of central-level planners, from command and control to guidance and facilitation. It is a shift that many have difficulty making.

In some countries, even ones that are highly decentralized in theory, grants from the central government are often earmarked for certain aspects of health, such as the core package of primary health care services or public health packages. It is important for the central authorities to define what decision-making freedom lies with the local government and the local health office.

Central authorities must reconcile and bring together various operational plans and ensure alignment with the overarching NHPSP. Clear guidance on the standards and services that decentralized levels of the government are expected, or required, to provide, is necessary here. In addition, the MoH should ensure that sub-national health authorities have key roles to play in the strategic national-level planning process – harmonization and alignment of local operational plans with overarching NHPSPs is then more likely to occur.[VII]

VII For more detailed information on planning in a decentralized context, please see Chapter 11 "Strategizing for health at sub-national level" in this handbook.

Keep in mind that newly decentralized authorities may not immediately have the necessary capacities and experience to adequately conduct the operational planning. Especially at the beginning of a decentralization process, heavy technical support and guidance should be provided and central-level authorities should set aside time and resources to build capacity at sub-national levels. The MoH should ensure that its guidance and support is temporary only and that over time, sub-national levels will completely take over.

Box 6.7

District health profile

A district health profile can be a useful tool at local level to establish an understanding of the health situation locally and build from there to do operational planning according to local needs. At a minimum, a district health profile will contain:

1. basic geographical information, including a map and catchment area;

2. demographic information, including population broken down by sex, age and ethnicity where relevant;

3. epidemiological information;

4. resources available, including health workers, facilities and finances; and

5. baseline service delivery information such as immunization rates, water and sanitation coverage, numbers of hospital beds, and outpatient visits, among others. Additional socioeconomic information on topics such as education, the state of the local economy and most common livelihoods, ethnicity, and special problems – such as conflict or environmental disruption – may be useful. The district health profile should not be excessively time-consuming in preparation.

When describing the district health profile it is important to decide how to account for, or at least acknowledge, health providers outside the government health sector. These may be formal providers, such as private practitioners and pharmacies, or informal providers, such as traditional healers and itinerant drug sellers. If there is dual practice, where government workers also work privately, that should also be acknowledged in the profile. Even if not a formal part of the operational plan, these types of practices have a large influence on the total amount of services provided in the health sector. Ideally, they would be part of the plan, although that is unrealistic in many, if not most, settings.

The amount of analysis done by each district or unit will depend to a large degree on the amount of autonomy or decision-making authority it has, and also to a certain extent on the amount of variation from the national norms. It is important to ensure that relevant data are collected at district level to allow data analysis at regular intervals for operational planning purposes.

6.6.2 What if fragmentation and/or fragility is an issue in your country?

Fragile states often refer to states that are in the midst of a conflict or disaster, or recovering from one. In such a situation, the operational planning process is even shorter term, often needing to be reworked in a matter of weeks or months, rather than a full year. Also, the services will focus on those things appropriate for emergencies. In such a context, flexibility and an eye for the likely political and economic evolution of the situation is crucial. Indeed, in fragile contexts, the environment and health situations are constantly evolving; this constant evolution calls for new actors with specific skills in emergency or disaster response to act in the field. This frequently creates a confusing overlap of responsibilities, with multiple agents, both internal and external, entering the service provision field. As difficult as it is in an emergency, it is key that a few talented and experienced individuals take on the role of coordination and planning. Ideally, the lead in this process is the government health care system, aided by external partners, not the reverse.[VIII] The most important aspect is that a solid process is put in place to track the changing situation and the new actors who come into play, and to engage multiple stakeholders in a productive dialogue. The operation plan must be flexible to adapt to these factors rapidly and effectively.

In some contexts, when the crisis is in its acute phase, stakeholders will most likely focus the majority of efforts and resources on vertical health programmes for the population subgroups in most need. However, if a crisis situation becomes more protracted and chronic, it is advisable to rely more on existing national or local structures, and their set-up to provide all types of health services for the whole population, and seek to strengthen them. In such a case, systematic involvement of local actors should be emphasized in order to ensure sustainability of jointly planned activities and smoothen the transition back to normalcy. In post-Ebola Guinea, for example, the three-year health systems recovery plan was designed based on input from 38 district operational plans, demonstrating the MoH's strong emphasis on sub-national levels as the operational unit of implementation. It should also be noted that the health systems recovery plan was explicitly made the first phase of the 10-year national health plan, instead of it being a separate or parallel plan – evincing the MoH's resolve to keep existing plans, structures and stakeholders as the foundation of the health system.

Operational planning in fragile states requires a shorter-term framework and an ability to be flexible in the midst of political and economic evolution.

Another major challenge in fragile states is human resources for health, as they tend to be more unstable, with health workers and their families often missing or on the move. The operational plan should include means of protecting the safety of health workers and their families to the extent possible.

VIII For a more detailed discourse on health planning in a fragile state context, please see Chapter 13 "Strategizing in distressed health contexts" in this handbook.

6.6.3 What if your country is heavily dependent on aid?

In some countries, the majority of funds for public health services come from sources outside the country. Even though these resources should all come from donors who follow the principles and practices of the Paris Declaration, it may unfortunately not reflect reality. This has been demonstrated in cases where third-party financers reserve the right to approve the part of the operational plan that they are financing before funds are released. This may occur not only with external donor support, but also when a national disease control programme reserves the right of approval for sub-sections of the plan.

Health planning stakeholders need to be informed in a transparent manner of the resources that can be expected and obligations that come with those resources.

An operational planner at local level needs to be informed in a transparent manner of the resources that can be expected and the obligations that come with those resources with regard to activities, time deadlines and reporting. Donor-funded services, especially those implemented by the district team, should be part of the district operational health plan. It may be necessary to add an additional column to the planning spreadsheet or database to reflect funds from sources other than the government budget. Ideally, the reporting would be on the same schedule as the government reporting, but that is not always possible. A means of easing reporting is planning in three-month blocks, so that one can mix and match the various reporting dates of the government and donors, if they are different. The central health planning authority can greatly aid districts or other operational health units in providing a format for planning that can be easily sorted for reporting activities by donor and by reporting period.

This means that it is essential to have a planning matrix or database that allows individual programmes, and their donors, to extract the information they need to monitor activities and keep resources flowing. If not, they will either bypass the general health planning process, or add programme- and donor-specific planning exercises, separate from the general health plan, neither of which is desirable. The planning processes must try to accommodate the reasonable needs of all stakeholders.

In fact, there have been cases where individual donors, or their implementation units, call in members of district health teams for planning exercises for their individual interest, separate from the over-all district operational plan or NHPSP. These individual programme plans have often been developed as a separate exercise from the unified district health plan with separate dates, budgets and lines of authority. There has been some progress on unifying the different planning exercises, but it is far from universal. Managers should try to avoid fragmented programme-driven or donor-driven plans and aim at integrating them in a unified district plan as much as possible.

The planning process becomes even more complicated if the operational plan has to be produced in more than one language. This can happen in situations where external partners require a copy of the plan in an international language, or when the country does not have a single national language. It is preferable to allow people to work in their own language for planning, but it can leave a large and difficult translation issue as deadlines are approaching. If translation is needed, time and resources will need to be allocated. It is important that it be an accurate translation so there are not multiple versions of the plan in circulation, something that can lead to a loss of confidence in the transparency of a health system.

6.6.4 What if your country has strong vertical health programmes?

The discussion in this situation is essentially the same as the discussion that occurs with donor dependence, but is also relevant when funding for vertical programmes comes from domestic sources. It is helpful if the central health planning office and the heads of the various vertical programmes, have agreed on formats and timetables for planning and reporting.

A key decision is whether reporting on activities will go through the general health programme and be consolidated as an entire health plan, or whether it goes through the individual vertical programmes and is consolidated by them and then reported to the broader health sector.

When there are relatively few vertical programmes it is manageable to have the reporting go through them. When there are multiple programmes, it becomes progressively more burdensome and problematic for lower-level implementers.

However, central health planners cannot be excessively dogmatic on this issue, particularly where funding flows are specifically earmarked for certain programmes. A task of the central health planning authority is to help the lower level operational planners cope with multiple programmes by providing clear guidance on a national strategic direction (as spelled out in the NHPSP) for the health sector, with norms for the health district and its facilities, and tools and procedures in place to implement those norms. Otherwise, it is likely that some vertical health programmes, at least those that are well-funded, will just ignore the general health planning process.

Guidelines on how to include vertical programmes in the operational plans should be provided, where to fit their activities and funds into the matrix, and how to ease the reporting requirements. If at all possible, planning processes for the vertical programmes and the overall district health plan need should be unified in both time and place.

If the national planning processes do not make it easy to have a unified district operational health plan, a proactive district health management team can do it, to at least a partial extent, on their own. A proactive district management team can gain trust and recognition if the process of integrating the various plans is participatory (and using existing coordination mechanisms), accountable and transparent for everyone.

Searching for synergies between different programmes in the health sector has been a common topic of discussion.[15] Where the national authorities have been unable to build a guidance framework, the local level can do it, mainly because it is often the same individuals or team who are implementing the various vertical programmes. In such cases, putting resources (human or material) from vertical programmes in common and integrating activities is possible at the level of the operational plan.

Coordination and cooperation in developing a unified plan can be achieved. Then the various component plans can be grouped out of the matrix and sent off to the approvers as required. It is not an ideal situation, but one that can produce a positive benefit for the community. For example, mosquito nets can be delivered during immunization outreaches with mutual benefit to both programmes. Sometimes the operational problems can be solved on a local level more easily than in the capital.

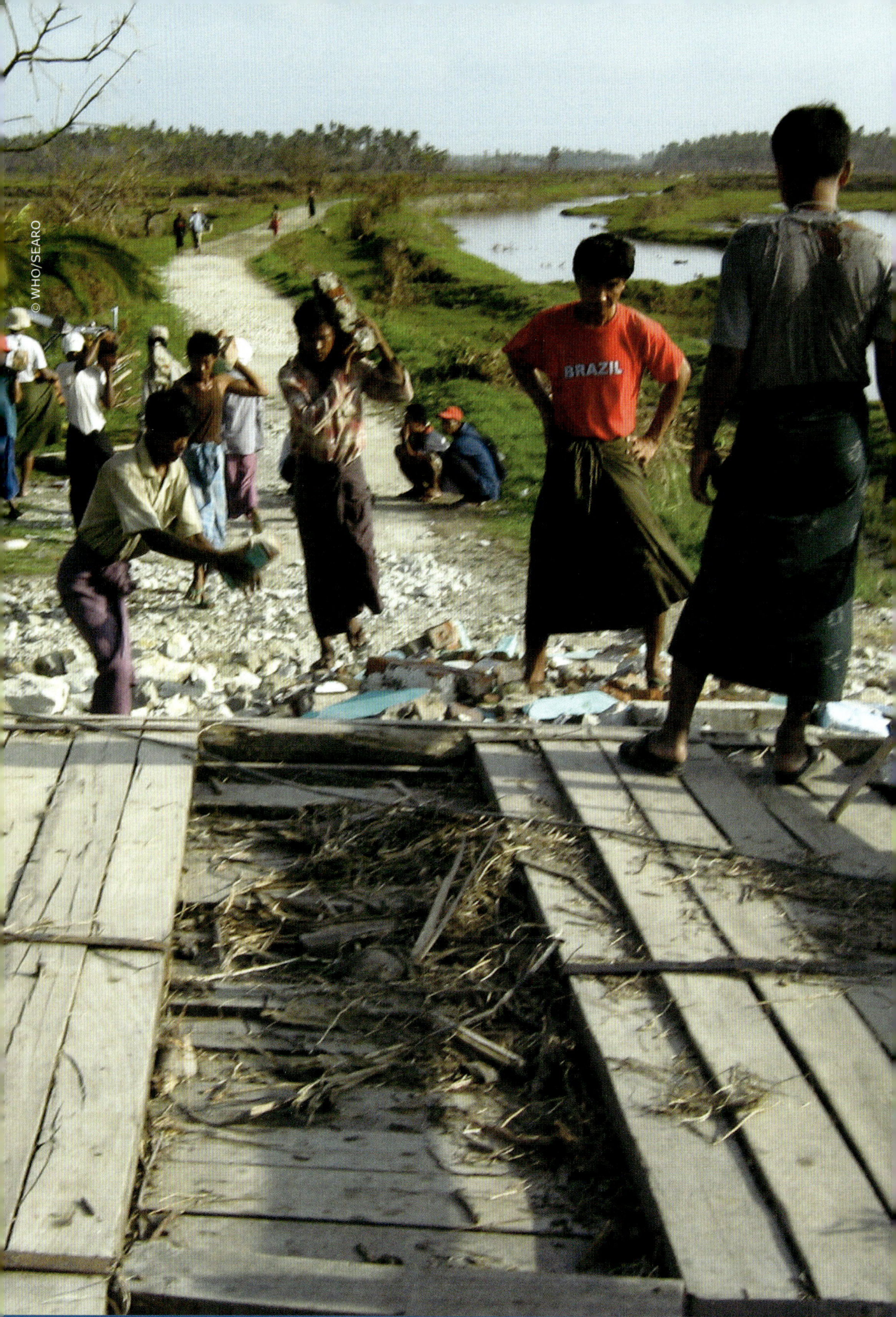

© WHO/SEARO

6.7 Conclusion

Operational planning, as the term indicates, "operationalizes" a strategic plan that defines the vision, goals and objectives for the health sector. Operational planning is managerial and shorter term, and deals with day-to-day implementation. It is where concrete activities are planned for at the operational level.

The operational planning process has the potential to greatly assist stakeholders in gaining a better understanding of the NHPSP target population and its needs, as well as stakeholders' own capabilities and limitations in implementation. Especially when defined jointly, an operational plan is critical for the clarity it offers as to what needs to be done, by whom, how and with which monies.

In this chapter, the core content of the operational plan is discussed, as well as the steps in the plan development process. The various roles and responsibilities of stakeholders are also examined. For two of the principal stakeholder groups, the main take away messages are below.

6.7.1 Key take away messages for the central health planning authority

(a) Operational health planning is the connection between strategic objectives and activity.

(b) The best operational plans are written by the people who carry them out.

(c) The central health planners have an obligation to provide clear guidelines to operational planners with regard to operational plans. It is important that deadlines are known, formats are clear, the degree of decision-making authority is known to all, and the approval process is transparent.

(d) A clear guidance framework, with orientation on the content, in an easy to use form of information technology should be provided by the central planning unit.

(e) The central health planning unit should aim to facilitate and assist operational planners rather than taking over the process.

(f) The weakest operational planning units should not be penalized for not producing their plans. Rather, adequate resources should be dedicated to support them in the operational planning process.

6.7.2 Main points for operational planners to keep in mind

(a) Everyone is an operational planner.

(b) Operational plans are a necessary management tool.

(c) Operational planning should involve a wide range of people rather than be dictated by the manager/boss. At the minimum, all those who are expected to implement the plan should be involved in the process.

(d) Operational plans should be open to revision as circumstances change.

(e) Coordination and cooperation can occur at the local, operational level, even if the methods for doing so are not yet well worked out at the centre.

References

1 Green A. An Introduction to health planning in developing countries. Oxford: Oxford University Press; 1992.

2 Surbhi S. Difference between strategic planning and operational planning. In: Key Differences [website]; 2015 (http://keydifferences.com/difference-between-strategic-planning-and-operational-planning.html, accessed 28 September 2016).

3 Cambodia Ministry of Health. Health Strategic Plan 2008–2015. Kingdom of Cambodia; April 2008 (http://apps.who.int/medicinedocs/documents/s18360en/s18360en.pdf, accessed 28 September 2016).

4 Annear PL, Grundy J, Ir P, Jacobs B, Men C, Nachtnebel M, et al. The Kingdom of Cambodia health system review.Health Syst Transit. 2015;5(2) (http://www.wpro.who.int/asia_pacific_observatory/hits/series/cambodia_health_systems_review.pdf, accessed 28 September 2016).

5 Universal health coverage in action at European Development Days. In: Universal Health Coverage Partnership [website]. Geneva: World Health Organization; 2016 (http://uhcpartnership.net/universal-health-coverage-in-action-at-european-development-days/, accessed 28 September 2016).

6 Department of Planning and Health Information. Volume 7: The planning process for provinces with 1 operational district. Phnom Penh: Kingdom of Cambodia Ministry of Health; March 2003.

7 A framework for national health policies, strategies, and plans. Geneva: World Health Organization; 2010 (http://www.who.int/nationalpolicies/FrameworkNHPSP_final_en.pdf, accessed 28 September 2016).

8 Schiavo-Campo S. Of mountains and molehills: "the" medium-term expenditure framework. Paper presented at "Conference on Sustainability and Efficiency in Managing Public Expenditure": Honolulu; September 2008 (blog-pfm.imf.org/pfmblog/files/MTEFpaperFinal.doc, accessed 28 September 2016).

9 The Ministry of Health and Social Welfare Tanzania. Planning of District Health Services. Core Module Four; Dar es Salaam; 2007 (http://www.tgpsh.or.tz/fileadmin/documents/JAST/Module_CM4.pdf).

10 Ministry of Health and Social Welfare. Guidelines for District Health Planning and Reporting. Pretoria; 2003.

11 Ibid.

12 Sport and Recreation Tasmania. Strategic and operational planning toolkit. Hobart: Government of Tasmania; 2015.

13 Chatora R, Tumusiime P. Planning and implementation of district health services. Brazzaville: World Health Organization Regional Office for Africa; 2004 (District Health Management Team Training Modules: Module 4; http://www.who.int/management/district/planning_budgeting/PlanningImplementationDHSAFROMd4.pdf, accessed 28 September 2016).

14 Tsofa B, Molyneux S, Goodman C. Health sector operational planning and budgeting processes in Kenya—"never the twain shall meet". Int J Health Plann Mgmt. 2016:31(3);260–76 (https://www.ncbi.nlm.nih.gov/pmc/articles/PMC4988384/, accessed 28 September 2016).

15 Maximizing positive synergies between health systems and Global Health Initiative. In: WHO/Health Systems [website]. Geneva: WHO; 2016 (http://www.who.int/healthsystems/GHIsynergies/en/, accessed 29 September 2016).

Further reading

Chatora R, Tumusiime P. Planning and implementation of district health services. Brazzaville: World Health Organization Regional Office for Africa; 2004 (District Health Management Team Training Modules: Module 4; http://www.who.int/management/district/planning_budgeting/PlanningImplementationDHSAFROMd4.pdf, accessed 28 September 2016).

Kirigia JM, Sambo LG, Agu VU, Lambo E. How to develop an operational plan for health. East Afr Med J. 2001;78(3 Suppl):S14–9. pmid:12002062.

Chapter 7

Estimating cost implications of a national health policy, strategy or plan

Karin Stenberg
Dheepa Rajan

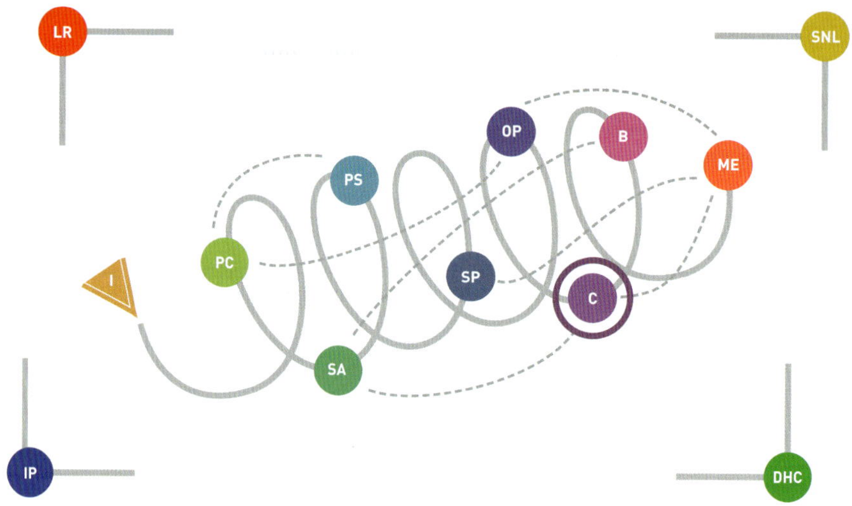

Cross-cutting topics relevant to national health planning

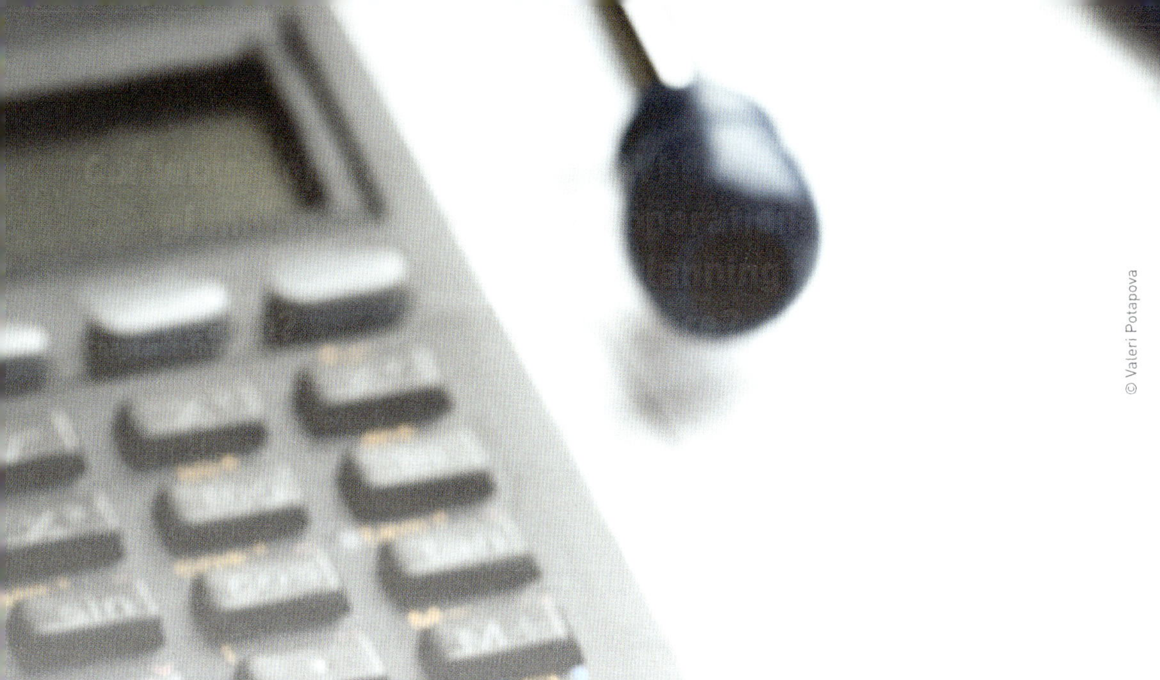

Overview

This chapter discusses the estimation of costs in relation to a national health policy, strategy or plan (NHPSP). The process of estimating costs can be a crucial step within the NHPSP formulation process which allows decision-makers to consider the extent to which policy objectives and strategic orientations are feasible and affordable. The process of costing a strategy should be considered an essential part of the planning process and not something to be undertaken after the overall plan has been completed and presented as a finalized document.

Several rounds of fine-tuning the cost calculations may be needed as the priorities are discussed and matched to the available resource envelope – potentially through scenario analysis.

Within this chapter, we outline key steps and principles to follow when estimating cost implications of the strategies outlined within a NHPSP. We provide an overview of methodological issues, along with recommendations on the various stakeholder groups which should be involved and the type of accompanying documentation that should be produced.

The focus of this chapter is thus a cost estimation in relation to an overarching vision for the entire health sector, as opposed to disease-specific estimates.

Summary

What is meant by "cost implications" of a NHPSP?

- Estimating the costs of a strategy serves to indicate the financial resource needs of planned activities. Broad policy objectives can be translated into activities and targets by year, to quantify the resources needed for implementation, estimate the related costs, and then assess aspects related to feasibility, affordability and efficiency.
- Costing is an iterative process and several rounds of discussion and calculation can be necessary to fine-tune the numbers. The aim is to inform the user of the potential overall magnitude of the costs and the main cost drivers.
- Costing results can inform the budget exercise.
- The estimated costs should be compared with the projected available financial resources, to assess affordability and potential resource gaps.

Why is it important?

- To improve the soundness of the NHPSP in terms of setting feasible and financially attainable targets, thus improving accountability.
- Affordability and therefore "cost" being key criteria in the priority-setting process, information on costs should inform the discussion on priorities in the health sector, which may include considering different sequencing of activities and reforms to match the resource availability. Strategies should also focus on increasing efficiency of current spending to make progress toward universal health coverage.
- Cost projections for the NHPSP can be used for advocacy to mobilize additional resources.
- The estimated NHPSP costs can feed into a Medium-Term Expenditure Framework (MTEF) and annual budgeting process and help gear resource allocation towards strategic priorities in order to improve health system performance and overall health outcomes.

When should costs be estimated for the NHPSP?

- Costs can be estimated as part of the planning process. A rough estimate of costs can start as soon as the major policies and overall direction of the health plan are agreed upon.
- Costing should match planned policies to the likely resources available, and closely follow discussions around the policy scenarios and strategies proposed for the NHPSP. Several rounds of refining the costing may be needed as the priorities are discussed and matched to the available resource envelope – potentially through scenario analysis.
- The cost estimates should not be interpreted as fixed resource needs but rather as an initial projection of resources needed, acknowledging that the environment is dynamic with a certain level of uncertainty related to population risks, and where best practice strategies and prices of goods and services constantly evolve.

Who should contribute to the costing of an NHPSP?

The costing of a NHPSP relates to the entire health sector. As such, it is led by the MoH, but must be relevant to all stakeholders involved in the planning process. The role of civil society, development partners and other government ministries is crucial when it comes to providing input data, ensuring consistency with government policies and plans put forth in other sectors, and validating the final estimates in terms of targets, costs and related projected outcomes such as accessibility to care and overall population health impact.

How is costing of the NHPSP carried out?

The cost estimation should be integral to the overall planning process. An initial scoping analysis gathers information on likely trends in available financing and fiscal policy "ceilings" over the planning period, along with planned reforms – including those that may impact on the cost structure, such as civil servant reforms, health provider payment reforms, etc. For example, what strategies are being considered to increase efficiency of current spending and make progress toward universal health coverage?

A costing team can form the liaison between the broader planning discussions and the cost estimation process. The team is often headed by specialists in the ministry of health (MoH) planning department, along with cadres from the MoH department of finances, but works closely with a range of stakeholders (e.g. various technical agencies and departments including the ministry of finance (MoF), district managers, development partners) to promote participatory processes and gain buy-in.

Inputs are gathered from a range of technical planning units (e.g. health workforce, maternal health, mental health) regarding their planned activities and targets, while taking into account the expected outcomes of their activities in relation to broader policy objectives and planned health reforms.

Scenarios on costs are presented and discussed through a series of consultations, including data validation processes with technical counterparts. Presenting cost data compared with estimated financing projections informs discussions on priority-setting as needed.

Multi-year cost projections[l] are continuously updated as required in a dynamic planning environment, and linked to mid-term reviews and annual plans.

Anything else to consider?

- decentralized environment;
- fragile environment;
- highly aid-dependent context.

l Multi-year cost projections for the health sector are often used as a basis for the expenditure targets calculated for a MTEF.

7.1 What do we mean by "estimating the cost implications" of a NHPSP? How does it fit into the broader health financing context?

Health planning, costing and budgeting are critical activities to inform policy development and implementation. Priority-setting, transforming priorities to operational plans – all crucial steps in the health policy and planning cycle – are covered in previous chapters of this handbook. The budget process is the subject of the subsequent chapter, Chapter 8.

This chapter serves to address the issue of projecting costs for a multi-year health plan to reflect planned results and investment. Estimating costs for a NHPSP should not be confused with the budgeting process. The multi-year projection of costs may reflect aspirational goals set out within the strategy, often reflecting commitments that have been agreed upon through broad consultative processes. In some instances the cost projections for the NHPSP exceed available resources. Those NHPSPs cannot be considered a realistic platform for planning. The combination of ambition and realism is a hard balance to maintain. Thus, the costing exercise needs to be combined with realistic projections of available financing, and adjusted accordingly, in order for the analysis to be credible. Countries may use frameworks such as the MTEF or other approaches to organize and present the information (Box 7.1).

NHPSP cost projections can open political opportunities. When the cost estimates have solid buy-in, they can be strongly leveraged as an overall reference for the implementation process, which is ultimately shaped by the annual budgeting process.

Box 7.1

What is an MTEF?

An MTEF is a comprehensive, government-wide spending plan that links policy priorities to expenditure allocations within a fiscal framework (linked to macroeconomic and revenue forecasts), usually over a three-year planning horizon.[II] The MTEF process facilitates the combination of cost projections with the projections on available resources, helps to discuss inter- and intrasectoral trade-offs, and informs ceilings that are set for expenditures in different government sectors. An MTEF covers all public expenditure and revenues from all source. In the context of a NHPSP with political targets for the entire health sector, the resource estimates for NHPSP activities may be broader and beyond the MTEF public sector resource envelope (private sector domestic financing for health, contribution of other sectors to health sector goals, etc.).

Projecting costs for investment strategies associated with a multi-year health plan is a critical component of strategizing for health.

II For more detailed information on MTEFs, see Chapter 8 "Budgeting for health" in this handbook.

7.1.1 What do we mean by costing in the context of this handbook?

"Costing" can be defined as a process of identifying the resources required to produce something or undertake an action, and then valuing these in monetary terms. There are multiple policy uses of cost data.[III] This chapter addresses the development of multi-year cost projections on the resources needed to implement strategic activities linked to the NHPSP objectives in the medium term (3–10 years) and for the entire health sector. Such estimates would generally include resources needed both for the various health system areas (health workforce, governance, supply chain, etc.); as well as for different public health programmes, curative care, outbreak response and disease control. A common preoccupation concerns the inclusion of activities that may fall outside the traditional definition of the health sector. In the spirit of the Sustainable Development Goals (SDGs), health planning authorities can foster a multisectoral response to address those health issues which require it – the question of *who* (which sector) should pay for this and *why* is addressed in more detail in the chapter on intersectoral planning.[IV] Suffice it to summarize here that a certain level of investment still must be made by the health sector to foster better collaboration with other sectors. This should thus be reflected as a strategic orientation in the NHPSP and as a specific activity in an operational plan.

To a large extent the costing process will entail translating broader policy goals (which can include benefits or "outputs" such as "increase in the utilization rate of health facilities") into concrete activities. The transformation of high-level policy objectives expressed in the NHPSP into specific activities and targets is a process which should be informed by a thorough situation analysis and studies on feasibility. For example, programme-specific targets (e.g. those related to malaria or HIV/AIDS) should be set taking into account the overall capacity of the health system (availability of trained nurses etc.), reflect the most recent evidence on effective interventions and investment strategies, and then set targets against which decision-makers can be held accountable. An integrated approach across health programmes is particularly important when planning the utilization of shared resources (such as health workers), and is equally crucial when considering programme-specific approaches that could more effectively be shared (such as separate laboratories versus joint laboratory facilities). The costing process can be helpful in fostering an in-depth reflection on the details of operationalizing a plan, and helps to identify areas where more strategic thinking is required.

A large part of the costing work thus relates to:

(a) strategic thinking around what resources would be required to implement policy objectives, i.e. strategic reforms and innovation within the health system;

(b) more detailed definition around the kinds of inputs required (staff time, materials, vehicles, medicines, etc.) for the specific activities. The details are required in order to subsequently attach a quantity and a price to each input.

The discussion on the broader policy goals and the associated activities takes part during the

III "Costing" can have multiple objectives and refer to many different kinds of analysis. Annex 7.1 provides an overview of different situations in which a cost analysis can inform strategizing for health.

IV Please see Chapter 12, "Intersectoral planning for health and health equity" of this handbook.

planning process. So bringing together those who plan and those who cost at an early stage is critical, as it ensures that the national health plan does not end up becoming a wish list of activities or goals for which resources are insufficient, or capacity is lacking – meaning that they cannot be implemented. The costing process can help to provide a realistic, financial feasibility assessment as an important element in the decision-making process.

The costing should also be used to look at potential duplication of activities among different actors in the health system. One of the conclusions from the analysis carried out in Sudan to develop NHPSP cost projections is that the exercise helped to highlight duplication in areas such as monitoring and logistics.[1] Similar findings regarding duplication of activities became evident during the costing of Angola's Plano Nacional de Desenvolviento Sanitario 2012–2025.[V]

Box 7.2

How much does a NHPSP cost? A valid question

Some may argue that estimating the overall cost of a NHPSP serves little purpose, and that efforts would be better addressed at estimating costs of more discrete financing-related strategies, such as "how much financing is required for extending my benefit package", or "what cost assumptions should be used when reimbursing different providers?". While these two more specific questions are certainly extremely valid and useful, the process of costing a NHPSP can serve to inform decision-making on strategic directions. The crux lies in the definition of "costing" and the approach taken for the analysis. In the case of NHPSP costing, the costing should not be approached as a mere mathematical exercise of attaching numbers to activities; it should be used strategically as a policy instrument to discuss issues around feasibility, financial sustainability, and the need for prioritization when resources are limited. The NHPSP costing can also be most useful in specific contexts to bring various technical programmes and planners together in a joint discussion.

Bringing the costing element into the process of strategic planning at an early stage helps ensure that the national health plan is accompanied by a realistic projection of resource needs, and not an unaffordable "wish list".

V Tania Lourenco, MoH Angola, personal communication (29 March 2016).

The objective of a NHPSP costing exercise often evolves into an analysis with a very broad and visionary question: what resources are required, and how should they be organized, in order for the health sector to meet the priority health needs of the population? The key word here is priority, because overall health needs will be infinite, and in the end, resources are scarce in relation to needs.

Scenario analysis – i.e., alternative projections for how the strategic vision outlined within the plan could be implemented, along with the associated costs – can be a useful tool to inform the planning dialogue.

There is seldom a single answer to this question, and within this chapter we refer to "scenario analysis" – i.e. the development of alternative projections for the strategic vision outlined within the plan. While the overall vision for the health system may be long-term over the next 20–30 years (Box 7.3), the medium-term scenarios (3–10 years) that are the subject of an NHPSP and thus, this handbook, can refer to more specific scenarios, for example:

- different strategies for health system investment – i.e. boosting the "backbone" or "hardware" of the system;
- different service delivery platforms for packages of health services;
- different scope of services to be delivered – whether the existing set of services will be expanded to include, for example, more tertiary care or a greater number of mental health services;
- the focus on prevention and public health interventions vs treatment;
- demonstrating cost savings that can arise as a result of shifting care models and from focusing on high impact preventive interventions;
- considering strategies for differentiated geographical targeting, or focusing on vulnerable groups, where relevant, and what this would require in terms of resource planning;
- different models of providers' payment (which ultimately alters their incentives, their behaviours, and the related resource use);
- different assumptions as to how care-seeking could change with (i) investments in the health system and (ii) changes in incentives for both patients and providers, and thus coverage of health services and predicted health outcomes;
- changing policies on essential medicine lists and pharmaceutical prices (e.g. reference prices);
- different assumptions around economic growth and estimated available health budget.

We will see throughout this chapter how scenario analysis is proposed as an approach to help examine the feasibility and affordability of different policy reforms or strategic investments in the medium term.

Box 7.3

Long-term projection models: Australian health care expenditure 2003 to 2033[2]

Many member countries of the Organization for Economic Co-operation and Development (OECD) with a primarily tax-funded health care model undertake expenditure predictions over the longer term in order to assess the fiscal future of health specifically. Modelled projections for Australia combine demographic data on population ageing and population growth, with non-demographic factors such as changes in disease rates, volume of services per treated case, access to treatment, and health price inflation. The analysis applies assumptions around what shares of expenditure will be funded by the government, as out-of-pocket, or through other private means. Estimates produced in 2008 indicated that total health and residential aged care expenditure is projected to increase by 189% from 2003 to 2033, representing an increase from 9.3% of gross domestic product (GDP) in 2002–2003 to 12.4% in 2032–2033. The largest projected increases in volume of care and related costs concern diabetes and dementia. **The report concludes that projection work is relevant, not so much for the accuracy of the numbers produced, but because it assists in an understanding of the drivers of health care expenditure, and the place of the health sector in the economy, which can subsequently be used to inform policy to address the anticipated changes.**

7.1.2 How does NHPSP costing fit into the broader health financing context?

Many health plans suffer from a weak situation analysis, unclear prioritization and poor rationale for target setting, combined with limited thinking about financing and sustainability.[3] A major challenge is that planning and costing are often not truly participatory and based on a multi-stakeholder dialogue. The consequence is a plan which does not adequately reflect what stakeholders want and are willing to implement. Such plans then do not properly serve to inform the budgeting process and actual implementation on the ground. It is a repeated observation that policy-making, planning, budgeting and costing take place independently of each other (often by different technical units within the MoH). Another challenge is ensuring coordination between central-level and regional/district/community-level planning (top-down vs bottom-up processes).[VI]

Development assistance brings further distortions in low-income countries.[4,5] First and foremost, the costing of the NHPSP needs to consider what the anticipated policy changes are, and what resources can be better used. Should there be a reprogramming of current resources towards other priorities, or can a change in the governance institutions and processes lead to changes in the way that activities take place, towards more efficient strategies? The costing process also requires consideration of the fixed costs that are firm commitments and do not change vis-à-vis the number of services produced.

The cost projections should also consider anticipated changes in the supply and demand for health services. Changes on the supply side (e.g. how services are provided and purchased)

VI See also Chapter 11 "Strategizing for health at subnational level" of this handbook.

can also have implications for the demand side (lower copayments may result in increased care-seeking) (see Box 7.4).

Box 7.4

Costing benefit packages and provider payment[6]

Many NHPSPs contain a strong link to a benefit package of services, whether these are implicitly or explicitly defined. In order to advance the policy dialogue around a benefit package, in most political settings, an estimation of the cost implications can be helpful. While there are few guidance documents available on how to estimate costs for a benefit package, such processes tend to be geared towards benchmarking and setting rates for provider payments. Estimations of benefit package costs are therefore narrower than a NHPSP costing which considers activities that need to occur across the health planning spectrum. When costs have been estimated for extensions of the benefit package, such analysis forms an essential component of the scenarios for the NHPSP and must be considered.

7.2 Why estimate costs for the NHPSP?

This section discusses why estimating costs for the NHPSP can help to inform health policy dialogue. Other types of cost analyses which can inform health planning are described in Annex 7.1.

7.2.1 Because a NHPSP cost estimation is a necessary basis for policy dialogue on the affordability of the NHPSP

Costing can be seen as a foundation of a good and comprehensive national strategy. This view is reflected in the International Health Partnership (IHP+)'s five core attributes of a national health strategy, formalized and applied through the Joint Assessment of National Health Strategies (JANS) processes. Box 7.5 illustrates two attributes referring to the estimated costs and budgetary framework for the strategy.

Box 7.5

Criteria used to assess comprehensiveness of cost and budget frameworks for NHPSPs

IHP+ has identified core attributes of a national health strategy.[7] Attributes 8 and 9 specify characteristics for the costs and budgetary framework.

Attribute 8: The national strategy hs an expenditure framework that includes a comprehensive budget/ costing of the programme areas covered by the national strategy.	The strategy is accompanied by a sound expenditure framework with a costed plan that links to the budget. It includes recurrent and investment financing requirements to implement the strategy, including costs of human resources, medicines, decentralized management, infrastructure and social protection mechanisms. When appropriate, the framework includes costs for activities and stakeholders beyond the public health sector.
	Cost estimates are clearly explained, justified as realistic, and based on economically sound methods.
Attribute 9: The strategy has a realistic budgetary framework and funding projections. If the strategy is not fully financed, there are mechanisms to ensure prioritization in line with the overall objectives of the strategy.	Funding projections include all sources of finance, specify financial pledges from key domestic and international funding sources (including lending), and consider uncertainties and risks.
	Funding projections are realistic in the light of economic conditions, medium-term expenditure plans, and fiscal space constraints
	If the level of funding is unclear or there is a gap, then the priorities for spending are spelled out with the consequences for results (either by showing the plans and targets under high-, low-, and most likely- funding scenarios, or by explaining the process for determining spending priorities).

With the Sustainable Development goals there is increased emphasis on the role of domestic resources, even in low-income countries. The concept of "affordability" should be grounded in projections of locally raised resources

The overall cost estimate can be considered a reference point to inform the planning and financing dialogue. Understanding the costs and resource implications informs the policy dialogue on the affordability of the NHPSP, including whether targets are feasible and realistic. The notion of "affordability" is highlighted in the discussions around the Sustainable Development Goals, where the central financing component is increasing countries' capacity to raise domestic resources through improved tax administration and overall policies to combat mismanagement of funds and illicit financial flows.[8]

A strong link between planning and costing should exist from the onset of any discussion on planned reforms and targets, including on the resource requirements. The process is iterative because planning decisions must take into consideration operational and financial feasibility, while the cost projections need to adjust between planned activities and available fiscal space.

The challenge for the NHPSP costing is thus to go beyond a mere quantification of stated targets. In many countries the NHPSP costing team is a technical team, adjacent to the general NHPSP planning team, which receives information from the NHPSP. A key challenge is to ensure a two-way dialogue, to use the costing exercise to unlock dialogue on strategic priorities and reforms that should be reflected in the NHPSP. Such a process requires three things that are in short stock: technical capacity, power to influence, and time. The second challenge is to move the planning and costing work beyond the technocratic government sphere and ensure a real multistakeholder process and participatory dialogue. Even if the actual calculation work might be left to those who are trained to perform complex computations, the assumptions behind the numbers and the details of the activities that the numbers represent must be based on multistakeholder policy dialogue.

Fig. 7.1 Costing a national health policy, strategy or plan

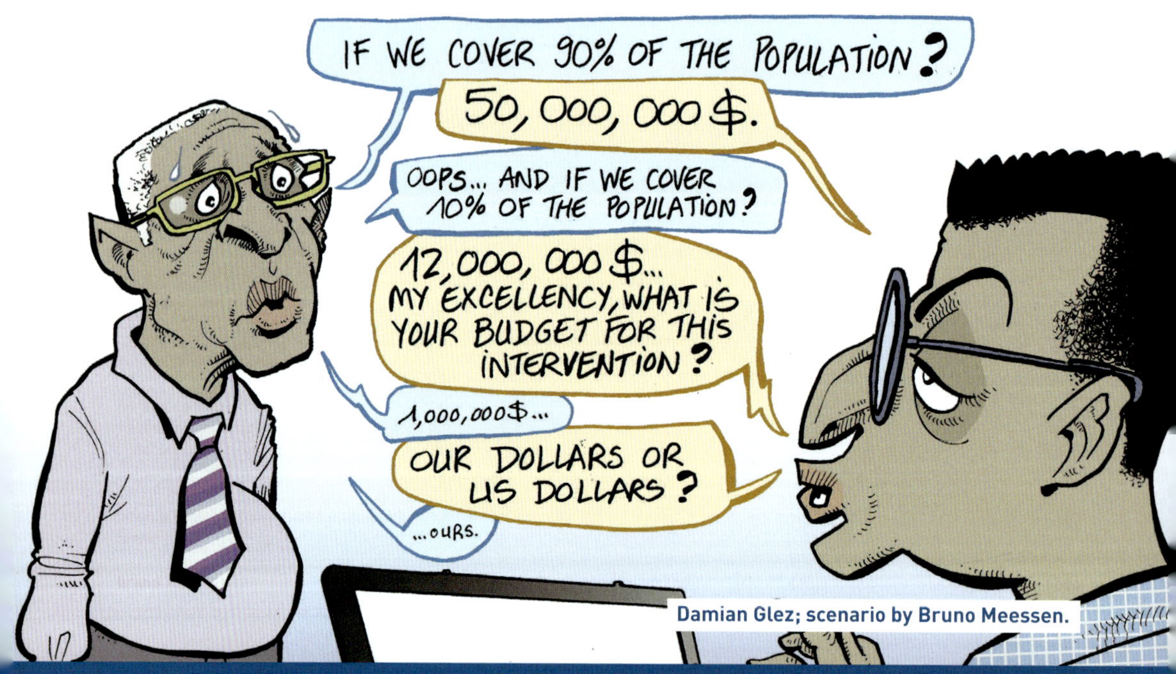

Damian Glez; scenario by Bruno Meessen.

Table 7.1 Estimating costs for NHPSP implementation: challenges and potential strategies to overcome the challenges

CHALLENGES	POTENTIAL STRATEGIES
Costing team is disconnected from planning dialogue	Develop scenarios with whatever data is available (e.g. salaries, anticipated commodity costs for key health services), present these to gain policy-makers' attention regarding the power of cost projections. The cost scenarios (based on the best available evidence) can be leveraged to stimulate a rational, multistakeholder policy dialogue on health sector priorities.
Costing exercise is perceived as externally owned	Foster local understanding of how the costed NHPSP can be useful for policy dialogue. When local capacity is constrained, focus on fostering the more critical roles related to ensuring MoH quality assurance of the data estimation process and final results.
Time constraint for analysis	Focus on cost drivers. Avoid going into too many details and losing the interest/momentum.
Limited interest by various technical programmes and data managers to participate in the process	Conduct outreach with the health programmes and health system departments; explain the objectives of costing; discuss how previous NHPSP estimates were developed and used and what can be improved this time around. Look explicitly into the costing that might have been done for their own programme planning and show linkage/limitations.
Challenges finding local data; reliance on global/default data	Use global/default data but document assumptions and data sources explicitly. Define data collection agenda for next costing round.

The link between planning and costing must be very strong from the beginning – any discussion on planned reforms and targets should take into consideration resource requirements.

7.2.2 Because costing can help promote cohesive support for the NHPSP

In countries where health programmes (e.g. health workforce, maternal health, mental health) or the broader health community (other line ministries, professional associations, academia, civil society, etc.) may have had limited involvement in the overall NHPSP process, the process provides an opportunity for these stakeholders to get engaged and feel their issues are taken on board. These processes often have greater value than just the technical generation of numbers and indicators, since they also help establish overall ownership of the NHPSP. In many settings, however, the individual specific health programmes have limited interest in the NHPSP process as they may not see the benefits of engaging in a sector-wide discussion. This is where the central planning unit of MoH needs to make a concerted effort to reach out to individual programmes and engage their interest. This is easier when planning cycles are aligned.

The first lesson of economics is scarcity: there is never enough of anything to fully satisfy all those who want it. The first lesson of politics is to disregard the first lesson of economics.
— Thomas Sewell

7.2.3 Because NHPSP cost projections put the MoH in a stronger position during the budget negotiation stage

Scarcity of resources is the first lesson of economics, in that there will never be enough to undertake everything that policy-makers wish to do. Health expenditures typically constitute around 6–15% of public spending, making health one of the largest sectors in most countries.[VII] Health sector planning requires information on the costs of planned policies precisely because they need to be examined in light of the scarce resources available.

NHPSP discussions with stakeholders can include a debate on the financial implications of the NHPSP. Having resource needs estimates readily available can help to advocate and mobilize additional resources from government and partners in support of the health plan. It is also important to remain in continuous dialogue with the ministry of finance (MoF) to discuss what information they are most interested in having when making resource allocation decisions for the health sector. This often includes concrete information on health system outputs or health outcomes (Box 7.6). The presentation of estimates should be carefully developed so that it provides information in a language which MoF staff can understand and relate to, which then makes it a good tool for lobbying and negotiating with the MoF.

VII In 2014, low-income countries on average spent 10.4% of their general government expenditure towards health. The values for lower middle-income and upper-middle-income countries were 6.3% and 10.5% respectively. High-income countries on average give higher priority to health with a share of 16.9%. Source: WHO Global Health Expenditure Database (http://who.int/health-accounts/ghed/en/,accessed 10 July 2016)

Box 7.6

More money for health in Ethiopia following MoH–MoF negotiations[9]

"It was a result of a revolution in the way we started planning for health that impressed the MoF to allocate more budget [to health]," says Nejmudin Bilal, former Director-General for Policy, Planning and Financing, MoH, Ethiopia.

In Ethiopia, the health sector progressively received large national budget allocation increases during the decade 2000–2010. Ceilings were shifted to accommodate increases for the health sector – quite a revolution, considering that usually, MoHs in many countries tend to be one of the least successful line ministries in government to argue for increased budget allocations.

How did the MoH in Ethiopia manage such a feat?

A detailed costing exercise was undertaken for the Ethiopian Health Sector Development Plan III 2005/6–2009/10 which included a fiscal space analysis and several financing scenarios to convince the MoF to prioritize the health sector. A crucial MoH strategy was demonstrating to the MoF that health sector goals were not only linked to, but critical to, the achievement of National Development Strategy goals and Millennium Development Goals (MDG) targets; and that scaling-up one of the flagship programmes of the health sector – the Health Extension Programme (HEP) – could have a decisively positive impact on those commitments. The various financing scenarios were linked to plausible impact, for example, the MoH was able to demonstrate that full financing of the HEP would ensure achievement of MDG4 to reduce child mortality for Ethiopia, which translated into reality five years later.

The Ethiopia example (Box 7.6) is powerful testimony to the potential a MoH has to leverage rational health planning and costing results, especially when it is ably linked to a realistic fiscal space analysis and financing. The Ethiopia example also demonstrates the need to link the costing to a policy direction (here the health extension worker programme) and strong arguments to link the investments to improved health system performance, in this case a reduction in under-five mortality.

7.2.4 Because costing strengthens accountability

Costing can facilitate an open and transparent presentation of the investments and activities needed to achieve the stated goals; in effect, a detailed NHPSP costing strengthens accountability.

A detailed NHPSP costing can strengthen accountability for the strategy. This is particularly the case when the costing process requires an open and transparent presentation of the concrete investments and reforms needed to achieve the stated aims as well as an informed estimate of the resources required to achieve them. Depending on the scope of the NHPSP, accountability will encompass mainly the government implementing institutions but potentially also the full range of stakeholders in the health sector, including the private sector. A NHPSP costing exercise will help clarify who will fund what and how far partnerships with other stakeholders (such as public-private partnerships) are necessary to fulfil the goals of the plan.

Within the government policy space, a costed plan helps map out the envisioned policy changes and ensures that the amount allocated to health is adequate to undertake the planned policies. Estimating the costs of an NHPSP also requires getting down to the details of those policies. What activities should be undertaken in what year, and with what specific targets and inputs, in order to reach the objectives? How would the structure of costs be expected to change over time, e.g. through innovative delivery strategies, a transition towards the use of a more cost-effective mix of services and improved service efficiency, or through modified purchasing strategies?

Accountability and transparency are strengthened when NHPSP objectives are aligned with the planned reforms, and the planned inputs are clearly spelled out and linked to outputs and outcomes (Fig. 7.2). Targets for an NHPSP often centre on outputs, outcomes and impact. The necessary investments for achieving those targets will be input-based. This is where the NHPSP costing process can emphasize strong links between inputs, processes/strategies and the longer-term anticipated impact.

Fig. 7.2 From inputs to outputs: a conceptual framework[10]

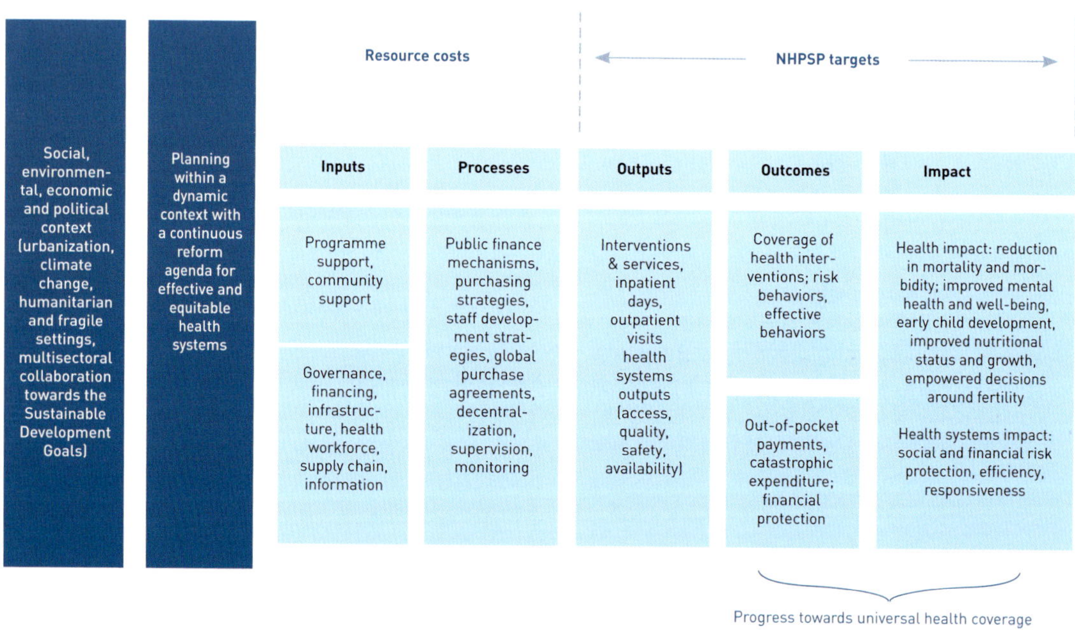

A well-costed plan allows a range of stakeholders – including civil society, private sector, parliamentarians and the media – to have insight into the rationale for resource allocation decisions, and to hold policy implementers accountable to the same. The essential next step, however, is the extent to which this information transparently feeds into the budget formulation process. In order to aid this process, information around the NHPSP multi-year cost estimates should be simplified enough for a range of audiences including those not working in the health sector. This can require three or four layers of messages (for technical health specialists, health policy-makers, non-health policy-makers, the general public, etc.). Box 7.7 provides an example of how examining projected costs for a strategy allows stakeholders such as civil society to challenge targets and standards set for service provision.

Box 7.7

Using cost estimates to influence resource allocation: an example demonstrating the influence of civil society in South Africa[11]

In South Africa in the 1990s the government health budget was only partially covering HIV/AIDS prevention and treatment drugs. There was limited access to drugs that prevent mother-to-child transmission (PMTCT) of HIV, as well as antiretroviral therapy (ART) in general. This led to the creation of a Treatment Action Campaign (TAC) in the mid-1990s. The TAC became a mechanism that allowed civil society to examine targets, assumptions and budget calculations, and to challenge them openly.

In 1998, the government suspended trials on PMTCT, stating high costs as the primary reason. The TAC was able to demonstrate that costs would be lower than the government had estimated, and show that public funds spent on a PMTCT programme would actually save money by reducing future HIV infections and associated costs. The discussion ended in court, where the judge ruled in favour of TAC, stating that a country-wide programme using Nevirapine (a common HIV drug) was affordable. As part of the legal process, the judge drew attention to the provincial health departments' underspending of their HIV/AIDS budgets, and argued that resources should be available. Between 2000 and 2003, a similar process was followed for ART.

7.2.5 Because the costing can help in the selection of relevant priorities according to available funds

Historically, many NHPSP processes estimated costs, compared these with estimates on available financing to demonstrate a financing gap, and then stopped short of taking the analysis further. While the demonstration of a funding gap can serve an advocacy purpose, in most settings it will not lead to an increase in resources. A necessary subsequent step will therefore be to set priorities for the medium-term investment framework. Here, information on costs is highly useful. The process of priority-setting is politically delicate and success relies on the adoption of a transparent process with clear criteria. In the priority-setting chapter of this handbook,[VIII] one of the possible criteria to be used for priority-setting within the national health planning process is cost. There are different types of cost analyses which can be used to feed into the priority-setting process; one of them is certainly the costing of the NHPSP since cost implications of planned activities will affect how those activities are prioritized. The generation of multiple scenarios may be particularly useful to highlight how there may be trade-offs – for example, extending service coverage vis-à-vis improving quality of care for existing services. The use of scenarios can also be done to identify a key set of priorities which will remain the core of the NHPSP implementation plan should there be unexpected shocks such as funding cuts.

The projected costs can be used to inform the policy dialogue on more efficient use of health sector resources.

An increasing number of countries also use "budget impact analysis" to consider the incremental economic impact that a new technology would have on the health sector, as part of priority-setting through health technology assessment processes.[IX] Such studies model the budgetary resources incurred due to illness with the current situation, and compare with those of the introduction of a new technology.[12] While such models can be very useful for informing decisions on the margin concerning new technologies, this chapter does not consider single intervention assessments, but deals with multiyear projections for the entire health sector.

7.2.6 Because costing can be a useful approach to inform discussions around efficiency

Costing can also be used to inform a dialogue on how to evaluate the current use of available resources, and whether these can be more efficiently spent. In many settings fiscal constraints make it difficult for any increase in resource allocation towards the health sector, and there may even be a reduction in available resources. Efficiency gains are thus the most available route to create fiscal space. Discussions on efficiency may be organized around the following:

Allocative efficiency. This concerns the "what" – i.e. the health service package that is being provided, and whether changing the composition of services within the package (subsidized by public funds) would bring more value for money. Here, cost-effectiveness analysis[X] is a useful tool to assess efficiency. In the case of a budget reduction for health, important decisions would need to be made whether to restrict access and/or increase co-payment for some services and/or populations and if so, which ones.

VIII See Chapter 4 "Priority-setting for national health policies, strategies, and plans" of this handbook.

IX Health technology assessment is the systematic evaluation of the properties and effects of a health technology, addressing the direct and intended effects of this technology, as well as its indirect and unintended consequences, and aimed mainly at informing decision making regarding health technologies. (Definition of The International Network of Agencies for Health Technology Assessment: http://www.inahta.org/, accessed 19 July 2016).

X See Chapter 4 "Priority-setting for national health policies, strategies, and plans" of this handbook.

Technical efficiency. This relates to "how" resources are used, and whether the same set of services could be delivered more efficiently. Potential strategies may include shifting tasks from one type of health worker cadre to another, changing purchasing strategies for drugs and medicines in order to obtain lower prices, and shifting from inpatient to outpatient care where this can be safely and effectively done.

Specifically in the context of an NHPSP, key issues include the inefficiency of parallel systems (e.g. supply chain systems for specific disease programmes), and how improved integration across the health system can bring increased value for money. Again, scenarios that highlight the resource implications of different investment strategies and compare these with the expected outcomes will help inform discussions.

7.2.7 Summary of rationale for costing of the NHPSP

The purpose of estimating costs of implementing strategies as outlined in the national health plan is therefore to examine:

- the overall envelope required; as well as
- how resources should be distributed to support different policy objectives, including allocation by areas of health intervention/ geographical regions, etc.

The results of the above should serve to inform, in an iterative way, priority-setting when the overall envelope is insufficient and while keeping in mind that certain costs are fixed and cannot be reallocated in the short term (e.g. health worker salaries).

The NHPSP costing process therefore provides key input into the policy dialogue on feasibility, efficiency, affordability and financial sustainability as follows:

1. to assess whether the plan is realistic in terms of what it sets out to achieve (the link between activities/inputs, resource needs, and projected policy outcomes);
2. to ensure that the plan is realistic in terms of the funding available (costs are aligned with the likely financial resources available);
3. to facilitate evidence-informed negotiations with the social health insurance agencies and other fundholders on expected outcomes and efficiency gains;
4. to generate clear and transparent information to inform the health budget formulation process.[XI]

XI For discussions on the use of cost and budget projections to strengthen accountability, please see chapter 8 "Budgeting for health" in this Handbook.

7.3 Timing of NHPSP costing

The projection of costs should start early on in the planning process, ideally as soon as the potential priority reform areas and strategic directions are known. Preliminary costing should take place to put approximate price tags on these priorities and assess to what extent they are feasible. Too often, costing work is undertaken after an overall plan has been completed and presented as a finalized document. Sometimes the costing is taken out as something done "on the side", neglecting the power of the costing process to transform and refocus the policy dialogue. The problem with such practices is that they de-link the strategy from the overall financing needs.

There have been instances where the retro-active costing demonstrated that the targets set in the NHPSP would require investments that are unaffordable within the medium-term time-frame. This then may call into question the overall validity of the NHPSP in the first place. A cost estimation is an opportunity to bring the NHPSP back to the reality of what can be actually operationalized on the ground, within a certain budget envelope.

De-linking costing from planning neglects the power of the costing process to transform and refocus the policy dialogue.

Moreover, the added value of scenario analysis will be minimal if the planning process is already concluded. If there is no longer any scope to discuss different policy scenarios, then the costing becomes a mechanical and mathematical exercise of multiplying activities by prices without being able to influence the policy debate. Of course, this is a false dichotomy and depends on the targets and strategies outlined in the NHPSP. If the targets remain diffuse, there is still scope to use the costing to model different implementation scenarios and discuss the benefits of one versus the other.

A general rule, however, is to limit the notion of "plan first, then cost" as it will set a divide between those who plan and those who cost. Instead, costing should be integral to the planning process. Below in section 7.5.2 we present an outline of how cost projections for a NHPSP can be produced through an iterative process where the validity of estimates increases as numbers are fine-tuned with each round of iteration.

The time-frame for the costing process as well as the necessary resources to undertake a solid costing depend primarily on three things:

(i) the approach chosen in terms of scope and methodology/tools;
(ii) the availability of data to inform the costing; and
(iii) the political willingness and participation of knowledgeable planners to provide inputs into the process.

When costing is produced for an overall national health plan, taking into account all major diseases, health areas and service providers, along with systems building, it is not unusual to spend between three and six months estimating costs on the first attempt. It should be emphasized that an extended timeline of three to six months does not imply full-time work on the costing, but allows for consultation processes and for an iterative process that dynamically feeds into discussions around the ambition of target set within the strategic plan (see Fig. 7.3 for a country example from Mozambique where the process in total was estimated to have taken six months, due to periods of inaction between the three phases of preparation, analysis, quality assurance and finalization). A costing that links strategic policy changes to costs requires a wide range of assumptions, data and information inputs, especially in comparison to traditional (historical) line item budgeting. For this reason, various software-based tools (see Box 7.11) come equipped with defaults to aid in reducing the time spent on data collection so that planners can focus on overall resource allocation questions, at least for the first round of estimates.

Fig. 7.3 Process of costing the national health sector plan in Mozambique[XII]

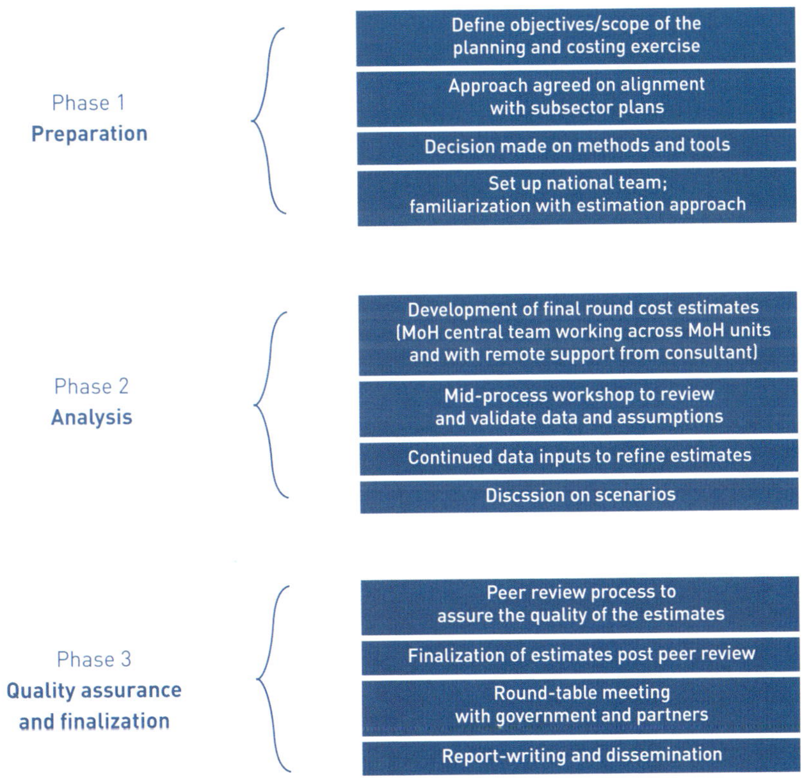

XII Costing team for the Plano Estratégico do Sector Saúde, 2014–2019, personal communication, [June 2013].

7.4 Roles and responsibilities of NHPSP stakeholders in the costing process

While led by the public administration, the scope for the NHPSP costing should to the extent feasible cover the entire health sector, and not only publicly financed services. Different stakeholders will play different roles in this process. The following list of stakeholders to be engaged in the process mirrors the overall list of organizations to be involved in the overall planning process, as emphasized throughout this handbook.

7.4.1 Ministry of health

The estimation of costs related to the NHPSP is often best led by the MoH. It is often managed jointly by the department of finance or economics and the department of planning. This happens when the NHPSP itself is within the MoH's authority, and costing is a key input and key step in the overall planning process. The calculations may be overseen by an ad-hoc team or by an institutionalized unit. The technical costing work may be outsourced to an independent institute or external consultants, if necessary, but they benefit from being supervised and guided by the MoH.

The estimation of NHPSP costs is best led by the MoH, with early engagement of the MoF and in some countries, the ministry of planning or social welfare as well.

Costing is an iterative process and involves developing various scenarios for stakeholders to consider. The planning-costing iterative process as well as the scenario-building work involves making several assumptions and hypotheses for the health sector; these are clear decisions to be made by the MoH for its own sector, independently of whether the technical work around quantitative estimates is being carried out by external consultants or internal staff.

7.4.2 Other ministries, including those of planning and finance

Multisectoral partnerships are paramount to improving population health-related outcomes. The engagement of other ministries for public health outcomes is therefore critical. An example is in the area of noncommunicable diseases, where ministries relating to sport, youth, transport, energy, water, environment and agriculture play a critical role in ensuring an enabling environment for favourable public health outcomes. Similarly, the role of the ministry of education in improving overall health is unquestionable, whether through direct efforts (such as school health, and academic institutions for training health workers) or through indirect efforts (a better-educated population is likely to engage in more effective preventive behaviour and seek timely care when needed). Involvement of the ministry of army and defence is often important because of their management of military health facilities.

The role of other government ministries is also crucial when it comes to providing input data, ensuring consistency with government policies and plans put forth in other sectors, validating the final estimates in terms of targets, costs and related projected outcomes, such as accessibility to care and overall population health impact. Engagement of the MoF, health insurance funds and other major fundholders in the NHPSP costing process is beneficial to promoting alignment with overall budget and financing processes.If done well, the cost estimates can be a basis for a common language between the MoH and the MoF. In particular:

- reaching out to the MoF at the start of the process to gather macroeconomic data around gross domestic product growth projections and other financing indicators, to inform projections around likely available domestic financing for health;
- inviting fundholders and the MoF to join the NHPSP process as active stakeholders and share in discussions around the estimated resources required, how to finance these, and what health outcomes they will buy;
- keeping fundholders informed about the process of the NHPSP costing, and linking this to the overall budget planning initiatives like MTEF;
- inviting fundholders to the final stages of discussion around draft costs and discussing affordability and sustainability.

In some countries, there will be a separate ministry of planning, which will obviously play a key role in the process, not least because of its link to national institutes of statistics and other units that collect and manage data and research.

7.4.3 Sub-national health authorities, including community level

Regional and district health authorities have an important role in providing complete data and information to the central level for a consolidated central exercise such as the NHPSP costing. Good, reliable data from district and regional level are critical for informing the national health planning process, including the situation analysis.[XIII] The situation analysis documents and analyses can be a good starting point from which extracts can be used to start building scenarios. Moreover, they can help ensure that projected estimates reflect planned activities to overcome regional bottlenecks.

In addition, issues around the challenges and bottlenecks faced at the local level should be communicated clearly to those who are developing the NHPSP and related costing as they need to be reflected in the underlying assumptions made when discussing policy reforms and building costing scenarios. In any case, since planning and costing are so closely linked, the same regional and district health authorities who are part of the overall national health planning process should also contribute to the costing (Box 7.8). The process whereby this will be done differs between countries and depends on the extent to which health policy and planning are decentralized.

Transparent data and information that reflect how the health system and health needs differ between geographical regions is critical for informing the national health planning process, especially the situation analysis and costing.

7.4.4 Parliamentarians

The national budget is generally brought to the legislature for discussion and subsequent passing into law. This is when public hearings and debates may take place on specific parts of the budget and/or the budget on the whole, with specific legislative committees engaging in discussions of specific topics. Here, the health committee of the parliament will be active in studying the health sections of the overall budget and preparing an analysis and response, often in the form of amendments.[XIV] The legislature is thus an important partner for the MoH here and it can increase support for its costed plan by engaging with parliamentarians early on in the planning and costing process to inform, explain and clarify why certain strategic directions have been selected and how their cost implications were estimated.

XIII For more detailed information, see Chapter 3 "Situation analysis of the health sector" in this handbook.

XIV For more information on health budgets and the budget process as a whole, see Chapter 8 "Budgeting for health" in this handbook.

Box 7.8

Aligned priority/target-setting and costing in a federal system – Ethiopia [XV]

Due to the highly decentralized structure of the Ethiopian health system, an aligned approach to priority-setting and costing across different levels of administration is necessary to inform the health budget. The country is divided into nine regional states and two city administrations, which are further divided into woredas (districts)—a basic decentralized administrative unit—and kebeles—which consist of 2500–4000 population. All these levels have their own two types of plans: strategic and operational plans. Therefore, to ensure alignment of plans prepared at all levels (vertical and horizontal alignment), the Ethiopian health sector redesigned its planning and monitoring and evaluation (M&E) process in 2007, and now implements with the principles of "one plan, one budget and one report" of harmonization and alignment. The planning process follows the top-down and bottom-up approach in order to align priorities and targets. A top-down approach means an indicative plan produced at higher level with high-level priorities and disaggregated targets are cascaded to lower levels. Based on the cascaded-down priorities and targets (indicative plan), lower level (districts and health facilities) prepare their comprehensive plan, which will be aggregated to the upper-level (region and then national level) bottom-up approach.

To ensure harmonization and alignment, the sector uses the same costing and planning methodology at all levels. Aligned costing techniques across different levels of government allow for assumptions in Ethiopia's national health plan to accurately reflect bottlenecks faced in local health sectors.

7.4.5 Private sector

Ideally, the private sector should be a full-fledged partner in the cost estimation process. In many countries, a large proportion of health care is directly provided by the private sector; in addition, much of the supply-side inputs for the health sector come from the private sector. The contributions of the private for-profit, private non-profit, private practice within the public sector, and public-private partnerships need careful consideration. Input directly from the private sector is essential in getting the data and information right.

A general approach may be adopted for NHPSP costing.

(a) Focus on those activities that relate to government-incurred costs:

- regulating service delivery, e.g. regulation and accreditation of private providers;
- regulating activities related to public health determinants in the broader sense, e.g. regulation of private manufacturers of foods and beverages, employers overseeing workers' health.

XV Kahsu Bekuretsion, Federal MoH, Ethiopia, personal communication (18 May 2016).

(b) Be explicit about private sector service delivery in terms of assumptions. It should be noted that information regarding private sector activities (quality, prices) may not be readily accessible and the costing team will need to carefully consider what assumptions to make and/or how to gain access to quality data. The decision to estimate and include the related costs depends on the scope of the NHPSP costing, and the provider payment structures.

- When private providers are paid by the government for service provision, such costs can be presented separately.
- The inclusion of private sector costs for which prices are unknown should be carefully considered: such estimates will have high uncertainty and will push NHPSP cost estimates upwards.[XVI]
- An option is to present costs for public-sector related activities, along with a description of anticipated engagements of the private sector.

(c) Model available financing

- The role of the private sector is critical for the assumptions on estimated available financing (the role of out-of-pocket spending, contributions by other private sector sources).

7.4.6 Development partners

The development partners' role revolves around providing relevant data and information on the projects and programmes in which they are involved, in relation to the projected NHPSP activities. Such information relates both to (i) planned activities (for the costing), and (ii) anticipated financing (for estimating available financing). Development partners may support the government directly in its programmes (on-budget funding) or may act outside the budgeting space of the government and undertake independent activities (off-budget funding). Note that the Paris Declaration (2005), the Accra Agenda for Action (2008), and the Busan High-Level Forum on Aid Effectiveness (2011) all encourage on-plan and on-budget activities of the development partners. In some low-income countries, external resources may make up more than half of the public budget for health. The external resources may have an impact on the costing of the health plan (for example, some commodities are provided as part of development assistance and internally procured at international price rates rather than local prices), but also with respect to the anticipated financing to be made available to the government over the planning period. In some countries, district-level health sector activities are being undertaken by development partners so their participation in the costing process is very important also for sub-national considerations. Development partners should be held accountable to provide the data/information on planned investments in an acceptable and understandable format.

The private sector plays a key role in implementation of the NHPSP, so its cost estimations should take this into account when strategically important.

XVI When it is difficult to access private sector data, the public sector cost can be used as a placeholder in order to generate an idea of the expected total resource requirement. Assumptions should be clearly documented.

7.4.7 Civil society, professional associations, academic institutions, think tanks and special interest groups

Civil society works directly with the populations in need of the services, and represents their demands. Professional associations represent health workers and know in practical terms which resources they need to provide services. Academic institutions are important with regards to their knowledge of any databases and studies (costing, cost-effectiveness, etc.) which could be of use in the NHPSP costing. As with other stakeholders, it is important for civil society to be transparent in providing relevant data and information and, through their critical input into the overall planning process, ensure that the assumptions made for costing scenarios are realistic and feasible, and relevant to the populations they represent (Box 7.9).

Box 7.9

Civil society organizations (CSOs) and costing in Uganda

Since the mid-1990s, CSOs have increasingly contributed to policy discussion and health policy formulation in Uganda.[13] Uganda has taken a comprehensive approach to strategizing for health, in which all governments, donors and stakeholders from the health sector are brought together; this allows the government to understand more fully the resource needs and costs based on the input of different parties, such as CSOs. NHPSPs in Uganda have benefited from CSOs proximity to health services and local knowledge.

Many CSOs in Uganda are directly involved in service delivery, hence their input is critical in the planning and costing process.[14] For example, information on district-level resource needs or facility-level intervention costs are often provided by CSOs, and cost estimation assumptions are discussed in detail with all service providers, including CSOs.

7.5 How to estimate NHPSP costs: methodological approaches

7.5.1 Getting started: setting objectives and defining an approach for the NHPSP costing

One of the initial steps in any costing exercise will be to determine the objectives and expected outputs. For the multi-year NHPSP projections, the scope of costing should be defined in relation to the policy reforms that are envisioned. There are multiple approaches.

Goal-oriented projections. The key question is "which strategies will bring us closer to attaining our goals?" Note that some targets may be fixed at an international level such as the SDGs.[16] The analysis should carefully investigate the potential related activities, and what would be the estimated associated funding requirements.

Resource-driven costing. The key question is "how can we maximize returns within a fixed budget envelope?" This ultimately considers policy reforms that will help make progress towards policy goals and targets within a financially constrained context, with a set spending target.

Bottleneck analysis. This considers current bottlenecks within the system and what would bring about a reduction in these, thus resulting in improved overall health-system (see Box 7.11) performance, and subsequent progress towards policy goals.

Many times, all three above approaches are relevant to the country context. While resources are limited, NHPSPs should consider the existing system bottlenecks and how best to invest to move towards health targets. Here again, scenarios can be a powerful tool to allow a discussion around how to bring goal-oriented planning closer to an assessment of resource constraints, through modelling different policy reforms. It will be useful within the analysis to consider allocative efficiency (what to do) as well as technical efficiency (how to do it) – and to consider both dimensions when discussing what can be changed within the current system as well as within a possibly expanded resource envelope.

Costing exercises can adopt multiple approaches such as goal-oriented projections, resource-driven costing, and bottleneck analysis. These approaches are not mutually exclusive and all three examples here may be relevant at country level.

Box 7.10

NHPSP costs (in USD) presented by strategic objective: country example from the Democratic Republic of the Congo National Health Plan 2011–2015

		Strategic directions					
RESULTS	**PROGRAMMES**	**2011**	**2012**	**2013**	**2014**	**2015**	**TOTAL 5 YEARS**
		I. Development of health districts					
Expected result #1: The population covered by quality health care services has increased by 30%	1. Improvement in health service coverage	33 222 600	24 803 400	23 113 400	23 173 400	23 233 400	127 546 200
	2. Streamline health facility functionality at all levels of the health system	68 465 400	84 476 420	108 297 020	117 089 420	158 467 840	536 796 100
	3. Support to health districts to provide basic interventions	53 776 800	49 830 000	43 255 500	39 945 900	37 754 400	224 562 600
	4. Improvement in health service quality	201 520	160 436	257 050	222 961	178 367	1 020 334
Expected result #2: The curative health service utilization rate has increased by 25%	1. Promotion of community participation in the health sector	6 455 715	806 315	821 915	829 715	825 115	9 748 775
	2. Health promotion	88 500	166 500	244 500	283 500	310 500	1 093 500
	3. Improvement of financial access	–	–	–	–	–	–

There should be a clear and joint decision by all stakeholders concerning the scope of the costing and the extent to which the costing covers public services only, or the full sector. Overall it is recommended (for example in the JANS guidelines, Box 7.5) that NHPSP costing should be broad and cover the full implementation needs for both health and other sectors. Ultimately, however, this will depend on information available and how the end results will be used.

A first step is to identify the types of outputs which one expects to have as the end result of the costing, since these will influence the scope of the analysis, the level of detail required in the final results, and how the information is gathered, analysed and presented. If a pre-developed template or software tool is used to inform the costing, the types of outputs that the tool can produce should be assessed based on the actual policy needs. Annex 7.2 provides some suggestions for standard presentation formats. As mentioned above, it is useful to consider early on how the costed NHPSP should link to the country's budget formulation process and how costs should be presented to facilitate such a process.

Box 7.11

Bottleneck analysis

Given the importance of contextual factors influencing health-care seeking patterns as well as the supply of quality health services, a concept which has proven effective at identifying and costing implementation barriers is bottleneck analysis. A systematic analysis of health system performance at decentralized level often reveals that many weaknesses in implementing effective health activities and strategies are related to service delivery bottlenecks at the district level.[18]

Bottlenecks among lower levels of implementation can exist at various levels and for an array of reasons. For instance, demand-related constraints may involve community norms and household behaviour, whereas at the provider level issues may concern local government financial management, and at the district level the constraint may be poor monitoring practices.[19] The first step of a bottleneck analysis is to identify those bottlenecks at district level, and to develop strategic action plans through consensus building activities, following which marginal costing can be performed under different scenarios to inform subnational plans and eventually a national level strategy.

The concept of bottleneck analysis was successfully developed into a practical tool for situation analysis, strategic investment scenarios, and marginal cost estimates in the Marginal Budgeting for Bottlenecks (MBB), developed by the United Nations Children's Fund (UNICEF) and the World Bank.

The MBB tool assists the user to consider what high-impact interventions could be used in existing health plans, what major health system bottlenecks are impeding on effective service delivery, what is the potential cost of alternative plans to alleviate a system's hurdles, and what are the additional financial resource needed. Importantly, the tool also indicates what could be achieved in terms of health outcomes by removing the bottlenecks.[21] While the MBB tool primarily focuses on maternal and child health, it has successfully been used in many settings to inform cost scenarios for national health sector strategies.[21] A notable example is the Ethiopia plan described in Box 7.6. These bottlenecks are usually linked to: availability of essential commodities and human resources, accessibility and utilization of health services, quality of services and continuity of services.

7.5.2 Costing the NHPSP in 20 steps

The NHPSP costing process involves iterative exchange between those who plan and those who cost; early engagement and constant dialogue on the different cost scenarios are essential.

The estimation of costs can be part of processes related to a new plan but also the revision of pre-existing plans and estimates, such as a mid-term review of a NHPSP or a multi-year operational plan, or during any other milestone events in a country's health policy and planning cycle.

The 20 steps listed below describe the costing of activities that relate to a new NHPSP under development. The list of steps is not meant to be prescriptive, but serve as an example only.

1. **Early engagement.** Bring up the topic of costing at the initial stages of planning the development of the NHPSP. In a context where those who are costing are part of the national health planning process from the beginning, they will be privy to and have access to the situation analysis data and discussions to get a sense of the key interventions that need to be costed. Make the point that even the initial discussions of the planning process can be informed by a discussion around the resource implications of the various overall policies considered (e.g. a changing composition of the health workforce, or a shift towards a stronger primary health care model) and whether these would fit within the anticipated resource envelope.

2. **Prepare.** Identify the scope of the costing and the expected outputs, the intended audience (primary users of the cost estimates) and the time frame, in relation to the overall strategic planning process. Note the deadline: by when do you need the estimates in a preliminary format and in a final format?

3. **Team formation.** Set up a coordinating team (typically two to ten people). The team size will depend on the scope of the costing, the anticipated detail of analysis and the time given to complete the work. All members do not necessarily need prior costing experience but there should be at least two or three members who have experience of costing and understand the data requirements. Ensure that the coordinating team will have access, within the period of the costing exercise, to key experts within the different departments of the MoH as well as within the major national health priority programmes.

4. **Budget envelope.** Gather information on likely trends in available financing and financial "ceilings" over the planning period (including projections for macroeconomic growth and allocations to health).

5. **Discuss alternate strategies for coverage.** Undertake a review of current health system bottlenecks. Map and consider planned reforms that may impact the cost structure (e.g. civil servant reforms, health provider payment reforms). Get a good sense of what the main strategic areas of investment will be over the planning period. What alternate strategies are being considered to address bottlenecks, increase efficiency of current spending, and to make progress toward universal health coverage? What can be the expected impact of these strategies on coverage for health services? How would the unit in charge of the NHPSP define the key reforms that will impact on service delivery, governance structures, accessibility to care and overall health system performance?

Based on discussions to date, what alternative scenarios could be considered for the plan itself and the related costs?

6. **Get buy-in.** Conduct an initial briefing to explain the process to various decision-makers and planners (e.g. department heads, district managers, MoF, parliamentarians, private sector representatives, donors) in order to gain their buy-in. Present findings of the budget envelope analysis. Discuss and get agreement on the directions for the costing and how it relates to the plan, including if possible, several scenarios to discuss the financial implications of emphasizing different policies within the NHPSP. Discuss the importance of health system investments and how to address existing service delivery bottlenecks.

7. **Develop a data collection plan** for making the cost projections (see Box 7.12).

8. **Gather specific inputs** from various technical planning units (e.g. health workforce, maternal health, mental health) regarding their planned activities and objectives, and where possible, taking into account the expected outcomes of their activities in relation to broader policy objectives and planned health reforms. Where relevant, these discussions should consider possible scenarios that link the programme-specific investment plans to the overall investment strategies for the NHPSP. An example might be a reallocation of resources, and an accompanying health financing reform that restructures the way resources are allocated and providers receive payment. In this context the strategies put forth by specific units such as health workforce and mental health should reflect the same broader move. At this stage, this is to inform the first rough costing, focus on getting the assumptions right for cost drivers such as human resources (salaries and other costs), and investments in infrastructure and logistics. Quick methods can be used for deriving cost for medicines – for example, through applying inflation measures to past years' estimates, or potentially using tools with pre-populated standards for drugs per case treated (see Table 7.2 below).

9. **Analyse the resource implications** of the planned activities and assess overall financial needs. This is the time to assess the potential scope for synergies and increased coordination and/or integration between specific programmes and departments, and likely constraints (e.g. health system constraints to deliver programme-specific targets).

10. **Modelling impact.** When modelling the expected health impact, review the expected outcomes. If a limited health impact is projected, discuss with programme experts and consider how investments could be geared towards more effective interventions.

11. **First-round.** Finalize the first-round analysis of costs, identify the main cost drivers and cross-check the validity of the data relating to cost drivers.

12. **Refine fiscal space projections.** Obtain and/or develop projections for macroeconomic growth and allocations to health, in order to project fiscal space and overall financial

space for the duration of the plan (the term "financial space" is used here to define the broader financing context, to include not just the government's expenditure but also that of the private sector and development partners). This step would be done in collaboration with the MoF.

13. **Conduct a mid-term consultation** to discuss first-round results, various scenarios for adjusting policies and plans, and assumptions on likely effectiveness of strategies in addressing bottlenecks. Brainstorm on cross-cutting issues – e.g. overcoming potential health worker shortages; the role of the private sector in service delivery. Discuss the need for prioritization in view of anticipated resource constraints. This could be a three- or four-day workshop involving a broader group of stakeholders in order to get buy-in and involvement, and to further discuss the production of implementation scenarios.

Data validation is an essential step to ensure the quality of the cost estimates; it also greatly facilitates the buy-in of technical counterparts.

14. **Prioritization.** Following the workshop, adjust the cost projection as needed, given the discussions on prioritization.

15. **Data validation.** Engage in overall quality-control processes, including subjecting the cost projections to peer review. Organize a data validation workshop to validate the coverage, inputs and outputs for the scenarios with technical counterparts. Fine-tune the projected costs with inputs from planning units.

16. **Map costs** to various presentation frameworks, including the country budget formats, to inform future budget allocation discussions.

17. **Write a report** to document the assumptions, process and results.

18. **Organize a consultation workshop** with a broader set of stakeholders (technical and policy) and discuss the NHPSP objectives and the costs at the same time – along with scenarios for priority-setting in different contexts of growth and/or financial austerity.

19. **Update** the estimated resource projections as may be needed post the consultation workshop. Undertake updates to the estimates as needed within a dynamic planning environment, and link these processes to midterm reviews and annual plans.

20. **Support institutionalization** of the above processes.

Box 7.12

Developing a data collection plan for the cost projections

In order to facilitate data collection, a mapping of relevant documents and resource persons should be undertaken upfront. It is helpful to indicate which team members will be responsible for retrieving each data source.

Examples of information data sources, used to project costs for the NHPSP activities[XVII]

TYPE OF DATA	DOCUMENTS AND RELATED INFORMATION	INSTITUTIONS AND RESOURCE PERSONS
General planning documents	▸ Previous NHPSP and related costing, if any ▸ Mid-term and/or final review of previous NHPSP ▸ Situation analysis to inform new NHPSP ▸ Health sector reviews ▸ National health accounts ▸ Demographic and health survey/multiple indicator cluster survey for coverage of health services ▸ Budget framework	Name and contact for each document
Health workforce	▸ Health workforce projections and existing plans ▸ Research studies that assess health personnel efficiency and time allocation ▸ Salaries and incentives	
Medicines	▸ Essential medicines list ▸ Prices of drugs and consumables ▸ Logistics and supply chain arrangements, including cold chain	
Malaria programme	▸ National strategic plan for malaria ▸ Global Fund proposal ▸ Evaluation of programme performance ▸ Treatment protocols	
Maternal health	▸ Health indicators related to maternal health (coverage, health outcomes, etc.) ▸ Various strategic plans and road maps and associated evaluations ▸ Emergency obstetric care assessments	

The level of detail provided and the quality of data in these systems and documents will differ from country to country. In a decentralized setting, reporting systems may be set up such that data are mostly to be managed at the regional level. For example, few facilities may report to the central level. In this case, it may be necessary to conduct data collection at the regional level.

XVII Andre Zida, Abt Associates, formerly with Ministry of Health, Burkina Faso, personal communication, [24 April 2016].

Sector reviews and updating cost estimates

During a NHPSP review (mid-term or annual), progress made towards the objectives should be analysed in relation to whether the budget allocation was sufficient or if there are other, non-financial constraints. The sector review process may reveal a need to reorient the NHPSP and/or to consider alternative implementation strategies. It may also reveal a change in the estimated available financial resources compared to what was initially predicted. This provides an opportunity to review the plan and to revise the costing in an inclusive and transparent manner. The review is also an opportunity to validate the assumption using actual data.

Iterative costing

The process to estimate costs is iterative by nature, and the level of accuracy will increase over time. The first production of cost estimates should rely on broad assumptions so as to be able to produce an overall estimate that can feed into the policy discussions around financial affordability at an early stage. Table 7.2 illustrates this further.

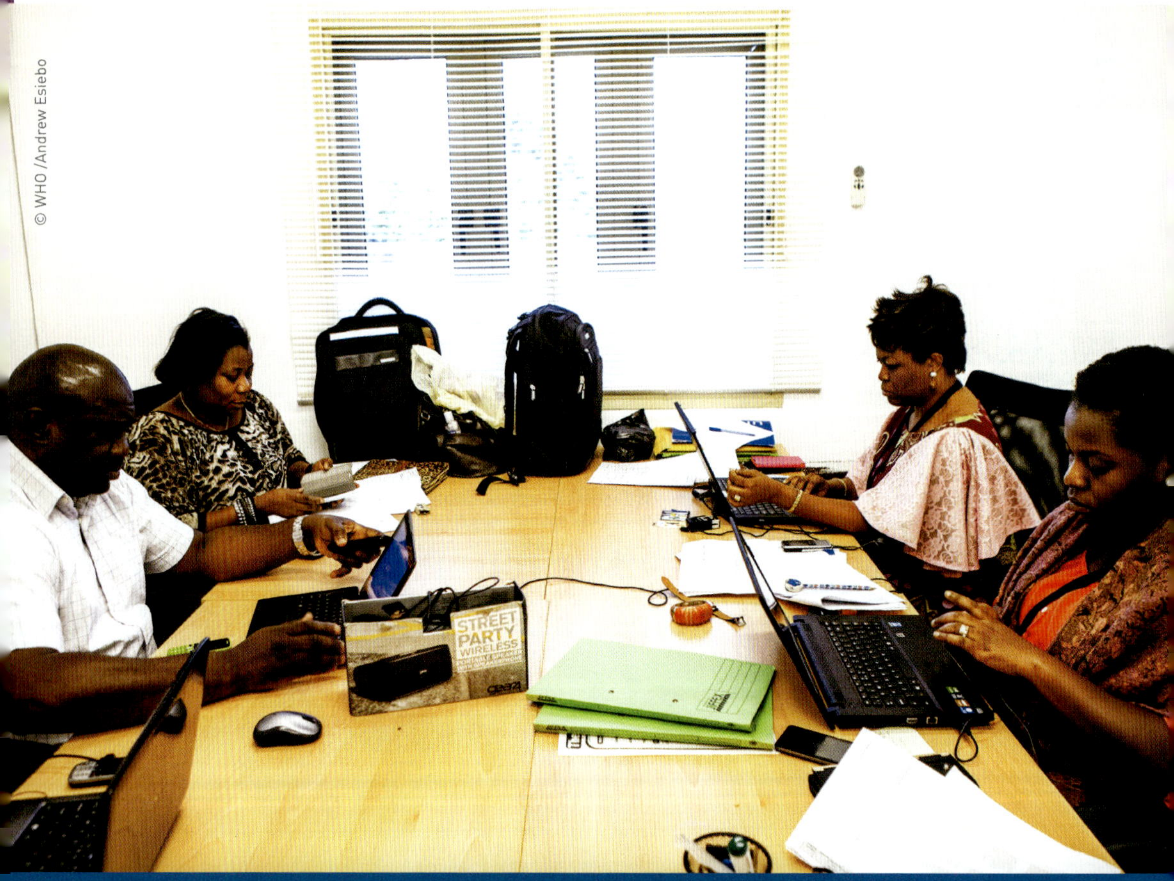

Table 7.2 A progressive approach to costing a NHPSP

	PURPOSE	APPROACH
First-round estimates	▸ Using broad assumptions, assess the overall resource envelope required and compare this with financial resources likely to be available, to assess general affordability.	▸ Focus on overall health systems needs and on the major programmes and areas likely to drive the costs (such as health worker salaries). ▸ Use simplified assumptions for intervention inputs and drug prices based on status quo, unless there are known differences likely to impact the overall costs. ▸ Adjust medicine costs for anticipated coverage increases.
Second-round estimates	▸ Derive an estimate that is more specific to the planned increase in coverage and the support activities required, that allows for discussion around relative costs of different programme areas/ strategic objectives.	▸ Having examined cost drivers and discussed potential reallocations within an affordable envelope, fine-tune some of the assumptions related to the cost drivers to ensure that they are correct (e.g. price of drugs for multidrug resistant TB; price of vaccines; targets for vehicles and equipment). ▸ Adjust some of the more prominent activity objectives and related costs to fit into the available envelope, if needed. ▸ Estimate likely gains in service coverage triggered by strategies addressing bottlenecks. ▸ Consider undertaking a scenario analysis without yet fine-tuning all of the cost input assumptions.
Close to final estimates	▸ Derive an estimate that is specific to (the adjusted) planned targets and activities, taking into account financial sustainability.	▸ Ensure that all relevant health services and activities are included in the costing, including those with smaller budgets. ▸ Prioritize as needed to take into account financial/ fiscal constraints. ▸ Fine-tune further as needed by reviewing input assumptions. ▸ Submit to peer review.
Final estimates	▸ Produce a final cost estimate that can later be used to inform the budget.	▸ Finalize assumptions and related documentation.

7.5.3 Different approaches, methods, and tools to inform NHPSP costing: some issues to consider

As a general point the benefits of cost information must be balanced against the cost of producing it. When developing a costing methodology, there is a need to balance elements such as level of detail, timeliness, accuracy and complexity with the cost of producing the cost information. The adopted costing practice must meet the stated needs, but the practices must also be sustainable. The investment made to produce cost information should not exceed the benefits the information provides.[20]

This section outlines approaches and concepts with respect to measuring and estimating costs. The first part considers overarching issues. The second part considers specific methods – such as unit costs, input-based costing, historical budgeting – and discusses the context of their application, including advantages and disadvantages. A third part considers different classifications of costs and benefits of presenting these separately. The fourth part covers the topics of inflation, exchange rates, and using specific pre-developed tools.

Overarching issues

Listed below are some of the issues to consider when selecting a methodological approach for costing the NHPSP.

Answers to policy questions will determine the scope of the costing and the link to other ongoing policy processes (such as benefit package reforms).

Expected outputs of the costing exercise, including stakeholder expectations, should be ascertained. If the expectation is to have a detailed activity-based plan which links inputs to outputs, this determines the approach to be taken.

It is important to establish a timeline: the time available to undertake the costing (if limited, one may opt for historical budgeting for smaller cost categories and focus on the main cost drivers for the detailed estimations).

Available resources to undertake the costing (human, financial and information) will affect the approach taken.

Another determining factor is the capacity to access the required information, and resource persons/experts to undertake the costing.

Medium- and long-term sustainability of the proposed practices will enhance their value. Devising scenarios: modelling efficient systems vs actual practice.

A NHPSP resource needs projection may be based on norms (such as, "a health worker should be in the facility eight hours per day, providing the correctly prescribed drugs according to national guidelines") or actual observed behaviours (such as, "health workers are on average in the facility four hours per day, often not following the national guidelines for drug prescriptions"). The approach taken for the analysis reflects a philosophical perspective. If it is not expected that inefficient behaviours will change in the short- to medium-term, the costing team may want to discuss how to take account of some inefficiencies or slack in the system (Box 7.13). The bottleneck analysis should address how to reduce inefficiencies over time, and to model:

(i) the costs of activities that would add incentives to be more efficient, and
(ii) adjust the assumptions in the cost model such that efficiency increases over time.

Box 7.13

Scenarios for health worker projections in Mozambique and Sierra Leone

The costing of the Mozambique NHSP (Plano Estratégico do Sector da Saúde, PESS)[21] considered two scenarios for human resource projections. A first scenario assumes a highly efficient work force that achieves high productivity based on the use of clinical equipment and high skill levels. A second scenario assumes more intensive labour inputs expressed as longer duration of patient encounters, especially among the "basic" nurse cadres and mid-level staff. The technical team considers that the second scenario reflects actual service delivery conditions more closely, and the use of scenarios here allowed for policy discussions that were based on concrete modelling.

In Sierra Leone, the costing of the Health Sector Recovery Plan 2015–2020[22] allowed for an examination of the predicted health worker capacity utilization and inpatient bed capacity utilization. These outputs facilitated a discussion on current staff distribution, in particular on obvious shortages of key health care providers in comparison to the predicted requirements as corresponding to implementation of the plan. The modelling led to concrete policy commitments by the government to review the planned health worker production and hiring strategies for the health sector.

Alignment of programme-specific estimates with NHPSP costing

By programme-specific plans we refer to sub-sector plans such as a malaria strategic plan or a maternal health roadmap. Overall it is recommended that programme/sector-specific plans should be fully aligned with – and ideally completely incorporated into – the NHPSP. It is often assumed that the sum of all programme plans is equal to an overarching NHPSP. This assumption completely ignores the significant health system investments usually spelled out in NHPSPs – all the more reason why programme plans need to carefully consider the underlying health system capacity to deliver health services, both under current capacity as well as with planned improvements for the future.

In general, the costing methods and health system assumptions used across the different programme areas and NHPSP need to be comparable. If the costing for one area (e.g. malaria) assumes a health system that is inefficient and with significant wastage rates, but another area (e.g. immunization) assumes that the health system is working optimally, the underlying assumptions are different. Standardizing assumptions across programmes is therefore important. This includes price assumptions used across programmes. If resources are supposed to be shared (e.g. health workers), then assumptions around the prices of shared resources need to be consistent across different areas in the plan.

Assumptions on prices and health system capacity used in the cost estimations across the different programme areas and for the NHPSP need to be comparable.

Methods

Bottom-up assessment versus historical allocation

As discussed above, costing a plan can/may link the plan's policy targets to activities, and the activities to specific costs. The level of detail by which costs are estimated may vary. To some extent, a historical allocation approach (or "inertia budgeting") may be used, whereby an amount is allocated to a specific area in the plan based on the previous year's budget, often with a small percentage increase to account for inflation. This may be justifiable if the amount spent in previous years was considered to be appropriate in achieving the specific functions, and if a similar level of activity and related (or nominally higher) budget is expected to suffice for the coming years as well. Examples may include the cost for overhead functions such as maintaining a national cancer registry or the salary bill for MoH central-level programme management staff.

Bottom-up costing relies on detailed information regarding inputs, quantities and prices. Historical allocation is an allocation method based explicitly on the previous year's budget. While there are situations for which historical allocations are necessary, a more detailed and nuanced costing methodology can better meet the needs for NHPSP costing.

The use of inertia budgeting should be carefully considered. However, this approach is less useful when the purpose is to cost a strategy which envisions a health system which is likely to be quite different from the status quo; for example, comprising significant new investments or different types of services, a change in the way services are provided and financed, and a subsequent explansion of health service coverage. Here, a more detailed bottom-up approach to the costing would more adequately capture the resources needed in reflecting such changes in the system.

The analysis may use a combined approach, and while inertia budgeting may be deemed sufficient for some areas, the focus can be on more detailed costing in other areas.

Bottom-up costing/activity-based costing: using unit costs or an input-based approach?

Bottom-up costing relies on detailed information regarding inputs, quantities and prices. The starting point is the identification of specific activities and annual targets, such as the population in need of specific services, by year. This is then multiplied by the average inputs – e.g. as required per person and service, and their respective prices. Such an approach may also be referred to as activity-based costing. The bottom-up approach is useful in that it allows for modelling how cost structures may change for existing activities if new reforms are implemented (for example, when output changes based on a specific input mix, or when the prices of inputs change).

Both unit costs and and input-based approaches can be used to inform bottom-up costing. Unit costs refer to the cost incurred to produce one unit of "output", for example, the cost per fully vaccinated child. Applying unit costs to volumes required can help provide a quick appraisal of the funding required, but has certain limitations in that unit cost estimates are very dependent on the specific assumptions that went into producing them. For example, Adam et al.[23] showed that the estimated cost for one outpatient visit was very sensitive to the assumptions made on how many patients are seen by a provider per day (see Box 7.14 for more information on unit costs).

Input-based costing tends to take a more detailed approach, with costs derived through the multiplication of quantities and prices. The input-based approach keeps the prices and quantities, seen as the key "inputs" of a cost, separate and distinct. For example, providing pregnant women with malaria treatment may require an outreach strategy to raise awareness, effective diagnostics, antimalarial drugs, the time of the health worker, and the use of the health facility. Using unit costs, on the other hand, means bundling the quantity and price into one – for example, the cost for treating a pregnant woman with malaria would include assumptions on the type of treatment provided and the cost for that treatment that are not usually disclosed to those wishing to understand what the unit cost is based on. Table 7.3 summarizes advantages and disadvantages of these two approaches.

A bottom-up costing approach is resource intensive but allows for modelling how cost structures may change as new reforms are implemented.

Table 7.3 Input-based costing vs. unit cost approach

	INPUT-BASED COSTING	UNIT COST APPROACH
Advantages	▸ Being able to separate out different components (e.g. health workers, medicines, transportation costs) and thus estimate these separately, allowing for greater transparency and predicting how the cost structure, and cost drivers, changes over time. ▸ Being able to adjust costs if quantities or price levels change, due to changes in factors such as treatment guidelines or procurement strategies.	▸ Can be used to provide quick estimates of resource needs, particularly when done at high level (e.g. unit cost per inpatient care multiplied by the projected increase in inpatient care utilization during NHPSP). ▸ Provides estimates that reflect part of a shared system, when not wishing to estimate the full cost of the system.
Disadvantages	▸ Resource-intensive, requires assumptions around the extent to which resources are used or left "idle".	▸ Relies on good quality data through cost studies, which are resource intensive in themselves. ▸ If data is inaccurate, may provide wrong estimates. ▸ Challenging to know how representative unit costs are. ▸ Challenging to compare unit costs across services when derived through different studies. ▸ Costs structures will change with evolving health system, making unit costs quickly outdated.

Estimates derived from an an input-based approach can be transformed into unit cost estimates but the reverse is not always true. Within an NHPSP costing, both approaches may be combined.

Box 7.14

Top-down derived unit costs

Unit costs are typically derived using a "top-down approach". This refers to a process whereby the total amount of resources is known, and is then allocated to different cost functions, using specific allocation algorithms. An example is assessing costs for hospital care, where the total expenditures of the hospital are allocated to the different departments, in order to assess the cost of each specific department, and the average cost per patient seen for different types of care. The unit costs derived from actual practice will reflect the existing system, including current capacity utilization of resources and associated inefficiencies (for example, if there is a lot of slack time by certain types of health worker, their capacity is underutilized and unit costs will generally be higher than in a more efficient system).

The concept of economies of scale implies that unit cost should decrease with an increase in coverage as the fixed costs are spread over more units of output. However, once a certain level is reached, corresponding to full capacity, unit costs may increase again (step increase). They will likely not decrease again until a certain level of hospital activity and turnover is achieved. In most settings it is difficult to know where the "average facility" or delivery programme sits within the cost curve.

Illustration of a typical "unit cost curve" reflecting published data

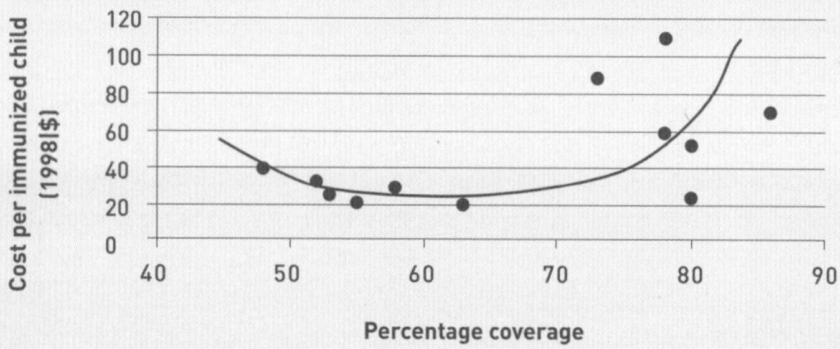

Source: adapted from Johns B and Tan Torres T. Costs of scaling up health interventions: a systematic review. Health policy and planning. 2005. (http://heapol.oxfordjournals.org/content/20/1/1.long, accessed 18 October 2016)

Given that unit costs derived from a top-down allocation reflect the current system, they do not necessarily indicate the resources needed to guarantee quality outputs, especially in chronically underfunded health systems. When unit costs are used, there needs to be careful consideration around how one would expect unit costs to vary over time and across populations, and whether the data gathered as the reference point reflects the anticipated resources needed in the system.

Lump Sums

Lump sums refer to a cost figure which includes several inputs, quantities, and cost lines bundled into one. The lump sum cost would generally cover more items than a unit cost, but with less transparency – such as an overall lump sum cost required for pandemic or emergency preparedness. Lump sums are inferior to unit costs and inputs-based costing because of their lesser detail, but again the analyst needs to consider the resources available for the costing and whether to use lump sums in some instances, especially for those items that constitute a small part of overall costs. In certain settings general rules of thumb may be applied, for example any costs anticipated to constitute 1% or less of the overall resource envelope can use less sophisticated methods.

The lump sum amount should nevertheless be sufficient and proportional to the expected outputs. Some categories of costs, such as utilities, may seem fixed in nature and thus make a case for lump sum costing, but in fact they may hide inefficiencies in resource use. An example is in former Soviet Union countries where utility costs make up a large share of the budget, partially due to the infrastructural setup. High density of facilities incur large fixed costs for electricity and heating, and utility costs may be used to subsidize other resource use. In the Republic of Moldova for example, in 2000, over 25% of government health expenditure was spent on utilities.[24] A few years later, expenses for water, heating and electricity fell by 6.8%.[25]

Treatment of various types of costs

Capital versus recurrent costs

The costing should generally present a breakdown of capital and recurrent costs separately. Capital costs are those which last for more than a year (for example, an X-ray machine) whereas recurrent costs, once the good is consumed, last for less than a year (e.g. the electricity costs related to running the X-ray machine).[26] The purpose of separating these is to allow planners to understand what share of the costs are one-off capital investments. The model used for costing should also have clear links between capital and recurrent costs. Every additional unit of capital invested will incur additional recurrent costs. For example, in many states of the former Soviet Union, the government incurred significant recurrent costs for running hospitals, the capital investments of which were made 30–40 years ago. Closing down hospitals could free up resources currently used in running inefficient structures, reallocating those resources to lower-level, close-to-patient services. In other settings there may be an expressed need within the NHPSP for significant investments in tertiary care, and when this includes building new hospital structures, such investments should be accompanied by increases in recurrent investments in relation to salaries, commodities and operating costs. Please note that the investment plans and related funding may be accessed through different ministries and/or departments for recurrent vs capital costs.

Different types of costs need to be treated differently, and sometimes separately: capital vs. recurrent costs, intervention vs. programmatic costs, direct vs. indirect costs.

Intervention versus programmatic costs

When working with technical disease programmes in the MoH, many programmes set objectives both for health interventions (e.g. skilled delivery at birth) as well as for programmatic (programme-specific) activities (e.g. conduct demand generation activities such as information and outreach into communities, or organizing training courses to improve midwives' skills to provide quality care at birth). Ensuring and managing a sufficient budget for actual service delivery is usually out of the influence of the specific technical programme; however, arguing for and managing the budget specific to "programmatic" activities is directly within its influence. It is often necessary, therefore, to estimate and present intervention and programmatic costs separately.

Total versus marginal costs

The NHPSP will require estimations around its total cost, to inform MTEF and budget discussions. Marginal costs are those that refer only to additional resource needs above the current health system setup, including those incurred to reform and increase the efficiency of the system. It is possible to estimate marginal costs and then add those to the current health spending, with or without modelled modifications to the latter in view of anticipated reforms, but the caveats need to be well known and documented in terms of whether the current level of investment and expenditure should be expected to remain as is, for the duration of the NHPSP.

Additional issues

Inflation

The costing may incorporate inflation or not. In either case, the decision should be clearly communicated, and the assumptions for inflation made explicit. The primary reason for not presenting costs that take inflation into account is that inflation is an uncertain factor, and future trends may digress considerably from what was presented for the NHPSP. The recommendation is, therefore, for those countries wishing to present estimates that consider inflation to include several output tables, where at least one has constant price levels, while others present scenarios for constant inflation, IMF-predicted inflation, reduced and/or increased inflation levels. Another option is to initially present costs in constant prices and then whenever estimates are updated and/or presented to various funding partners, to convert costs into inflation-sensitive numbers, taking into account the latest available data on inflation

Exchange rates and traded goods

The costs of drugs and diagnostic tests are influenced by whether they can be purchased locally or are imported using foreign exchange. If there is a reliance on imports, the affordability measured in the local currency will rely on favourable exchange rates. It may be important to reflect this when estimating and presenting the costs, and to indicate:

- which type of investments are most affected by assumptions around exchange rates;
- present multi-year estimated costs both in local currency as well as in USD or another global currency.

Costing tools

There are multiple tools available to inform priority-setting and cost projections, whether for specific diseases or for broader health sector planning. Using pre-developed costing tools has several advantages and disadvantages. Some of these are listed in Table 7.4.

Table 7.4 Potential advantages and disadvantages of pre-developed costing tools

POTENTIAL ADVANTAGES	POTENTIAL DISADVANTAGES
▸ Tools provide a checklist of recommended inputs for different activities or interventions, often populated for a list of high-impact priority interventions that are globally recommended. The provision of a checklist can help reduce the risk that critical but less visible activities are unaccounted for (such as administrative costs and maintenance of equipment and vehicles).	▸ Users may use the checklist as an absolute guide and be tempted to fill in every section without carefully considering what is most relevant within the national context.
▸ Tools provide calculation algorithms, thus simplifying the mathematics of calculations.	▸ Calculation algorithms may hide details from the user, thus limiting transparency.
▸ Tools facilitate the use of standardized methods/prices across calculation areas (such as different disease programme areas). ▸ Tools help to provide an evidence base with which to explain the health system implications of programme-level investments.	
▸ Tools often provide global default prices of inputs such as medicines, vaccines and vehicles, and sometimes even local prices, such as wages of health workers. The defaults often come from similar contexts or countries and can be used to inform an initial rough costing and serve as checks for local data. The added value of defaults is that: ▸ after a quick feasibility check, they can be used for the first round of rough costing; ▸ they can be used as a check against which local data can be measured.	▸ Users may apply default data uncritically without looking for local alternatives. ▸ If default data are not kept up to date, they may reflect outdated numbers and prices.
▸ Tools may provide a standard template format for activities, such that users can easily enter data related to target-setting for training courses, vehicle purchases, etc. ▸ Less probability of making calculation mistakes ▸ Formulae are pre-tested and validated ▸ A standard, validated template makes it more easily accessible for review.	
▸ When tools include an epidemiological impact component, they will allow for calculations of the predicted impact of the plan.	▸ Epidemiological impact estimates need to be considered as indicative estimates, and not as an absolute given.
▸ Tools provide output data quickly and automatically, including tables and graphs. ▸ An analysis of the health system as a whole may be easier with all costing-associated data in one database	
▸ Adjustments can be made over time in one single consolidated database, which can be monitored.	▸ The use of tools requires local capacity to be built and maintained to ensure that projections can be updated as needed.

The OneHealth Tool was developed by a group of UN agencies on request by countries for a health sector-wide planning and cost estimation tool.

The OneHealth Tool (developed by an interagency working group consisting of costing experts from WHO and other United Nations [UN] agencies) is one of the available instruments that can be used to generate overall costs and scale-up targets for a costing that supports strategic planning and budgeting. The OneHealth Tool was designed to enable the user to assess to what extent targets set within the plan are feasible, and to consider programme goals and health systems jointly. The tool can also be used to produce estimates of health impact related to changes in coverage and service delivery initiatives (Box 7.15).

Box 7.15

The OneHealth Tool[27]

The OneHealth Tool is a software tool designed to inform national strategic health planning and costing in low- and middle-income countries. Its development was overseen by an interagency working group with representatives from WHO, UNAIDS (Joint United Nations Programme on HIV/AIDS), UNDP (United Nations Development Programme), UNFPA (United Nations Population Fund), UNICEF, World Bank and UN Women.

The OneHealth Tool was developed as a complement to disease-specific tools which neglected to take into account health systems costs. The tool links strategic objectives and targets of disease control and prevention programmes to the required investments in health systems, and provides a platform for analysing the costs of a full health sector plan. It provides planners with a single framework for scenario analysis, costing, and health impact analysis of strategies for major diseases and health system components.

In addition to calculating costs, the tool estimates the likely reduction in mortality and morbidity based on targets identified by the user. Furthermore, for strategic planning, a useful feature is the possibility to design scenarios to develop "what if" plans and examine their costs and impact.

The tool is pre-populated with defaults for disease prevalence and incidence, intervention protocols for promotive, preventive and curative care, and prices of drugs, supplies and equipment – all of which can be changed by the user.

The first official version of the OneHealth Tool was released in May 2012. Since then the tool has been applied in more than 30 countries to inform planning and costing.

Summary recommendation

When resources allow, the recommendation is to use bottom-up (input-based) costing to:

- link inputs to outputs, thus enhancing accountability;
- link the costing (specific cost items) to categories in the national budget;
- use realistic assumptions on implementation pace and impact of strategies on health intervention coverage on the basis of a bottleneck analysis.

A NHPSP costing need not be based on detailed inputs down to the exact number of gloves and cotton balls required by each facility in the coming years, but does benefit from a costing that links inputs to outputs at a level that is context-specific and population-driven enough, yet minimizes the need for detailed planning. The key point is that the selected approach should be evidence-informed, and that the planning unit should be able to justify indicated amounts, whether based on historical data or a bottom-up forecast.

7.5.4 Assuring high quality cost estimates

It is crucial that steps are taken to ensure that the NHPSP costs meet the required standards. Guidance on standards and criteria are included in the JANS (Box 7.5), which primarily focuses on the comprehensiveness of the costing (includes all types of resources and stakeholders), transparency (estimates are clearly explained), realism (limited specific guidance is provided through JANS, but the "reality checks" below may serve as a guide) and methodological soundness (input data must be as accurate as possible, as must the calculation algorithms).

First, some initial "reality checks" should be done early on in the costing process:

- calculate per capita estimates, which are more readily interpreted than aggregate estimates;
- compare per capita estimates with current spending, with past projections, and with estimates available through the global public literature and/or those produced by neighbouring/similar countries;
- compare costs with current expenditure.

Check cost drivers (Box 7.16) and compare with commonly known current cost drivers from current budgets or health accounts.

Secondly, it can also be helpful to send the costing for peer review. Such review processes may involve internal or external experts' feedback, or both. Feedback will allow the team to improve the calculation and presentation of estimates.

Third, setting up processes for data validation and overall stakeholder consultation as described above in the sequence of proposed steps, will support validation of assumptions used, priorities set and outputs produced. One of the processes of reviewing the costing is through a comprehensive JANS process, but there are also other ways of peer review, such as inviting costing experts to comment remotely.

Box 7.16

Examining cost drivers within the estimated projected resource needs for Angola's Health Sector Development Plan 2013-2025[28]

	Programme	Costs 2013–2025 (USD million)	% of cost 2013–2025
1	Prevention and disease control	24 472	30.2
2	Primary health care and hospital care	851	1.1
3	Health workforce	20 517	25.3
4	Research	7	0.0
5	Health facility network	33 001	40.7
6	Logistics, medicines and medical devices	2130	2.6
7	Health information and management systems	53	0.1
8	Governance and institutional framework	20	0.0
9	Financing and sustainability	26	0.0
	Total	**81 077**	**100.0**

The Plano National de Desenvolvimento Sanitário (PNDS), or the Health Sector Development Plan, is a strategic and operational tool for realizing the political targets outlined in the long-term national development strategy "Angola 2025" and the national health reform policy. The PNDS vision positions health at the centre of national development and social justice, promoting universal equitable access to quality health care, in view of combating poverty and improving well-being of the population. The plan for 2012–2025 sets ambitious targets to achieve these goals, and projected costs for the planned investments would equate an increase in health spending per capita from USD 186 in 2011 to USD 276 in 2025.

The table above shows sample results from the cost projections for the plan. USD 81 billion over 13 years of the plan equates on average USD 6.2 billion per year, although costs are estimated to increase over the period and reach USD 9.4 billion in 2025.

The main cost driver is extension of the health facility network (40.7%), which primarily entails building and maintaining infrastructure for health, as needed after the Angola civil war which destroyed much of the available facility network. The second largest cost driver (30.2%) is prevention and disease control, which is where the various national programme estimates fall, including significant cost drivers such as (in order of magnitude, not shown here): nutrition, cancer control, chronic kidney disease, HIV/AIDS, and child and maternal health. These five programme areas jointly account for over 80% of the projected cost within the category of prevention and disease control. The health workforce accounts for 25.3% of the overall projected PNDS costs.

7.6 What if...?

This section outlines costing issues in specific settings such as decentralized contexts, highly donor-dependent countries, and fragile states.

7.6.1 What if your country is decentralized?

If health is a mandate for a decentralized entity, the full health policy and financing cycles may fall under a decentralized authority. A decentralized process may have in place institutional arrangements for coordination, planning, budgeting, financial reporting, and implementation across government ministries/institutions, as well as between the different administrative levels of the country. These coordination bodies are important mechanisms for health-planning stakeholders to discuss specific issues linked to cost estimations and underlying assumptions as well as review initial calculations and cross-check and compare.

In decentralized settings, it is important to harmonize and align costing assumptions and methodologies across sub-national entities to avoid a diverse and heterogeneous set of data which makes aggregation of country-wide national estimates very difficult.

The MoH or other central planning authority should give strong guidance as to the standards and methodologies to be used for costing – without it, a diverse and heterogeneous set of data from the various decentralized structures will make aggregating countrywide data and producing national estimates very difficult. For example, the cost of a community outreach campaign is not comparable between two regions if the underlying costing assumptions and methodology used are not harmonized.

In many large countries, the majority of public spending on health takes place at subnational level. Local governments tend to have better access to context-specific data such that the cost estimates can be fine-tuned and really relevant to the local setting. These estimates are extremely useful to feed into national averages and aggregates and form a critical basis for NHPSP costing.

Some questions to consider for costing and budgeting in decentralized settings are given below. Since cost estimations are linked to budget allocations, these issues are relevant for both.

What does decentralization actually mean in practice in your country? How far are structures, responsibilities, and budgets actually decentralized?

The more power and authority actually vested in local authorities, the more scope there is for rational costing and budgeting that is close to the real needs of the local population.

Does the central-level authority need to aggregate costing and budgeting nationally?

If so, guidance and templates from a central authority would be useful and necessary to reduce the burden and error margins of reformatting and restructuring in order to compare and aggregate. In addition, technical support from a central authority might be recommended.

The central-level authority should take into account revenue generation at different levels for more accurate fiscal space projections.

How transparent are health system costs, budgets, and expenditures reported at decentralized level?

A low level of transparency may indicate a lack of accountability to the population coming under the decentralized authority and a subsequent lost opportunity to leverage the planning and budgeting advantages of being close to the population.

7.6.2 What if your country is heavily dependent on aid?

In an aid-dependent context, vertical programmes may receive large amounts of funding as earmarked budgets. Specific programmes (e.g. HIV or malaria) often have multi-year projections that have been estimated as part of development proposals. These projections should be aligned with the overall NHPSP analysis. A few key points should be noted.

First, the relative role of externally funded disease-specific or life cycle-specific strat- egies within overall sector priorities is often an issue in low-income countries.[29] Here an analysis of the impact of programme objectives and their projections on overall shared health systems resources can be extremely useful to stimulate discussion on alignment of donor-supported projects with NHPSP goals.

Second, sustainability becomes an issue when a large share of resources is external. This should be kept in mind when undertaking a NHPSP costing exercise in view of (a) the volatility of external aid flows,[30] and (b) the planned transition from external donor support to domestic financing as countries "graduate" from donor eligibility.

Third, externally funded projects may run through different service delivery models from government funded systems, thus resulting in inequitable care.

The costing work can be leveraged as a powerful instrument to inform the dialogue on the above-mentioned issues and strengthen harmonization around health sector activities by different stakeholders.

Fourth, cost can be significantly higher in programmes directly funded by donors.

7.6.3 What if fragility is an issue in your country?

Fragile or post-conflict states will have a reduced tax base and limited revenue generation compared to other countries, translating into an increasing reliance on informal payments and on donor funding. In addition, the transition from short-term emergency relief to longer-term development means a shift in funding models for the health sector – usually, there is some government takeover of basic services with heavy donor assistance. In most cases, this will be accompanied by the continued presence of emergency services as well, creating several parallel funding streams for different types and levels of services which necessitate strong steering capacity and management by the MoH. This, almost by definition of a fragile state, rarely exists, which makes rational planning and costing extremely complex and challenging. Moreover, investment needs are often higher in fragile states than in other more stable but similar states, due to the need to rebuild the health system.[31]

In a fragile, post-conflict setting, time constraints may not allow high levels of costing detail but a focused emphasis on ensuring that the costing work is done swiftly by experienced experts is crucial. The results of a realistic costing of recovery and reconstruction can be leveraged to influence donor commitments and pledges.

An additional dilemma lies in the highly politicized environment within which transition governments interact with their populations. Unrealistic expectations may be raised, with no adequate capacity and budget to back up their implementation. This vicious cycle can further threaten security. In such a situation, it is important to:

- undertake a solid and realistic costing of what a post-conflict/emergency health system will cost – time constraints may not allow high levels of detail, but a focused emphasis on ensuring that the costing work is done by experienced experts is crucial;
- attempt to use the realistic costing of recovery and reconstruction to link to and influence donor commitments and pledges – rather than the other way around, i.e. not allowing donor commitments and interests drive the recovery planning and costing.

Scenario analysis can be an extremely useful tool in fragile contexts to account for the uncertainty of the situation.

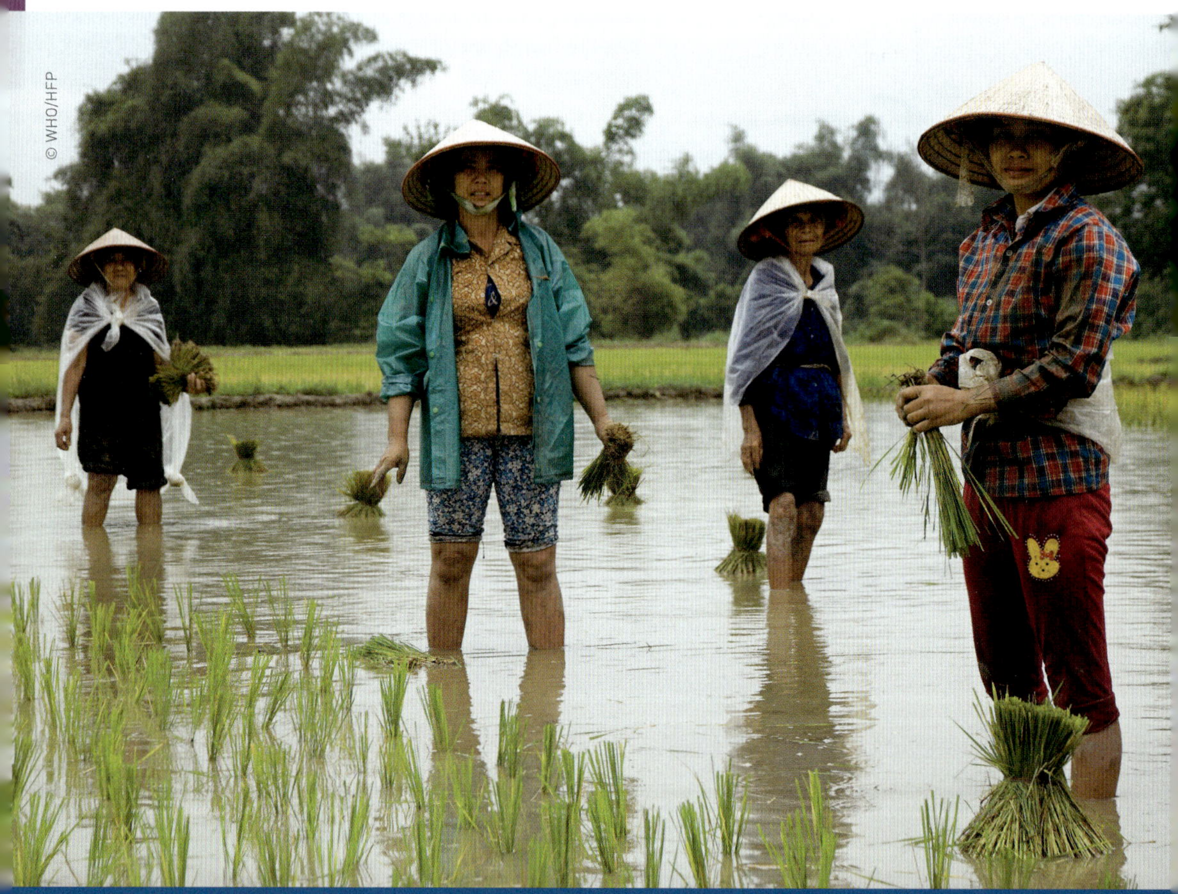

7.7 Conclusion

This chapter has discussed key issues to consider for multi-year cost projections in relation to developing a NHPSP.

The chapter has emphasized the need for NHPSP costing to be an integral part of the planning process, and for costing to be considered within a broader context of budgeting and financing processes. The estimation of costs is crucial as it can help underline the need to set priorities, and to inform the prioritization process.

The cost projections should be interpreted as reflective of a dynamic and uncertain context, thus necessitating updates over time. The advantages of a bottom-up approach – linking inputs to outputs, which support accountability and transparent information sharing – have been put forward.

The most important factor affecting the cost estimations are the estimates of the impact on coverage gains of the implementation approaches of specific strategies and activities outlined in the NHPSP. These estimates of gains in coverage need to be spelled out in studies such as the bottleneck analysis.

The use of scenarios can be a powerful tool to demonstrate which implementation strategies may be more feasible and affordable than others within the short- to medium-term planning period. Scenarios can help inform policy-makers that the cost estimates are not to be interpreted as absolute "static" numbers, but should be considered as indicative estimates for which a considerable uncertainty interval applies.

Finally, NHPSP cost analysis is an essential component to feed into the decision-making dialogue at all levels. The process of estimating resource needs through a participatory approach can in itself strengthen buy-in to the NHPSP process among national stakeholders and external partners.

In summary, it is essential for the NHPSP costing process to be:

- an integral part of planning;
- locally owned;
- reflecting the planned policy reforms;
- subject to validation and review processes;
- a tool for feasibility and efficiency analysis;
- a tool for accountability.

References

1 Waddington, C. Lessons from the JANS on Sudan's national health sector strategic plan. Lessons learnt paper prepared for the International Health Partnership+. Geneva: Joint Assessment of National Health Strategies (JANS); 2013 (http://www.internationalhealthpartnership.net/fileadmin/uploads/ihp/Documents/ Results___Evidence/JANS_Lessons/Lessons%20from%20JANS%20in%20Sudan%20July%202013%20-%20%20FINAL%20AUGUST%202013.pdf, accessed 7 July 2016).

2 Goss J. Projection of Australian health care expenditure by disease, 2003 to 2033. Canberra: Australian Institute of Health and Welfare; 200 8 (http://www.aihw.gov.au/publication-detail/?id=6442468187, accessed 8 July 2016).

3 Green A. An introduction to health planning for developing health systems, 3rd edition. Oxford: Oxford University Press; 2007, 18–20.

4 Tsofa B, Molyneux S, Goodman C. Health sector operational planning and budgeting processes in Kenya: "never the twain shall meet". Int J Health Plann Manage. 2015. doi:10.1002/hpm.2286.

5 Stierman E, Ssengooba F, Bennett S. Aid alignment: a longer term lens on trends in development assistance for health in Uganda. Global Health. 2013; 9(1):7 (http://www.ncbi.nlm.nih.gov/pmc/articles/PMC3599223/, accessed 8 July 2016).

6 Özaltın A, Cashin C, editors. Costing of health services for provider payment: a practical manual based on country costing challenges, trade-offs, and solutions. Washington (DC): Results for Development Institute, Joint Learning Network for Universal Health Coverage; 2014.

7 International Health Partnership (IHP+). Joint assessment of national health strategies and plans: combined joint assessment tool and guidelines. Version 3, August 2013 (http://www.internationalhealthpartnership.net/fileadmin/uploads/ihp/Documents/Tools/JANS/JANS_updated_guidelines_August_2013.pdf, accessed 9 July 2016).

8 Inter-agency Task Force on Financing for Development. Addis Ababa Action Agenda: monitoring commitments and actions. Inaugural report: 2016. New York: United Nations; 2016 (http://www.un.org/esa/ffd/publications/inaugural-2016-iatf-report.html, accessed 09 July 2016).

9 Ethiopia Federal Ministry of Health. Health sector strategic plan (HSDP-III) 2005/6-2009/10. Addis Ababa: 2005 (http://www.etharc.org/index.php/resources/download/finish/33/81, accessed 17 July 2016); Omaswa F, Boufford JI. Strong ministries of health for strong health systems: an overview of the study report: supporting ministerial health leadership: a strategy for health systems strengthening. African Centre for Global Health and Social Transformation (ACHEST)/The New York Academy of Medicine; 2010 (http://unpan1.un.org/intradoc/groups/public/documents/unpan/unpan038593.pdf, accessed 8 July 2016).

10 Adapted from Figure 1 of: Monitoring, evaluation and review of national health strategies: a country-led platform for information and accountability. Geneva: World Health Organization/International Health Partnership; 2011 (http://www.who.int/healthinfo/country_monitoring_evaluation/1085_IER_131011_web.pdf, accessed 17 July 2016).

11 Overy N. In the face of crisis: the Treatment Action Campaign fights government inertia with budget advocacy and litigation. International Budget Partnership: 2011 (From Analysis to Impact, Study No. 7; http://internationalbudget.org/wp-content/uploads/LP-case-study-TAC.pdf, accessed 11 July 2016).

12 Mauskopf JA, Sullivan SD, Annemans L, Caro J, Mullins CD, Nuijten M et al. Principles of good practice for budget impact analysis: report of the ISPOR Task Force on Good Research Practices — Budget Impact Analysis. Value in Health. 2007:10(5);336–47 (http://www.ispor.org/workpaper/research_practices/Principles_of_Good_Research_Practices-Budges_Impact_Analysis.pdf, accessed 8 July 2016).

13 Thue N, Makubuya AN, Nakireunda M. Report of a study on the civil society in Uganda: for the Royal Norwegian Embassy in Uganda. July 2002. Norwegian Agency for Development Cooperation (NORAD) (https://www.norad.no/en/toolspublications/publications/2009/report-of-a-study-on-the-civil-society-in-uganda-for-the-royal-norwegian-embassy-in-uganda/, accessed 12 July 2016).

14 Kruse SE. CSO and SWAps in Uganda: the role of civil society organisations in Uganda's health sector programme. June 2003 (NORAD Report 5/2004; https://www.norad.no/globalassets/import-2162015-80434-am/www.norad.no-ny/filarkiv/vedlegg-til-publikasjoner/052004.pdf, accessed 12 July 2016).

15 Muhangi D. Study of civil society organizations in Uganda: phase II report. September 2004. Uganda Program for Human and Holistic Development (UPHOLD); 2004 (http://uphold.jsi.com/Docs/Resources/Research/CivilSociety/civil_society_organisation_mapping_study_phase2.pdf, accessed 12 July 2016).

16 A listing of the Sustainable Development Goals can be found on the website of the Unite d Nations Department of Economic and Social Affairshttps://sustainabledevelopment.un.org/topics/sustainabledevelopmentgoals, accessed 18 July 2016.

17 Republique Democratique du Congo. Plan National de Developpement Sanitaire PNDS 2011–2015. Kinshasa: Ministère de la Santé Publique; 2010 (http://www.who.int/pmnch/media/events/2014/drc_pnds.pdf?ua=1, accessed 14 July 2016).

18 Soucat A. Health systems for the Millennium Development Goals: country needs and funding gaps. Un-edited conference version 29–30 October 2009 (http://www.foresightfordevelopment.org/sobipro/55/359-health-systems-for-the-millennium-development-goals-country-needs-and-funding-gaps, accessed 19 July 2016).

19 Soucat A, Netsanet Walelign N. Reaching the MDGs evidence on high impact interventions. Kigali; June 23–27, 2015 (https://www.youtube.com/watch?v=SX-jLovHbXFE, accessed 31 July 2016).

20 Guidelines on costing. In: Policies, directives, standards and guidelines [website]. Ottawa: Government of Canada; 2016 (https://www.tbs-sct.gc.ca/pol/doc-eng.aspx?id=30375, accessed 10 July 2016).

21 Dutta A, Perales N, Silva R, Crivillé C. Estimated resource needs and impact of Mozambique's Plano Estratégico do Sector Saúde, 2014–2019: results from the OneHealth model. Washington (DC): Futures Group, Health Policy Project; 2014 (http://www.healthpolicyproject.com/pubs/242_MozambiqueRelat%C3%B3riodeCustosparaPESSEglish.pdf, accessed 18 July 2016).

22 Nsofor E. Mission report on the costing of the multi-year Sierra Leone Health Sector Recovery Plan 2015–2020: February 16–March 27, 2015. Freetown: Human Support Services; 2015.

23 Adam T, Ebener S, Johns B, Evans DB. Capacity utilization and the costs of primary care visits: implications for the costs of scaling up cost interventions. Cost Eff Resour Alloc. 2008;6:22 (http://resource-allocation.biomedcentral.com/articles/10.1186/1478-7547-6-22, accessed 7 July 2016).

24 Haazen DS, Hayer AS. Financing capital costs and reducing the fixed costs of health systems. In: Kutzin J, Chasin C, Jakab M, editors. Implementing health financing reform: lessons from countries in transition. Copenhagen: WHO Regional Office for Europe; 2010 (Observatory Studies Series, 21; http://www.euro.who.int/__data/assets/pdf_file/0014/120164/E94240.pdf, accessed 8 July 2016).

25 Atun R, Richardson E, Shishkin S, Kacevicius G, Ciocanu M, Sava V, et al. Moldova: health system review. Health Systems in Transition. 2008;10(5):1–138 (http://www.euro.who.int/__data/assets/pdf_file/0004/95161/E91756.pdf, accessed 9 July 2016).

26 Creese A, Parker D, editors. Cost analysis in primary health care: a training manual for programme managers. Geneva: World Health Organization; 1994.

27 For more information on the OneHealth Tool see: Cost effectiveness and strategic planning (WHO-CHOICE) (http://who.int/choice/onehealthtool/en/, accessed 18 July 2016); OneHealth Tool (http://www.internationalhealthpartnership.net/en/tools/one-health-tool, accessed 19 July 2016); PC Applications: OneHealth Tool (http://www.avenirhealth.org/software-onehealth.php, accessed 19 July 2016).

28 República de Angola. Plano Nacional de Desenvolvimento Sanitário 2012–2025 (PNDS). Luanda: Ministério da Saúde (website).

29 Stierman E, Ssengooba F, Bennett S. Aid alignment: a longer term lens on trends in development assistance for health in Uganda. Global Health. 2013; 9(1):7 (http://www.ncbi.nlm.nih.gov/pmc/articles/ PMC3599223/, accessed 8 July 2016).

30 Ibid.

31 Witter S. Health financing in fragile and post-conflict states: what do we know and what are the gaps? Soc Sci Med. 2012:75(12);2370–7. doi: 10.1016/j.socscimed.2012.09.012.

Further reading

Creese A, Parker D, editors. Cost analysis in primary health care: a training manual for programme managers. Geneva: World Health Organization; 1994.

Green A. An Introduction to health planning for developing health systems, 3rd edition. Oxford: Oxford University Press; 2007.

Guidelines on costing. In: Policies, directives, standards and guidelines [website]. Ottawa: Government of Canada; 2016 (https://www.tbs-sct.gc.ca/pol/doc-eng.aspx?id=30375, accessed 10 July 2016).

The OneHealth Tool [website]. Washington (DC): Avenir Health; 2016. (http://www.avenirhealth.org/software-onehealth.php, accessed 10 July 2016).

The world health report. Health systems financing: the path to universal coverage. Geneva: World Health Organization; 2010 (http://apps.who.int/iris/bitstream/10665/44371/1/9789241564021_eng.pdf, accessed 10 July 2016).

Annex 7.1

Examples of purposes of estimating and analysing costs, at different levels of the health system

LEVEL OF ANALYSIS	EXAMPLES OF TYPE OF ANALYSIS AT THIS LEVEL	COMMON OBJECTIVES
individual health centre/hospital	Estimate the cost per patient for different diagnoses.	▶ Assessing efficiency ▶ Set user fees ▶ Develop cross-subsidization strategy ▶ Facility resource planning
Specific health service project/ delivery strategy	Estimate costs related to delivering community based nutrition interventions.	▶ Economic evaluation (cost-effectiveness) ▶ Assess financial sustainability of new/existing programme/project
Provider payment scheme	Setting new reimbursement rates for health providers	▶ Health financing strategy ▶ Inform payment mechanisms
National programme	Costing a maternal and newborn health roadmap	▶ Advocate for greater resource allocation to programme-specific goals. ▶ Analyse the effect of changing program goals, inputs or delivery strategies upon the overall estimated resources required. ▶ Estimate costs for proposal development (Global health initiatives, other donors).
Intervention-specific implementation cost	▶ Budget impact analysis	▶ Calculate and compare scenarios for modifying clinical practice, including both costs and savings from the provider perspective
	▶ Cost-effectiveness	▶ As part of priority-setting and decision-making processes, examine cost effectiveness as explicit criteria
District-level plan	Estimate budget for all planned health activities in the district.	▶ Inform the district annual operational budget.
NHPSP	Estimate costs related to planned health activities in the country.	▶ Inform priorities within the national strategic health plan and related budget. ▶ Advocate for greater/different resource allocation / mobilize resources.

Annex 7.2

Sample content to be included in a report for costing an NHPSP

Acronyms

Acknowledgments

Executive summary

Background

Background/context of analysis, including health financing context (macroeconomic parameters)

Study objectives

Methods

Process for decision on methodology used for costing

Description of methodology/tools used

Data sources

Where relevant, top-down ceilings or allocation mechanisms vs bottom-up costing

Assumptions

Assumptions around:

- how to model certain policy reforms;
- changes in utilization patterns;
- multisectoral approaches;
- private vs public sector involvement;
- a description of the parameters used to predict availability of financial resources.

Results (where possible, present multiple scenarios)

Standard results for costs:

(Note: all results should clearly state whether inflation is included or not)

- total costs, and per capita costs;
- recurrent vs capital costs;
- breakdown of costs between different categories (e.g. drugs, salaries, programme activities);
- breakdown by disease/programme;
- identification of cost drivers and discussion around cost how these may change due to policy reforms;
- comparison of estimated costs with estimated resources available;
- a comparison of estimated costs with current health expenditure per capita.

Additional results, when possible

- Estimated health impact
  e.g. number of maternal deaths prevented, number of child deaths prevented, if the plan is implemented as intended.
- Progress towards national health goals, including the SDGs

Discussion

- Gaps in the comprehensiveness of the costing
- Data limitations
- Uncertainty

Overall notes

- Use pie charts, graphs and summary tables in the main report
- Include more detailed tables as annexes if appropriate

Chapter 8

Budgeting for health

Dheepa Rajan
Helene Barroy
Karin Stenberg

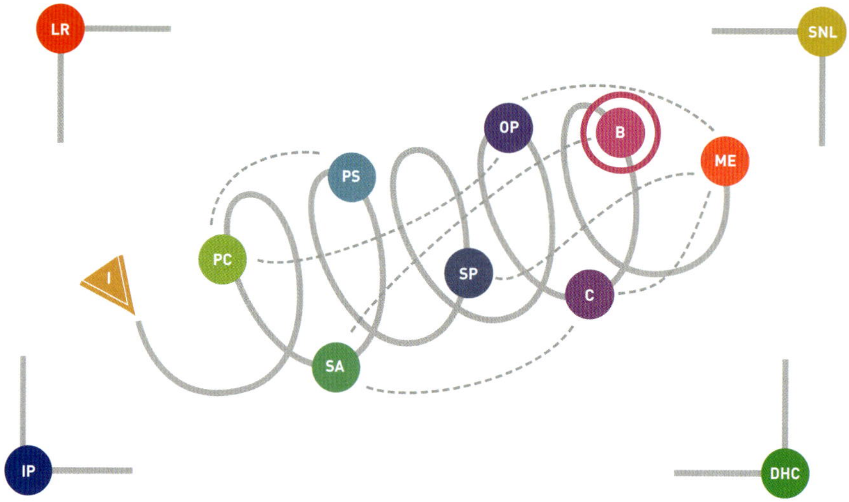

Cross-cutting topics relevant to national health planning

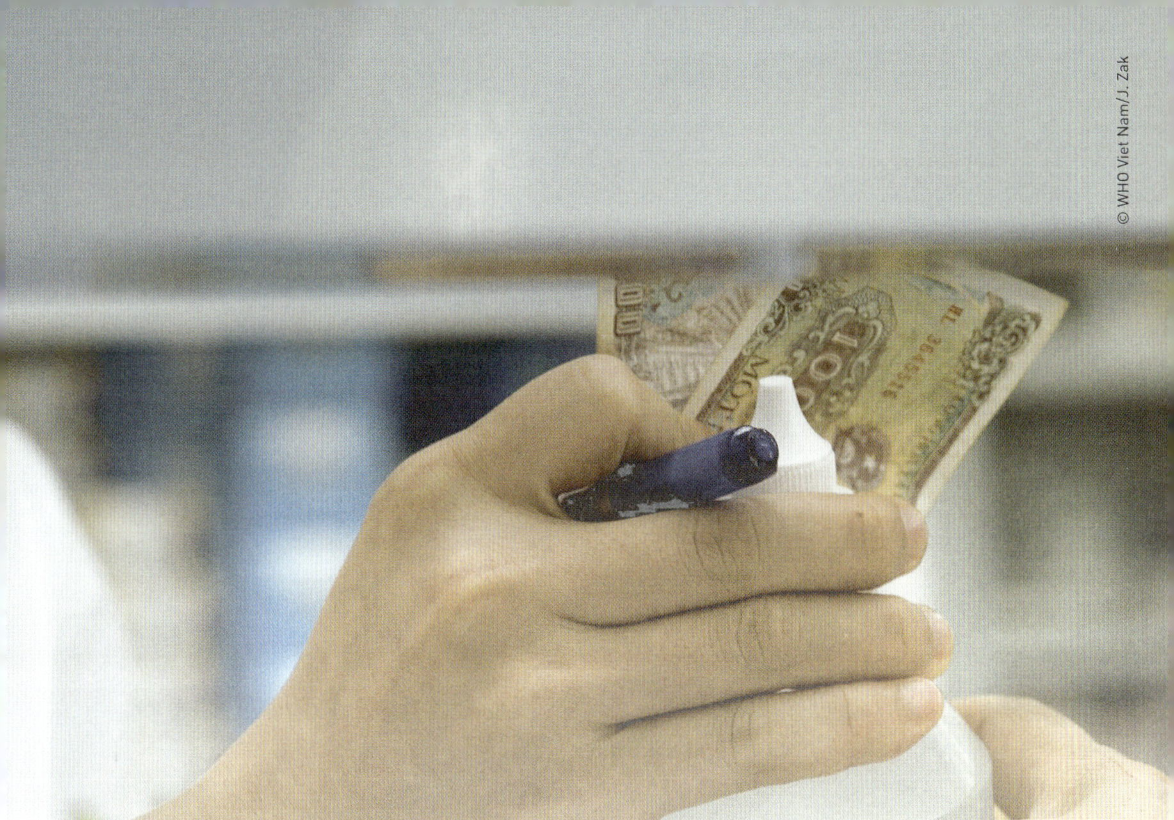

© WHO Viet Nam/J. Zak

Overview

Engaging in budget preparation, understanding guiding principles of budgeting as well as the political dynamics that enable the budget elaboration and approval process, is essential for health planners and managers. In many countries, the consequences of not doing so means that health policy-making, planning, costing and budgeting take place independently of each other, leading to a misalignment between health priorities and allocation and use of resources.

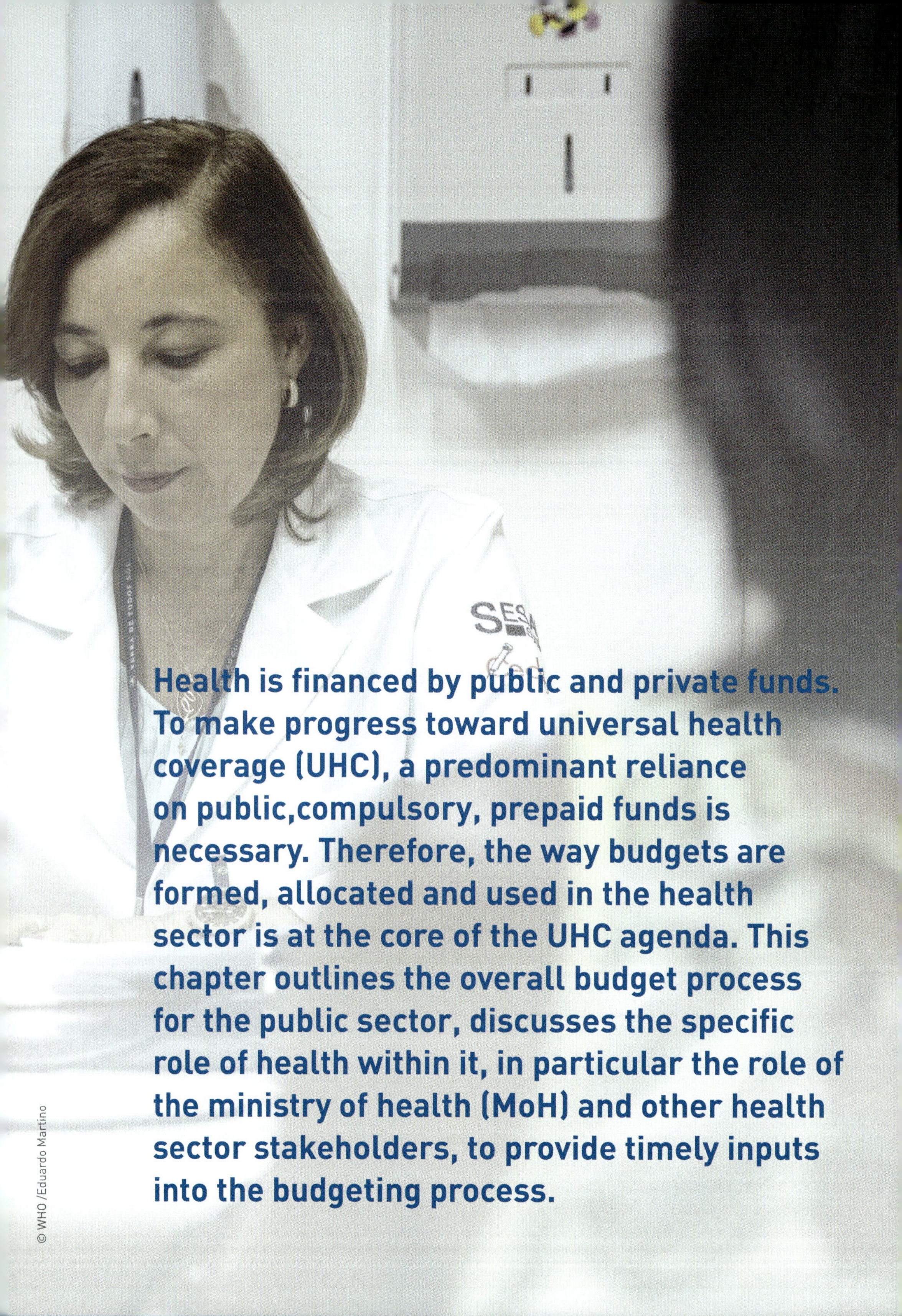

Health is financed by public and private funds. To make progress toward universal health coverage (UHC), a predominant reliance on public,compulsory, prepaid funds is necessary. Therefore, the way budgets are formed, allocated and used in the health sector is at the core of the UHC agenda. This chapter outlines the overall budget process for the public sector, discusses the specific role of health within it, in particular the role of the ministry of health (MoH) and other health sector stakeholders, to provide timely inputs into the budgeting process.

Summary

What is meant by budgeting for health?

Budgeting is related to the process of defining the allocation of resources to produce the best outputs given the level of revenues. A health budget, typically included in the general government budget, is more than a simple accounting instrument to present revenues and expenses – rather, it is a crucial orienting text, declaring key financial objectives of the country and its real commitment to implementing its health policies and strategies. While every implementing health organization develops a budget, in this chapter we discuss the national government budgeting process, which includes inputs from a wide range of health sector stakeholders.

Why is it important to understand the health budgeting process?

For those who seek to influence resource allocation in country, a good understanding of the guiding principles of budgeting as well as the political dynamics that enable the budget elaboration and approval process is essential. In many countries, a lack of understanding of budgeting issues results in delinked processes such that health policy-making, planning, costing and budgeting take place independently of each other. This leads to a misalignment between the health sector priorities outlined in overall strategic plans and policies and the funds that are ultimately allocated to the health sector through the budgeting process. This misalignment has negative consequences: resources are not used as intended, and accountability is weakened. On the other hand, a good understanding of the budget process and engagement by MoH and other health sector stakeholders at the right time during the budget cycle will increase the chances that the final resource allocation matches planned health sector needs.

When does the budgeting process take place?

The budgeting process starts with a preparation/formulation stage of budget proposals, which includes a negotiation phase between MoH and ministry of finance (MoF) and ends up with parliamentary review and approval. In many countries the fiscal year follows the 12-month calendar year, beginning on 1 January; in some countries, the fiscal year may start at a different date (e.g. 1 October in the United States of America, 1 July in Australia and New Zealand). In a given year, there are three cycles potentially taking place at the same time: the implementation of the current budget, which essentially takes place throughout the year, at any given time; budget preparation for the next year; and audit or review of the previous year.

Who are the people involved and engaged in the health budgeting process, in particular the budget preparation phase?

Ministries of budget/finance and related entities are the leading agents for budget development. Ministries of health play a critical role to prepare, present and negotiate credible, priority-oriented budget proposals for the sector. Civil society and the general public can seek to influence health budget definition by engaging with the executive or the legislature.

How does the budgeting process work from the point of view of national health policy/strategy/plan (NHPSP) stakeholders?

The budget cycle starts with the government planning for the use of the coming year's resources. To allow this to be done in accordance with health priorities, health planning stakeholders have to engage strategically in this process and be prepared to support it. This chapter takes the reader through the steps of the budget cycle and some practical issues for the health community to consider.

Anything else to consider?

- decentralized environment;
- fragile environment;
- highly aid-dependent context.

8.1 What is meant by budgeting for health? Some key concepts

8.1.1 What is a budget?

Narrowly defined, the budget is the government's forecast of revenue and planned expenditure, usually provided on an annual basis. A health budget is the portion of the national budget allocated to the health sector, including all ministries and agencies involved in health-related activities. A health budget is more than a simple accounting instrument to present revenues and expenses – rather, it is a crucial orienting text, declaring the country's key financial objectives and its real commitment to implementing its health policies and strategies.

8.1.2 Public financial management

Public financial management (PFM) rules govern how budgets are formulated, funds disbursed and accounted for. This is centrally important to UHC because PFM is the interface that helps ensure that increases in public spending translate into expanded health coverage.

National health authorities should aim to effectively engage with national budgetary authorities to foster credible, priority-oriented health budgets, and ensure efficient fund flows and budget execution in order to ultimately strengthen accountability.

8.1.3 Medium-term expenditure framework (MTEF)

An MTEF is a comprehensive, government-wide spending plan that is expected to link policy priorities to expenditure allocations within a fiscal framework (linked to macroeconomic and revenue forecasts), usually over a three-year forward-planning horizon. Mid-term budgeting can help connect revenue forecasts, sectoral allocations and health policy priorities, and strengthen the overall quality and credibility of annual budget envelopes.

A health budget allocates national funds to the health sector, declares key financial objectives of the country, and represents a commitment to health policy and strategy implementation.

In order to do that well, governments need to be able to generate robust forecasts of forward macroeconomic conditions and revenue flows, as well as of the forward cost of existing and new policies. While the former is usually the responsibility of the central government,[I] the latter can only be done well using the specialized knowledge at sector level. Some countries have also initiated the development of sector/health-specific MTEF (see Fig. 8.1) that fit into the overall framework, which can help define more credible annual allocations.

I This is exercised through the introduction of good macroeconomic models and mechanisms to consult on forecasts with stakeholders such as the central bank, the revenue authority and independent research agencies.

Fig. 8.1 Key stages of a comprehensive MTEF[1]

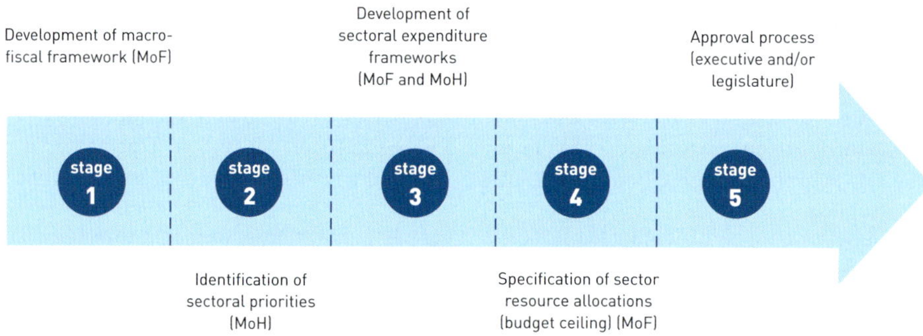

8.1.4 Line-item budgeting for health

Line-item budgeting is a way to manage budget information according to the types of expenses or cost categories. While this approach aims to increase transparency and accountability, it may often in fact restrict flexibility and lead to inefficient resource allocation.

Line-item budgeting has been the norm in many countries, in which the budget information is organized according to the types of expenses or cost categories. For health, these generally focus on staff, supplies (operational costs), and capital investment/equipment, all of which can be characterized as inputs for health systems. Providers receive a fixed amount for a specified period to cover specific input expenses (e.g. personnel, medicines, utilities).

The existence of many line items is a way for the legislature to retain control, but provides little flexibility to operationalize and manage health funds because the expenditure must follow strictly defined budget lines. In many countries, line-item budgeting has been a major deterrent to a functioning health purchasing system, which would require setting up appropriate payment mechanisms to enable funds flow to the right services and maximize efficient use of public funds.

8.1.5 Performance budgeting

"Performance budgeting", "performance-based budgeting", "programme-based budgeting" and "budgeting for results" are similar terms, with a common unifying feature: they are all concerned with introducing performance information into budget processes. The Organisation for Economic Co-operation and Development (OECD) has defined performance budgeting as a form of budgeting that links allocated funds to measurable results.[2] These alternative budget classifications present advantages for managing funds through increased autonomy for funds managers. Specifically for the health sector, it ensures that funds flow to the priority services and enables the purchasing of health services to be operational. By making explicit the purposes and results of budget spending, budget managers can also be held to account by the legislature and citizens.

8.1.6 Fiscal space and fiscal space for health

Fiscal space is typically defined as "the availability of budgetary room that allows a government to provide resources for a given desired purpose without any prejudice to the sustainability of a government's financial position".[3] Tandon and Cashin's conceptual framework to assess fiscal space for health in countries include factors such as macroeconomic conditions, the extent to which health is re-prioritized within the government budget, whether new earmarked funds for health have been introduced, the amount of external aid and increased efficiency of existing government health outlays.[4]

Health planning stakeholders have variable influence over these five factors. Some are directly outside of their control, such as the macroeconomic conditions. Others are in the direct domain of the health sector and therefore require particular attention from health planning stakeholders – namely the efficiency of current health expenditures and the amount of external aid for health. Furthermore, there are those factors which are not directly in the hands of health planning stakeholders but for which the health sector can play an important role in terms of advocacy – namely the prioritization of health within the overall government budget, and whether there are efforts to introduce new earmarked funds specifically for health.

Fiscal space for health analysis could be better mainstreamed and systematized into the budgeting process in many countries to enhance budgeting decisions. Health planning stakeholders would do well by leveraging the fiscal space analysis to take a closer look at the political and institutional enabling factors which can actually support improved formulation, allocation and use of health budgeted resources.[5] A better use of existing public resources toward UHC helps expand the fiscal room for the sector.

Line-item budgeting is a way to manage budget information according to the types of expenses or cost categories; however, this budgeting system does not provide the required flexibility to operationalize health plans and maintain a well-run health purchasing system.

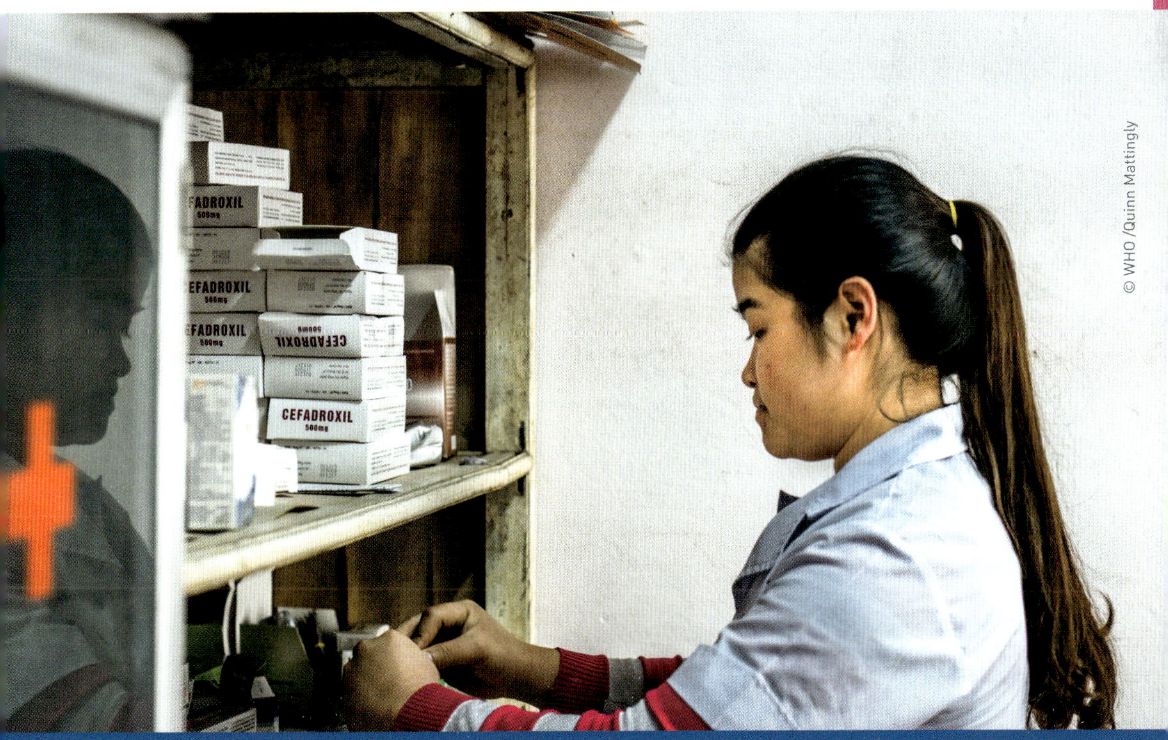

© WHO /Quinn Mattingly

8.1.7 Strategic purchasing

Purchasing involves three sets of decisions: identifying services to be purchased, choosing service providers based on certain criteria, and determining the modalities of payments to providers.

As one of the generic sub-functions of health financing,[II] purchasing refers to the allocation of resources to health service providers. Purchasing involves three sets of decisions, namely:

1. **identifying the interventions** or services to be purchased, taking into account population needs, national health priorities and cost-effectiveness;

2. **choosing service providers** based on criteria such as service quality, efficiency and equity;

3. **determining how services** will be purchased, including contractual arrangements and provider payment mechanisms.[6]

Purchasing is undertaken by a purchasing organization which can be, for example, an insurance scheme, a MoH, or an autonomous agency. Purchasing should not be confused with procurement, which generally only refers to buying medicines and other medical supplies.

There is a growing consensus, backed by efforts being made by countries, to move away from a passive approach to purchasing (no selection of providers, no performance monitoring, no effort to influence prices, quantity, or quality of care) to an active or strategic one.

Strategic purchasing with general budget revenues involves linking the transfer of funds to providers, and, at least in part, to information on aspects of their performance and the health needs of the population they serve.

II Health financing functions include: revenue raising, resource pooling and strategic purchasing.

8.2 Why is it important to understand the health budgeting process?

During the budgeting process, health planning stakeholders and managers will inevitably be requested by MoF to provide information on sectoral priorities and an associated price tag. Understanding the guiding principles of budgeting as well as the political dynamics that enable the budget elaboration and approval processes is essential to make the case for health. In many countries, a lack of understanding of these budget-related issues results in delinked processes such that health policy-making, planning, costing and budgeting take place independently of each other. This leads to a misalignment between the health sector priorities outlined in overall strategic plans and policies and the funds that are ultimately allocated to the health sector through the budgeting process. This misalignment has negative consequences: resources are not used as intended, and accountability is weakened (see Box 8.1). On the other hand, a good understanding of the budget process and solid engagement by MoH and other health sector stakeholders at the right time during the budget cycle will increase the chances that the final resource allocation matches planned health sector needs.

In reality, the allocation of resources to different institutions and purposes is essentially a political, rather than a purely technocratic process.[III] After having analysed needs and determined the most equitable and efficient policies and plans, health planning stakeholders must proactively engage in this politically-influenced process, as it determines the details of the national health budget, which impacts on effectiveness and efficiency of public spending for health. How health managers will be able to spend their money largely depends on what the budget allocation is. Not only is the budget envelope amount relevant, but so too is how that total amount is structured, how it flows into the system, timing of disbursements and how it will enable health financing to function in practice and to purchase the needed health services.

Understanding the guiding principles of the health budgeting process minimizes the chance of misalignment between health sector priorities outlined in strategic plans and the funds that are allocated to the health sector.

Understanding and influencing the budget formulation for the health sector is also a matter of efficiency and equity, two key health policy objectives linked to UHC, a principle increasingly enshrined in many countries' NHPSPs. How a budget is formulated and allocated, including to lower levels of government, has a direct impact on how well and how efficiently funds can and will be used. Supporting a fair distribution of resources across populations and/or geographical areas is likely to have a direct impact on health sector outputs.[7]

III For more information, please see Chapter 4 "Priority-setting for national health policies, strategies and plans" in this handbook.

Box 8.1

Côte d'Ivoire: understanding the root causes for misalignment between health planning and budgeting[8]

Several factors can explain the misalignment between health planning and budgeting at both central and decentralized levels in the Ivorian context.

At central level, first, there is a noticeable lack of a general framework and aligned calendar between health planning and budgeting. There is no specific mechanism to align the budget formulation and national health planning processes. Operational plans are often developed for the ongoing year, while the budget is formulated for the next year. In addition, there is no alignment on the objectives and goals between the two documents. The budget elaboration is solely driven by the logic of facility-based funding through inputs, while the existing strategy sets a different approach through well-identified programmes and expected results. Also, when the programme-based budgeting process was introduced, it was used more as a means to reflect externally financed programmes than to fit with nationally defined priorities as set out in the NHPSP. Finally, weaknesses also resulted from the fact that the processes were relatively top- down, without considering local sector needs in a post-war context.

8.3 When does the budgeting process take place?

8.3.1 Budget cycle steps – a brief overview

The various public finance processes are structured around the budget cycle. This annual cycle aims to ensure that public expenditure is well planned, executed and accounted for. A standard budget cycle incorporates four distinct stages:

(a) budget definition and formulation;

(b) budget negotiation and approval;

(c) budget execution;

(d) budget reporting, auditing and evaluation.

The MoH is expected to translate government policy goals (as described in the NHPSP) into cost[IV] estimates to fit into the suggested budget ceiling for the sector. The budget ceiling is given by the MoF based on its revenue forecast outlining the country's macroeconomic prospects in the medium term.

The MoF and MoH engage in negotiations over these requests which culminate in the formulation of a formal health budget proposal that is supposed to typically reflect revenue and expenditure plans for the budget period (most often one year). The budget proposal (which includes the health budget component) is typically presented for budget approval to parliament, which can propose amendments, before formal adoption.

Budget execution, or spending, consists of a set of processes that lead to effective fund flows/transfers from the treasury to the MoH, and onwards to sub-recipients (for example, districts, health providers, etc). The principal issues that the MoH will be faced with during the budget execution phase are the actual delivery/purchase of health services by those on the front line (e.g. health service providers) and the financial management function that supports the former.

A standard budget cycle incorporates four distinct stages: budget definition and formulation; budget negotiation and approval; budget execution; and budget reporting, auditing and evaluation.

Budget evaluation refers to internal and external control processes which are designed to ensure compliance with predefined targets and procedures. Governments also have accounting and reporting procedures which help keep records of financial and/or non-financial flows;[9] these need to be respected and cross-checked.

An important point to note here is the issue of budget amendments that can be passed by parliament during the course of the fiscal year. This can happen when, for example, budgetary resources are lower than expected and overall spending needs to be reduced. Negotiations will determine whether the health-specific budget will be maintained or changed. It is often at this stage of budget renegotiation that the prime minister or president may play a key role in arbitrating between different priorities and sectors. Health leaders need to maintain a sufficient level of advocacy to ensure that the sector remains a budget priority throughout the year.

IV See Chapter 7 "Estimating cost implications of a national health policy, strategy or plan" in this handbook.

8.3.2 Fiscal vs. calendar year

Not all countries use the calendar year to determine a fiscal year; either way, the budget steps remain the same.

Some countries' budget cycles, referred to as fiscal years, follow the calendar year and others do not. A fiscal year refers to a consecutive 12-month period which may or may not follow the January to December calendar. That being said, the most common fiscal year countries use is the calendar year. Other commonly used fiscal years are 1 July of one year to 30 June of the following calendar year and 1 April of one year to 31 March of the following calendar year.[10] Fig. 8.2 depicts the budget cycle steps according to a fiscal year which is identical to the calendar year.

Fig. 8.2 Budget steps during a fiscal year starting on 1 January

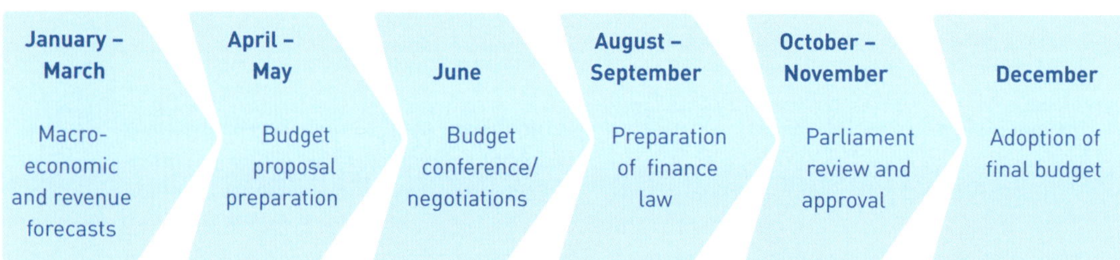

January – March
Macro-economic and revenue forecasts
April – May
Budget proposal preparation
June
Budget conference/ negotiations
August – September
Preparation of finance law
October – November
Parliament review and approval
December
Adoption of final budget

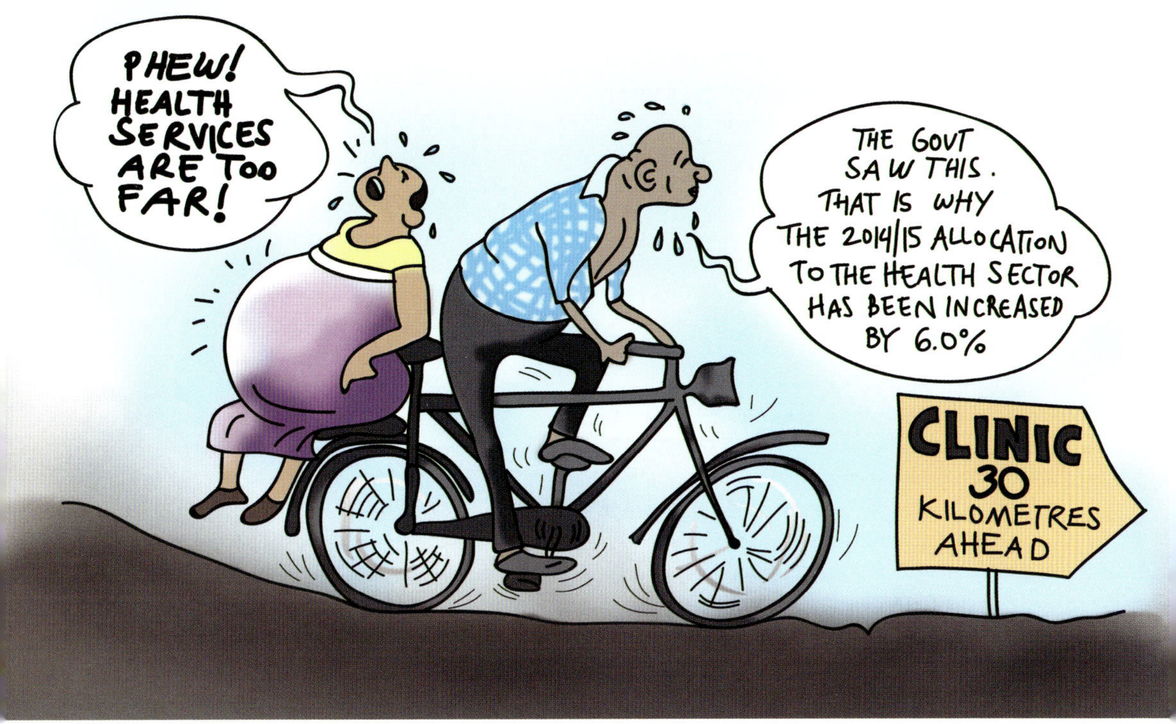
PHEW! HEALTH SERVICES ARE TOO FAR!
THE GOVT SAW THIS. THAT IS WHY THE 2014/15 ALLOCATION TO THE HEALTH SECTOR HAS BEEN INCREASED BY 6.0%
CLINIC 30 KILOMETRES AHEAD

Fig. 8.3 How important is budget prioritization for health?[11]

8.4 Who are the people involved and engaged in the health budgeting process? Roles of different stakeholders

8.4.1 MoH: engaging in health budget formulation and execution

(a) MoH's role in health budget formulation

Developing robust health budget envelopes requires strong engagement by health ministries with national budget decision-makers – first, because progress toward UHC is often associated with increased public funding for health, and secondly, because the latter also demands a functioning public finance system to align revenues with services and to manage expenditure better. Thus, the dialogue with MoF/treasury must involve not just the level of funding but also the PFM rules that govern their use (forming budgets, distributing them, expenditure management, reporting).

In particular, the MoH's role in the process of budget formulation boils down to three key inputs.

(i) Analysis of expenditure forecasts against expected revenues; the aim here is to estimate the potential for increased health spending. Institutionalizing fiscal space for health analysis within MoH will be an important step in this direction;
(ii) Drafting of credible, well-defined health budget proposals; systematizing costing and priority-setting exercises within the defined envelope;
(iii) Engaging in budget negotiations and advocating for a sound health budget allocation.

The Ministry of Health (MoH) must engage strongly with national budget decision-makers during health budget formulation. Credible, well-defined expenditure forecasts and systematized costing and priority-setting exercises can put MoH in a sound negotiating position with the Ministry of Finance.

(b) MoH's role in health budget execution

The budget execution stage is a pivotal process for all ministries including health, as it is the one which enables the actual implementation of NHPSP activities. MoH's key role here is one of supervision, support, and oversight of budget execution as this is often the deciding factor for implementation rates – poor technical and administrative support and oversight capacity generally results in a low health budget execution rate, and in more unused fiscal margins. Evidence shows that fiscal space expansion for the health sector is largely possible simply by increasing effectiveness in government health spending.[12]

For purposes of health budget execution, MoH's role includes understanding PFM systems, and in particular, expenditure rules and regulations. In many countries, MoH's capacities require strengthening in this area, as expenditure management is often not well known or understood by those who do not have specialist skills in public finance. For example, in many countries, the MoH is not the final decision-making authority on spending (MoF is). This means that payment requests for services already rendered end up with the MoF (see Box 8.2). If the expenditure is not in line with expenditure rules, MoF may decide not to pay, especially in a circumstance where funds are not sufficient to cover all payment requests coming in from all sectors. Another challenge linked to a lack of understanding of the PFM system is the funds disbursement schedule. In many countries, it does not necessarily follow the needs of sector plans; instead, funds may be disbursed only at specific times of the year in specific amounts. Health ministries should take this into consideration when planning activities and health budgets for more effective implementation.[13]

Early engagement on the part of MoH with the MoF can provide better understanding of the financial management rules and the system within which expenditures must happen. Closer cooperation and inclusion of MoF representatives in key MoH consultations can help both sides better understand each others' needs and challenges.

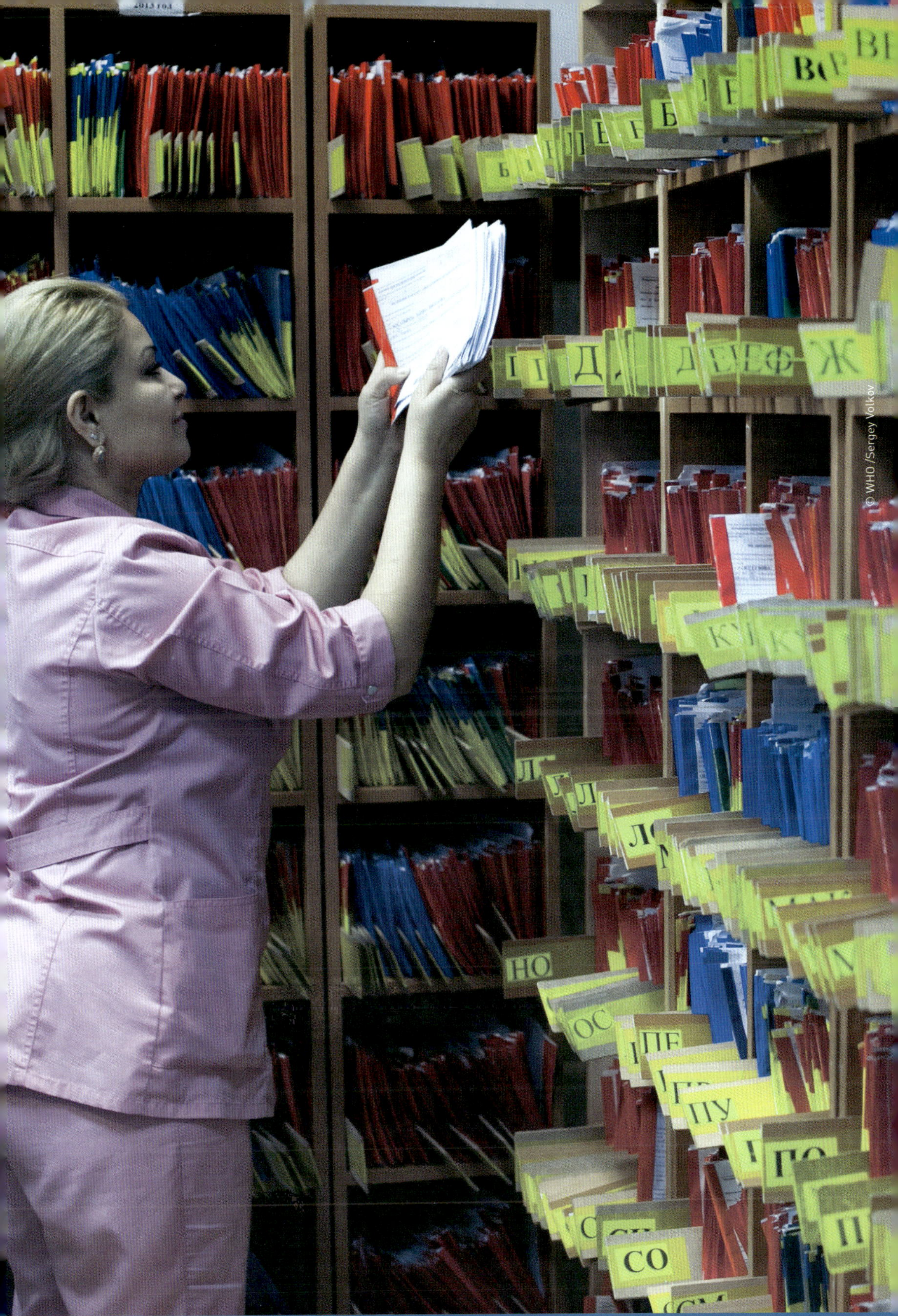
Ж
НО
ОС
ПУ
СО

Box 8.2

Low execution levels of the health budget: where does the problem lie?[14]

In many countries, health budgets are poorly executed, but little is known about the underlying causes of under-execution. A detailed analysis of the Democratic Republic of the Congo context reveals that the responsibilities lie on many fronts; many weaknesses and delays at both MoH and MoF explain low execution of the health budget envelope, with one major systemic bottleneck being the fact that the MoF still holds the final spending decision-making authority above all line ministries.

A closer look at the budget execution process in the Democratic Republic of the Congo in recent years demonstrated that the principal impediments were:

(i) MoH's estimation of necessary resources for health was finalized too late; the calculations have been of varying quality over the years;
(ii) MoF releases funds directly to those who are expecting payment from MoH (final spending decision-making authority is with MoF) and often does not do so in a timely manner.

Over 2011–2013, MoH's forecasted necessary resources on equipment, services, and other discretionary expenditure respectively came to 14%, 21%, and 59% of the funds finally requested from the Treasury, evincing an unambiguous disconnect between the estimation of resource needs and actual resources used. It was, however, noted that the MoH's estimation of necessary resources were more in line with funds spent for personnel expenditure (94%).

On the MoF side, monies paid out directly to suppliers/service providers on behalf of MoH came to only 55% for goods and equipment and 40% for construction. This implies that roughly half of MoH's suppliers received late payments. In addition, when the budget cycle closed at year end, these late payments remained as arrears in MoH's name and needed to be transferred to the following year's budget.

All in all, the bottlenecks are clearly systemic in nature and imply weaknesses on various fronts and a need for a more comprehensive, long-term reform in government processes and government capacity.

A core element of effective health budget execution and expenditure management is strategic purchasing,[15] referring to the arrangements in place, and mechanisms used, to allocate funds to health service providers. MoH is the entity that must think through and design how health services should be purchased, in harmonization with existing PFM rules. This MoH task of improving the strategic purchasing of health services is central to strengthening health system performance and progressing towards UHC, as it determines the way services are funded and providers incentivized (see Table 8.1).

Table 8.1 What can health planners do/help to foster PFM and health financing system alignment?

PUBLIC FINANCE CYCLE	TYPE OF ACTIONS /SUPPORT NEEDED FROM HEALTH PLANNERS
Mid-term budget planning	Elaboration of robust health MTEF
	Systematized fiscal space for health assessment
	Investment case for health sector to support budget prioritization
Budget formulation and negotiation	Elaboration of sound annual sectoral envelopes
	Refined budget structure
	Costing for specific policy change (provider payment mechanisms, benefit package)
Execution process	Good understanding of PFM rules Harmonizing PFM rules and health purchasing arrangements
Reporting, auditing, evaluating	Unified reporting and auditing system, and financial management information system
	Institutionalized public expenditure for health assessments and national health accounts, with a particular focus on public expenditure

8.4.2 Role of civil society organizations (CSOs) in the health budgeting process

Other stakeholders such as CSOs and the general public can seek to influence the budget by engaging the executive or the legislature in various ways: analysing budget proposals from the angle of grassroots needs, advocating for more transparency in budget processes, and taking part in local budget-setting processes.[V]

Civil society engagement in the budget process should be welcomed and encouraged by government, parliament and other stakeholders.

The reality is that, in most cases, time for budget negotiations is short and budget sessions are not long enough to make the process as participatory and effective as it should be. Nevertheless, MoH can play its part in encouraging and ensuring more citizen and CSO involvement by producing or endorsing best-practice documents on citizen/CSO engagement in budgeting and collaborating with civil society to get nuanced citizen feedback (beneficiary assessment surveys, citizen scorecards, opinion polls, etc.) for planning, budgeting, and monitoring.[VI]

Civil society engagement in the budget process should thus not only be welcomed but also encouraged by government, parliament, and other stakeholders. Several countries report low legislative capacity to analyse budgets, and thus they are dependent on line ministries as well as civil society, academia, and other bodies to support their study of the budget. An example from Mexico demonstrates that civil society engagement with legislatures on budget analyses can be cardinal even if it is not easy, does not happen overnight, and is mostly characterized – at least in the initial stages – by building up relationships and credibility with government and parliament (Box 8.3).

Even in fragile settings, case studies from Asia and Africa demonstrate that systematized citizen assessments of budget proposals can indeed be conducted and can add great value to the budget formulation process. More importantly, they have the potential to strengthen overall governance and accountability practices between citizens and public authorities.[16]

A few countries have moved a step further by introducing a "participatory budget", in which citizens are involved in budget priority-setting processes at local levels. The example of the Democratic Republic of the Congo shows the interesting lessons learned (Box 8.4).

Once the budget is formally presented to the legislature, public hearings and debates may also create space for civil society to express itself on specific issues and/or the budget as a whole. Often legislative committees engage in discussions with civil society and other stakeholders before voting.

V Beyond the preparation phase, citizens and civil society platforms can also play an active role in the oversight phase. Good practices in country experience include: citizens' report cards and social accountability mechanisms.

VI In the Philippines, for example, the government obliges departments and agencies to consult and partner with CSOs when preparing agency budget proposals in the budget preparation stage.

Box 8.3

Civil society participation in health budgeting: the case of Mexico[17]

In Mexico, the NGO FUNDAR (Centre for Research and Analysis) monitors public policies in social sectors, especially health. One of the policies it has been monitoring for many years is the Seguro Popular (SP – People's Insurance) programme as it is one of the most important health policy programmes for those who would otherwise be uninsured. The SP is thus Mexico's solution to right-to-health legislation and is endowed with a generous budget. FUNDAR spent many years concentrating on research and analysis of the SP's policies, and learning how to package and present its analysis for legislators and other CSOs.

Health policy in Mexico is decentralized; the federal government transfers up to 85% of allocated health resources to the state authorities for SP services. In several states, decentralized budget information is unavailable and there is little transparency as to which agency or entity is actually implementing SP services. The consequences at health service delivery level are dire, with constant shortages of medicines, high out-of-pocket payments by households, and low investment in health infrastructure. In addition, the SP has proven to be a "golden egg" for many states, with its large budget, large flexibility in spending, and little oversight and control. Opposition politicians have criticized it bitterly, stating that it has not lived up to expectations.

Through its budget analysis work, FUNDAR first gained credibility and built trust with various legislators and state-level civil society actors. Over several years, FUNDAR began to make suggestions to modify Mexico's article on social protection spending to become more transparent – this involved meeting with the executive and the legislative branches, mainly the Health Committee and the Budget and Public Accounts Committee. The suggestions were not taken into consideration in the following budget decrees but after much perseverance, seven amendments, all influenced by FUNDAR, were incorporated into the 2012 Federal Budget Decree. These amendments touched at the heart of accountability and transparency issues and, at least in theory, seek to improve expenditure control and evaluation of the SP budget, and increase the legislature's capacity to supervise spending via the National Audit Office. The lesson to be learned here is that influencing national budgets is a long-term process and both civil society and parliamentarians, as well government, and ultimately the population, can greatly benefit.

Box 8.4

Participatory budget: lessons from pilot experiences in the Democratic Republic of the Congo[18]

Rural and urban citizens' recent participation in the formulation and management of local budgets has helped to strengthen governance in the Democratic Republic of the Congo. How does participatory budgeting work in practice? The local authority presents its budget to the public, specifying the share of the budget to be allocated to local investment. Through a process of dialogue, community members are able to choose for themselves which priorities should be addressed and funded under the local budget. The population is also involved in monitoring the implementation of the activities selected through this participatory process. Using mobile phones, which most Congolese now own, stakeholders in the Participatory Budgeting Project can easily obtain, from wherever they happen to be, useful information on the date, time, and place of meetings. They can also find out what was decided at meetings, vote by SMS (short message service) and, importantly, monitor and evaluate the decisions made through voting – all while going about their daily lives. This participatory approach has enabled the decentralized territorial entities involved in the pilot project to improve local governance through social accountability, effective participation of citizens in the management of public affairs and citizen monitoring of public investments.

8.5 How does the budgeting process work from the point of view of NHPSP stakeholders?

Fig. 8.4 Aligning budget and strategic priorities: a core challenge [19]

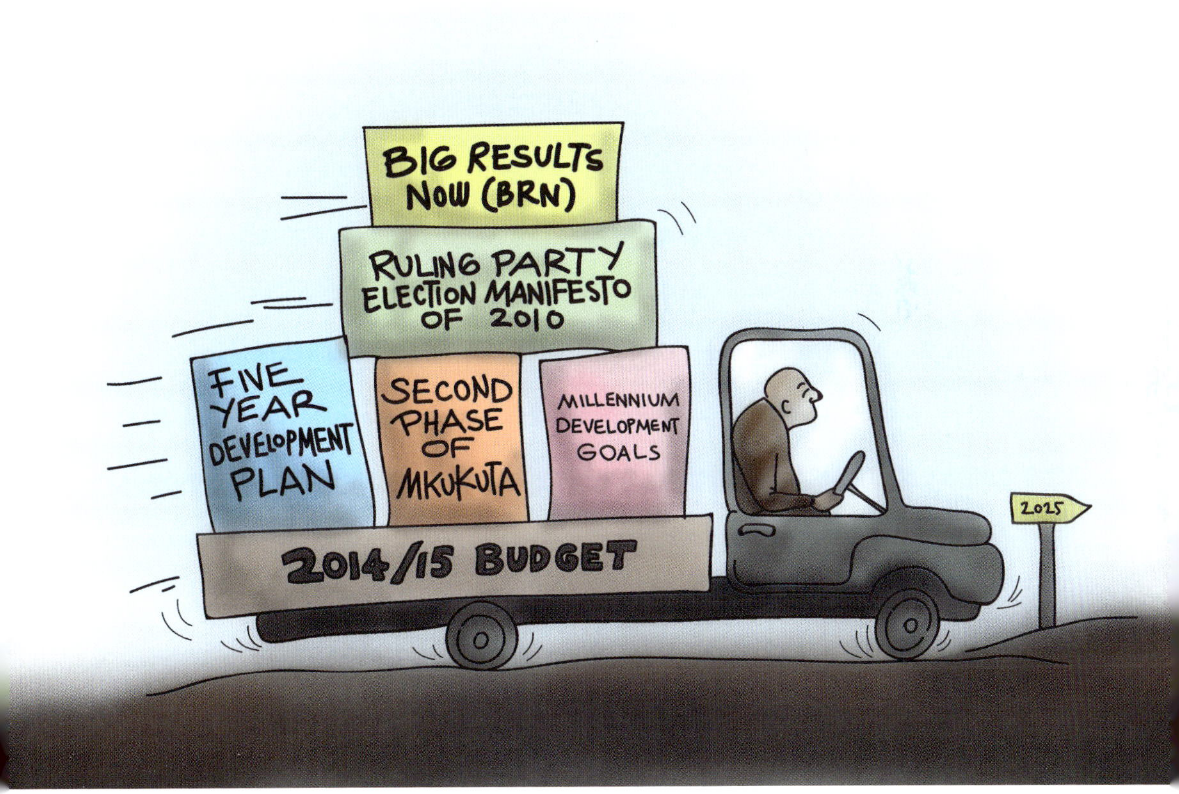

The budget cycle starts with the government planning for the use of the coming year's resources. To allow this to be done in accordance with health policy priorities, health planners have to engage strategically in the process and be prepared to support it.

8.5.1 Budget formulation

The macroeconomic projections, calculated usually by a macroeconomic unit in the MoF, enables the budget office within the MoF to determine the global level of expenditure that can be allowed without adverse macroeconomic implications, given expected revenues and a safe level of deficit.

It is important to keep in mind that the MoF must accommodate various government priorities and make decisions on trade-off. MoH thus must come with a solid evidence base and arguments which have been thought through carefully to make the case for health.

In many countries, the prime minister or the president and/or the cabinet will be directly involved in budget formulation and preparation, especially in influencing the main strategic orientations and modalities of implementation.

The initial formulation of the national budget happens within the budget office of the MoF, with input from the various sectors. The degree of openness and interaction with the other sectors is very specific to each country, and this process will determine how long it takes to come up with a budget (weeks or months). The MoF will certainly request clear, transparent, and concrete information from its own individual departments or from other ministries directly. Some MoFs issue budget circulars to give instructions to line ministries, with the indicative aggregate spending ceiling stated for each ministry. This circular will also include information on how to prepare spending estimates in a way that will be consistent with macroeconomic objectives. It will spell out the economic assumptions to be adopted on wage levels, the exchange rate and price levels (and preferably differentiated price levels for different economic categories of goods and services).

MoH negotiations could be with the budget office directly or with an individual from a different MoF department assigned to the health sector. The MoF must accommodate various government priorities and make decisions on trade-offs in order for budget expenditure totals to tally up to what is available with the country's fiscal space. There will also be negotiations between central-level management MoH and the district-level budget holders.

In reality, a lot of the budgeting processes make use of historical budgeting, i.e. the budget is based on last year's allocations. Unless there are major changes to the economic situation or government priorities (e.g. the 2014 Ebola crisis in West Africa), the broad contours of the budget should be generally known. They will be a combination of critical projections on economic growth, inflation, demography, revenue (all of this information should be included in the pre-budget statement) and overarching fiscal goals. Budgeted funds are often tied up with the fixed costs of staff and infrastructure, leaving limited flexibility, and perhaps even reduced budgetary scope for key patient treatment inputs, such as medicines and other disposable items.

The MoH can bring itself into a strong negotiating position by having its costed plan and plan of negotiation ready before the MoF begins calling on the different sectors for information. Normally, simply requesting an increase in funds for the health sector will not be adequate to convince a finance ministry that is dealing with several competing priorities. A costed plan is a prerequisite to negotiations with the MoF; however, in addition, specific information such as, for example, who are the ultimate beneficiaries of this plan, what are the expected health outcomes, and if necessary, how this will affect the country's economy and government goals as a whole, should be deliberated upon beforehand, calculated and analysed, for discussion with the MoF. This is a critical stage for engaging in the budgeting process, including budget advocacy and negotiating with various stakeholders. Working hand in hand with civil society organizations and think-tanks can be useful here, especially in specific areas of expertise (Box 8.3).

Once budget negotiations have been finalized, the cabinet endorses the proposals for inclusion in the budget that will go to parliament.[20]

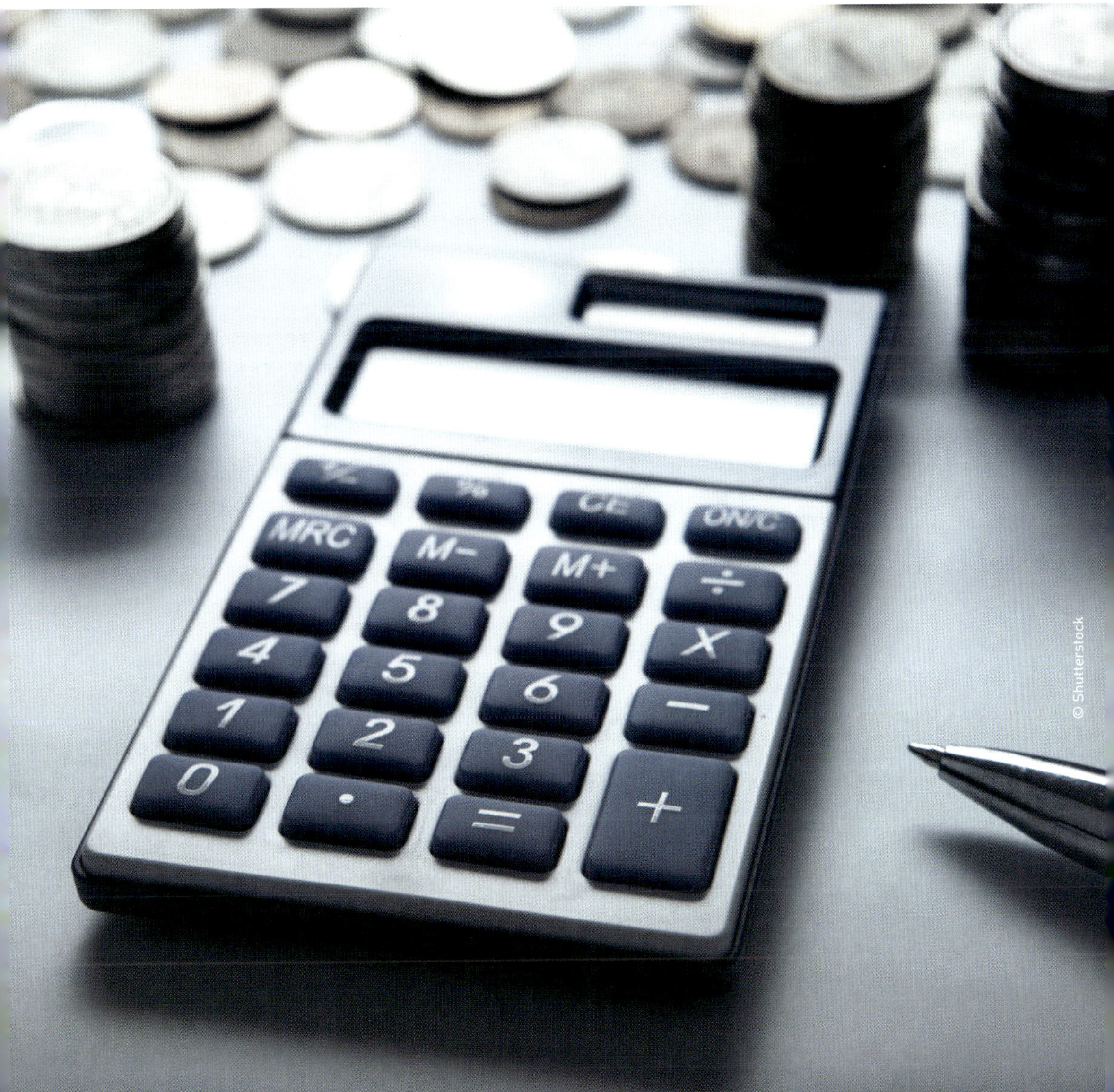

© Shutterstock

Box 8.5

Key steps of Liberia's budgeting process[21]

Using the illustrative example of Liberia helps us understand in practice how budget preparation involves a large range of stakeholders at each and every step of the process.

In Liberia, the MoF leads planning and budgeting process. The MoF calculates revenue projections and then disseminates this information to the respective line ministries, sometimes in the form of a workshop. The line ministries are then responsible for submitting budget proposals, following which budget hearings, debate, and revisions of the original revenue projections take place between MoF and the line ministries. The MoF must accommodate various government priorities and make decisions on trade-offs in order for budget expenditure totals to add up to what is available with the country's fiscal space. There will also be negotiations between central-level management MoH and the district-level budget holders.

The process culminates in a draft budget which the MoH officially submits to the President and the Parliament. Once the Parliament has adopted the national budget, the line ministries are supposed to adjust their internal budgets according to final budget allocations.

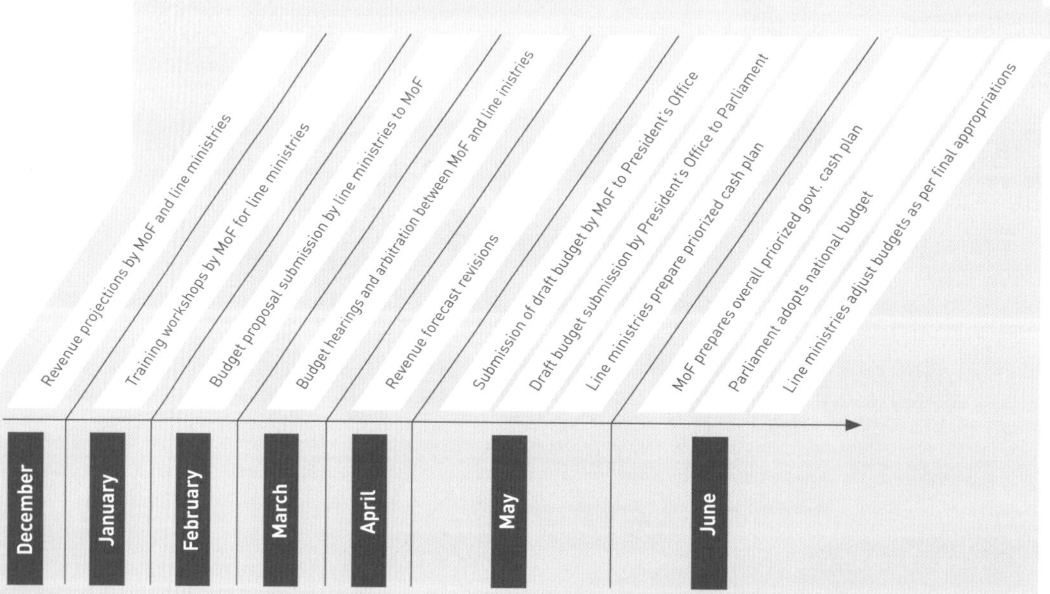

Box 8.6

The budget preparation process in Ghana[22]

The budget process in Ghana is an annual event which includes top-down setting of ceilings and broad priorities and bottom-up prioritization and allocation. Key steps in the process are listed below.

1. A request for inputs from the general public, including civil society and private sector groups.
2. An update of the macroeconomic framework, including overall expenditure ceilings and the distribution of government and donor funds.
3. An early policy review by ministries, departments and agencies, including costing of objectives, policies and activities.
4. Cross-sectoral meetings to identify: areas of overlap and duplication in outcomes, objectives and key outputs; areas where collaboration and coordination are required in the planning and implementation of activities; and comments and feedback on prioritization of objectives.
5. Review and finalization of ceilings in view of predicted cost forecasts.
6. Final ceilings are approved by Cabinet.
7. Development of more detailed first-year operational plans. These are developed bottom-up including regional and district plans, reflecting the policy direction and priorities set out in the NHPSP.
8. Discussion of operational plans in policy and technical hearings with the Ministry of Finance and Economic Planning. After finalization the Ministry consolidates the national budget.
9. Final allocation of ceilings between cost centres and objectives.

8.5.2 Budget approval or enactment

The budget enactment process is a vital time for the MoH to liaise with the legislature health committees and support budget analysis and cross-verification with the costed health plan.

The budget is said to be "enacted" when it is brought to the legislature for discussion and subsequent passing into law. The (budget) appropriations committee usually has the power to vote on financial issues here as the leading legislative body making spending recommendations and decisions on behalf of the legislature. In the budget approval stage, public hearings and debates may take place on specific parts of the budget and/or the budget on the whole, with specific legislative committees (or subcommittees) engaging in discussions of specific topics. Here, the health committee (which may be organized as a subcommittee of the appropriations committee, or a separate standing committee)[VII] will be active in studying the health sections of the overall budget and preparing an analysis and response, often in the form of amendments. It is here that the MoH has the vital opportunity to liaise with the legislature and support the technical analyses and cross-verification with the costed health plan. During this stage of the budget cycle, media attention to the country's budget is high and this forum can be used to bring attention to specific issues, in partnership with advocacy organizations and civil society.

8.5.3 Budget execution

The supreme audit institution's (SAI) mandate is to monitor public spending against stated budgets and spending targets and ensure accordance with relevant laws and regulations.

This stage of the budget cycle includes the actual implementation of the planned budget, which rarely is executed exactly as the budget dictates. The decisive issue is whether unplanned spending is adequately justified by policy decisions, changes in macroeconomic projections, or other reasons, and is well documented.

In many countries, budget implementation and oversight capacity is weak, which exacerbates problems of a poor budget system, and thus budget execution that is further away from the planned budget. For the MoH, and any line ministry for that matter, it is essential that its own sector costing and MTEF work has made explicit where funds should go and for which activities. This can help in a situation where the budget is unclear or where reporting systems do not provide adequate information to monitor expenditure.

8.5.4 Budget evaluation

Budget evaluation and oversight for the full national budget is usually undertaken by a supreme audit institution (SAI). Its mandate is to monitor public spending against stated budgets and spending targets, and ensure accordance with relevant laws and regulations. SAIs are among the most important agencies for ensuring that money is spent in the appropriate way, in the way it was intended.

Increasingly, SAIs are tasked with auditing the efficiency of fund utilization, examining value for money, and assessing performance of public services.[23] Normally, the task of following up on and enforcing audit results and recommendations is within the remit of the legislature. Ideally, the legislature and the SAI (and where relevant, with civil society organizations) should collaborate closely to ensure that SAI findings are acted upon.

Specifically for the health sector, health budget execution can be evaluated during periodic sector reviews. This would fall within the health policy and planning cycle and is separate from national-level budget audits, although health-specific audits can and will certainly be undertaken by a country's SAI.

VII Not all health-related committees in a legislature will have influence over the budget. The exact committee or body which has a health mandate and influence over the budget will differ in each country.

8.6 Important operational issues for health planning stakeholders to consider during the health budgeting process

8.6.1 Legal considerations

Although the precise legal framework for government budgeting varies from country to country, it is usually spelled out in some form or other, be it through a law or decree or regulatory directive or other means. Health planning stakeholders should be aware of how to source information relevant to the budget and where to position their technical inputs and influence.

The constitution is at the top of the legal hierarchy. Although it usually deals only with broad principles, the constitution may clarify three important aspects:

1. the relative powers of the executive and legislative branches with respect to public finance;
2. the definition of the financial relations between national and sub-national levels of government; and
3. the requirement, for example, in common law systems, that all public funds be spent only under the authority of a law.

The organic law is usually the main vehicle for establishing principles of public financial management. This may take the form of a single law that guides budget formulation, approval, execution, control, and auditing, or there may be several general laws covering specific areas of public finance management that may also relate to national and sub-national levels of government. The organic budget law also gives to the government, or the minister responsible for public finance, the authority to issue detailed regulations and instructions.

The constitution, the budget organic law, and financial regulations are permanent and form the legal framework within which the annual budget law/finance law, which includes the revenue and expenditure estimates for a given year, is prepared, approved, executed and audited. The annual budget law can take different shapes depending on the system.

The legal framework that impacts budget formulation and execution is made up of the constitution, organic budget law, and financial regulations.

In the francophone and Latin American systems, the coverage of the annual budget law (budget or loi de finances in francophone countries and ley anual de presupuestos in Latin America) is rather far-reaching, since it stipulates the amount and details of revenue and expenditure, the balance amounts, any new tax legislation measures and any permitted changes to spending. Brazil, for example, has minimum health spending thresholds in place at municipal, state and federal levels of government that require a certain percentage of the annual budget be dedicated to health services.[24] Under the common law system, only revenue and expenditure estimates need to be presented to the parliament. By contrast, the annual budget in many transition economies has often been rather summary in format as no detailed legislation stipulates the contrary: prior to any recent reforms, budget estimates were presented in aggregate format, by budgetary institution – typically only the major supervisory institutions and not their subordinate units – and broken down only by broad "functions".[25]

8.6.2 How can countries introduce and effectively undertake multi-year budgeting?

MTEFs in the health sector were borne out of the need to ensure financial affordability and operational feasibility of health policy proposals.

Since the mid-1980s, budgeting reforms worldwide have been concerned in a significant way with engineering a shift from planning and approving budgets for one year at a time to a multiyear perspective to improve predictability and sustainability in sector funding. The need to ensure the financial affordability and operational feasibility of policy proposals has been a major factor behind the introduction of medium-term perspectives. Given that the disconnect between health policy-making, planning, and budgetary processes was recognized as a common factor of several countries' governance, the health MTEF has increasingly come to be regarded as a central element of public expenditure management reform programmes (see Box 8.7).

Box 8.7

Introducing health MTEF in Africa: the case of Malawi and the Democratic Republic of the Congo

Malawi[26]

In 1993, a Budget Management Review in Malawi revealed real weaknesses in the country's budgeting system; it especially highlighted the fact that both sector-specific as well as overall spending objectives of the government were unclear. In 1995, the World Bank assisted in introducing the MTEF process in Malawi in four sectors, including health, in response to the review's findings. The first year of implementation focused very much on adequately costing sector-specific priorities to reflect the sector strategic plans. All of the other sectors joined in the following year, with the MoF providing overall guidance and management. After the initial years of implementation, it was clear that the Budget Division needed more staff and provisions were made for an increase in personnel. The MTEF in Malawi was seen as a process to support improved decision-making and to better link policies, priorities, resources, and budgets. It has involved both a top-down and bottom-up joint approach – top-down meaning a macroeconomic analysis looking at total revenue and allocation of budget ceilings to different sectors. At the same time, a bottom-up approach at sector level consisted of formulating a sector strategy and breaking the strategy down into activities and costs. In Malawi, a special emphasis was given to involving a wide range of stakeholders in the design and implementation of the process and presenting the budgeting process as a management tool for all sectors. With the MTEF work, the MoF has taken on a less controlling role and is more of a supervisor of performance, ensuring accountability and transparency in resource use. An evaluation in early 2014 demonstrated good improvement for Malawi's budget credibility and stronger links between policies and budgets. However, significant improvements were still necessary for budget execution and control as well as accounting procedures.

Democratic Republic of the Congo[27]

From 2011 the Research and Planning Division at the Ministry of Public Health (MoPH) has run a programme to improve the budget process via a results-oriented management concept that uses the MTEF as a tool. Since 2012, the national MoPH and provincial ministries have compiled a national and provincial MTEF each year. This tool is featured in the roadmap for government expenditure reform initiated by the Ministry of Economy and Finance, making the health sector a trailblazer for a reform to be extended to all other sectors. The benefits are twofold. First, results-based management practices are picked up by provincial planning and budgeting teams. These teams will play a central role in allocations of resources for health. Second, the tool makes it easier to develop arguments in defence of the health budget when choices are being made for the annual budget. In 2014, sound arguments helped the MoPH obtain a 20% increase in the budget initially announced for non-wage expenditure. This represents an additional USD 10 million in the health allocation.

However, the unpredictability of external resources and uncertainty surrounding decentralization makes the medium-term budget process an especially delicate exercise that often has little link to macroeconomic realities. The MTEFs in the Democratic Republic of the Congo are developed using incomplete and patchy data: the provinces have no clear idea of the domestic and external resources that they will receive the following year. Therefore, MTEFs are hardly ever used to manage resources and are more of a theoretical exercise. The MoPH's efforts to improve the budget process are hampered by the uncertainty surrounding decentralization and the fragmentation of external financing. Recent efforts by the MoPH to strengthen their financing strategy should enable the government to set out its official vision of the health financing and decentralization architecture, which will improve the budget process.

To date, MTEFs have seen a mixed impact on increased budgetary predictability for health ministries, but there is some evidence that they have led to budget reallocations to the sector.[28] It is a common observation that the quality of forward spending estimates, as well as revenue forecast, is generally poor. For the former, they tend to consist far too frequently of the proposed budget for the first year of a multiyear framework, followed by inflation adjusted projections of cost for the later years: multiyear incrementalism, in other words. On the latter, revenue projections are sometimes judged as unrealistic and do not allow for adequate strategic planning.

The process and quality of health and overall MTEF need strengthening in most countries, more specifically:

- more realistic resource scenarios;
- better alignment of MTEF ceilings with annual sector allocations;
- more support to MoH for developing sound health expenditure scenarios;
- more participatory processes.

Box 8.8

Barriers to medium-term budgeting[29]

Legacy systems in francophone and anglophone countries in Africa may affect the implementation of standard reforms such as a medium-term budgeting. While francophone systems have budget control benefits and offer some mechanisms that are not out of keeping with a medium-term perspective (such as allowing for capital programming to have a multiyear legal basis in the financial laws), they also present important challenges. The central control over spending ministries discourages spending agencies from taking strategic responsibility for better spending and the budget format does not help either. With a strong emphasis on law in francophone systems, the lack of legal provisions for modern budget management mechanisms such as MTEFs and programme budgeting mean that reforms to these effects have very little impact. On the plus side, the requirement to adhere to the West African Economic and Monetary Union directives, however, has driven successful reforms of key parts of the PFM systems.

In anglophone Africa, the United Kingdom-based financial management tradition can clash with the constitutional form of modern states. The role of parliament in undermining comprehensive, medium-term budgeting that is affordable and effective is among the key concerns. In anglophone countries the strong legal emphasis on the accountability of the spending agency (in this case, MoH) accounting officers in turn undermines a strong finance ministry mandated to run a disciplined budget process. The weak role of parliaments and inadequate capacity for medium-term forecasting, particularly at sector level, further affects the impact of these reforms.

Fig. 8.5 Introducing performance-based budgeting: from concept to practice[30]

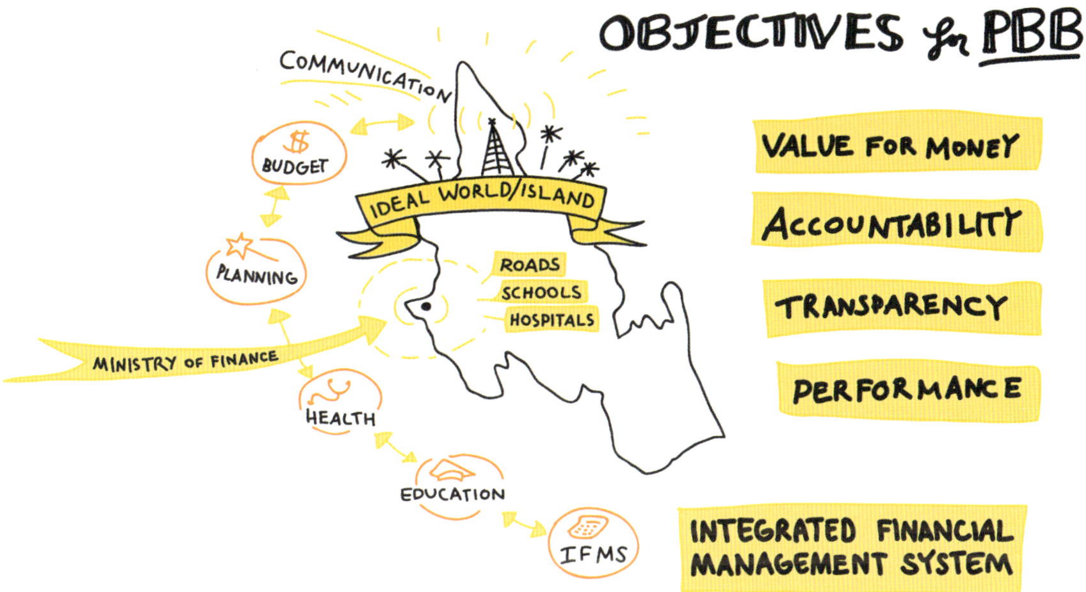

8.6.3 How can countries move from a line-item to a programme-based budget?

Many countries are progressively moving away from activity-based or line-item budgeting towards a system that is more focused on outputs and places emphasis on results. The shift from traditional budgeting to alternative budgeting methods with results and performance at its focus is noted to be more useful as a policy or decision-making tool. It assures elected and administrative officials of what is being accomplished with the money, as opposed to merely showing that it has been used for the purchase of approved input.[31] At the end of the budget cycle, a review of performance is supposed to help planners allocate and spend more effectively toward the set targets in the following years (see Box 8.9). In moving towards performance budgeting, countries adopt a system of planning, budgeting and evaluation

The move towards performance-based budgeting creates a system that emphasizes the relationship between money budgeted and results expected. However, caveats include the increased risk of new budget silos and initial confusion in weak PFM systems.

that emphasizes the relationship between money budgeted and results expected.

However, there are caveats. While performance-based budgeting seems to have been effective to better inform resource allocation decisions and in supporting higher quality of negotiation processes between MoF and line ministries like health, systematic evidence has been lacking on the actual effects on health sector performance. Performance-based budgeting requires considerable budget management capacity within the spending institutions. Providing more autonomy to such institutions (such as MoH) would require that accountability systems are in place and functioning to ensure that more flexibility indeed leads to better sector results.

However, in weak PFM systems, the introduction of an alternative budget classification is likely to create more confusion and to reduce accountability, at least initially. Budgets may therefore need to be presented using several different formats in a transition phase.

Specifically for the health sector, the introduction of programme budgets can increase risks of creating new silos (programme budgets are often disease-specific vertical programmes). Modifying the budget structure will not be sufficient to drive flows to expected results. Just as equally important as budget structure are personnel management and structure of government that provide incentives and accountability for improved health sector performance.

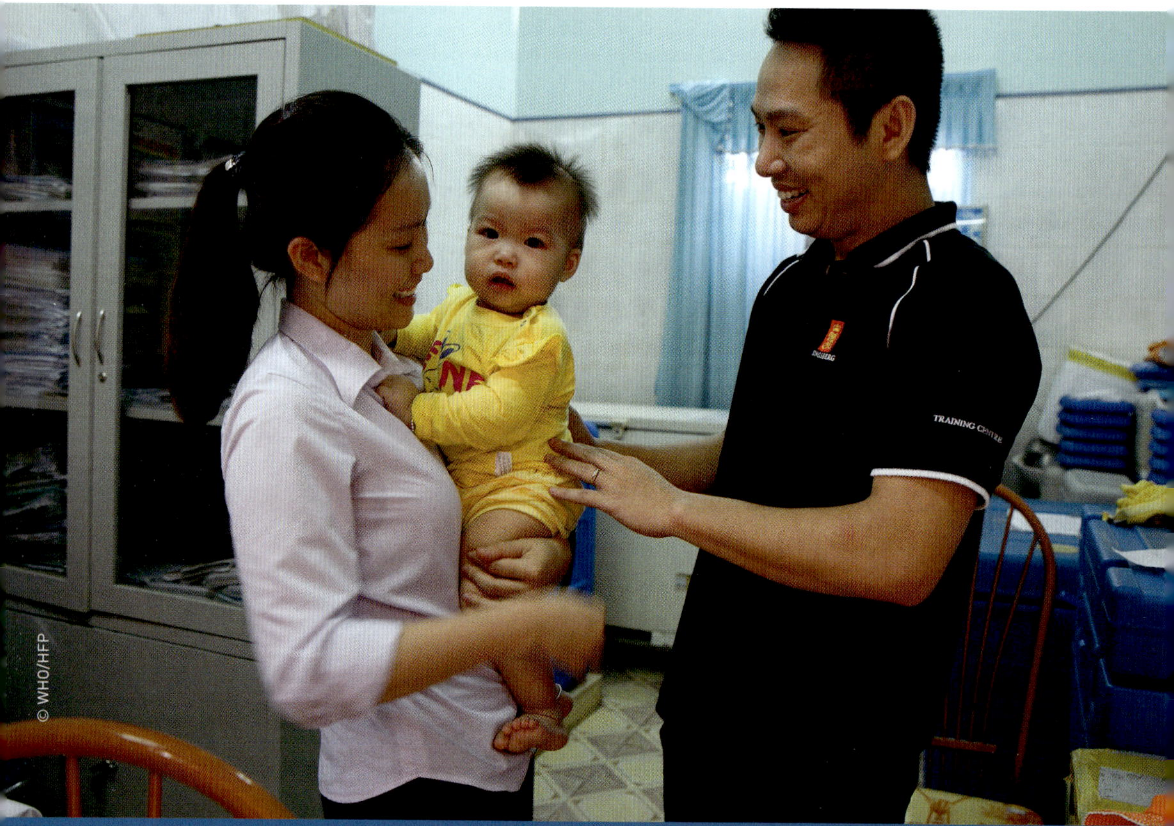

Box 8.9

From line-item to programme budgeting: the case of the Republic of Korea[32]

The Republic of Korea's budget system revealed that the most problematic feature of the budget classification system was that it placed primacy on classifications by organization (ministries and agencies) and, most of all, by budget account. As a result, programme or activity level expenditures were fragmented over different accounts. Conversely, even when a programme or activity was funded solely through a single budget account, it took considerable cross-checking to verify that there are no other expenses in another account. The opacity of spending information for programmes or activities was compounded by the fact that there were more than 6000 activities. Thus the solution demanded that the budget classification system be simplified in order to make the spending information more transparent and accessible. Furthermore, this streamlining of the classification system should be accompanied by greater discretion granted to spending ministries like health. This would also allow the budget office and the legislature to concentrate on the broader resource allocation decisions while harnessing the expertise of front-line managers in spending within their sectors, in order to raise the efficiency of lower-level spending decisions.

With this general direction in mind, the Government decided on several basic principles for restructuring its line-item budget into a programme budget:

1. a programme cannot span multiple ministries;

2. all activities that have the same policy objective must be grouped under a single programme, regardless of revenue source;

3. programmes must be clearly differentiated from one another both in policy objective and programme name.

Further guidelines have been set to ensure that the programme classification matches that of the National Fiscal Management Plan (NFMP – the country's MTEF) and that the final number of activities is reduced to a level that is practical for resource allocation decision-making. Additionally, the Government decided that all indirect costs (salaries, facility maintenance, etc.) for each ministry would be aggregated into a separate programme, as would simple transfers among different budget accounts, rather than trying to distribute such costs or transfers into other programmes.

8.6.4 When and how should countries assess fiscal space for health?

The move towards performance-based budgeting creates a system that emphasizes the relationship between money budgeted and results expected. However, caveats include the increased risk of new budget silos and initial confusion in weak PFM systems.

The quest for fiscal space for health should be mainstreamed into the budgeting process (see Fig. 8.6 and Box 8.10). Situating fiscal space for health analysis in the overall budget forecast process is essential. It is likely that the analysis will be best placed at the medium-term budget formulation stage. It is a critical moment, largely unexploited, which should allow aligning realistic revenue forecasts with government priorities and associated expenditure ceilings. Sector-specific fiscal space assessment, if conducted prior to and as a support for the elaboration of a sound MTEF, will maximize impact on change. With such an assessment, health planners will bring useful technical value and support for exploring the actual potential fiscal space, rather than focusing on historical frameworks and ceilings.

A more realistic sense of the actual potential fiscal space for health can also aid health ministries to better plan for a possible reduction of resource allocations to health during the year – which can happen in times of financial difficulty due to fluctuations in external aid, a reduction in domestic resources, or other reasons. In such circumstances, NHPSP implementation can be deeply undermined if potential resource reductions are not adequately planned for and taken into account from the very beginning.

Box 8.10

Taking stock of fiscal space for health: main lessons from assessments in developing countries[33]

Lessons from country evidence have shown that in contexts with very limited public spending for health (all standards included), fiscal space for health projections have helped to identify feasible scenarios for expanding resource availability on both the revenue generation and the expenditure side. They signalled existing margins from clearly untapped resources (e.g. taxation, mineral resources), from misalignment with government priorities and international commitments (e.g. low health prioritization) and from effectiveness and efficiency-related losses (e.g. low execution, skewed allocations, technical inefficiencies).

In more advanced countries (i.e. higher revenues and health prioritization within the budget envelope), evidence has shown that further gains are likely to derive from the expenditure side through improved management of the existing health budget envelope. In the short and medium term, a strategic combination of improved execution and modified allocation within the budget envelope is likely to drive fiscal space expansion for the sector. In such contexts, successful country experiences have focused on how to align an existing budget envelope with the UHC goals (i.e. reduce inequalities in service use and spending), rather than delaying or derailing the sequence of their reform process and expecting sizeable gains from the resource side.

Fig. 8.6 Positioning fiscal space for health analysis in the budgeting process[34]

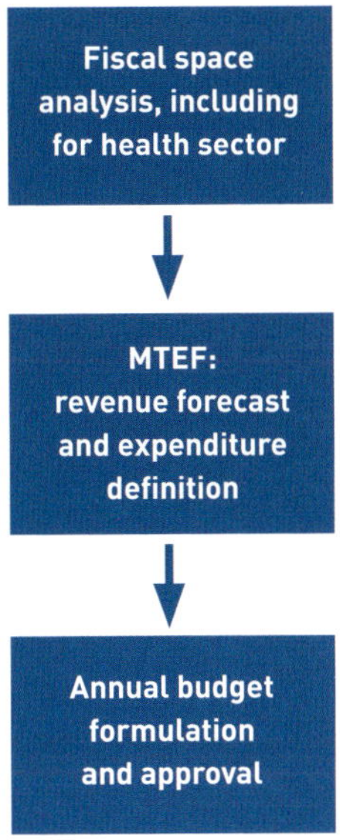

8.6.5 How can the necessary data be collected?

Accessing and effectively using quality budget and financial data is critical for health planners and managers, especially to drive future investment decisions. In many countries, MoH and other stakeholders cannot rely on good quality budget and financial data, for the following reasons:

- lack of access to and use of data by relevant MoH units;
- poor classification of public expenditure for health;
- weak financial management reporting and consolidation systems within MoH and across ministries.

Over the past decade, the systematized production of national health accounts has helped to monitor overall health expenditure from different sources at country level and to provide globally a systematic description of the financial flows related to the consumption of health care goods and services (see Box 8.11). MoH is encouraged to make use of health accounts outputs in a more systematic manner to further inform health planning and budgeting. There is also a need to institutionalize and systematize public expenditure assessments, as well as national health accounts, within MoH to strengthen their ability to inform and influence budget

Good quality budget and financial data are essential to inform health planning and budgeting. Expenditure assessments should thus be institutionalized, not the least because countries are encouraged to move towards a dominant reliance on public expenditure to make progress towards UHC.

decision-makers. As countries are encouraged to move toward a dominant reliance on public expenditure to make progress toward UHC,[35] more efforts shall be put on strengthening production and effective policy use of good quality public expenditure for health data. In doing so, three main aspects can be annually monitored:

1. how much is allocated to the health sector compared to the overall budget;
2. how much of the allocated budget is actually executed;
3. reasons for under or over-spending.

Box 8.11

Role of national health accounts in informing budget formulation and expenditure tracking[36]

Health accounts cover actual expenditure and not budgets or commitments. Health accounts track health expenditure from all sources (including nongovernmental) to different types of providers (for example, hospitals vs providers of ancillary services) and different uses (for example, inpatient vs outpatient care or curative care vs preventive care).

Health accounts address five basic questions.

1. Where do resources come from (through which financing mechanisms have the revenues/resources been pooled)?
2. Who is managing those resources and under which financing arrangements do people get access to health care goods and services?
3. What kinds of goods and services are consumed?
4. Which health care providers deliver these goods and services?
5. Who benefits from the expenditures (by age, gender, regions, diseases)?

A new System of Health Accounts was issued in 2011 to allow comparison across countries and to accommodate a number of changes and improvements.

8.6.6 How should countries understand and influence the political economy of budgeting for health?

Overall, the budget elaboration process is a site for contestation of power and resources, and therefore not just an outcome of economic rationality. It is above all a political exercise (Box 8.12). Central to health planners is the acknowledgement that the budget preparation phase is fundamentally political, because it is about making real policy choices based on societal preferences and linking them to practical health sector strategies.

In order to understand the political economy of the budgeting process, it is necessary to understand the accompanying processes of health policy and planning.[37]

- The process of allocating resources to different goals, priorities or institutions is essentially a political, rather than purely technocratic one. In addition to analysing health needs, health planning stakeholders should pay sufficient attention to understanding political processes pertaining to budgeting prior to and during the budget formulation process.
- The process of budget allocation does not occur in isolation from macroeconomic and revenue issues, and efficiency/effectiveness concerns in the use of funds for health and in the other sectors. A holistic understanding of public expenditure systems – and the institutional cultures that condition them – is important in order to formulate strategies for change and improvement (i.e. an increased allocation to health).
- It should never be automatically assumed that health allocations translate accurately into spending. What money actually gets spent by whom, on what items and for what purpose is often determined during the process of budget execution, which in itself implies political, financial and technical interactions within a large range of interests and powers.

The budget process is fundamentally a political exercise, an acknowledgment that must be understood by health planning stakeholders.

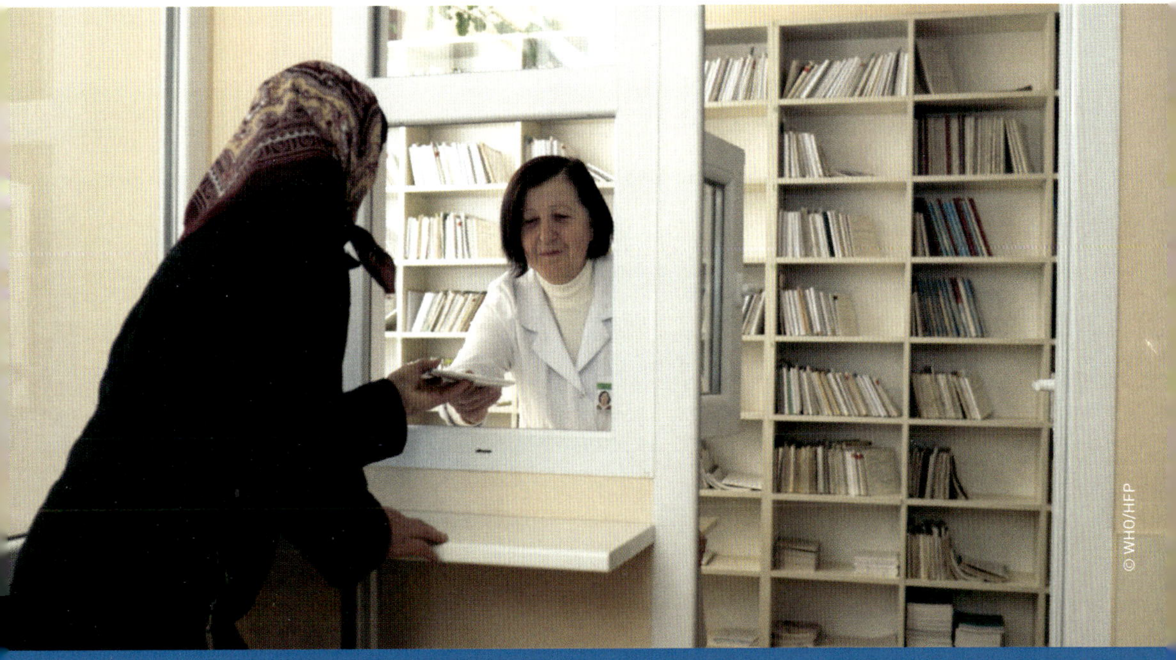

© WHO/HFP

Box 8.12

The politics of budget formulations[38]

To guarantee meaningful change in budget allocations, it is recommended to have information about the following:

(a) the formal structure of roles and responsibilities within the budget process;

(b) the formal rules governing decision-making, political choice and accountability within the public expenditure management system;

(c) the networks of stakeholder power and influence (outside the formal allocation of roles and responsibilities), which influence the outcomes of the budget process;

(d) incentives for action (covert as well as overt) affecting the decision-making of politicians and officials during budget formulation and execution;

(e) the latitude for independent discretionary action of bureaucrats at all levels of the budget execution process;

(f) the norms and values prevailing in key institutions within the budget formulation and execution process.

The experience of budget initiatives with social/health goals suggests a number of broad lessons that can help guide practice, including the following: Firstly, budget processes which are successful in relation to social/health goals often involve a broad range of actors with different positions and skills – including NGOs, researchers, parliamentarians, members of political parties, technocrats and members of the social groups in question themselves. Secondly, many successful social initiatives on the budget process in developing countries have benefited from donor support. Sometimes this has been through support to civil society groups, sometimes through support to building capacity in government, and sometimes through the provision of extra resources (e.g. through Heavily Indebted Poor Countries debt relief). Thirdly, successful initiatives (such as the participatory budgeting movement in Brazil, or the gender budget initiative in South Africa) are often facets of a broader popular political movement or project. Where governments have particularly strong frameworks of policy goals, or other frameworks for accountability (such as constitutional provisions related to economic and social rights), the space for pro-poor engagement in the budget process is stronger.

8.6.7 Looking beyond budget: importance of public finance systems for health financing and UHC

From a public finance perspective, the key objectives of PFM are to maintain sustainable fiscal discipline, ensure strategic and effective allocation of resources and the efficient delivery of public services. On the other hand, health financing is typically characterized by functions that guide the collection, allocation and pooling of resources, as well as the purchasing of services, with the ultimate goal being universal health coverage (UHC). Fostering mutual understanding and further alignment between PFM and health financing systems is critical, and health planning stakeholders have a critical role to play here.

PFM systems shape the level and allocation of public funding (budget formulation), the effectiveness of spending (budget execution) and the flexibility in which funds can be used (pooling, sub-national PFM arrangements, purchasing). While PFM is sometimes considered a bottleneck for effective health spending due to rigidities in the way budgets are formulated and executed, PFM rules also provide the sector with a domestic, integrated platform to manage resources irrespective of their sources (i.e. a core attribute of pooling) and their levels (i.e. across national and sub-national entities).

From a PFM perspective, health is perceived as one of the spending sectors that deliver key public services and goods but overall lacks a good understanding of the PFM roles and rules for public sector effectiveness and financial accountability. In some countries, health is seen as a sector with less capacity, vis-à-vis other sectors, to adequately formulate its priorities and needs and define credible budgets. Often, actual health sector spending is far from initially defined targets. In most low-income countries, actual health spending is typically lower than budget allocations, which ultimately reflects the sector's difficulties to plan, commit and disburse according to national PFM rules. The perception of lack of measurable, immediate health outputs of public resources tends to also reinforce a common perception of the sector's ineffectiveness and inefficiencies.

The key objectives of public finance systems are to maintain sustainable fiscal discipline, ensure strategic and effective allocation of resources and efficiently deliver public services.

Overall, health has been both a distorting and innovating sector for PFM systems. Over the past two decades, the health sector has sometimes generated the development of parallel PFM systems to secure investments and limit fiduciary risks for external investments. Earmarked allocations and parallel budgeting, pooling procurement, reporting arrangements have become a strong attribute of the sector's development aid. At the same time, several low- and middle-income countries have also embarked on alternative health financing reforms that have been mutually beneficial for both the sector and PFM as a whole, through, for example, the development of sectoral MTEFs, the strengthening of domestic procurement mechanisms, the tracking of resources and expenditures up to the sub-national levels, a sound management of domestic pooled funds, the introduction of purchasing agents and strategic payment mechanisms to control expenditure and expand coverage at the same time. In this respect, the health sector can help leverage domestic PFM efforts.

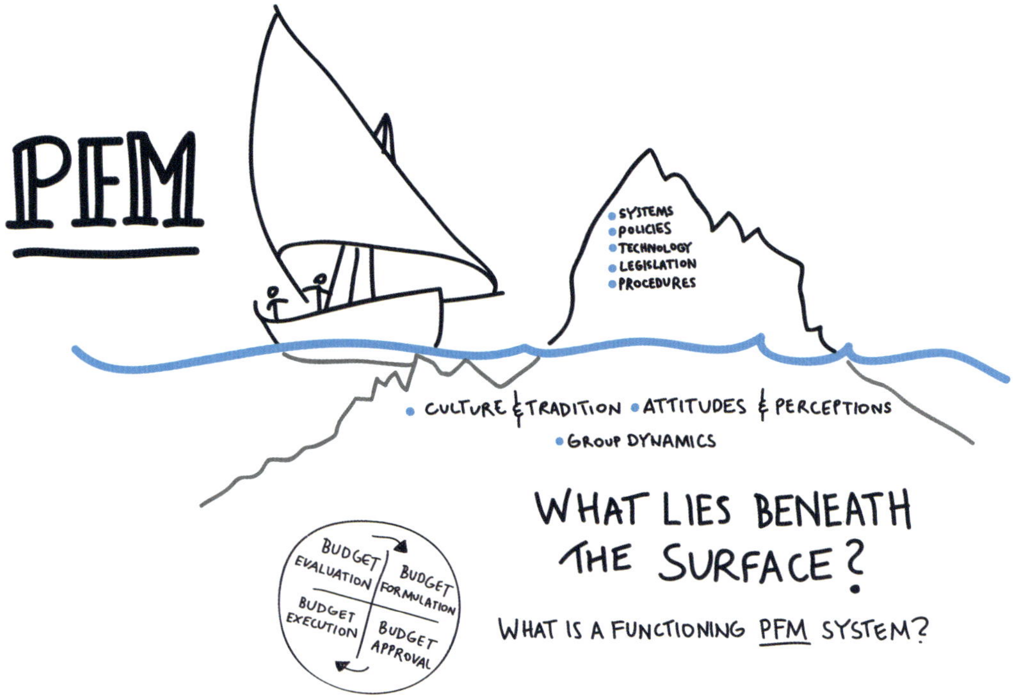

Fig. 8.7 What does it mean to have a functioning PFM system?

8.7 What if...?

This section outlines budgeting issues in specific settings such as decentralized contexts, highly donor-dependent countries, and fragile states.

Fiscal decentralization involves shifting some responsibilities for expenditures and/or revenues to lower levels of government; this can have an impact on health sector funding, as well as how funds flow to the health system.

8.7.1 What if your country is decentralized?

If health is a mandate for a decentralized entity, the full health policy and planning cycles may fall under a decentralized authority. Fiscal decentralization involves shifting some responsibilities for expenditures and/or revenues to lower levels of government; this can have an impact on health sector funding, as well as how funds flow to the health system. In particular, it is important to clarify where local governments can determine the allocation of health expenditures themselves versus those where the centre mandates expenditures and decentralized entities simply execute those health expenditures.

For health planners, it is critical to understand at which level revenue and expenditure decisions are taken (see Box 8.13). Decentralization can make health budgeting processes more complex in that sense, even more so in contexts with weak governance systems. In addition, care must be taken to avoid new inefficiencies due to decentralization, such as separate procurement by each region when it would make most sense to procure together as a single purchaser.

Three main challenges have been observed across decentralized countries or those in the process of decentralization.

(a) Resource mobilization mechanisms can end up being competing and fragmented, leading to inefficiencies in collection and pooling efforts;

(b) Health sector priorities (often set at national level) may be misaligned with sub-national-level budgets and spending targets (e.g. health can de-prioritized in sub-national budgets);

(c) Financial record management is more complex, with resulting poor national consolidation of financial data and limited financial accountability.

A well-managed decentralization process will have in place institutional arrangements for coordination, planning, budgeting, financial reporting, and implementation across government ministries/institutions as well as between the different administrative levels of the country. These coordination bodies are important mechanisms for MoH and health planning stakeholders to discuss specific budget-related issues linked to specific rules (e.g. the design of fiscal transfers) as well as review budget execution against sector priorities.[39]

Box 8.13

Caveats in a decentralized setting: the case of Zambia[40]

The catch in decentralized settings comes when the decentralization process is not prepared adequately or does not function as it should. This might mean that some structures and responsibilities are decentralized but not others, limiting the empowerment truly given to local district managers and communities, and also limiting its benefits. An example of the problems that may arise in such a situation can be seen in Zambia, where an evaluation of decentralization after about a decade of implementation found that health districts had only a moderate range of choice over expenditures, user fees, contracting, targeting and governance. Their choices were even more limited over salaries and allowances and they had no control over additional major sources of revenue, like local taxes. Health system performance indicators also showed no major change compared to before decentralization, suggesting that the expected advantages for the health system did not come into play. This is a particularly difficult situation, since expectations are often raised with the introduction of a decentralization policy but cannot be matched with action on the ground when not adequately implemented. This situation is usually linked to power and decision-making in some areas still being held centrally, leading to tensions between top-down central-level policy decisions and more locally driven agendas.

The central planning authority should give strong guidance as to the methodologies to be used for costing, budgeting, and expenditure tracking – without it, a diverse and heterogeneous set of data from the various decentralized structures will make aggregating countrywide data and producing national estimates very difficult. For example, an additional layer of analysis must be conducted for national health accounts data in countries with highly decentralized health financing systems with little central-level guidance or authority. Getting comparable and consistent figures is often a challenge that may necessitate external expertise. Many countries may not have the time or resources to make this extra effort. At a global level, there is a definitive drive to establish centralized District Health Information Software (DHIS2) and Hospital Management Information Systems to strengthen consistency in reporting.

Finally, an issue which can arise in a decentralized setting is a relative lack of reporting and transparency on money flows. Often, it is the central level that is held to closer scrutiny and is subject to political pressures on the funds it allocates and disburses to decentralized authorities. After that, as Box 8.3 illustrates in the case of Mexico, access to regional or district budget and expenditure data may be considerably more difficult. Low levels of transparency at regional or district levels may reflect a lack of accountability to the population on matters related to health budgets and expenditures. This would imply that the advantages and added value of a decentralized system close to population needs are not being leveraged and that budget-related problems have simply been relocated from central to decentralized level. As Box 8.3 also demonstrates, civil society groups can be key partners of the government and population to ensure better accountability and transparency at lower levels of the health system and advocate for the objectives of decentralization to be fulfilled.

Some questions to consider for costing and budgeting in decentralized settings

What does decentralization actually mean in practice in your country? How far are structures, responsibilities, and budgets actually decentralized?

- The more power and authority actually vested in local authorities, the more scope there is for rational costing and budgeting that is close to the real needs of the local population.

Does the central level authority need to aggregate costing and budgeting nationally?

- If so, guidance and templates from a central authority would be useful and necessary to reduce the burden and error margins of reformatting and restructuring in order to compare and aggregate. In addition, technical support from a central authority might be recommended.
- The central-level authority should take into account revenue generation at different levels for more accurate fiscal space projections.

How transparent are health system costs, budgets, and expenditures reported at decentralized level?

- A low level of transparency may indicate a lack of accountability to the population coming under the decentralized authority and a subsequent lost opportunity to leverage the planning and budgeting advantages of being close to the population.

Box 8.14

Budgeting and health expenditure management in a decentralized state: Nigeria[41]

Nigeria is a federal state with three tiers of government, namely, the federal government, 36 state governments, and 774 local governments. The principal actors in the Nigerian public health sector are the Federal MoH (FMoH), the 36 State Ministries of Health (SMoH), the 774 Local Government Authorities (LGA) Departments of Health, and the authorities of the Federal Capital Territory, as well as various government parastatals and training and research institutions that are concerned with health matters.

The FMoH, the SMoH, and the LGA Departments of Health are responsible for planning and managing health spending in their respective jurisdictions. Public expenditure streams for the three levels of government are largely uncoordinated. Federal, state, and local allocation and expenditure decisions are taken independently, and the federal government has no constitutional power to compel other tiers of government to spend in accordance with national priorities.

The complexity of fiscal transfers and financial flows in Nigeria between federal, state, and local agencies makes it difficult for the government to reconcile and track resource flows across the different levels and agencies of the health system. In general, the absence of accurate and detailed records on budgets and expenditures indicates that government administrations at all levels do not have the means to ensure that health resources are distributed equitably, efficiently, and effectively.

A further complication to Nigeria's decentralized setting came with the creation in thirty states only, of a new agency, the State Primary Health Care Development Agency. This agency is now responsible for primary health care in the state and is tasked to bring all primary care facilities and staffing under its control. In the 30 states where this Agency exists, the LGA Health Authorities are also under its direct control, creating much confusion as to the delineation of tasks and funding mechanisms.

This example from Nigeria demonstrates that decentralization does not always solve existing problems; in fact, when not organized and managed properly, decentralization can create unintended hurdles.

8.7.2 What if your country is heavily dependent on aid?

Budget transparency is a key principle of the Paris Declaration on Aid Effectiveness (2005), whereby donors and recipient countries agreed that greater budget transparency is necessary to ensure that resources are allocated towards effective poverty reduction strategies. The Accra Agenda for Action (2008) and the Busan Partnership Agreement (2011) also included additional commitments for donors to provide timely information on aid flows to recipient governments, such that country budgets can rely on predictable financial flows.

However, in reality, countries that rely more heavily on donor funds are especially vulnerable to the unpredictability of external funds. Donor dependence is a tricky concept as the definition as to what constitutes dependence is not clear – in particular whether dependence is more an issue of influence rather than an amount or share of the budget provided through external assistance. Nevertheless, it is acknowledged that external fund inflows may not only be positive. Donor grants may be earmarked and there may be a lack of reliable projections for future planning years.[42] In addition, there are indications that increases in development assistance is not necessarily associated and matched with an increase in government health spending from domestic sources.[43]

A review of 16 highly aid-dependent countries (countries with an Open Budget Index [OBI] aid dependency index averaging more than 10% over the years 2000 to 2006) revealed that although the presence of donors can promote reforms to strengthen budget transparency, the effects may be offset by other characteristics of donor activity, such as fragmentation and limited use of aid modalities for broader government support and pooled sector funding.[44]

The 2012 Open Budget Survey Report measures the state of budget transparency, budget participation and budget oversight in 100 countries. One of the principal findings was that budget transparency in low-income countries is affected by the choice of aid modalities (i.e. the ways in which aid is provided) and the type of donor interventions, rather than the overall level of aid dependence. In short, the greater the proportion of aid channelled through recipient country budget systems, the more those systems will be strengthened and the more likely they are to become transparent.

"Rather than being linked to the level of overall aid dependence, the transparency is more correlated with an index of donor engagement which tries to capture the quality rather than the quantity of donor flow."[45]

The effect is not just from the amount of aid and the modalities, but also from the number of donors present. The greater the number of donors there are, the greater the fragmentation. In many countries, health remains the most fragmented sector, thus complicating sector-wide planning.

The most common budget-related challenges in aid-dependent countries include:

- problems with predictability of donor funds and alignment, harmonization, and coordination with sector strategies and sector strategy budgets;
- a disconnect between the pledged and actually disbursed monies from donors to aid-dependent countries;
- the timing of fund release – this impacts on budget credibility and ability to implement activities;
- donor conditionalities tied to specific funds.

Overcoming some of the above-mentioned challenges involves constant dialogue with donors on these issues. It can help considerably to gather and document evidence demonstrating the kinds of difficulties encountered by the budget-related challenges, including implementation delays or lack of implementation altogether.

Common budget-related challenges for aid-dependent countries are the limited predictability of donor funds, the disconnect between pledged and disbursed donor monies, the timing of fund release which may be in line with need, and donor conditionalities tied to specific funds.

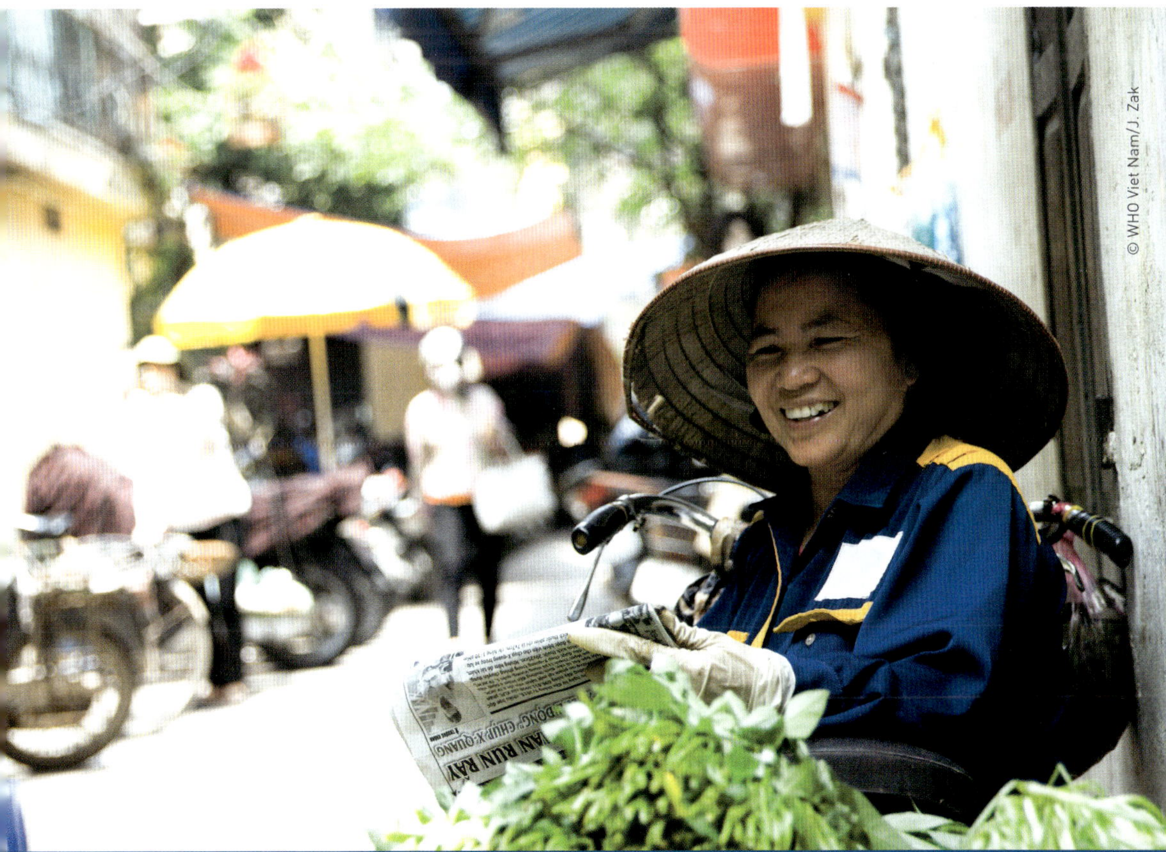

© WHO Viet Nam/J. Zak

8.7.3 What if fragmentation and/or fragility is an issue in your country?

Fragile or post-conflict states will have a reduced tax base and limited revenue generation compared to other countries, translating into an increasing reliance on informal payments and on donor funding. In addition, the transition from short-term emergency relief to longer-term development means a shift in funding models for the health sector – usually, there is some government takeover of basic services with heavy donor assistance. In most cases, this will be accompanied by the continued presence of emergency services as well, creating several parallel funding streams for different types and levels of services that necessitate strong steering capacity and management by the MoH. This is – almost by definition of a fragile state – rarely existent, which makes rational planning and budgeting extremely complex and challenging. (See, for example, Box 8.15).

Private expenditure, remittances from abroad, and aid inflows end up attaining larger totals than expected for health in fragile state situations. Estimates from Afghanistan, Liberia, and the Darfur region of Sudan demonstrate that private health spending soars when public financing is largely absent.[VIII] High levels of private spending means that only those with money can pay to have access to health services.

A good basis for policy dialogue during the national health planning process would be a basic estimation of the total future resource envelope to be expected for health. Due to the uncertainty of estimations, various scenarios can be developed, i.e. low levels of financing vs high levels of financing. If possible, a special study examining the level of private expenditure would be warranted, given the weight of private expenditure in the health sector.

Box 8.15

Health accounts in a conflict-affected or emergency setting

In conflict-affected countries the health accounts activities remain logistically and methodologically challenging because of the inherent insecurity, governance and institutional weaknesses. Usually government investments are very limited, out-of-pocket expenditures may increase and the access to health care services and goods is limited, which may lead to an increase of risk-taking behaviour and impoverishment. These countries rely heavily on international aid for health care provision but at the same time the absorptive capacity in the recipient government institutions may be very low. The health accounts in post-conflict settings usually focus on resource tracking of external funds. It is important to validate the health accounts results internally (with the data authorities and stakeholders), but also to cross-check the data with other sources (donor reports and international databases) as well as analyse the data, comparing them with general economic and health indicators. The findings from health accounts reports can help improve donor accountability and coordination, ensure more equitable distribution of development aid, and lead to better reallocation of health care funds.

VIII More information can be found in Chapter 13 "Strategizing in distressed health contexts" in this handbook.

8.8 Conclusion

A health budget should be viewed as a crucial sectoral orienting text, declaring key financial objectives and its real commitment to implementing health policies and strategies.

During the budgeting process, health planning stakeholders and managers will need to understand the guiding principles of budgeting as well as the political dynamics that enable the budget elaboration and approval processes; not doing so will be a huge missed opportunity to make the case for health. If MoH and other health sector stakeholders are actively and knowledgeably engaged with MoF and others during the budget cycle, resource allocation will more likely match planned health sector needs, and execution is more likely to follow allocations.

The various public finance processes are structured around the budget cycle. In this chapter, the four distinct budget cycle stages (budget definition and formulation, budget negotiation and approval, budget execution and budget reporting, auditing and evaluation) are elaborated upon, with an emphasis on health sector stakeholders' specific role in each, possible entry points for engagement, and particular issues to consider when doing so.

In essence, developing robust health budget envelopes requires strong engagement by health ministries with national budget decision-makers, to make the standpoint of the health sector clear, comprehensible and compelling. This requires MoH and planning stakeholders to think through the operational details and costs of health sector needs and how health services should be purchased within the framework of existing PFM rules.

References

1 Adapted from: World Bank. Public Expenditure Management handbook. Washington (DC); 1998 (http://www1.worldbank.org/publicsector/pe/handbook/pem98.pdf, accessed 17 August 2016).

2 This definition of "performance budgeting" can be found in the Budgeting and public expenditures section of the OECD website at: http://www.oecd.org/gov/budgeting/seniorbudgetofficialsnetworkonperformanceandresults.htm, accessed 17 August 2016.

3 Heller PS. The prospects of creating 'fiscal space' for the health sector. Health Policy Plan. 2006;21(2):75–9 (http://www.ncbi.nlm.nih.gov/pubmed/16415338, accessed 17 August 2016).

4 Tandon A, Cashin C. Assessing public expenditure on health from a fiscal space perspective. Washington (DC): World Bank; 2010 (HNP Discussion Paper; http://siteresources.worldbank.org/HEALTHNUTRITIONANDPOPULATION/Resources/281627-1095698140167/AssesingPublicExpenditureFiscalSpace.pdf, accessed 17 August 2016).

5 Barroy H, Sparkes S, Dale E. Fiscal space for health: from concept to practice, Brief summary of findings and key messages, Background paper for the WHO meeting on "Fiscal space, public financial management and health financing: sustaining progress towards universal health coverage" held at Montreux, 26–28 April 2016. Further information on this meeting at: http://www.who.int/health_financing/topics/public-financial-management/montreux-meeting-2016/en/.

6 Resilient and Responsive Health Systems (RESYST). What is strategic purchasing for health? Topic 4: Financing research theme; 2014 (http://resyst.lshtm.ac.uk/sites/resyst.lshtm.ac.uk/files/docs/reseources/Purchasing%20brief.pdf, accessed 17 August 2016).

7 Cashin C. Health financing policy: the macroeconomic, fiscal, and public finance context. Washington (DC): World Bank Group; 2016 (A World Bank study; http://documents.worldbank.org/curated/en/394031467990348481/Health-financing-policy-the-macroeconomic-fiscal-and-public-finance-context, accessed 17 August 2016).

8 Bassalia D. Misalignment between health planning and budgeting in Cote d'Ivoire. (unpublished), Harmonization for Health in Africa, Community of Practice; 2016.

9 Andrews M, Cangiano M, Cole N, de Renzio P, Krause P, Seligmann R. This is PFM. Boston: Harvard University; 2014 (CID Working Paper No. 285; https://www.hks.harvard.edu/content/download/69282/1249938/version/1/file/285_Andrews_This+is+PFM.pdf, accessed 17 August 2016).

10 Fiscal year: country comparison to the world. In: The world factbook. Washington (DC): CIA (website) (https://www.cia.gov/library/publications/the-world-factbook/fields/2080.html, accessed 17 August 2016).

11 United Republic of Tanzania. Government budget for financial year 2011/2012: citizens' budget edition. Dar es Salaam: Ministry of Finance in collaboration with Policy Forum (http://www.opengov.go.tz/files/publications/attachments/CITIZEN_ENGLISH_2011_12_FINAL_en_sw.pdf, accessed 30 August 2016).

12 Mathonnat J. Disponibilité des ressources financières pour la santé dans les pays d'Afrique subsaharienne. CERDI. Agence Française de Développement. 2010 (http://www.ffem.fr/webdav/site/afd/shared/PUBLICATIONS/RECHERCHE/Archives/Notes-et-documents/52-notes-documents.pdf, accessed 18 August 2016).

13 Public financing for health in Africa: from Abuja to the SDGs. Geneva: World Health Organization; 2016 (WHO/HIS/HGF/Tech.Report/16.2; http://apps.who.int/iris/bitstream/10665/249527/1/WHO-HIS-HGF-Tech.Report-16.2-eng.pdf, accessed 30 August 2016).

14 Barroy H, Andre F, Mayaka S, Samaha H. Investing in universal health coverage: opportunities and challenges for the Democratic Republic of Congo. 2014 Health public expenditure review. Washington (DC): World Bank; 2016 (http://documents.worldbank.org/curated/en/782781468196751651/pdf/103444-WP-P147553-PUBLIC-Health-PER-Investing-in-Universal-Health-1608488.pdf, accessed 18 August 2016).

15 The world health report: health systems financing: the path to universal coverage. Chapter 4: More health for the money. Geneva: World Health Organization; 2010 (http://apps.who.int/iris/bitstream/10665/44371/1/9789241564021_eng.pdf, accessed 18 August 2016).

16 Petrie M, Shields J. Producing a citizens' guide to the budget: why, what and how? OECD Journal on Budgeting. 2010;2:1–13 (https://www.oecd.org/gov/budgeting/48170438.pdf, accessed 18 August 2016).

17 de Renzio P, Krafchik W. Lessons from the field: the impact of civil society budget and analysis and advocacy in six countries: practitioners guide. Washington (DC): International Budget Project; 2005 (http://www.internationalbudget.org/wp-content/uploads/Lessons-from-the-Field-The-Impact-of-Civil-Society-Budget-Analysis-and-Advocacy-in-Six-Countries.pdf, accessed 18 August 2016).

18 Participatory budgeting: an experience in good governance. Washington (DC): World Bank; 10 September 2012 (http://www.worldbank.org/en/news/feature/2012/09/10/participatory-budgeting-an-experience-in-good-governance, accessed 18 August 2016).

19 United Republic of Tanzania. Government budget for financial year 2011/2012: citizens' budget edition. Dar es Salaam: Ministry of Finance in collaboration with Policy Forum (http://www.opengov.go.tz/files/publications/attachments/CITIZEN_ENGLISH_2011_12_FINAL_en_sw.pdf, accessed 30 August 2016).

20 Potter B, Diamond J. Guidelines for public expenditure management. Washington (DC): International Monetary Fund; 1999 (https://www.imf.org/external/pubs/ft/expend/, accessed 30 August 2016).

21 Improving health sector resource allocation in Liberia: towards developing a resource allocation formula. Washington, (DC)/Monrovia: World Bank/Ministry of Health and Social Welfare; [2012].

22 Health dialogue case study: maternal and child health in Ghana. Centurion: Collaborative Africa Budget Reform Initiative (CABRI); 2011 (http://www.cabri-sbo.org/uploads/files/Documents/report_2011_cabri_value_for_money_health_1st_dialogue_english_cabri_health_dialogue_ghana_case_study.pdf, accessed 18 August 2016).

23 van Zyl A, Ramkumar V, de Renzio P. Responding to challenges of supreme A audit instituions: Can legislatures and civil society help? U4Issue. 2009:1(http://www.u4.no/publications/responding-to-the-challenges-of-supreme-audit-institutions-can-legislatures-and-civil-society-help/, accessed 18 August 2016).

24 Cashin C. Health financing policy: the macroeconomic, fiscal, and public finance context. Washington (DC): World Bank Group; 2016 (A World Bank study; http://documents.worldbank.org/curated/en/394031467990348481/Health-financing-policy-the-macroeconomic-fiscal-and-public-finance-context, accessed 17 August 2016).

25 Potter B, Diamond J. Guidelines for public expenditure management. Washington (DC): International Monetary Fund; 1999 (https://www.imf.org/external/ pubs/ft/expend/, accessed 30 August 2016).

26 Malawi: public expenditure review. Washington (DC): World Bank; 2013 (Poverty Reduction and Economic Management 4; http://documents.worldbank.org/curated/en/568641468048896702/Malawi-Public-expenditure-review, accessed 18 August 2016)

27 Barroy H, Andre F, Mayaka S, Samaha H. Investing in universal health coverage: opportunities and challenges for the Democratic Republic of Congo. 2014 Health public expenditure review. Washington (DC): World Bank; 2016 (http://documents.worldbank.org/curated/en/782781468196751651/pdf/103444-WP-P147553-PUBLIC-Health-PER-Investing-in-Universal-Health-1608488.pdf, accessed 18 August 2016).

28 Gottret P, Schieber G. Health financing revisited: a practitioner's guide. Washington, DC: World Bank; 2006 (http://documents.worldbank.org/curated/en/874011468313782370/Health-financing-revisited-a-practitioners-guide, accessed 18 August 2016).

29 Are we asking the right questions? Embedding a medium-term perspective in budgeting. Centurion: CABRI; 2007 (http://www.cabri-sbo.org/en/publications/are-we-asking-the-right-questions-embedding-a-medium-term-perspective-in-budgeting-4th-annual-seminar, accessed 18 August 2016).

30 Programmed-based budgeting: experiences and lessons from Mauritius. Centurion: CABRI. 2010 (CABRI Joint Country Case Study; http://www.cabri-sbo.org/uploads/files/Documents/ report_2010_cabri_capable_finance_ministries_budget_practices_and_reforms_english_cabri_budget_practices_and_reforms_-_mauritius.pdf, accessed 18 August 2016).

31 Ibid.

32 Kim JM, editor. From line-item to program budgeting: global lessons and the Korean case. Seoul: World Bank/Korea Institute of Public Finance; 2010 (http://www1.worldbank.org/publicsector/pe/bookprogrambudget.pdf, accessed 18 August 2016).

33 Barroy H, Sparkes S, Dale E. Fiscal space for health: from concept to practice, Brief summary of findings and key messages, Background paper for the WHO meeting on "Fiscal space, public financial management and health financing: sustaining progress towards universal health coverage" held at Montreux, 26–28 April 2016. Further information on this meeting at: http://www.who.int/health_financing/topics/public-financial-management/montreux-meeting-2016/en/.

34 Ibid.

35 Jowett M, Kutzin J. Raising revenues for health in support of UHC: strategic issues for policy makers. Geneva: OECD/Eurostat/World Health Organization; 2015 (Health Financing Policy Brief No 1; http://apps.who.int/iris/bitstream/10665/192280/1/WHO_HIS_HGF_PolicyBrief_15.1_eng.pdf), accessed 16 August 2016).

36 OECD, Eurostat, WHO. A system of health accounts 2011. Paris: OECD Publishing; 2011 (http://www.who.int/health-accounts/methodology/sha2011.pdf, accessed 18 August 2016).

37 Norton A, Elson D. What's behind the budget? Politics, rights and accountability in the budget process. London: Overseas Development Institute; 2002 (https://www.odi.org/sites/odi.org.uk/files/odi-assets/publications-opinion-files/2422.pdf, accessed 18 August 2016).

38 Ibid.

39 Kakhonen S, Lanyi A. Decentralization and governance: does decentralization improve public service delivery?. Washington (DC): World Bank; 2001 (PREM Notes No. 55; https://openknowledge.worldbank.org/handle/10986/11382, accessed 30 August 2016).

40 Bossert T, Chitah MB, Bowser D. Decentralization in Zambia: resource allocation and district performance. Health Policy Plan. 2003;18(4):357–69 (http://www.ncbi.nlm.nih.gov/pubmed/14654512, accessed 18 August 2016).

41 Ohadi E, El-Khoury M, Williamson T, Brinkerhoff D. Public budgeting and expenditure management in three Nigerian states: challenges for health governance. Bethesda (MD): USAID/Health Systems 20/20; 2012 (https://www.hfgproject.org/wp-content/uploads/2015/02/Public-Budgeting-and-Expenditure-Management-in-Three-Nigerian-States-Challenges-for-Health-Governance.pdf, accessed 18 August 2016); input from Ogochukwu Chukwujekwu, WHO, unpublished observations, 2016.

42 de Renzio P, Angemi D. Comrades or culprits? Donor engagement and budget transparency in aid dependent countries. Barcelona: Institut Barcelona d'estudis internacionals; 2011 (IBEI Working Papers 2011/33; http://www.internationalbudget.org/wp-content/uploads/Donor-Engagement-and-Budget-Transparency.pdf, accessed 18 August 2016).

43 Lu C, Schneider MT, Gubbins P, Leach-Kemon K, Jamison D, Murray, CJ. Public Financing of Health in Developing Countries: A cross-national systematic analysis. Lancet. 2010;375(9723): 1375–87. doi: http://dx.doi.org/10.1016/S0140-6736(10)60233-4.

44 de Renzio P, Angemi D. Comrades or culprits? Donor engagement and budget transparency in aid dependent countries. Barcelona: Institut Barcelona d'estudis internacionals; 2011 (IBEI Working Papers 2011/33; http://www.internationalbudget.org/wp-content/uploads/Donor-Engagement-and-Budget-Transparency.pdf, accessed 18 August 2016).

45 Tandon A, Cashin C. Assessing public expenditure on health from a fiscal space perspective. Washington (DC): World Bank; 2010 (HNP Discussion Paper; http://siteresources.worldbank.org/HEALTHNUTRITIONANDPOPULATION/Resources/281627-1095698140167/AssesingPublicExpenditureFiscalSpace.pdf, accessed 17 August 2016).

Further reading

Andrews M, Cangiano M, Cole N, de Renzio P, Krause P, Seligmann R. This is PFM. Boston: Harvard University; 2014 (CID Working Paper No. 285; https://www.hks.harvard.edu/content/download/69282/1249938/version/1/file/285_Andrews_This+is+PFM.pdf, accessed 17 August 2016).

Barroy H, Andre F, Mayaka S, Samaha H. Investing in universal health coverage: opportunities and challenges for the Democratic Republic of Congo. 2014 Health public expenditure review. Washington (DC): World Bank; 2016 (http://documents.worldbank.org/curated/en/782781468196751651/pdf/103444-WP-P147553-PUBLIC-Health-PER-Investing-in-Universal-Health-1608488.pdf, accessed 18 August 2016).

Cashin C. Health financing policy: the macroeconomic, fiscal, and public finance context. Washington (DC): World Bank Group; 2016 (A World Bank study; http://documents.worldbank.org/curated/en/394031467990348481/Health-financing-policy-the-macroeconomic-fiscal-and-public-finance-context, accessed 17 August 2016).

Le Houerou P, Taliercio R.(2002): Medium term expenditure frameworks: from concept to practice: preliminary lessons from Africa. Washington (DC): World Bank; 2002 (African Region Working Paper Series No. 28; http://www1.worldbank.org/publicsector/LearningProgram/Le%20Houerou-Taliercio.pdf, accessed 20 August 2016).

Kutzin J, Yip W, Cashin C. Alternative financing strategies for universal health coverage. In: Scheffler RM, editor. World scientific handbook of global health economic and public policy. Volume 1: Economics of health and health systems. World Scientific Publishing Company; 2016, 267–309 (http://www.who.int/health_financing/documents/alternative-strategies-for-uhc/en/, accessed 18 August 2016).

Norton A, Elson D. What's behind the budget? Politics, rights and accountability in the budget process. London: Overseas Development Institute; 2002 (https://www.odi.org/sites/odi.org.uk/files/odi-assets/publications-opinion-files/2422.pdf, accessed 18 August 2016).

Tandon A, Cashin C. Assessing public expenditure on health from a fiscal space perspective. Washington (DC): World Bank; 2010 (HNP Discussion Paper; http://siteresources.worldbank.org/HEALTHNUTRITIONANDPOPULATION/Resources/281627-1095698140167/Assesing-PublicExpenditureFiscalSpace.pdf, accessed 17 August 2016).

Tsofa B, Molyneux S; Goodman C. Health sector operational planning and budgeting processes in Kenya- "never the twain shall meet", International J Health Plann Manage. 2015;31(3):206–76 (http://onlinelibrary.wiley.com/doi/10.1002/hpm.2286/full, accessed 19 August 2016).

Wildavsky, A. Political implications of budgetary reform. Public Administration Review. 1961; 21;183–90 (http://www.jstor.org/stable/973628) [subscription required].

World Health Organization. Public Financing for Health in Africa: from Abuja to the SDGs. WHO/HIS/HGF/Tech.Report/16.2; 2016.

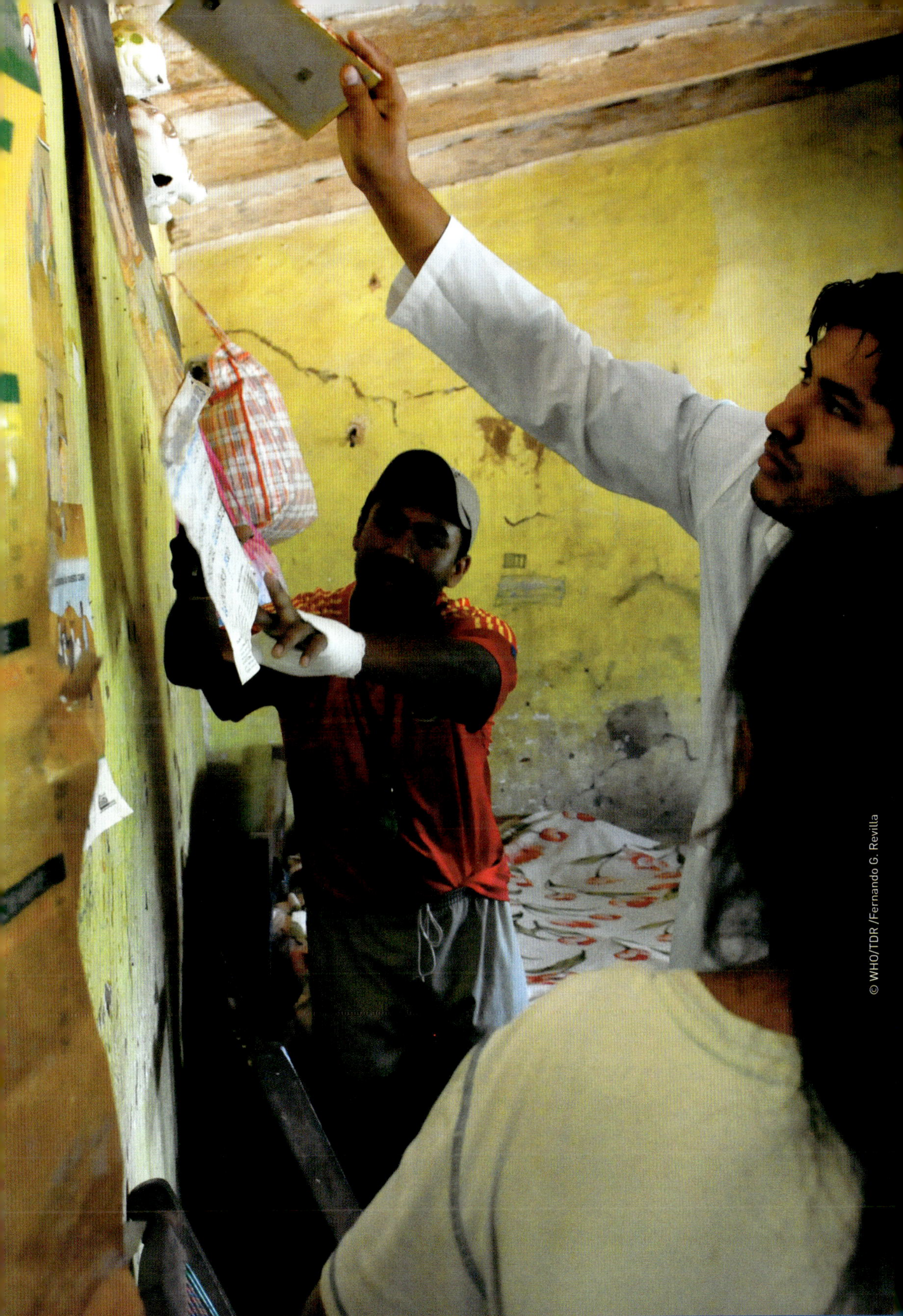

© WHO/TDR/Fernando G. Revilla

Chapter 9

Monitoring, evaluation and review of national health policies, strategies and plans

Kathryn O'Neill
Kavitha Viswanathan
Eduardo Celades
Ties Boerma

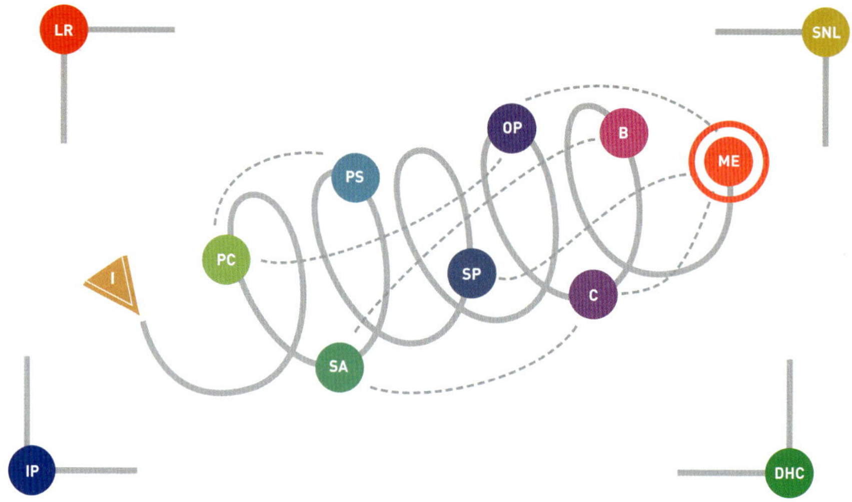

Cross-cutting topics relevant to national health planning

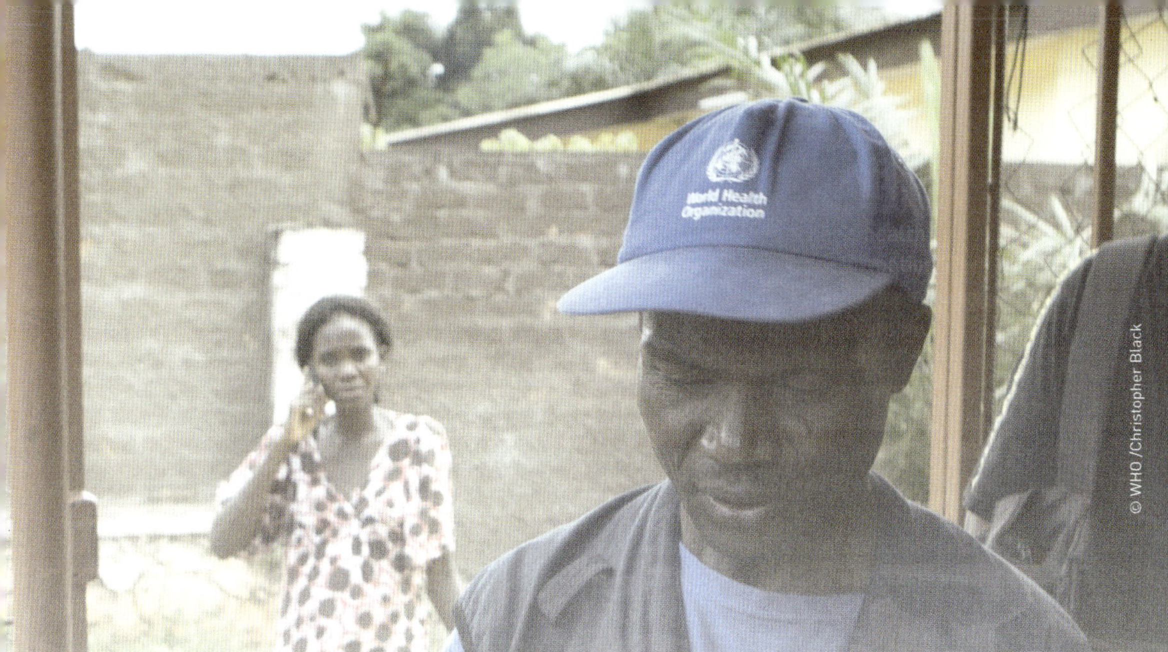

© WHO /Christopher Black

Overview

This chapter outlines the aim and importance of monitoring, evaluation and review as the basis for tracking progress and performance of national health policies, strategies and plans (NHPSP) and to inform the health policy dialogue. Monitoring, evaluation and review require an integrated approach that builds on a single country-led monitoring and evaluation (M&E) platform. Key components and attributes of a strong country-led platform for monitoring, evaluation and review are specified here; in addition, key recommendations are made for countries to move forward and strengthen the platform.

Summary

What do we mean by monitoring, evaluation and review of NHPSPs?

Monitoring, evaluation and review are essential functions to ensure that priority health actions outlined in the NHPSP are implemented as planned against stated objectives and desired results.

- Monitoring means bringing all data together to analyse the progress of implementation of activities.
- Evaluation builds upon monitoring and assesses whether the desired results of a NHPSP intervention have been achieved.
- Based on the evidence gathered through M&E processes, reviews are used to assess overall progress and performance, to identify problems and take corrective actions.

A single country-led platform brings together all the elements related to monitoring, evaluation and review of the health sector plan, including national policy and plans relating to M&E and country health information systems (HIS), well-functioning data sources, institutional capacity for data collection, management analyses and use, as well as the country review processes for planning and decision-making.

Why is it important?

Because:

- progress and performance of the national health strategy need to be tracked;
- country monitoring is the basis for regional and global monitoring of priority health issues;
- reporting progress on health-related Sustainable Development Goals (SDGs) requires sound M&E systems;
- health inequities need to be monitored;
- countries need functional surveillance mechanisms;
- accountability is a necessary basis for policy dialogue.

What are the components of an M&E platform

Monitoring, evaluation and review of the national health strategy require an integrated and comprehensive approach that builds on a single country-led platform as described in the IHP+ framework for monitoring national health strategies[1] that meets all country data needs and allows monitoring of progress towards the health-related SDGs, with high-level political commitment and investments by countries and international partners. The four main components of an M&E platform should be strengthened:

1. sound policy and institutional environment, including sound governance policies and multi-stakeholder coordination mecha-

nisms, a strong M&E plan as an integral component of the national health strategy, a comprehensive logical framework that guides selection of indicators and targets, use of international data standards, unified data architecture and innovations;

2. well-functioning data sources including civil registration and vital statistics (CRVS) systems, population-based surveys, routine facility information systems, facility surveys, administrative data sources such as national health accounts and health workforce registries, logistical information systems, disease and public health surveillance, research studies among others;

3. strong institutional capacity for data collection, management, analysis, use and dissemination;

4. effective country mechanisms for review and action, such as a regular and transparent system of reviews with broad involvement of key stakeholders and processes for translating results into decision-making.

How to strengthen monitoring, evaluation and review?

Key steps to strengthen the country-led platform include:

1. assess the key attributes of the M&E platform as required and identify priority actions to address key gaps and weaknesses;
2. review and select core indicators and develop baseline and targets for monitoring national priorities and health goals;
3. develop a comprehensive M&E plan, including alignment of disease-specific plans and identification of priority actions;
4. cost the M&E plan and develop a common investment framework as the basis for government and partner investments;
5. review and evaluate the M&E platform regularly.

Who are the key stakeholders?

Stakeholders include national and sub-national policy-makers, programme managers and planners, civil society and development partners.

When should monitoring, evaluation and review take place?

Monitoring, evaluation and review should be linked with the country planning cycles, when progress and performance of the sector are discussed and remedial actions are taken.

Anything else to consider?

- fragile environment;
- decentralized environment.

9.1 What do we mean by monitoring, evaluation and review of NHPSPs?

9.1.1 What are the differences between monitoring, evaluation and review?

Monitoring, evaluation and review are essential functions to ensure that priority health actions outlined in the NHPSP are implemented as planned against stated objectives and desired results.

Monitoring means collecting, tracking and analysing data to determine what is happening, where, and to whom. Monitoring uses a set of core indicators and targets to provide timely and accurate information in order to inform progress and performance reviews and decision-making processes. In the context of NHPSP, the indicators and targets should be linked to the strategic directions and key objectives for the health sector.

Evaluation builds upon the monitoring data but the analysis goes much deeper. Additional data are often needed to take into account contextual changes and determine if change is attributable to services.

Reviews gather evidence through monitoring and evaluation processes to assess progress and performance. Health sector reviews require national institutional mechanisms involving multiple stakeholders to provide the basis for mutual accountability. Reviews should link assessment to country follow-up action including prioritization, resource allocation and policy dialogue. Several characteristics are recommended to ensure a sound health sector situation analysis.

9.1.2 Monitoring, evaluation and review need a strong, country-led M&E platform

Monitoring, evaluation and review of the NHPSP requires an integrated and comprehensive health systems approach that builds on a single country-led M&E platform, as described in the IHP+ framework for monitoring national health strategies.[2] This platform should meet all country data needs and allow monitoring of progress towards national health sector goals as spelled out in the NHPSP as well as the international health-related SDGs, while enjoying high-level political commitment and investments by countries and international partners.

Monitoring is collecting, tracking and analyzing data to determine what is happening, where and to whom, while evaluation builds upon the monitoring data into a deep analysis.

A single country-led platform brings together all the elements related to monitoring, evaluation and review of the NHPSP, including specific policy and plans relating to M&E and country health information systems (see Fig. 9.1). In addition, the country's data sources and institutions for data generation, compilation, analysis, synthesis and dissemination form an integral part of the single platform. Country review processes should make use of the platform's evidence base as an anchor for planning and decision-making.

The platform covers health system components and major disease programmes; it serves as the mechanism for sub-national, national and global reporting, aligning health sector stakeholders at country and global levels around a common country-led approach.

The platform aims to be relevant for countries and for global health partnerships, donors and agencies alike, and to result in better alignment of country and global monitoring systems. The platform should reduce duplication of efforts, focus on health sector results monitoring, and result in better accountability and harmonization of M&E systems.

Fig. 9.1 M&E platform and its links with HIS

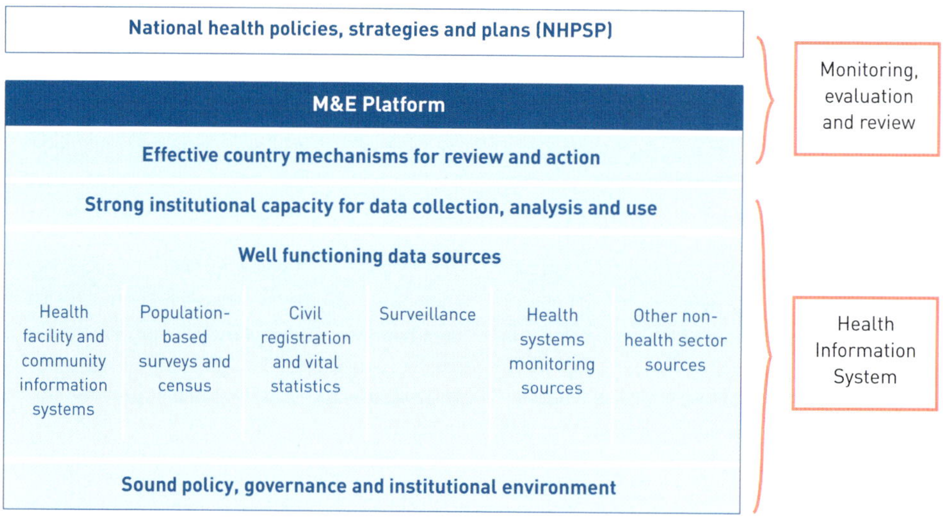

A single-led country platform for monitoring, evaluation and review should allow monitoring of progress towards national health sector goals as spelled out in the NHPSP and international health-related SDGs.

The platform is often described by the M&E plan and/or the HIS strategic plan. The M&E plan is normally developed in parallel to the development of the NHPSP, and reflects its priorities. In some countries, the national health strategy has a specific M&E chapter giving an overview of indicators and priorities for strengthening M&E systems. This is often accompanied by a separate detailed M&E plan. In some countries, the HIS strategy is used as an operational plan to strengthen data sources and the overall HIS, to respond to the monitoring needs of the national health strategy.

Both the M&E plan and the HIS strategic plan can help to align health partners, governments and other stakeholders around the national priorities to strengthen the systems that generate health information. They are complementary, and both M&E and HIS strategic plans can cover all functions outlined previously.

9.2 Why are monitoring, evaluation and review important?

9.2.1 Because progress and performance of the national health strategy need to be tracked

The NHPSP addresses the public health needs of the country and lays out a plan to address these issues. Monitoring, evaluation and review are important, as they provide the basic measurement systems and accountability mechanisms to plan, manage and account for the objectives and targets of the national health strategy. Indicators are required to support programme planning, monitoring, reviews and accountability for the health sector as a whole, and for specific programmes.

All countries need to be able to generate statistics on mortality by age, sex and cause of death; disease incidence and prevalence; coverage of interventions, including quality of services; prevalence of risk factors; financial protection; and data on health system inputs and outputs to manage and plan services. The data generated through the country information system allows a country to monitor the progress and performance of both the overall health sector plan and disease-specific subplans, such as those for HIV, tuberculosis, malaria, etc. at both national and sub-national level. By starting from a known baseline, progress can be paced appropriately given the available resources.

9.2.2 Because country monitoring is the basis for regional and global monitoring of priority health issues

Over 90 targets have been endorsed by Member States at the World Health Assembly and other governing bodies. There are also hundreds of recommended indicators to cover the wide array of health and disease programmes. WHO and partners have agreed on a Global Reference Set of 100 Core Indicators to be prioritized for the purposes of monitoring progress.[3]

Monitoring, evaluation and review provide the basic measurement systems and accountability mechanisms to plan, manage and account for the objectives and targets of the national health strategy.

9.2.3 Because reporting progress on health-related SDGs requires sound M&E systems

The overarching health goal is associated with 13 targets (or subgoals), including three related to the MDGs, three related to the emerging agenda of noncommunicable diseases and injuries, and three cross-cutting or health systems focused, including universal health coverage (UHC) (See Fig. 9.2). Additional health-related indicators are included in other SDG goals.

Reporting progress on the 13 targets of health-related SGDs, such as universal health coverage, requires sound M&E systems.

9.2.4 Because health inequities need to be monitored

Statistics should highlight health inequalities by major stratifiers, including demographic (age, sex/gender), socioeconomic status (wealth, education), and geography (province/district) or other characteristics (migration, minorities etc.). Data on levels and inequalities in financial protection and coverage of interventions are the core of UHC monitoring.

9.2.5 Because countries need functional surveillance mechanisms

All countries need active disease/public health surveillance for detecting, reporting and responding to specific notifiable conditions and events, in particular epidemic-prone communicable diseases. Surveillance systems draw upon multiple sources of information, including routine health and disease records and sentinel surveillance systems in specific populations.

9.2.6 Because monitoring, evaluation and review are a necessary basis for accountability

The monitoring of national priorities, including health-related SDGs, requires well-established mechanisms for accountability at country, regional and global levels. Such mechanisms need to be inclusive, independent, evidence-based and transparent, and lead to remedial actions.

Fig. 9.2 Health SDG monitoring framework[4]

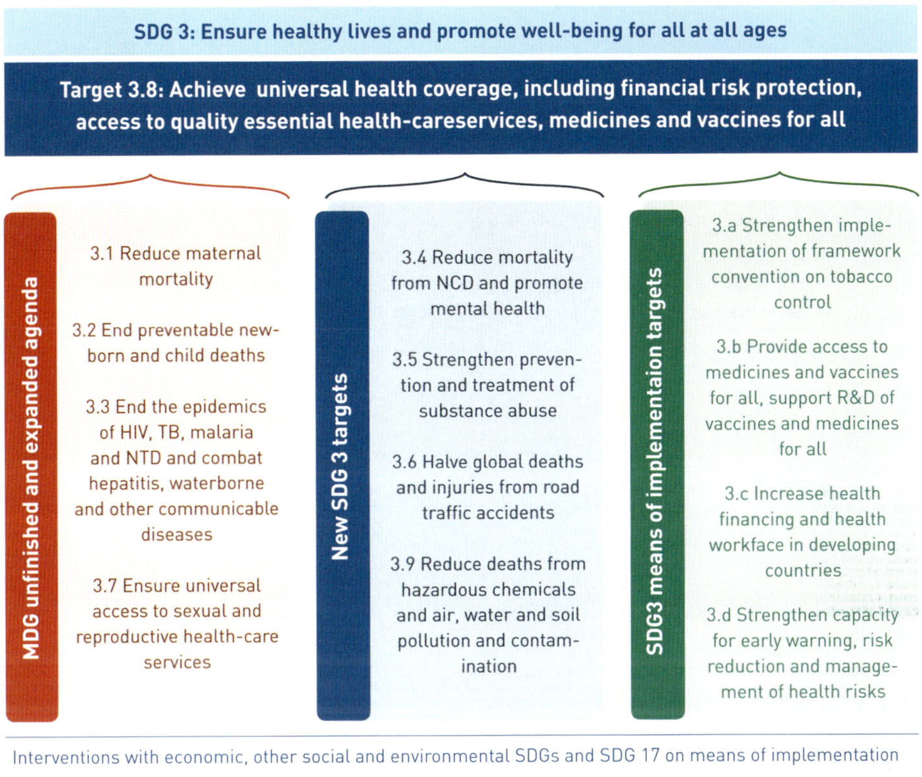

9.2.7 Because there is a growing interest and demand for quality data for decision-making and accountability

In the Summit on Measurement and Accountability for Results in Health in June 2015, over 600 global health leaders, decision-makers, thought-leaders and implementers from over 60 countries representing development partners, partner country governments, and civil society endorsed the Health Measurement and Accountability Post-2015 Roadmap[5] and 5-Point Call to Action.[6] The Call to Action identifies a set of priority actions and targets that aims at strengthening country data and accountability systems for the post-2015 sustainable development agenda. The Health Data Collaborative was formed as a result of a call from Global Health Agency leaders (September 2015) to do more together to support countries implementing the five point call to action. The value add of the Collaborative is collective and aligned action that aims to reduce fragmentation in country HISs, to maximize the impact of respective investments and to enhance sustainability.

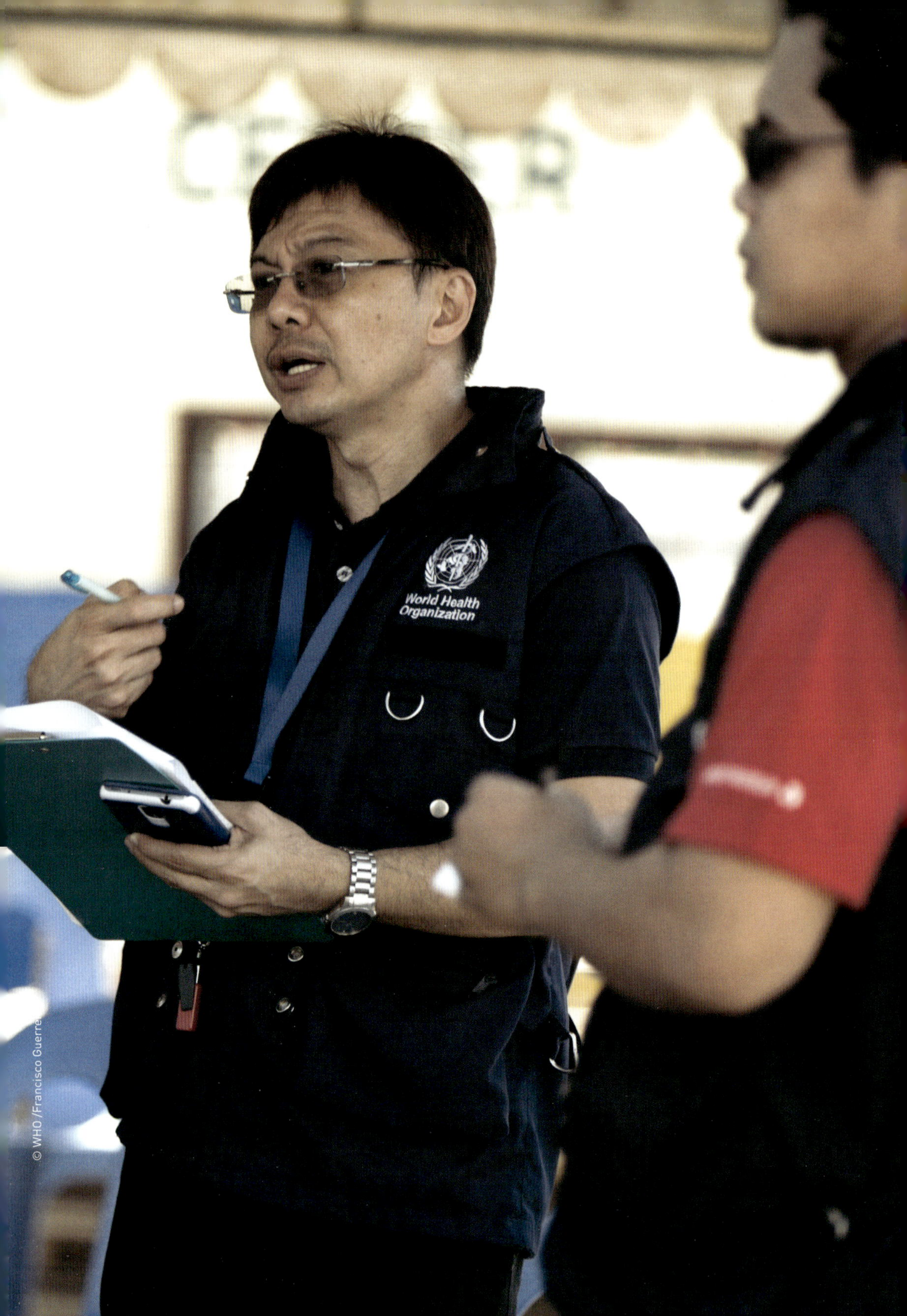
World Health
Organization

9.3 What are the components of an M&E platform?

In order for an M&E platform to be strengthened, it is important to understand the desirable end result: a sound country-led platform for monitoring, evaluation and review. It has four main components. These are:

- sound policy and institutional environment;
- well-functioning data sources;
- strong institutional capacity for data collection, management, analysis, use and dissemination;
- effective country mechanisms for review and action.

This section reviews the main components of the M&E platform.

9.3.1 Sound policy and institutional environment for M&E

A sound policy and institutional environment includes the following key elements.

Effective governance structure and coordination mechanisms

The monitoring, evaluation and review platform requires an effective governance structure, in which key institutions and stakeholders have clear roles and responsibilities in the process of collecting, analyzing and using data for decision-making. An effective governance structure includes a country-led coordination mechanism for conducting monitoring, evaluation, and periodic review of the health sector with active multi-stakeholder participation (government, development partners, and civil society). Typically this coordination mechanism is a sub-group of the overarching Health Sector Coordination Committee.

A strong M&E plan

A strong M&E plan addresses the goals and objectives of the NHPSP and is based on a sound situation analysis of the M&E system in the country. The M&E plan is comprehensive and addresses the selection of a balanced parsimonious set of core indicators with well-defined baselines and targets, identifies the data sources for each indicator and specifies plans for addressing data gaps and weaknesses and conducting data quality assessments, specifies analytical outputs, and plans for communication and dissemination of results. The plan also outlines ways to address institutional capacity-building in data collection, analysis and dissemination. Annex 9.1 provides a template outline for the development of a comprehensive M&E plan. The M&E plan can also be accompanied by a comprehensive national HIS strategy that provides additional details for strengthening the country HIS.

A comprehensive M&E framework guides the monitoring, evaluation and review work, including the selection of core indicators and targets. The IHP+ common M&E logical framework (see Fig. 9.3) provides a logical and results-chain representation of the M&E and review work, and shows how inputs into the health system (e.g. financing and infrastructure) and processes (e.g.

A sound country-led platform for monitoring, evaluation and review includes a sound policy and institutional environment; well-functioning data sources; a strong institutional capacity for data collection, management, analysis, use and dissemination; and effective country mechanisms for review and action.

supply chain) are reflected in outputs (such as the availability of services and interventions) and eventual outcomes (e.g. intervention coverage) and impact (e.g. improved health outcomes). The framework not only facilitates the identification of core indicators of the NHPSP along each link in the results chain, but also links indicators to data collection methods. The common M&E framework can be used by all stakeholders and government to demonstrate performance of both programmes and health systems.

Fig. 9.3 The IHP+ common M&E logical framework for a national health strategy

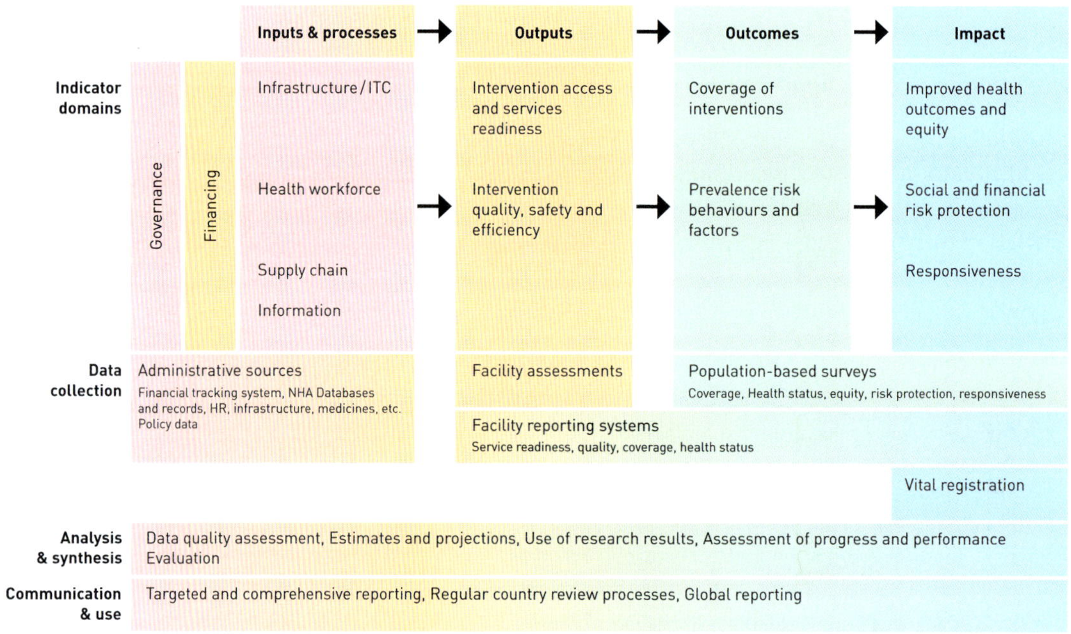

Source: Monitoring, evaluation and review of national health strategies: a country-led platform for information and accountability. Geneva: World Health Organization; 2011 (http://www.who.int/healthinfo/country_monitoring_evaluation/1085_IER_131011_web.pdf?ua=1, accessed 17 October 2016).

Core indicators and targets based on international data standards

Core indicators

Selection of indicators should be informed by considerations of scientific soundness, relevance, usefulness for decision-making, responsiveness to change, and data availability. The challenge is to ensure a balanced parsimonious set of core indicators with well-defined baseline and targets. The core indicator set should be responsive to the information needs for monitoring progress and performance towards the main objectives of the NHPSP, and there should be an appropriate balance across the logical framework (i.e. covering inputs, outputs, outcomes and impact) and across major programme areas (see Box 9.1).

It is important to keep in mind that quantitative indicators are intended to be indicative of reality, i.e. they are tracer indicators and they are not intended to describe the totality of what is happening.

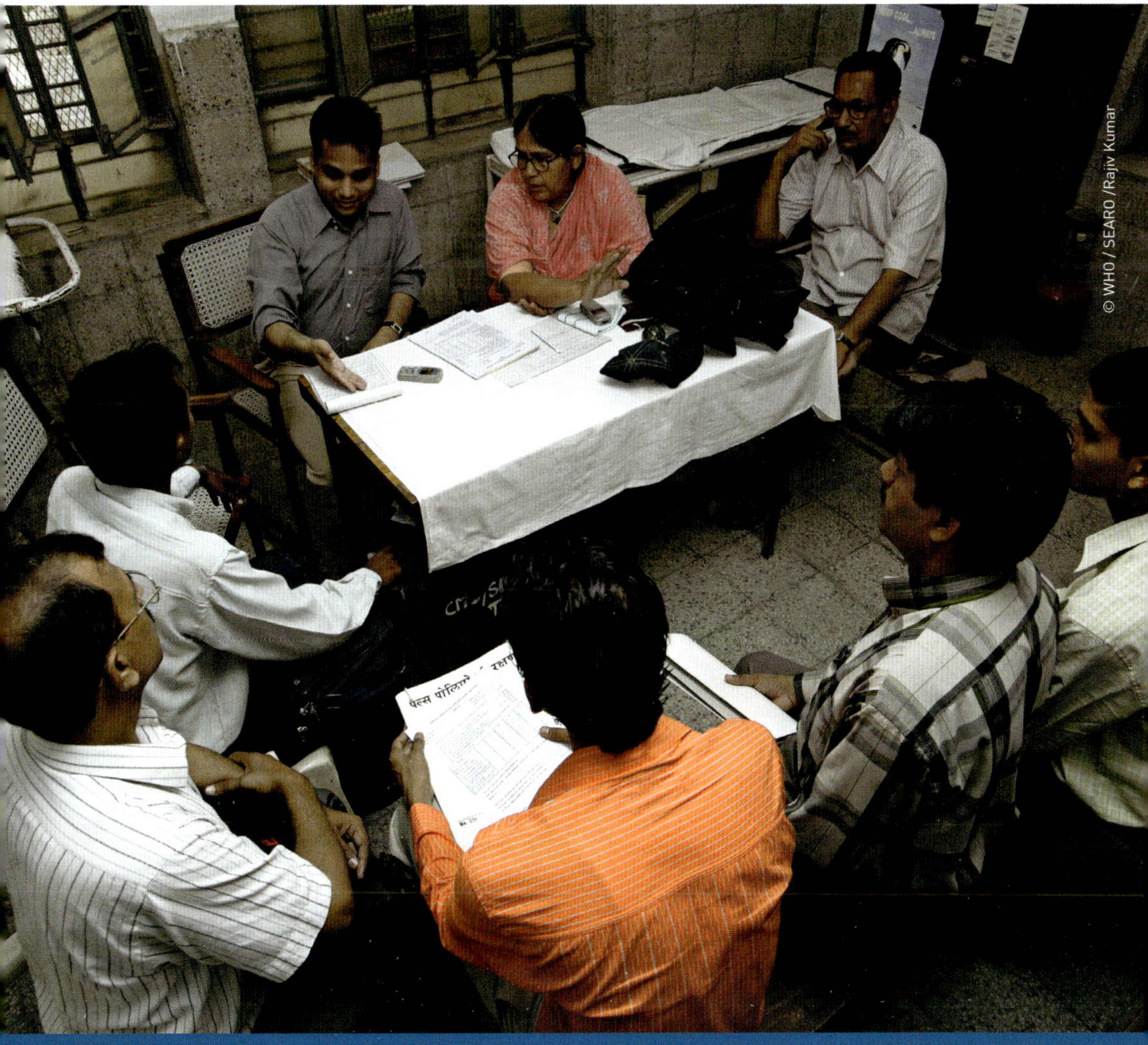

Box 9.1

Global Reference List of 100 Core Health Indicators[7]

Adopting international standardized indicators allows countries to benchmark their performance against similar countries in their region or income category. It also reduces the effort in generating separate reports for in-country and external stakeholders. The Global Reference List of 100 Core Health Indicators is a standard set of core indicators prioritized by the global community to provide concise information on the health situation and trends, including responses at national and global levels. The Global Reference List of 100 Core Health Indicators contains indicators of relevance to country, regional and global reporting across the spectrum of global health priorities, including the post-2015 health goals of the SDGs. Countries can choose the set of indicators that match their national health strategy's priorities and their capacity to collect the necessary data. Fig. 9.4 provides an overview of the Global Reference List of 100 Core Health Indicators.

Health status

Mortality by age and sex

- Life expectancy at birth
- Adult mortality rate between 15 and 60
- years of age
- Under-five mortality rate
- Infant mortality rate
- Neonatal mortality rate
- Stillbirth rate
- Mortality by cause

Maternal mortality ratio

- TB mortality rate
- AIDS-related mortality rate
- Malaria mortality rate
- Mortality between 30 and 70 years of age from cardiovascular diseases, cancer, diabetes or chronic respiratory diseases
- Suicide rate
- Mortality rate from road traffic injuries

Fertility

- Adolescent fertility rate
- Total fertility rate

Morbidity

- New cases of vaccine-preventable diseases
- New cases of IHR-notifiable diseases and other notifiable diseases
- HIV incidence rate
- HIV prevalence rate
- Hepatitis B surface antigen prevalence
- Sexually transmitted infections (STIs)
- incidence rate
- TB incidence rate
- TB notification rate
- TB prevalence rate
- Malaria parasite prevalence among childen aged 6-59 months
- Malaria incidence rate
- Cancer incidence, by type of cancer

Fig. 9.4 Global Reference List of 100 Core health indicators

Risk factors

Nutrition
- Exclusive breastfeeding rate 0-5 months of age
- Early initiation of breastfeeding
- Incidence of low birth weight among newborns
- Children under 5 years who are stunted
- Children under 5 years who are wasted
- Anaemia prevalence in children
- Anaemia prevalence in women of reproductive age

Infections
- Condom use at last sex with high-risk partner

Environmental risk factors
- Population using safely managed drinking-water services
- Population using safely managed sanitation services
- Population using modern fuels for cooking/heating/lighting
- Air pollution level in cities

Noncommunicable diseases
- Total alcohol per capita (age 15+ years) consumption
- Tobacco use among persons aged 18+ years
- Children aged under 5 years who are overweight
- Overweight and obesity in adults (Also: adolescents)
- Raised blood pressure among adults
- Raised blood glucose/diabetes among adults
- Salt intake
- Insufficient physical activity in adults (Also: adolescents)

Injuries
- Intimate partner violence prevalence

Service coverage

Reproductive, maternal, newborn, child, and adolescent
- Demand for family planning satisfied with modern methods
- Contraceptive prevalence rate
- Antenatal care coverage
- Births attended by skilled health personnel
- Postpartum care coverage
- Care-seeking for symptoms of pneumonia
- Children with diarrhoea receiving oral rehydration solution (ORS)
- Vitamin A supplementation coverage

Immunization
- Immunization coverage rate by vaccine for each vaccine in the national schedule

HIV
- People living with HIV who have been diagnosed
- Prevention of mother-to-child transmission
- HIV care coverage
- Antiretroviral therapy (ART) coverage
- HIV viral load suppression

HIV/TB
- TB preventive therapy for HIV-positive people newly enrolled in HIV care
- HIV test results for registered new and relapse TB patients
- HIV-positive new and relapse TB patients on ART during TB treatment

Tuberculosis
- TB patients with results for drug susceptibility testing
- TB case detection rate
- Second-line treatment coverage among multi-drug resistant tuberculosis (MDR-TB) cases

Malaria
- Intermittent preventative therapy for malaria during pregnancy (IPTp)
- Use of insecticide treated nets (ITNs)
- Treatment of confirmed malaria cases
- Indoor residual spraying (IRS) coverage

Neglected tropical diseases
- Coverage of preventive chemotherapy for selected neglected tropcial diseases

Screening and preventive care
- Cervical cancer screening

Mental Health
- Coverage of services for severe mental health disorders

Health systems

Quality and safety of care
- Perioperative mortality rate
- Obstetric and gynaecological admissions
- owing to abortion
- Institutional maternal mortality ratio
- Maternal death reviews
- ART retention rate
- TB treatment success rate
- Service-specific availability and readiness

Access
- Service utilization
- Health service areas
- Hospital bed density
- Availability of essential medicines and commodities

Health workforce
- Health worker density and distribution
- Output training institutions

Health information
- Birth registration coverage
- Death registration coverage
- Completeness of reporting by facilities

Health financing
- Total current expenditure on health (% of gross domestic product)
- Current expenditure on health by general government and compulsory schemes (% of current expenditure on health)
- Out-of-pocket payment for health (% of current expenditure on health)
- Externally sourced funding (% of current expenditure on health)
- Total capital expenditure on health (% current + capital expenditure on health)
- Headcount ratio of catastrophic health expenditure
- Headcount ratio of impoverishing health expenditure

Health security
- International Health Regulations (IHR) core capacity index

Baselines and targets

Each core indicator must have a defined, time-bound target. Setting targets requires a baseline measurement that provides the starting point from which achievements are defined. Targets describe a level of progress that is realistic but meaningful given the resource investment. Target definitions must also take into account the methods used for measurement and the feasibility and frequency with which measurements are taken (see Box 9.2 and Fig. 9.5).

Box 9.2

Target setting approaches

There are several approaches to framing targets, depending on the type of achievement and information available.

- Absolute targets: a specific numerical target citing a baseline value, e.g. measles vaccination coverage from 70% to 85% in five years.
- Relative targets: a relative change that is independent of the initial value of the starting point (for example, a reduction of the under-five mortality rate by two thirds (Millennium Development Goal 4). Relative target-setting is often used when baselines are uncertain.
- Annual rates of change: describes the pace of change expected, especially during a period of ramping up services, e.g. increase in expanded coverage from 2% per year to 4% per year.

Fig. 9.5 Core indicators of the United Republic of Tanzania Health Sector Strategic Plan (HSSP) III[8]

	Overall Progress	Achievement	Target 2015	Equity	Compare (rank)
HEALTH STATUS					
Life expectancy (years)		61 (F)/58 (M) (2011)	62/59		
Under-5 mortality rate		81/1,000 (2006-10)	54		1
Neonatal mortality rate		26/1,000 (2006-10)	19		1
Infant mortality rate		51/1,000 (2006-10)	-		1
Child stunting rate		35% (2011)	22%	GRW	3
Child underweight rate		14% (2011)	14%		5
Maternal mortality rate		454/100,000 (2004-10)	156	G	2
Total fertility rate		5.4 (2008-10)	5.1	GRW	4
Adolescent fertility rate		44% (2010)	39%	GRW	5
HIV prevalence among young people		2.0% (2011/2)	-	G	
HIV prevalence, pregnant women (15-24)					
TB notification rate		75% (2011) 52% (2012)	70%		
Leprosy cases diagnosed and treated					
Cholera incidence rate		343 cases	0		
Cholera case fatality rate		4.1%	<1%		
Malaria prevalence among OPD (lab)		33% (under 5)(2012)	-		
Parasitemia prevalence (children)		9.2% (2012	5%		
COVERAGE OF INTERVENTIONS					
Measles immunization coverage		100% (2012)	85%		1
DTP-Hb 3 immunization coverage		95% (2012)	85%		4
Vit A coverage (2 doses)		60% (2010)	-	GW	7
TT2 immunization coverage		88% (2011)	90%		
ANC first visit → 16 weeks		15% (2006-10)	60%		5
ANC at least 4 visits		36% (2009-10)	90%	R	7
Births in health facilities		58% (2011)	70%	GRW	
Skilled birth attendance		62% (2010-11)	80%	GRW	8
Postnatal care coverage		31% (2006-10)	-		
Contraceptive prevalence rate		27% (2010)	60%	GRW	5
ITN use (children/pregnant women)		73%/75% (2011/12)	80%		3
eMTCT coverage among pregnant women		77% (2011)	80%		
ART coverage among those in need		65% (2012)	60%		
TB treatment success rate		90% (2011)	85%		2
HEALTH SYSTEMS					
Government expenditure on health (%)		7.3% (2011)	15%		
Total health expenditure per capita		$37			
Insurance coverage (CHF/TIKA)		3% (2010)	80%		
Health worker density: doctors & AMO		0.9/10,000	-		
Health worker density: nurse-midwives		4.9/10,000	-		
Health worker density: pharmacists		0.12/10,000			
Outpatient visits per capita/year		0.73 per person	30		
Training institutes with full accreditation		56			
Stockouts of tracer meds & vaccine					

Unified data architecture

Countries benefit from instituting policies and enforcing commitment to implement a data architecture which is integrated with the national HIS. This includes providing comprehensive specifications on the content and accessibility of data sources. The availability of fully documented data standards for the national HIS fosters compatibility between data sources and across programme areas that maintain separate M&E systems.

Innovative Information technologies can play a role in strengthening data sources; for example, the use of electronic patient and facility records, application of hand-held devices for data collection, and data sharing and exchange through interoperable databases, which may be located at facility, district, regional and national levels. Countries should provide the overall legal and policy framework for technical and other innovations in health information. This includes use of electronic devices for web-based reporting of health events and feedback, which may occur at individual and aggregate levels. Development partners should support innovations that focus on scalable sustainable national approaches, and capacity development including public-private partnerships, collaborative arrangements with academia, and use of IT, as well as south-south and peer-to-peer collaboration.

The comprehensive M&E plan provides the basis for a multiyear costing/investment framework for M&E that government and development partners at all levels can commit to funding in order to monitor, evaluate and review the national health strategy.

A common investment framework

The comprehensive M&E plan provides the basis for a multiyear costing and investment framework for M&E that government and development partners at all levels can commit to funding in order to monitor, evaluate and review the national health strategy. Through a common investment framework, the government and its partners can identify shortfalls in funding, as well as avoid duplication of investment (see Box 9.3).

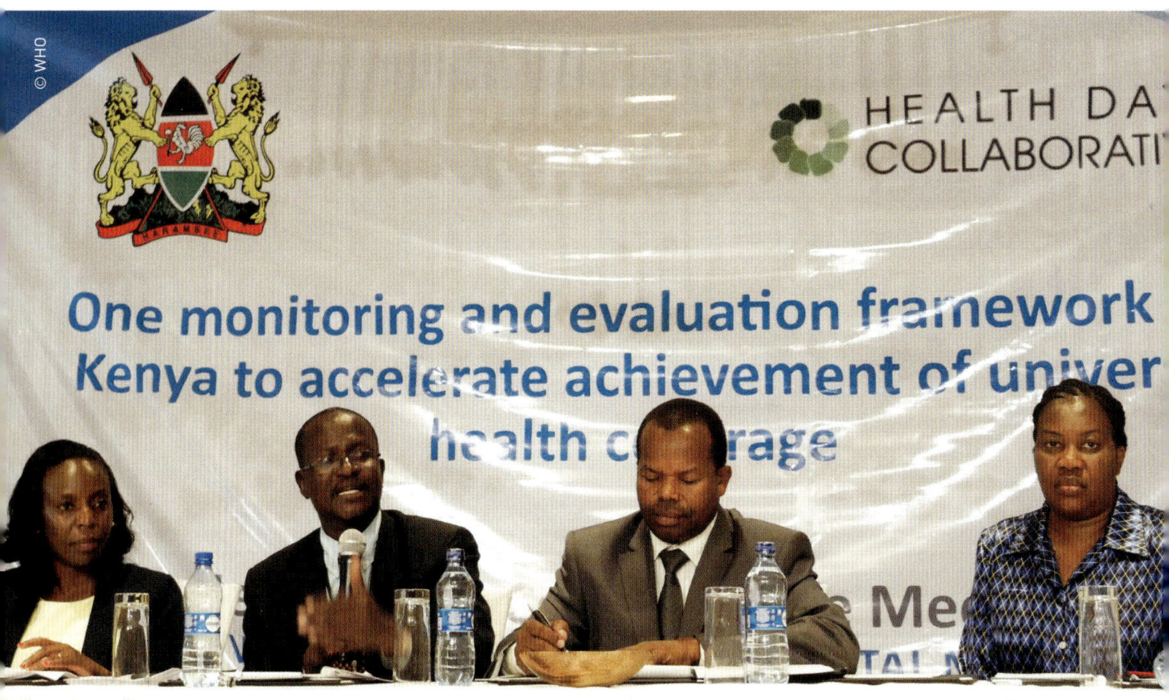

Box 9.3

Kenya case study: roadmap for one costed M&E Plan[9]

In many countries, single disease-focused M&E systems sometimes operate in isolation instead of talking to each other and linking up with government-led efforts. Some of these systems gather data on indicators that do not match up with those identified by countries in their national health plans. This creates inefficiencies and burdens health workers with reporting requirements.

In Kenya, to support the health ministry's leadership in integrating these M&E systems into a unified, more efficient framework, global health partners are now working together to harmonize their financial and technical resources and ensure they are in line with country priorities. During a four-day meeting in Nairobi in May 2016, various stakeholders signed a joint statement of commitments to support a unified "One M&E Framework" and launch the Kenya Health Data Collaborative. Partners in attendance included CDC (United States Centers for Disease Control and Prevention), GAVI (Global Alliance for Vaccines and Immunization), GIZ (Deutsche Gezellschaft für International Zasammenarbeit), Global Fund (Global Fund to fight AIDS, Tuberculosis and Malaria), PEPFAR (President's Emergency Fund for AIDS Relief), UNAIDS (Joint United Nations Programme on HIV/AIDS), UNICEF (United Nations Children's Fund), USAID (United States Agency for International Development), WHO, and World Bank Group.

The Ministry of Health (MoH) has drafted a detailed costed roadmap to be implemented by technical working groups focused on data analytics, quality of care, a new national health data observatory, civil registration and vital statistics, and informatics.

This collaborative approach will strengthen Kenya's HIS through a united front supporting and investing in one national M&E plan.

9.3.2 Well-functioning data sources

The broad array of health-related indicators that need to be monitored means that no single data source is able to meet all statistical needs. Country HISs should draw upon multiple data sources, led by competent country institutions for data collection, compilation and sharing, analysis and synthesis, and communication and use of results. The main data sources for health statistics as well as their predominant characteristics are outlined below (see also Fig. 9.6).

No single data source is able to meet all statistical needs; country HIS should draw upon multiple data sources.

Census of population and housing

This is the primary information source for determining the size of a population, its geographical distribution, and its social, demographic and economic characteristics. Censuses provide a denominator for the computation of vital statistics and many health indicators, especially in the absence of reliable information from the CRVS systems. Ideally the census should be conducted every 10 years, and it provides comprehensive vital statistical data.

CRVS systems

All countries should have CRVS systems that record the occurrence and characteristics of births, deaths and other vital events to produce fertility and mortality statistics. Statistics on causes of death are generated from the medical certification of cause of death according to the standards set out in the International Statistical Classification of Diseases (ICD). Where this is not possible, verbal autopsy can be used to estimate cause of death distributions in the population. Sample vital event registration systems are used as an intermediate measure to generate vital statistics using innovative methods.

Population-based surveys

Countries should have in place a multiyear programme of national health surveys for monitoring progress on key aspects on population health status, service coverage, health-related behaviours and risk factors, and out-of-pocket spending on health, including equity dimensions and the use of biomarkers. A survey programme identifies strategic priorities, periodicity and scope of data collection and enforces quality assurance, ethical practices, transparency and data sharing in accordance with stringent confidentiality protocols and in line with international standards for measurement to ensure comparability of results between populations and over time.

Health facility and community information systems

Timely and reliable statistics should be produced by health facilities (public and private) and communities to monitor health system inputs, disease patterns, health service provision and outcomes, including facility-based mortality and cause of death. Wherever feasible, electronic recording and web-based reporting systems should be used. The data are analysed and used in combination with other sources for planning, reviews and action at local, district and national levels of the health system. The facility information system includes verification through facility assessments to monitor quality of service delivery and care provided as well as data quality.

Public health/disease surveillance

Public health/disease surveillance systems detect, report, and respond to notifiable communicable diseases and other health events. Data generated by notifications should lead to immediate action for outbreak control. Wherever feasible, disease surveillance and response systems should be linked to routine facility and community information systems. Effective surveillance should improve detection and prediction of epidemics, as well as provide an objective assessment and efficient monitoring of intervention programmes. A well-defined set of core functions and surveillance capacities is monitored by WHO under the International Health Regulations.

Administrative data sources

All countries should have comprehensive databases and electronic tracking systems on health expenditures, logistics management, including commodities, medicines, equipment and supplies. An electronic health workforce registry can be used to track health workforce statistics. Systems of health accounts and health workforce accounts should be kept according to international standards.

Non-health sector data sources

Data sources from other sectors could also provide information related to the major causes of the global burden of disease or threats to health security, such as information on water and sanitation, air pollution, or the education sector.

Fig. 9.6 Preferred data sources for core health indicators

EXAMPLE OF CORE INDICATORS		PREFERRED DATA SOURCES
Vital events Noncommuniable disease mortality Suicide mortality rate Pollution-related mortality and illness Birth (death) registration	←	Civil registration and vital statistics system
Morbidity HIV incidence	←	Household surveys
Risk factors Malnutrition; insufficient physical activity; anaemia; tobacco use; acceptable diet; early breastfeeding; exclusive breastfeeding	←	
Health systems Financial protection; sexual and reproductive health (SRH) knowledge	←	
Coverage of interventions *Prevention*: skilled birth attendant; post-partum contact; syphillis *Screening*: immunization coverage; Insecticide-treated nets; family planning needs *Treatment:* Oral rehydration solution treatment; Skilled birth attendants; pneumonia care seeking; Anti-retroviral therapy;	←	Routine health faciltiy and community information systems Health facility assessments Household surveys
Policy environment Country's laws- SRH access	←	Administrative data sources

9.3.3 Strong institutional capacity for data collection, management, analysis, use and dissemination

All countries should have adequate institutional capacity for health data collection, compilation and sharing, data quality assurance, analysis and synthesis using all relevant data sources, and for communication and use of results. Capacity strengthening of country institutions, including MoH, national statistical office, and national public health and academic institutions are supported by global partners where relevant.

The specific areas in which capacity is required include the following.

Data collection

In general, the national statistics office (NSO) is responsible for household health surveys and vital statistics from birth and death registrations. However, the MoH often plays a major role as well. The MoH often leads on the compilation of administrative and clinical data, and may work with specific institutions to assess data quality. In addition, facility assessments are often conducted by the MoH, in which case, some degree of independence is needed for data collection, e.g. by employing staff from training schools for the field work.

Data compilation and storage

This involves bringing together data generated by the NSO, MoH, researchers, donors, development partners, nongovernmental organizations and others. This is usually the responsibility of the MoH or the NSO, but sometimes a semi-independent institution plays a major role. Providing public access to the health data is a critical element of transparency in a sound M&E system.

Data quality assessment, validation and adjustment

This should include independent assessments of the quality of data generated from clinical and administrative sources, ad-hoc surveys, and other data sources. This is ideally done by independent country institutions such as research and academic centres, working in collaboration with the MoH and the NSO.

Data analysis and performance reviews.

This involves synthesizing data from multiple sources for the purpose of reviews, planning, policy analysis, regional and global reporting, and evaluation. This work is ideally carried out by country institutions in collaboration with the MoH and NSO. Global partners may also provide technical assistance.

Estimation and statistical modelling.

Focusing on key health statistics, this includes the application of global standards, tools and methods to correct for bias and missing values; the generation of estimates; and forecasting for

All countries should have adequate institutional capacity for health data collection, compilation and sharing; data quality assurance; analysis and synthesis using all relevant data sources; and for communication and use of results.

planning purposes. Academic institutions as well as data analysis staff in the MoH or NSO have the main responsibility for estimation and statistical modelling.

Data presentation and dissemination to different target audiences.

The focus of data presentation and dissemination is on major decision-making processes, where effective communication of results may lead to an adjustment of implementation and revisions of plans. Global reporting should be aligned as much as possible with national reporting. Communicating to the general public and media is also critical and usually requires special skills. The responsibility for data presentation and dissemination often lies with data analysts in government and academic institutions, but special communication skills are required.

Box 9.4

Presenting data to assess equity

Achieving a goal such as UHC is fundamentally a question of equity. The figure below provides an example of how to display coverage inequity between the poorest quintile and richest quintile of a population for an array of essential health services.

Presenting measures of equity in health service coverage

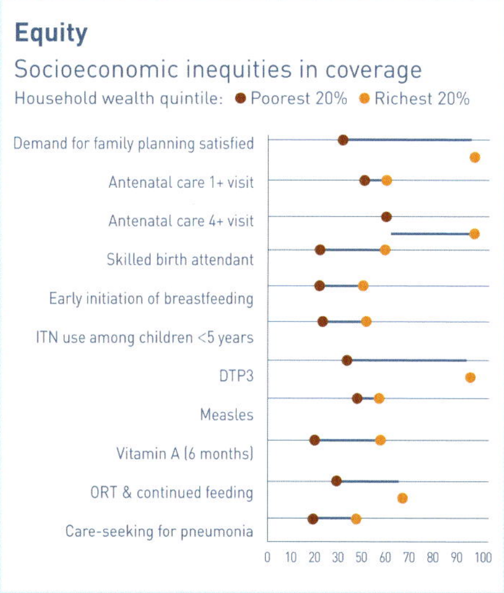

Source DHS 2007

Coverage levels are shown for the poorest 20% (re circles) and the ricket 20% (orange circles). The longer the line between the two groups, the greater the inequality. These estimates may differ from other charts due to differences in data sources.

The use of standard reports and graphics (such as above) help decision-makers to identify gaps easily and allow comparisons in performance between local areas and national level. Similar graphics can be used to assess equity in terms of other population characteristics such as geographical location, sex, and age.

9.3.4 Strong mechanisms for review and action

The value of an M&E platform depends on the extent to which data are reviewed, and used to take action to improve health outcomes (see Box 9.5). A clear indication that results from reviews do influence decision-making is when they are used to guide resource allocation and financial disbursement.

A clear indication that results from reviews do influence decision-making is when they are used to guide resource allocation and financial disbursement.

Box 9.5

Using health data in a situation analysis or sector review

Health data should be an integral part and parcel of any health sector situation analysis[I] or review. A health sector situation analysis is an in-depth look at all aspects related to inputs, processes, and outputs of the health sector, i.e. a full snapshot of the sector. This information is extremely relevant and useful to compare and contrast with existing data and information to better monitor progress. If existing data and information is sparse, a situation analysis can serve as a baseline to inform future monitoring and evaluation rounds. In a health sector review, the focus of the analysis is more on medium- to long-term trends, and on understanding root causes in order to propose feasible and viable solutions.

A health data analysis, combined with an examination of how activities in the health sector have been implemented and whether they are in line with the planned budget, can provide a solid evidence base for policy dialogue on why certain policies, strategies or plans have worked or not. The figure below demonstrates how health data is directly used and fed into the health sector policy dialogue.

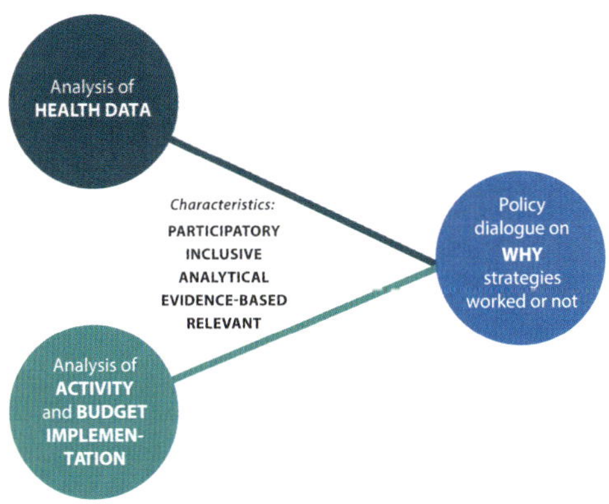

I For more information, see Chapter 3 "Situation analysis of the health sector" in this handbook.

Strong mechanisms for review and action have the following key attributes.

Mechanisms to provide routine feedback

Feedback loops should be bidirectional, allowing local service providers the information needed to address gaps in coverage or quality and for central level analysts to more effectively analyse and interpret data given local context and information needs. Open and transparent data systems are necessary to ensure all stakeholders can participate fully in the review and action planning process. This includes sub-national levels and nongovernmental stakeholders, among others. Service providers also benefit from benchmarking their performance against their peers as part of a supportive supervision approach, rather than a review system that penalizes open and candid examination of achievements and challenges.

A system of progress and performance reviews

There should be a system of joint periodic progress and performance reviews that involves a broad array of key stakeholders. The process must be a transparent system in which the measures of success and methods of measurement are documented and the results made available for public review. Reviews should take place at different intervals with different objectives (see Box 9.6).

Box 9.6

Types of reviews

Annual review: The annual review is focused on the indicators and targets specified in annual operational plans. These are mainly input, process and output indicators. If available, coverage indicators are also used. Annual reviews should help inform evaluation on a regular basis.

Mid-term review: This is normally conducted half way through implementation of the NHPSP. It covers all the targets mentioned in the strategy, including targets for outcome and impact indicators, and also takes contextual changes into account. The mid-term review should coincide with the annual review (e.g. the third year in a five-year plan). The results are used to adjust national priorities and objectives.

Final review: This involves a comprehensive analysis of progress and performance for the whole period of the NHPSP. The final review builds upon the annual and mid-term reviews, but also brings in results of specific research and of prospective evaluation that should be built in from the beginning.

Programme-specific reviews should not be conducted as separate, parallel activities – rather, they should be linked to the overall health sector review and contribute to it. This includes both the timing of the review and the methodology or analyses of data required.

Evaluation is planned in advance and implemented prospectively

A well-designed evaluation is planned at the same time as the development of the monitoring and evaluation plan for the national health strategy. Prospective evaluation combines data from routine monitoring systems for key indicators, complemented by in-depth studies – both quantitative (preferably longitudinal) and qualitative. These data are analysed together to draw conclusions about the attribution of changes to specific interventions and the contribution of contextual changes. Where possible, evaluations should use data from, and strengthen, health sector reviews. They should build upon existing country systems and include an explicit capacity-building and system-strengthening objective, where appropriate.

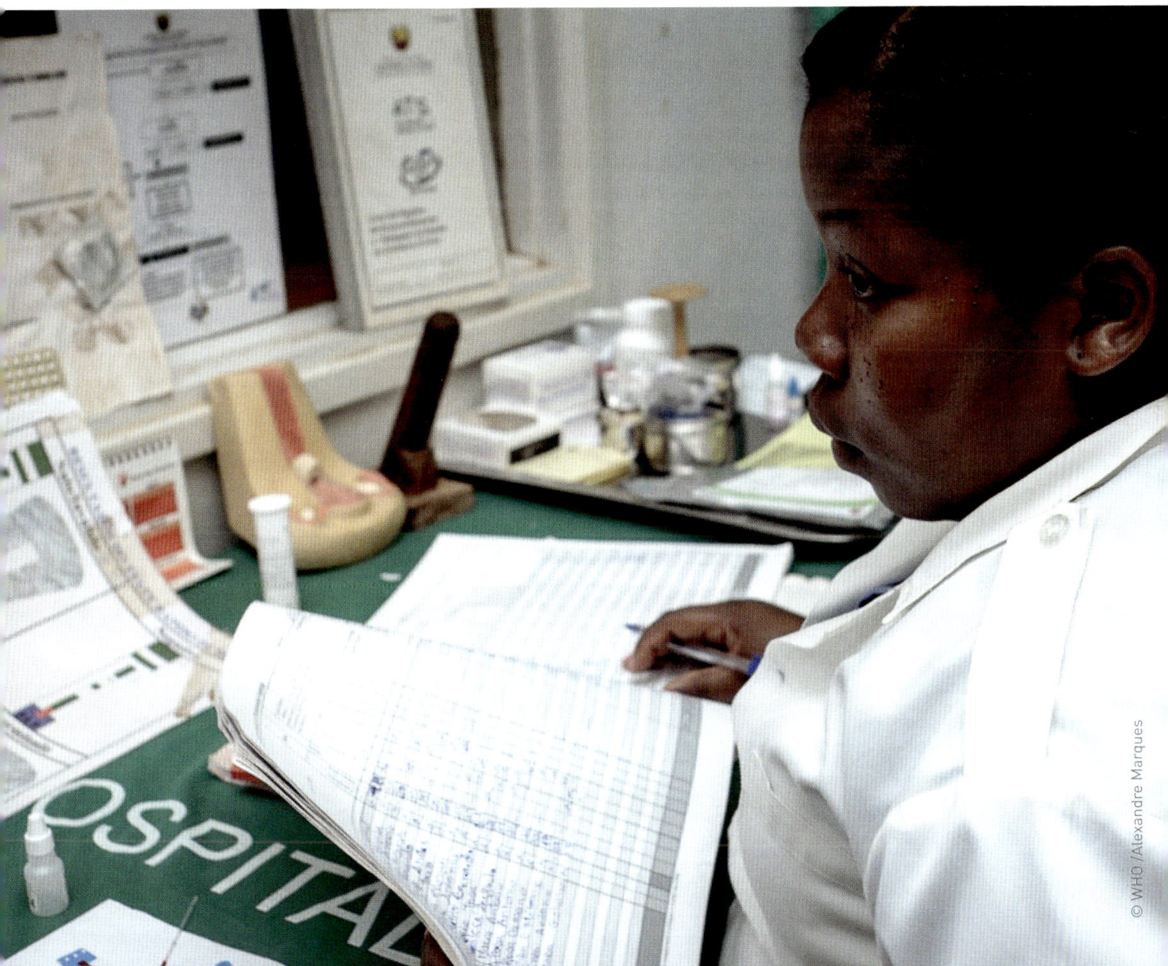

9.4 How can a country-led M&E platform be strengthened?

A country-led M&E platform can be strengthened by assessing key attributes of the platform and identifying priority actions, developing a comprehensive M&E plan and reviewing and evaluating the platform regularly.

1. **Assess the key attributes of the M&E platform as required and identify priority actions to address key gaps and weaknesses.**

   The country's M&E platform must be assessed according to the standards and attributes of a well-functioning platform in order to identify its gaps, strengths and weaknesses. Priorities should be identified based on the gaps.

2. **Review and select core set of indicators and develop baseline and targets for monitoring national priorities and health goals.**

   Based on the priorities set out in the national health strategy, MoH – jointly with stakeholders – must review and select a set of national core indicators. Programme-specific strategies should be reviewed alongside the overall NHPSP to identify and harmonize core indicators (see Box 9.7).

3. **Develop a comprehensive M&E plan, ensuring alignment of disease-specific plans and identification of priority actions.**

   The M&E plan should specify the coordination and alignment of M&E processes and mechanisms across specific programmes. The alignment of disease- and programme-specific plans with the NHPSP can be improved by ensuring that there is one comprehensive national M&E plan that specifies how it is linked to the disease-specific M&E plans in a logical and cascading manner.

4. **Cost the M&E plan and develop a common investment framework as the basis for domestic and partner investments.**

   A prioritized, costed action plan is the first step in garnering resources to strengthen the M&E platform. For each set of activities, domestic and partner investments should be identified and documented as a part of a common investment framework.

5. **Review and evaluate the M&E platform regularly.**

   Regular planned assessments of the M&E system are required in order to ensure that indicators are measuring what they are meant to; that data are generated according to standards; that data analysis and communication of results give the information needed by decision-makers; and that data management includes an assessment of overall data quality.

Malawi case study: "More can actually mean less"

Malawi's process for selecting the indicators included in the M&E framework of the country's second Health Sector Strategic Plan (HSSP II) began in late 2014. The list started with 195 indicators, and was progressively reduced. The Ministry of Health Department of Planning and Policy Development refined the list with collaboration of all MoH departments and in-country health partners. Stakeholders recognized that too many indicators place too much of a burden on data collection efforts and can obscure the view into the country's health priorities.

"We have a plethora of suggested indicators," says Dr Simon Ndira, a senior technical advisor on health information systems at the Ministry of Health. "But there is a general tendency to want to capture lots and lots of data without necessarily reflecting back to realize that more can actually mean less."

The criteria for selecting the core indicators considers several factors:

1. whether they are needed to track the new health-related SDGs;
2. whether they correspond with the list of 100 core indicators recommended by WHO;
3. whether they are included in the previous NHPSP, to allow tracking indicators over time;
4. whether they align with programme-specific indicators; and
5. whether they make sense in the context of Malawi's health priorities.

One major change in the list of core indicators included in HSSPII compared to HSSP I are measures to track newly emerging health problems, particularly noncommunicable diseases such as diabetes and hypertension; and multi-sectorial issues, such as sanitation, environment and nutrition.

As Malawi selects its core indicators, stakeholders also plan how to strengthen the relevant sources for collecting the data, such as the CRVS programme, and other administrative data sources.

9.5 Who should be involved in monitoring, evaluation and review?

At the request of the MoH, and under country leadership, key stakeholders – including different levels of government, civil society organizations (CSOs), international development partners, and local research institutions, among others – should be involved through the different steps to strengthen the M&E platform. Table 9.1 outlines some of their potential roles, which are country-specific and should be tailored to the context.

Table 9.1 Examples of the role of key actors in monitoring, evaluation and review

Actor	Regular monitoring	Evaluation	Review
MoH	Lead role in the periodic monitoring of the implementation of health policies, the utilization of health resources, and the attainment of health targets	Oversight of the process Identify processes, methods and tools to conduct the evaluation jointly with the implementer of the evaluation, if relevant	Coordination of the joint annual review, mid-term review, and others Oversight role
Other government institutions (ministry of finance, NSO, national registration bureau ...)	Collect, share and analyse relevant information for the health sector (e.g. births and death registration; population denominators; expenditure tracking ...)	Provide inputs (financial information ...) to the evaluation process	Provide inputs and contribute meaningfully to the review process, including making available the required information
National public health institute	Disease and programme-specific annual reviews, if relevant	Neutral and independent review of performance and analysis of barriers to progress in the sector	Findings from programme reviews and other studies and research should feed into the joint annual health reviews
International development partners	Promote and allow mutual accountability on delivering development partners' commitments and workplans in terms of funds, supplies or services	Promote mutual accountability, including evaluation of development partners' commitments, including reporting on indicators and behaviours set out in the compact or memorandum of understanding with MoH, if relevant	Promote mutual accountability, including demonstrating how any project support is aligned with the national strategy
CSOs	Monitor sector performance, highlighting shortfalls both to the authorities as well as the broader public	Advocate and communicate the results of the evaluation Provide CSOs' views at national/regional/provincial level	Be part of mutual accountability processes and discuss findings from the review
National research institutions	Analysis of progress and trends for coverage, utilization of services and health status	Act as independent body to conduct and/or complement an independent evaluation of the performance and progress of the sector	Findings from programme reviews and other studies and research should feed into the joint annual health reviews

9.6 When should monitoring, evaluation and review take place?

Monitoring, evaluation and review should be linked with the country planning cycles, when progress and performance of the sector are discussed and remedial actions are taken.

M&E should be linked with the country planning cycle, when progress and performance of the sector are discussed and remedial actions are taken.

Fig. 9.7 illustrates how a system of reviews may roll out over the course of a national policy and planning cycle.

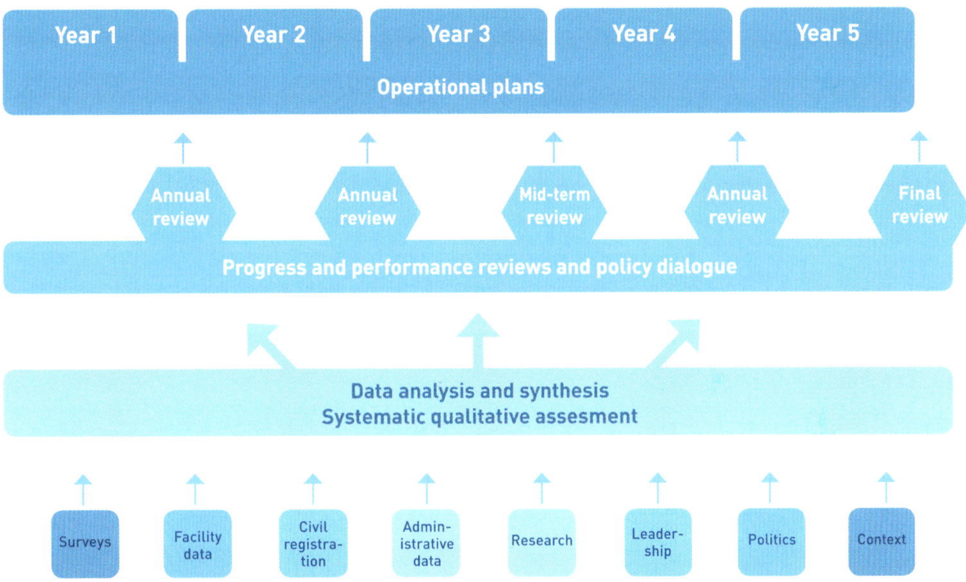

Fig. 9.7 Sample schedule for national health strategies' progress and performance reviews[10]

Ideally the annual reports or data products generated should meet the needs for country-level programme management, global reporting, and/or development partner reporting.

Box 9.8

Mozambique case study: Plan as One, to Deliver as One[11]

Joint annual planning based on the results of the monitoring and review processes is essential to identify effective evidence-informed actions, and to avoid duplication of efforts and funding for the same activities. In Mozambique's Zambezia province, for example, joint annual planning meetings follow evaluations and reviews, identifying effective approaches to prioritize investments in what works. These processes are led by the Provincial Directorate of Planning and Cooperation, and include all departments of the provincial health directorate, UNFPA (United Nations Population Fund), UNICEF, WFP (World Food Programme), donors, representatives from the districts and partners in the province, including CSOs. Results of the reviews inform planning, leading to synergistic results between partners and MoH.

In the immunization area, UNICEF and WHO have found ways to complement each other's work. UNICEF supports vaccine logistics, providing fridges and cold boxes for ensuring proper distribution and motorbikes for supervision. WHO provides training on its vaccine data management tool and technical support for supervision. Such complementary roles have helped to achieve the targets set by the MoH on three indicators related to immunization.

9.7 What if...?

9.7.1 What if fragmentation and/ or fragility is an issue in your country?

Monitoring, evaluation and review of NHPSPs in fragile contexts poses additional challenges to the regular monitoring process. Despite the variety of situations of fragility that have been described in previous chapters of the handbook, some common challenges to monitor, evaluate and review health progress and performance can be identified: dysfunctional policy and institutional environment; weak or inexistent data sources; significant data quality risks; weak institutional capacities to analyse and use data; inadequate operational capacity to monitor service delivery; ad hoc or changing planning and review cycles; limited stewardship capacities of the public sector; and rapidly changing health needs and priorities make difficult to standardize a monitoring and evaluation approach.

Health partners, donors and governments have been progressively adapting their monitoring, evaluation and review approach in these contexts. Various health partners have been working to address monitoring needs in fragile situations by focusing on a limited set of input and output indicators; adding indicators of conflict and violence to the monitoring framework; and supporting specific efforts of data collection, including working with local partners and international contractors.[12] Ebola-affected countries in West Africa have been also tailoring the planning and monitoring cycles to the post-Ebola recovery scenario. Sierra Leone has shortened the overall national planning cycle, has developed the 24-month Post-Ebola Recovery Strategy, spanning July 2015 to June 2017, which acts as an overarching frame for other sector strategies and plans. This has resulted in the development of specific sets of key performance indicators monitored on a monthly and quarterly basis.

Potential approaches to track progress and performance of NHPSPs in distressed health systems or fragile contexts include those listed below.

Adapt the monitoring, evaluation and review processes to the changing planning cycles (e.g. more frequent operational joint reviews could be relevant in contexts with insufficient and incomplete data generated by the routine health information system).

Include specific and priority-based indicators, such as gender-based violence indicators or conflict-related indicators.

Increase investments in health data systems, including verification and oversight processes, from a health systems strengthening perspective.

Engage local and non-state actors in the monitoring process, including data collection, analysis and use.

Gradually increase country system capacities, in coordination with partners, government and other actors.

Build capacity of the MoH for stronger oversight and monitoring.

In a fragile context, health partners can adapt monitoring and evaluation by focusing on limited sets of input and output indicators, adding indicators of conflict and monitoring to the framework, and supporting specific efforts of data collection.

9.7.2 What if your country is decentralized?

Monitoring and evaluation in a decentralized context requires alignment between different levels and feedback loops. Monitoring sub-national inequalities can inform targeted plans and policies.

Many countries have decentralized decision-making processes, including administrative and implementation functions of the health care system. Monitoring and evaluation in these contexts need to be tailored, taking in consideration some key aspects:

Monitoring and evaluation at *national* level in a decentralized context

- Alignment between national and sub-national strategies and plans

  The NHPSP should identify and lay out a sound and comprehensive monitoring and evaluation component.[13] However, the design of this component, or framework, needs to be coordinated and translated to sub-national documents for coherence. Likewise, sub-national strategies should form the basis for the national M&E framework. A constant interaction between the national and sub-national levels is crucial for the success, repeatability and reproducibility of monitoring, evaluation and review mechanisms.

- Review mechanisms and feedback loops to be comprehensive and inclusive to ensure accountability

  The review mechanisms chosen should be comprehensive – not just in terms of sectoral and programme related aspects but also in regard to national and sub-national levels. Thorough monitoring and evaluation activities require inclusive policy dialogue and systematic and regular assessments.[14] Those mechanisms – and the tools and methods to use them – need to be adapted to the formalized and non-formalized (especially in regard to dialogue processes) decentralization features that are prevailing in the country. Accountability towards the results of monitoring and evaluation needs to be claimed at every government level.

- Allowing reflections on the status of decentralization

  When undertaking monitoring and evaluation in a decentralized context, it is important to consider the ways in which decentralization has been integrated and used in all the previous planning steps. As a consequence of the breadth of evaluation, process-related issues might be considered as well – apart from health-related issues. It might be beneficial for the planning process to establish a link between health outcomes and decentralization. For example, the set of indicators related to health outcomes could be complemented by political, administrative and fiscal indicators for monitoring and evaluation purposes of the performance of sub-national planning features. Thus, routine data collection needs to be adapted, since those indicators are not always part of the collection set in many countries.[15] As a consequence of including decentralization in the evaluation, current responsibility, authority and accountability arrangements might need to be adapted.[II]

II Hutchinson and LaFond (see endnote reference 15) developed a "Conceptual Framework for Evaluating Decentralization", which offers a detailed guide for monitoring and evaluation of decentralization in the health sector, with an emphasis on conceptual questions and concrete options for action.

- Monitoring sub-national regional inequalities

Monitoring health inequalities between sub-national levels can inform targeted health programmes and policies, especially if disparities are substantial. Summary measures of inequality can condense disaggregated data into concise outputs, which could be used to show trends and make comparisons.[16] The selection of appropriate summary measures to quantify sub-national inequalities should be carefully chosen (i.e. pairwise differences and ratios), to provide a good understanding of sub-national-level inequalities to policy-makers, partners and civil society, among others, and thus to facilitate targeting and deploying interventions to disadvantaged subpopulations.

Special issues to consider for monitoring and evaluation at *sub-national* level

- Selection of tools and assessment methods

The analysis and assessment tools that will determine the success and validity of the M&E exercises, as well as increase accountability towards its results need to be selected according to the features of the health system. It is important to ensure consistency and comparability across the different sub-national levels and to support those levels (capacity and financial) to be able to analyse and use the data.

- Sub-national M&E plans

Countries that have been going through devolution processes, such as Kenya, have created a new layer of sub-national government, with allocated resources and prescribed functions. Access to sub-national-level data to monitor performance is paramount to track progress and performance of the sub-national health sector strategic and investment plans. Kenya has updated its M&E roadmap to ensure the M&E needs of its counties are identified and eventually addressed, including strengthening counties' analytical capacities.[17]

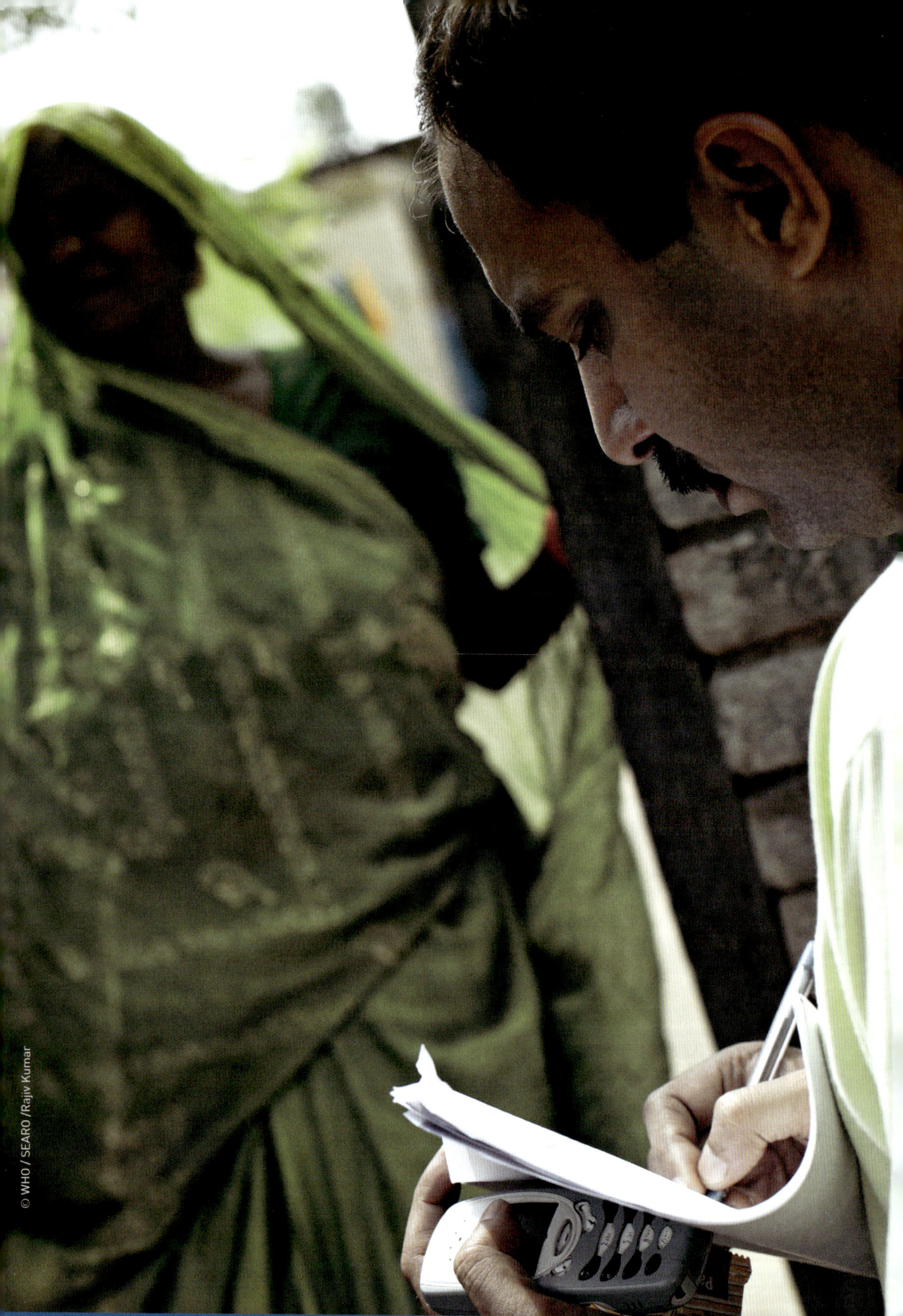

9.8 Conclusion

There is a growing interest and demand for quality data for decision-making and accountability. A strong monitoring, evaluation and review platform is needed to track progress and performance of the national health strategy; to report progress on health-related SDGs and regional and global monitoring of priority health issues, including health inequalities; and to provide the basis for accountability and policy dialogue.

A single country-led platform brings together all the elements related to monitoring, evaluation and review of the health sector plan, including national policy and plans relating to M&E and country HISs, well-functioning data sources, institutional capacity for data collection, management analyses and use, as well as the country review processes for planning and decision-making.

Aligning partners and governments around a country-led M&E platform is a unique opportunity to scale up enhanced technical support for strengthening country M&E capacities and data systems. A robust country-led monitoring and evaluation plan should form the basis for strengthening the country M&E platform and for improved alignment of domestic and partner investments. More on this approach can be found at: http://www.healthdatacollaborative.org/.

References

1 Monitoring, evaluation and review of national health strategies: a country-led platform for information and accountability. Geneva: World Health Organization; 2011 (http://www.who.int/healthinfo/country_monitoring_evaluation/1085_IER_131011_web.pdf?ua=1, accessed 17 October 2016).

2 Ibid.

3 Global reference list of 100 core health indicators. World Health Organization; 2015. (http://apps.who.int/iris/bitstream/10665/173589/1/WHO_HIS_HSI_2015.3_eng.pdf, accessed 17 October 2016).

4 Adapted from: Health in 2015: from MDGs, Millennium Development Goals to SDGs, Sustainable Development Goals. Geneva: World Health Organization; 2015 (http://www.who.int/gho/publications/mdgs-sdgs/en/, accessed 17 October 2016).

5 The roadmap for health measurement and accountability. Washington (DC): The World Bank Group; 2015 (https://live.worldbank.org/sites/default/files/roadmap_6-4-15_web.pdf, accessed 17 October 2016).

6 Health measurement and accountability post 2015: five-point call to action. 2015 (http://www.healthdatacollaborative.org/fileadmin/uploads/hdc/Documents/5-point-call-to-action.pdf, accessed 17 October 2016).

7 100 core health indicators. Geneva: World Health Organization; 2015 (http://www.who.int/healthinfo/indicators/2015/100CoreHealthIndicators_2015_infographic.pdf, accessed 17 October 2016).

8 Midterm analytical review of performance of the health sector strategic plan III 2009–2015. Dar es Salaan: United Republic of Tanzania Ministry of Health and Social Welfare; 2013 (http://www.who.int/healthinfo/country_monitoring_evaluation/TZ_AnalyticalReport_2013.pdf, accessed 17 October 2016).

9 One monitoring and evaluation framework for the health sector in Kenya: towards accelerating the achievement of universal health coverage in Kenya. The Kenya Health Data Collaborative Report. Republic of Kenya Ministry of Health; 2016 (http://www.healthdatacollaborative.org/fileadmin/uploads/hdc/Documents/Kenya_Health_Data_Collaborative_Conference_Report.pdf, accessed 17 October 2016).

10 Monitoring, evaluation and review of national health strategies: a country-led platform for information and accountability. Geneva: World Health Organization; 2011 (http://www.who.int/healthinfo/country_monitoring_evaluation/1085_IER_131011_web.pdf?ua=1, accessed 17 October 2016).

11 Support to the National Integrated Plan to achieve MDGs 4&5 in Mozambique. Lessons Learnt (2012-2015). UNICEF, UNFPA, WFP, WHO; 2015.

12 Review of the Global Fund in fragile states: final report. Euro Health Group; 2014 (http://www.theglobalfund.org/en/search/?q=global+fund+in+fragile+states, accessed 18 October 2016).

13 Monitoring, evaluation and review of national health strategies: a country-led platform for information and accountability. Geneva: World Health Organization; 2011 (http://www.who.int/healthinfo/country_monitoring_evaluation/1085_IER_131011_web.pdf?ua=1, accessed 18 October 2016).

14 Ibid.

15 See also: Hutchinson PL, LaFond AK. Monitoring and evaluation of decentralization reforms in developing country health sectors. Bethesda (MD): The Partners for Health Reformplus Project, Abt Associates Inc.: 2004 (http://www.phrplus.org/Pubs/Tech054_fin.pdf, accessed 18 October 2016).

16 Hosseinpoor AR, Bergen N, Barros AJD, Wong KLM, Boerma T, Victora CG. Monitoring subnational regional inequalities in health: measurement approaches and challenges. Int J Equity Health. 2016;15(1):18 (https://equityhealthj.biomedcentral.com/articles/10.1186/s12939-016-0307-y, accessed 18 October 2016).

17 Communiqué on commitments to support One Monitoring and Evaluation Framework for Kenya. Republic of Nairobi: Kenya Ministry of Health; 2016 (http://www.healthdatacollaborative.org/fileadmin/uploads/hdc/Documents/Kenya_Final_One_ME_Communique.pdf, accessed 18 October 2016).

Further reading

Policy and institutional environment

Global reference list of 100 core health indicators. Geneva: World Health Organization; 2015. Available in English and French (http://www.who.int/healthinfo/indicators/2015/en/, accessed18 October 2016).

Monitoring, evaluation and review: an assessment and planning tool, 2016. World Health Organization; 2016. In press.

Monitoring, evaluation and review of national health strategies: a country-led platform for information and accountability. Geneva: International Health Partnership (IHP+) and World Health Organization; 2011. Available in English, French and Spanish. (http://www.who.int/healthinfo/country_monitoring_evaluation/documentation/en, accessed 18 October 2016).

Monitoring progress towards universal health coverage at country and global levels: framework, measures and targets. Geneva/Washington (DC): World Health Organization /World Bank Group; 2014. Available in 6 UN languages (http://www.who.int/healthinfo/universal_health_coverage/report/2014/en/, accessed 18 October 2016).

Well-functioning data sources

Facility information systems

Creating a master health facility list. Working version. Geneva: World Health Organization; 2013 (http://www.who.int/healthinfo/systems/WHO_CreatingMFL_draft.pdf?ua=1, accessed 18 October 2016).

Data quality review: A toolkit for monitoring health facility data quality. Geneva, World Health Organization; 2016. In press.

Health facility & community data toolkit. Geneva: World Health Organization/USAID/University of Oslo; 2016 (http://www.who.int/entity/healthinfo/facility_information_systems/en/index.html, accessed 18 October 2016).

Performance of routine information system management tools package. Chapel Hill (NC): MEASURE Evaluation; 2016, Working document, April 2016.

Routine health information systems: a curriculum on basic concepts and practice. (Facilitators' guide, May 2016). Chapel Hill (NC): MEASURE Evaluation; 2016. In press.

Services availability and readiness assessment (SARA): an annual monitoring system for service delivery. Reference manual and implementation guide, version 2.2. Geneva: World Health Organization; 2015. Available in English and French (http://www.who.int/healthinfo/systems/sara_introduction/en/, accessed 18 October 2016).

CRVS

Strengthening civil registration and vital statistics for births, deaths and causes of death: resource kit. Geneva: World Health Organization; 2012 (http://www.who.int/healthinfo/CRVS_ResourceKit_2012.pdf?ua=1, accessed 18 October 2016).

Verbal autopsy standards: ascertaining and attributing causes of deaths. 2014 WHO verbal autopsy instrument. Geneva: World Health Organization; 2014 (http://www.who.int/healthinfo/statistics/verbalautopsystandards/en/, accessed 18 October 2016).

Rapid assessment of national civil registration and vital statistics systems. Geneva: World Health Organization; 2010 (http://apps.who.int/iris/bitstream/10665/70470/1/WHO_IER_HSI_STM_2010.1_eng.pdf, accessed 18 October 2016).

WHO application of ICD-10 for low-resource settings initial cause of death collection: the startup mortality list (ICD-10-SMoL), version 2.0. Geneva: World Health Organization; 2014 (http://www.who.int/healthinfo/civil_registration/ICD_10_SMoL.pdf?ua=1, accessed 18 October 2016).

Institutional capacity for data management, analysis and communication

Data analysis

Analysing mortality levels and causes-of-death (ANACoD) electronic tool. Geneva: World Health Organization; 2014. Available in English, French, Spanish and Russian (http://www.who.int/healthinfo/anacod/en/, accessed 18 October 2016).

A system of health accounts: 2011 edition. Geneva: Organisation for Economic Co-operation and Development (OECD)/Eurostat/World Health Organization; 2011 (http://who.int/health-accounts/methodology/sha2011.pdf?ua=1, accessed 18 October 2016).

Joint annual health sector reviews: why and how to organize them. Geneva/ Washington (DC):IHP+ and World Health Organization /World Bank Group; 2014 (http://www.internationalhealthpartnership.net/fileadmin/uploads/ihp/Documents/Results___Evidence/HAE__results___lessons/ihp_jar_oct2014_en_web.pdf, accessed 18 October 2016).

Progress and performance review and accountability

Handbook on health inequality monitoring with a special focus on low- and middle-income countries. Geneva: World Health Organization; 2013 (http://www.who.int/gho/health_equity/handbook/en/, accessed 18 October 2016).

Monitoring, evaluation and review in distressed health systems

The challenging operating environments policy. Board Decision. GF/B35/03 The Global Fund 35th Board Meeting 26–27 April 2016, Abidjan, Côte d'Ivoire (http://www.theglobalfund.org/en/board/meetings/35/, accessed 18 October 2016).

Thematic review of the Global Fund in fragile states. Final report. Global Fund; 2014 http://www.theglobalfund.org/documents/terg/evaluation_2013-2014/TERG_Evaluation2013-2014ThematicReviewFragileStates_Report_en/, accessed 18 October 2016).

Pooled funding to support service delivery: lessons of experience from fragile and conflict-affected states. London: Department for International Development (DFID); 2013. (http://r4d.dfid.gov.uk/pdf/outputs/misc_Gov/61050-PFs-Full_Volume(May2013).pdf. , accessed 18 October 2016).

Annex 9.1

Template/outline of an M&E plan

Chapter 1: National health strategy as basis for results and accountability

1.1 Goals and objectives of the national health strategy
1.2 Current status of the health information system
1.3 Process for development of the monitoring, evaluation and review component
1.4 Disease- and programme-specific monitoring, evaluation and review alignment

Chapter 2: Institutional capacity

2.1 Key country-led coordination mechanisms
2.2 Roles and responsibilities of key country institutions and stakeholders
2.3 Country capacity-building strategy

Chapter 3: Monitoring and evaluation framework

3.1 Monitoring and evaluation framework
3.2 Indicators
3.3 Data sources
- Data collection needs for all core indicators
- Critical data gaps and weaknesses and how to address these
- Data management

3.4 Data analysis, synthesis and quality
- Data analysis and synthesis work
- Regular assessments of progress and performance
- Processes for data quality assurance

3.5 Evaluation component
3.6 Data dissemination and use
- Analytical outputs and responsibilities

Chapter 4: Country mechanisms for review and action

4.1 System of joint periodic progress and performance reviews for use in decision-making
4.2 Links between programme-specific reviews and the general health sector review
4.3 Decision-making processes for remedial action and financial disbursement

Chapter 10

Law, regulation and strategizing for health

David Clarke

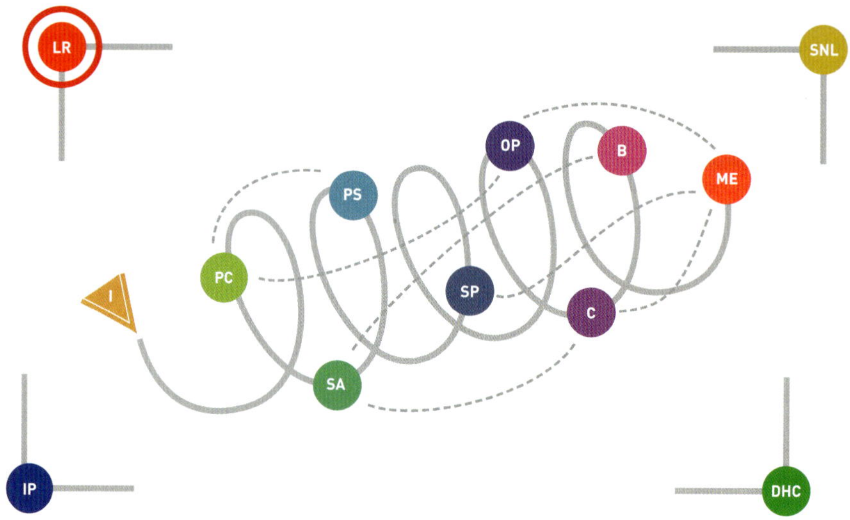

Cross-cutting topics relevant to national health planning

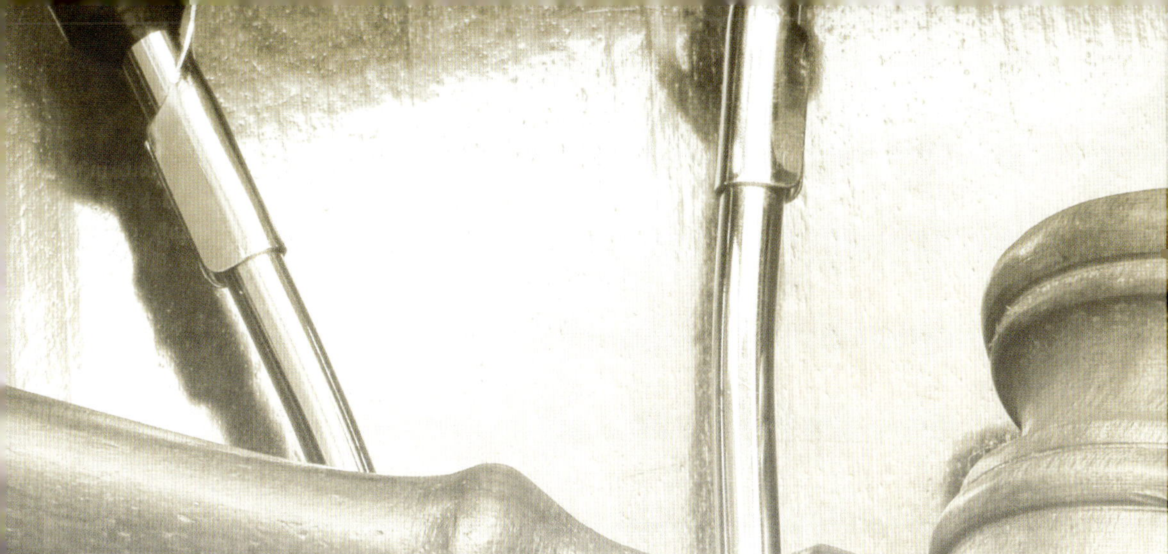

© WHO/Hyppolite Kalambay

Overview

For the national health planning process, regulation represents a key means by which a government gives effect to its health policy preferences, especially through the exercise of a government's law-making powers. The last 25 years have seen major changes to the way that governments organize themselves, provide services and make and implement policy. A range of decisions that were once taken by a health minister or a health ministry are now taken by regional and local government, autonomous public sector agencies, private firms, nongovernmental organizations and individuals. As a result, regulation has grown in importance as a key lever for governments to affect the quantity, quality, safety and distribution of services in health systems.

Summary

What is law and regulation?

The term "regulation" is commonly used in two ways.

First, it is used in a narrow sense to describe a category of delegated decision-making involving the use of secondary legislation.

However, in this publication the term is used in a second and broader sense to cover the use of instruments of various types for the implementation of socioeconomic policy objectives and includes laws.

Laws are rules that govern behaviour.

Laws can be made by a legislature, resulting in primary legislation (often called statutes or acts), by executive or local government through the issue of secondary legislation (including decrees, regulations and bylaws), or by judges through the making of binding legal precedent (normally in common law jurisdictions).

Why is law and regulation important?

National health planning process: Law and regulation set the ground rules for the health planning process.

National Health Policy/Strategy/Plan (NHPSP) implementation: Law and regulation are key implementation mechanisms for translating major health policy objectives into action through the setting of standards and requirements and the use of sanctions and incentives to exert leverage over the health system (and its participants).

When should work on law and regulation take place in the national health-planning process?

Thinking about law and regulation should take place at the start of the planning process. It is important for key actors involved to understand any legal rules and requirements that relate to how the process should be carried out.

Specific issues about law and regulation should be taken into account during the various planning activities; for example, regulatory analysis should take place as part of a country's work on its health-sector situation analysis, and when developing options for legal and regulatory interventions to give effect to the country's NHPSP.

Who should be involved in work on law and regulation?

The many people involved in work on laws and other forms of regulation, include political decision-makers, lawyers, policy analysts, health planners, health providers, health professionals and members of the public. The roles of the various actors vary, and encompass decision-making, resource mobilization and provision, contribution to the policy/regulatory dialogue, and implementation.

How do we go about work on law and regulation?

At the beginning of the process make sure that you understand any legal requirements to be met as part of running the planning process, including legal requirements relating to the budget process. Read any relevant laws and guides; get legal advice if necessary.

Meet with the ministry of health's policy and legal team to discuss your respective roles in any work on law and other forms of regulation, and discuss how this work might affect the planning process.

Identify other key people that you need to work with on law and other forms of regulation.

Map out any specific tasks that need to be carried out on law/regulation as part of your work on NHPSP implementation activities, and factor in work on these tasks as part of the process.

As it proceeds, assess at each stage in the process what issues, tasks and inputs you need to consider with regard to law and other forms of regulation.

Note: Work on law and other forms of regulation should not be regarded as a separate process, but should be an integral part of a country's health policy dialogue engaging stakeholders from health, finance and other ministries, civil society, nongovernmental organizations, international agencies, academic institutions, professional associations and communities. A similar approach should be taken when implementing law and regulation.

10.1 What do we mean by law and regulation?

10.1.1 Some key concepts

Regulation

Regulation is:

(a) the promulgation of rules by government accompanied by mechanisms for monitoring and enforcement (usually assumed to be performed through a specialist public agency);

(b) any form of direct state intervention in the economy, whatever form that intervention might take; or

(c) all mechanisms of social control or influence affecting all aspects of behaviour, from whatever source.

The first aspect, the promulgation of rules by governments, inevitably involves the exercise of a government's law-making powers, so the first dimension of the definition relates to the use of laws and legal tools to affect behavioural change. For example, a government may put in place mandatory rules requiring the operators of a health facility to obtain an authorization before they provide services, and impose sanctions where the rules are not obeyed.

The second aspect refers to other regulatory tools a government can use to control or influence conduct in the health system. Possible regulatory tools include economic tools and market instruments (such as tobacco taxes, nursing school quotas or drug pricing mechanisms) and disclosure regulation (such as requiring health providers to disclose certain information to consumers to empower them to make better choices).[1,I]

While all governments regulate, regulation is also made by non-state actors.

The third aspect of the definition reflects that increasingly, regulation is carried out by non-government actors as well as by government. This last aspect illustrates that governments have a choice: do they regulate themselves, or do they allow nongovernment actors to self-regulate? A good example is where a government has chosen to allow a health professional group to self-regulate and set the rules of conduct for its members.

I Disclosure regulation is designed to address information asymmetry. Health care organizations are required to provide open and transparent information to consumers and competitors on price, quality and quantity.

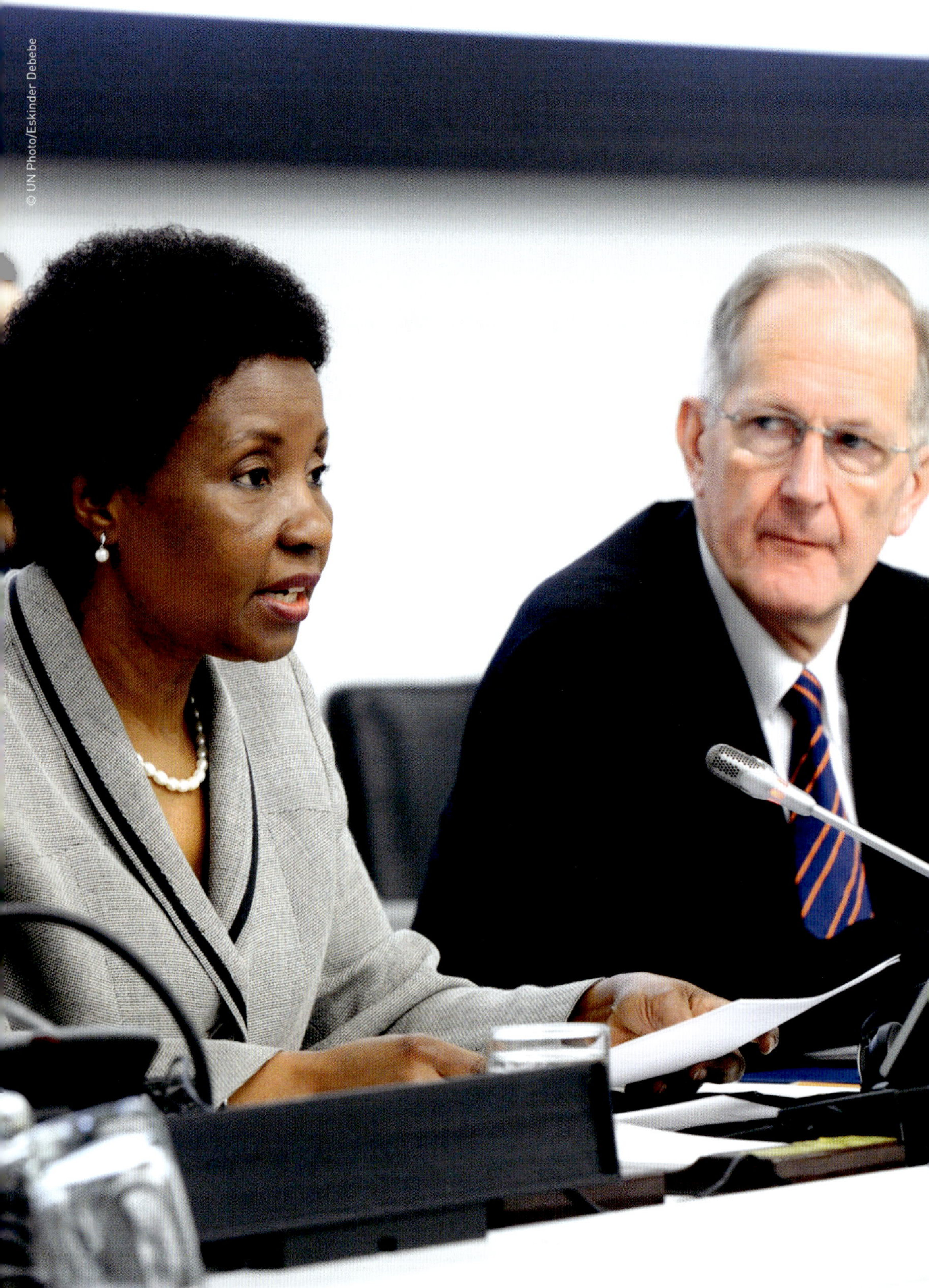

© UN Photo/Eskinder Debebe

Box 10.1

Examples of the different aspects of regulation

The promulgation of rules by government

Turkey provides a good illustration of how rules made by governments can lead to positive behavioural change (consistent with a government's policy intentions). To implement its policy to reduce smoking related diseases, Turkey introduced laws to impose tobacco taxation, ban tobacco product advertisements and smoking in public places. These interventions have led to a reduction in the proportion of tobacco smokers in the adult population.[2]

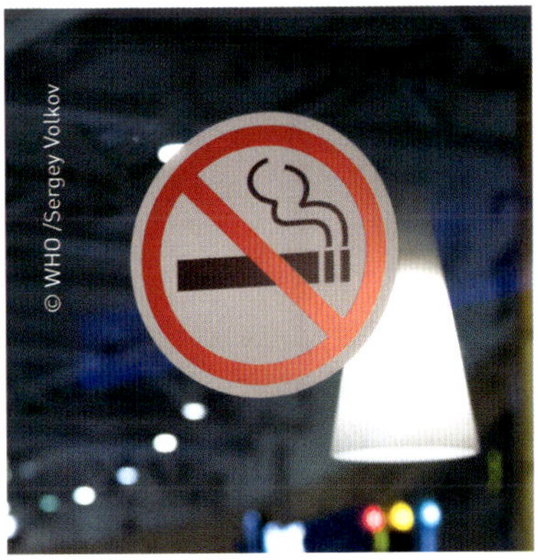
© WHO /Sergey Volkov

The use of other regulatory tools (e.g. incentive-based regulation)

Demand-side incentives, such as conditional cash transfers or vouchers to encourage the uptake of primary health care, are now being implemented in many Latin American countries and in Asia. These provide direct financial support to families for achieving specific targets, such as attending antenatal care or delivery in a health facility with trained professionals.[3]

Regulation by nongovernment actors

Many countries regulate their health workers using a self-regulatory model, e.g. the *Indian Medical Council Act*[4] allows the medical council to regulate professional conduct of medical practitioners by prescribing standards, and a code of ethics for medical practitioners.

Law

Law is one of the most important types of regulation.

Law is a key type of regulation and is used to encourage or change behaviour.

Laws are rules that govern behaviour, backed by coercive force and made by a legitimately constituted nation state.[5] Laws can be made by a legislature, resulting in primary legislation (often called statutes or acts), by executive or local government through the issue of secondary legislation (including decrees, regulations and bylaws), or by judges through the making of binding legal precedent (normally in common law jurisdictions).

Legislation

Legislation is a catch-all phrase to cover the different types of laws made by a country's legislature or other law-making body. The term legislation covers two main types of law: primary legislation and secondary legislation.

Primary legislation refers to statutes made by national legislatures (or by state legislatures in federal systems). Primary legislation usually defines broad powers and principles. However, as it is not always appropriate or possible for primary legislation to address all the technical details, systems and structures that are needed for implementation, these details are set out in secondary legislation.

Secondary legislation refers to laws made by executive or local government (examples include decrees, regulations, rules, orders and bylaws). Secondary legislation defines necessary technical details, as well as the systems and structures required to give full effect to primary legislation.

Box 10.2

Some examples to illustrate the differences between primary and secondary legislation

Nigeria

In 2014 Nigeria passed a National Health Act (an example of primary legislation) to provide a legal framework for the provision of health services. The Act ascribes health services roles and responsibilities to different tiers of government and to nongovernmental organizations. The operational details of the Act and its implementation have been left to secondary legislation, policy and administrative arrangements. For example, Part II of the Act provides a framework for regulating health establishments and technologies. The details of the framework are, however, left to secondary legislation, which will prescribe details about the classifications of health establishments and technologies under the Act, based on:

- their role and function within the national health system;
- the size and location of the communities they serve;
- the nature and level of health services they are able to provide;
- their geographical location and demographic reach;
- the need to structure the delivery of health services in accordance with national norms and standards within an integrated and coordinated national framework;
- and in the case of private health establishments, whether the establishment is for-profit or not.

Cambodia

In Cambodia's hierarchy of laws, matters of broad legal principle, key functions and powers and institutional arrangements are set in higher-level "laws" and royal decrees, with sub-decrees, ministerial orders, decisions, circulars and local regulation used to clarify meaning and intent and provide for practical implementation (see the diagram below).

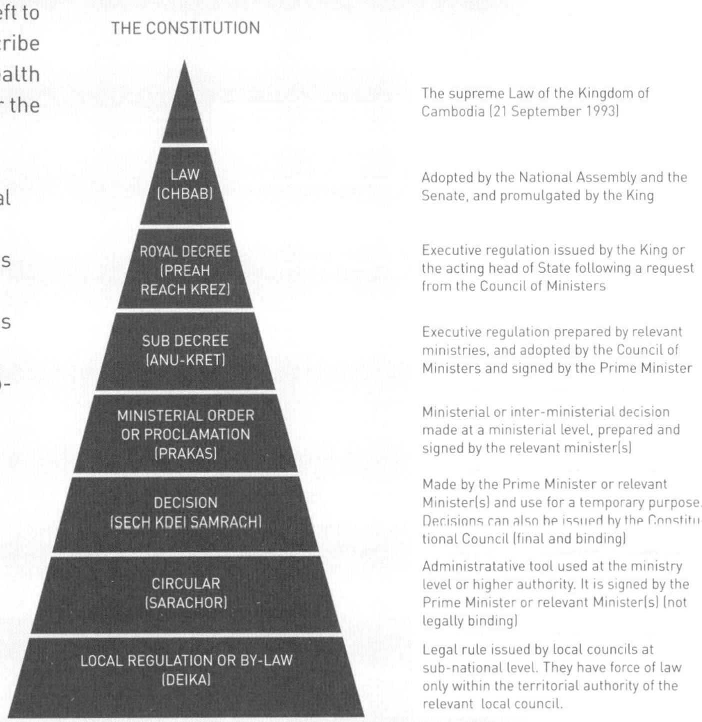

10.1.2 Ways in which law and regulation are used in the health sector

The strength of law and regulation comes from its power to:

- create and recognize rights;
- impose obligations and penalties;
- establish permanent institutions and institutional arrangements.[II]

Governments use laws and other forms of regulations in three broad ways.

Law and regulation help implement national health policy, establish rights, rules, and safeguards and help assure health security.

1. First, countries regulate to establish the legal architecture for the health system to ensure cohesion and efficiency. A health systems law establishes legal responsibility and accountability for the performance of key health-system functions (planning, priority setting, financing, service provision, integrity and supervision, etc.). For example, see Box 10.3 on the United Kingdom's National Health Services Act.

   In health systems where contracts are used to govern the provision and receipt of services, governments will also make laws to establish the legal basis for contracting in the system, and to establish the rights and responsibilities of buyers (patients) and sellers (health providers and insurers). This legal framework may be set out in a country's general contract laws and commercial laws (such as laws which prohibit anti-competitive behaviour) and in specific health laws (such as laws governing health insurance transactions).

2. Second, governments regulate in order to advance important policy objectives for their health systems, such as providing universal access to health services, establishing social protection floors, encouraging the efficient and equitable use of resources, or ensuring compliance with a country's international obligations - for example, the International Health Regulations.[III] For examples, see Box 10.4.

3. Third, governments regulate to protect members of the public from harm or from the adverse effects of unconstrained business activities in the health system (and to address market failure and inefficiencies in the health system). For instance, private providers might want to segment markets to concentrate on profitable market niches, such as patients with easy-to-treat conditions, or patients with higher incomes. In those circumstances, laws and other forms of regulation might be required to oblige (or incentivize) private providers to provide a broader range of services and allow service access regardless of patient income. For example, see Box 10.4.

II For example, see the discussion about the use of legislation to sustain and formalize the operation of Thailand's National Health Assembly (Box 10.9).

III The International Health Regulations 2005 are an international legal instrument that is binding on over 196 countries, including all of the member states of WHO.

Box 10.3

The structure for the NHS established by the Health and Social Care Act 2012[6]

The Health and Social Care Act 2012 provides for an extensive reorganization of the structure of the National Health Service in England (see the diagram below).

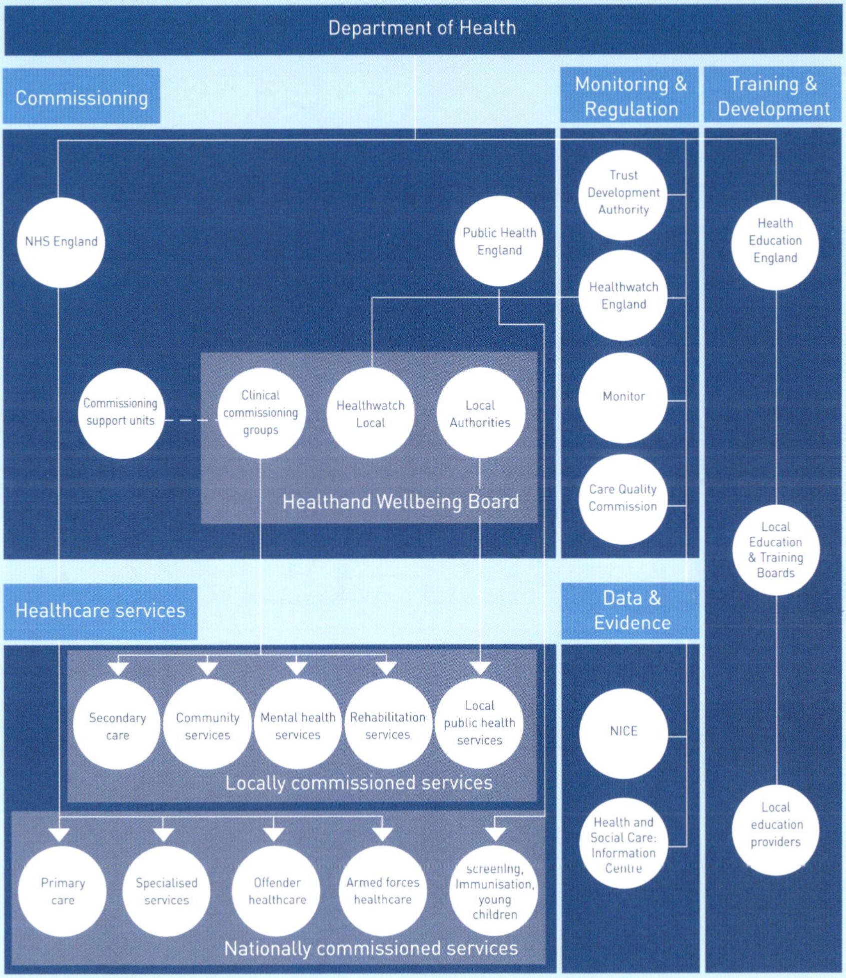

The Secretary of State for Health has overall responsibility for the work of the Department of Health (DH). DH provides strategic leadership for public health, the NHS and social care in England.

The Chief Medical Officer is the UK government's principle medical and scientific adviser, the professional lead for doctors in England, and the professional lead of all directors of public health in local government.

The National Medical Director of NHS England is responsible for clinical policy and strategy, promoting a focus on clinical outcomes, enhancing clinical leadership and promoting innovation.

The Chief Nursing Officer is the professional lead for nurses and midwives in England and oversees quality improvements in patient safety and patient experience.

The Chief Professional Officers (including the Chief Scientific Officer, Chief Dental Officer, Chief Pharmaceutical Officer and Chief Health Professions Officer) are the heads of their respective professions and provide expert clinical advice across the health system.

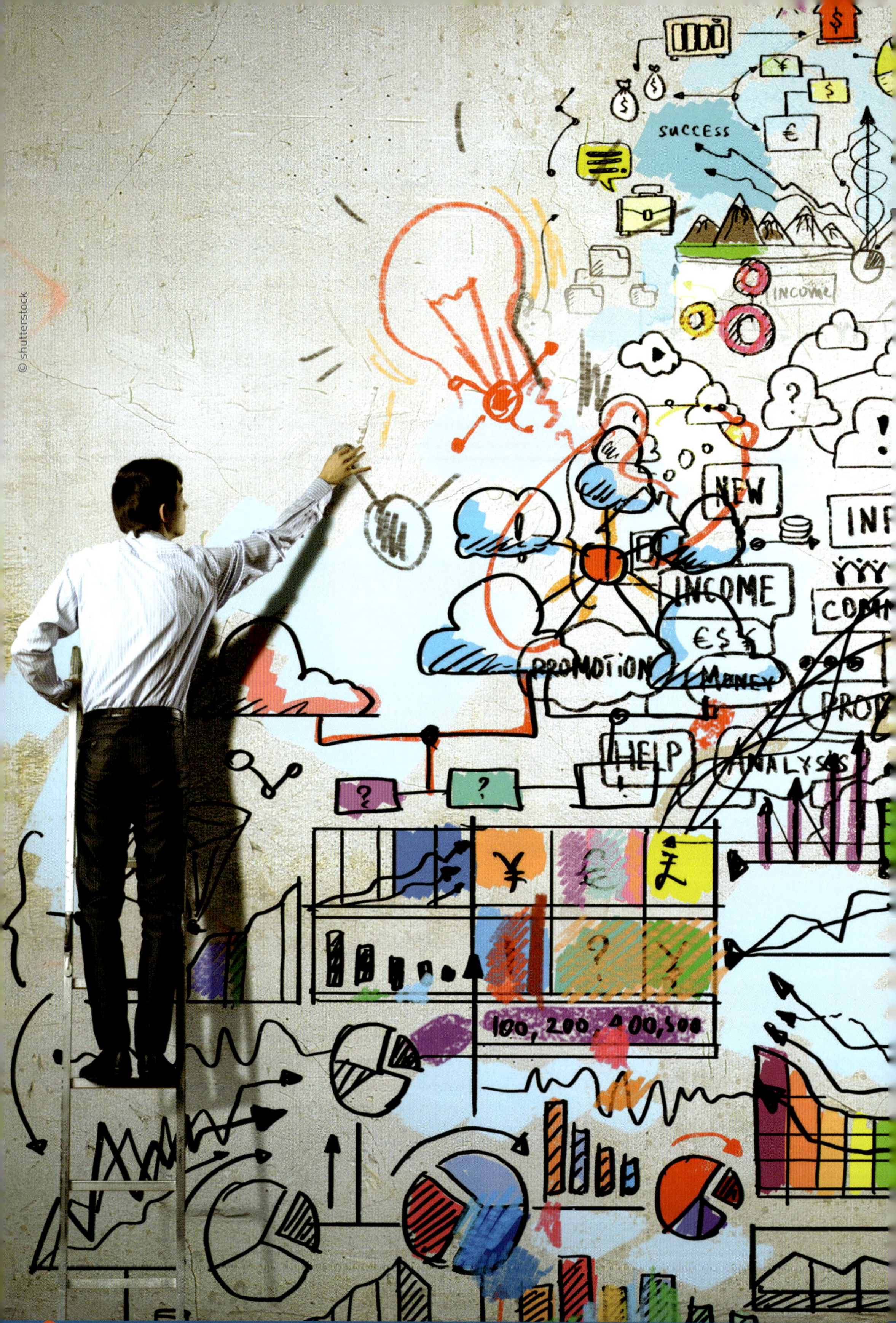
SUCCESS
INCOME
NEW
INCOME
PROMOTION
MONEY
HELP
100, 200, 400,500

Box 10.4

Examples of the different aspects of regulation

Health systems laws which establish the basis on which a country's health system is organized, governed and financed.

Laws which protect public health from communicable diseases or other public health risks, providing for public health surveillance and powers to take action to prevent the spread of disease or other public health risk. (These laws should be consistent with a country's obligations under the International Health Regulations 2005).

Laws which regulate the quality of health service provision.

Laws which provide for health system financing, such as social health insurance laws.

Laws which regulate the operation of hospitals, clinics or other health services.

Laws which establish social protection floors (a basic set of social rights derived from human rights treaties, including access to essential services – such as health, education, housing, water and sanitation, and others, as defined nationally – and social transfers, in cash or in kind, to guarantee income security, food security, adequate nutrition and access to essential services).

Laws which control the required training, qualifications and practice standards of health workers.

Laws governing the treatment and care of people with mental disorders.

Laws which regulate the safety and efficacy of medicines and medical devices.

Laws which regulate the manufacture, marketing and sale of food.

Laws which protect patient rights.

Laws which address noncommunicable disease risk factors including:

- tobacco consumption (where parties to the Framework Convention on Tobacco Control[IV] should ensure that their tobacco control laws comply with the Convention's requirements);
- the harmful use of alcohol;
- diet-related diseases (such as laws which control the marketing to children of foods and beverages which are high in fat, sugar or salt).

Laws which regulate the collection and use of health information (including protecting patient privacy).

IV The Framework Convention on Tobacco Control (FCTC) is an international treaty negotiated under the auspices of WHO to respond to the globalisation of the tobacco epidemic.

10.2 Why do we need law and regulation in the national health planning process?

Law and regulation in national health planning is used to establish a legal roadmap for the process and as a key implementation mechanism to translate policy objectives into action.

Law and regulation in the context of the national health planning process serves two key purposes:

(a) to establish a legal roadmap for the national health planning process; and

(b) as a key implementation mechanism, to translate major health policy objectives into action through setting standards and requirements and the use of sanctions and incentives to exert leverage over the health system (and its participants).

Box 10.5

An example of using law to give effect to health policy

As part of its policy of ensuring "health access for all", Burkina Faso passed a new law on universal health insurance in 2015. The passage of this law represents a major achievement as it enshrines the "right to health" in a legal framework designed to increase access to health services while reducing the risk of financial hardship for paying for them.

The key features of the new law are:

- the provision of basic health protection for the whole population via a pooled fund;
- mandatory enrollment in the fund based on a person's ability to pay and with government subsidizing the poor;
- benefits paid on the basis of health need rather than on the ability to pay.

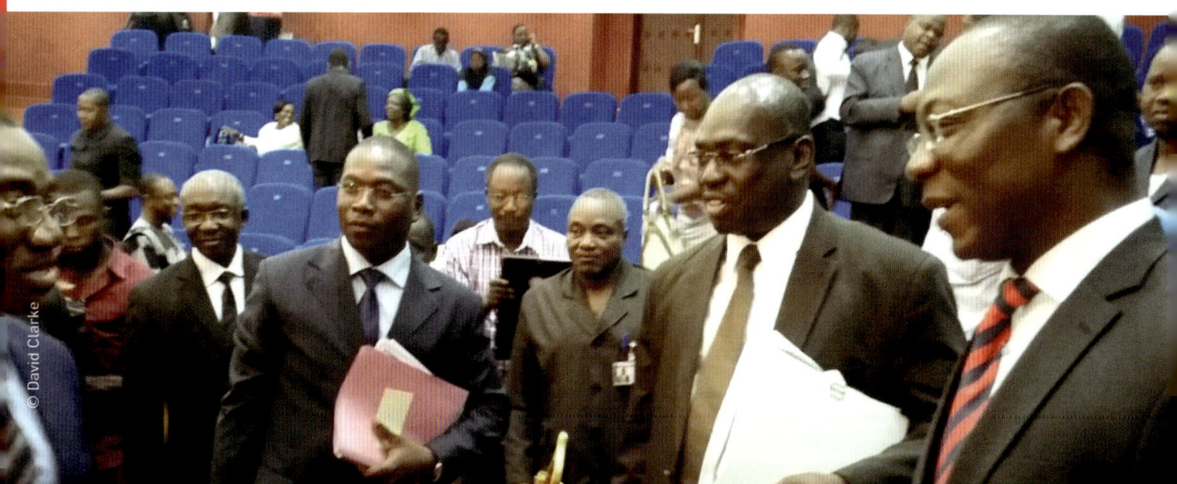

© David Clarke

10.2.1 A legal road map for the national health planning process

In some countries there are laws that set out what is in effect a legal road map for the national health planning process. This road map needs to be studied carefully to decide which issues are of most concern and require action with regard to a country's national health planning process.

This road map may consist of:

(a) law(s) which deal with the establishment of a national health plan or strategy;
and/or

(b) law(s) which establish the rules for establishing and approving a country's health budget.

Potential actionable issues within these two main road map areas are described further below.

Laws about national health policies, strategies and plans

For the national health plan/strategy a country may have a law that:

- requires the country to have a health strategic plan;
- tasks an agency or person with the making of the plan (e.g. a health ministry or a health minister);
- describes the key content that must be included in such a plan;
- prescribes who must be consulted on a plan and how;
- requires a certain process to be followed to finalize the plan;
- requires reporting against the plan to an oversight body (for example, a country's national assembly/legislature).

Laws help formalize and create a sustainable basis for the planning process.

The purpose of this sort of law is twofold.

- To provide a sustainable mechanism for national health planning (if the requirement to make a plan is a legal duty, it is far more likely to happen than if the requirement is an administrative matter).
- To provide a legal obligation to adhere to a mechanism that is designed to give national coherence for health policy (especially if a law provides that all sub-plans or activities should be consistent with the national health plan – an especially important issue in decentralized health systems).

Box 10.6

The New Zealand Public Health and Disability Act 2000 (NZPHD) – an example of a legal framework for health strategy formulation and planning

The NZPHD Act establishes the structure underlying public sector funding and the organization of health and disability services in New Zealand. It establishes district health boards (DHBs), and sets out the duties and roles of key participants, including the Minister of Health, Ministerial committees, and health sector provider organizations. DHBs are responsible for providing or funding the provision of health services in their assigned districts (with disability support services and some health services funded and purchased nationally by the Ministry of Health).

Setting a strategic direction

The NZPHD Act also sets the strategic direction and goals for health and disability services.

Section 8 of the Act requires the Minister of Health to determine a strategy for health services, called the New Zealand health strategy, to provide the framework for the Government's overall direction of the health sector in improving the health of people and communities. Section 8 also requires the Minister who is responsible for disability issues to determine a strategy for disability support services, called the New Zealand disability strategy, providing the framework for the Government's overall direction of the disability sector in improving disability support services.

Planning frameworks and requirements

Section 38 of the NZPHD[7] provides for the formulation of annual plans by DHBs. This section requires that every plan must address local, regional, and national needs for health services; how health services can be properly coordinated to meet those needs; the optimum arrangement for the most effective and efficient delivery of health services; and must reflect the overall direction set out in, and not be inconsistent with, the New Zealand health strategy and the New Zealand disability strategy.

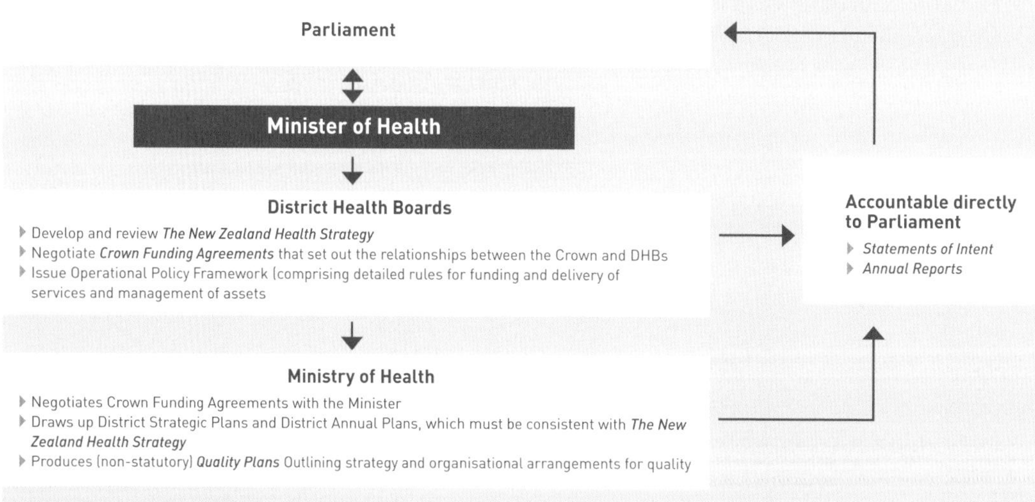

Laws governing the budget process

Another important category of laws which impact on the national health planning process are budget laws.

Most countries have norms governing the operation of their national budget process. In an increasing number of countries, the norms governing the national budget process (for historical reasons or because of budget reforms) have been made into legally binding rules (incorporated into a country's budget laws).[8]

There are a number of key reasons why countries establish the rules around their budget processes in their laws. For example, to:

- enhance the transparency of the budget system and its accountability for expenditure;
- clearly specify the financial powers of the legislature and the executive;
- provide clear operational rules for the budget system;
- ensure that budget rules have sufficient authority;
- elaborate on constitutional requirements for the budget system;
- reform the budget system;
- contribute to macroeconomic stability.

In countries where rules about the national budget process and budget system have been incorporated into the law, the legal approaches they have taken can vary widely though usually involve a hierarchy of laws made up of a country's constitution, an organic budget law and financial regulations.

The level of detail and specifications vary greatly
The constitutions of many countries specify the general roles of the legislature and executive, including a few essentials for budget processes; other countries' constitutions contain an entire chapter devoted to the budget and to public finance.

The details can be found in overarching laws as well as lower-level regulations
In some countries, the content of budget laws designed to support the annual budgeting processes is confined to setting out key principles concern to the legislature. The details of budget processes are then set out in lower-level regulations. In other countries, laws contain very specific provisions about all of the main stages of the budget process.

Budget laws can sometimes hold a special status
A few countries have given special status to budget-system laws. In these cases, constitutions require that a law specifies the schedule and procedures by which the budget should be prepared, approved, executed, accounted for, and final accounts submitted for approval (sometimes referred to as an organic budget law)

A legal framework for the health budget enhances good governance for the health sector, transparency and accountability.

Box 10.7

An example of a legal framework for budget laws

Rwanda has a legal framework for public finance management established by the Rwandan Constitution 2003 and the Organic Budget Law 2006.

The Constitution and the Organic law provide that the main institutions responsible for the budget are Parliament, Cabinet, the Ministry of Finance and Economic Planning and the Office of the Auditor General. Under the Constitution, the Chamber of Deputies is responsible for receiving and debating the annual finance bill before it becomes finance law with the concurrence of the Senate. The Cabinet, as the Executive, is responsible for the formulation, preparation and submission of finance bill to the Chamber of Deputies. The Executive is also responsible for budget execution, once the bill has become finance law. The Constitution also establishes the Office of the Auditor General. This Office provides independent assurance that governmental activities are carried out, and accounted for, consistent with Parliament's intentions. The Auditor General is required to submit an annual audited financial report to Parliament. The audit report indicates the manner in which the budget was utilized, unnecessary expenses that were incurred or expenses which were contrary to the law, and whether there was misappropriation or general misuse of public funds.

The Organic Budget Law and the accompanying Financial Regulations set out detailed procedures for the control and use of public funds.

10.2.2 Law and regulation as a key implementation mechanism for health policies and plans

Law and other forms of regulation are key tools for implementing health policy and plans.

Specifically law and regulation can support work on:

- achieving desired policy outcomes; and
- the management of specific inputs and processes which impact on health system performance (see Table 10.1 for examples of how law and regulation and contribute to elements of health system performance relevant to Universal Health Coverage [UHC]).

Laws and regulations are key tools for implementing health policy and plans.

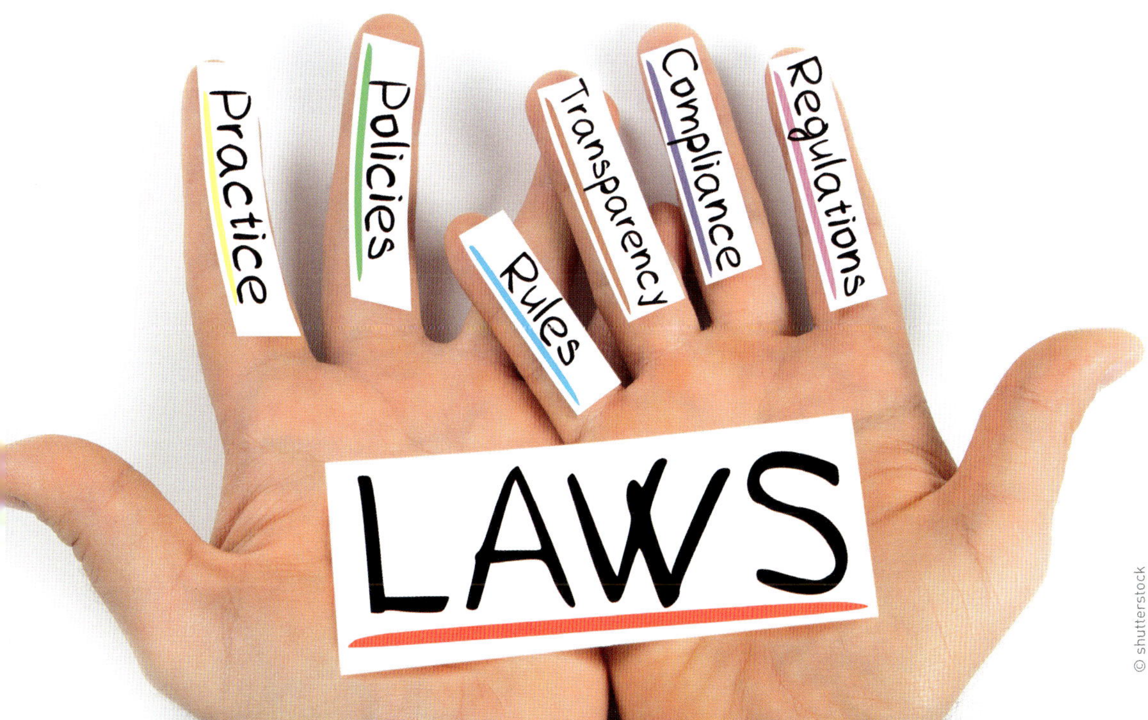

© shutterstock

Table 10.1 Law and regulation and health system performance

HEALTH SYSTEM OBJECTIVES	EXAMPLES OF REGULATORY STRATEGIES	EXAMPLES OF POSSIBLE REGULATORY TOOLS AND APPROACHES
Extend access to services relative to people's health needs	▸ Minimize barriers to service access ▸ Prevent discrimination (age, gender and disability) ▸ Focus on reducing inefficiency in the health system ▸ Develop equitable and transparent criteria for distributing health resources ▸ Empower service users to claim access rights	▸ Establish a list of essential health services and clear access criteria ▸ Establish mechanisms for ensuring access based on the criteria (e.g. through a law or through a contractual mechanism) ▸ Require the provision of information about health services and access criteria ▸ Legislate to prohibit specific activities which interfere with access rights ▸ Legislate to prohibit discrimination ▸ Establish patient-rights laws and charters ▸ Provide dispute resolution mechanisms to ensure access rights ▸ Use tax policy and subsidy ▸ Establish gatekeeping requirements
Financial risk protection	▸ Minimize inefficiency ▸ Develop mechanisms for pooling funds ▸ Promote the development of sustainable funding mechanisms ▸ Ensure transparency and accountability in the health financing system	▸ Provision of universal services funded through tax revenues ▸ Tax policy and subsidies ▸ Price controls ▸ Contracting and tendering processes ▸ Regulation of the health insurance market (for example licensing of insurers, prudential supervision, information provision, requirements to maintain reserves) ▸ Mandatory information disclosure (for example, freedom-of-information laws) ▸ Auditing and reporting mechanisms ▸ Mechanisms for addressing corruption and unauthorized charges for services

HEALTH SYSTEM OBJECTIVES	EXAMPLES OF REGULATORY STRATEGIES	EXAMPLES OF POSSIBLE REGULATORY TOOLS AND APPROACHES
Increase service coverage and quality and effectiveness relative to population need	▸ Ensure access to essential medicines ▸ Assure the quality, safety and effectiveness of services ▸ Focus on reducing inefficiency in the health system ▸ Promote the development of sustainable funding mechanisms ▸ Incentivize the private sector to align its goals with the government's desired social outcomes ▸ Improve clinical outcomes and effectiveness	▸ Generic substitution ▸ Price controls ▸ Maintenance of essential medicine lists and access criteria ▸ Control of prescribing practices ▸ Taxes and subsidies ▸ Contracting mechanisms ▸ Establishment of agreed priorities and outcomes for private sector service provision linked to incentives and sanctions for non-performance ▸ Control of noncommunicable disease (NCD) risk factors ▸ Use of clinical guidelines ▸ Regulation of services (e.g. licensing, certification, accreditation) ▸ Regulation of health professionals (entry criteria, competence and fitness to practice) ▸ Prohibition of anticompetitive behaviours ▸ Provision of incentives to work with at-risk or underserved groups ▸ Laws and mechanisms for controlling corruption

10.2.3 Law and constraints on government powers

As well as enabling government action, the law also provides the means, both constitutional and institutional, by which the powers of the government and its officials and agents are limited and held accountable under the law. Checks on government's powers take many forms. For example in some countries there is a formal separation of powers between the three branches of government: legislature, the executive government and the courts, where each branch is given powers to check and balance the other branches.

Governments are limited and held accountable by the law.

There may also be institutional checks and balances on the operation of executive government; examples include checks on government power by the legislature, the judiciary, and independent auditing and review agencies. In addition to these checks and balances, a country may also have controls which hold government officials accountable for misconduct.

What is important is that key actors involved in the planning process should understand any legal rules and requirements that relate to how the policy and planning process should be carried out. They should also ensure that in carrying out their work they act in accordance with any policies, procedures and rules that apply to their organization or to them individually.

10.3 When should legislation be used?

Legislation is a means to an end, one of a number of regulatory tools that can be used to achieve a particular policy outcome.

For example, a country may wish to establish a strategic health plan that binds government and nongovernment organizations to follow a particular approach. One way to meet this objective might be to pass a law to bind all these actors to act in accordance with the desired approach. However, this might not be necessary where these actors have incentives to follow the approach. For example, there may be a broad consensus about it or financial incentives which encourage the actors to follow it. In that situation passing legislation might not be necessary.

It follows that when deciding between the use of law, a regulatory approach or a non-regulatory approach to achieve a particular policy objective, careful consideration should be given to the advantages and disadvantages and the practicalities of implementing the different options. Here, Regulatory Impact Analysis (RIA) provides a systemic approach to critically assessing the positive and negative effects of the various alternative approaches (see Box 10.10).

10.4 Who should be involved in work on law and regulation? What are their roles and responsibilities?

Work on law and other forms of regulation covers technical health issues, policy dialogue, consideration of legal issues, political processes, planning and resource mobilization. It follows that many different actors are likely to be involved, including political decision-makers, lawyers, policy analysts, health planners, health providers, health professionals and members of the public.

To help health planners (and others) identify people with whom they may need to work on laws and other forms of regulations, a summary of the key actors and their roles is set out in Table 10.2.

Work on law and regulation should be well integrated into policy and planning processes.

Table 10.2 Key actors and their roles in health law and regulation

ACTOR	ROLE
Political decision-makers (e.g. ministers of health, other members of executive government)	▸ Advocate for the need for law or other forms of regulation ▸ Mobilize resources ▸ Make the ultimate decision on approach ▸ Provide political leadership and support for regulatory approach (whether laws or some other regulatory approach)
The health policy-maker	▸ Establish the policy objectives ▸ Coordinate the process ▸ Undertake analysis ▸ Provide advice to the ultimate decision-maker on how to proceed ▸ Evaluate the ultimate success of the chosen regulatory tool
The health planner	▸ Confirm that the objectives of the work are aligned with national plans for the health sector ▸ Ensure there is sufficient space within the health work programme to devote to a proposed law or other form of regulation ▸ Contribute data for the situation analysis ▸ Provide information about the costs and benefits of various alternative regulatory approaches (including the use of law) ▸ Help with planning for implementation

ACTOR	ROLE
The regulator	‣ Provide input during the situation analysis ‣ Help generate regulatory solutions (laws and others) that will work in practice ‣ Supervise and enforce the new regulatory approach
Other government agencies (for example the ministries of justice and finance)	‣ Ministry of justice to provide input on legal principles and legal policy It may also be involved in the drafting and making of any necessary laws ‣ Finance ministry will be involved in discussions about the economic impact of any new law or other form of regulation and its cost to government and the regulated sector
State, regional or local governments (in countries with decentralized health systems, national governments work with state, regional and local government on health sector regulation)	‣ Have input into the process of establishing policy objectives ‣ Provide input during the situation analysis. ‣ Help generate regulatory solutions (laws and others) that will work in practice ‣ Be part of the process of approving the preferred option ‣ Act as regulator, supervising and enforcing the new regulatory approach
The public	‣ Provide input for the situation analysis, for example: how does the current situation in a country affect the public in practice ‣ Help generate solutions
The subject of the proposed regulation	‣ Provide information for situation analysis, information about the impact of the chosen type of regulation (laws or otherwise) on the subject group (including costs) ‣ Help generate solutions ‣ Help to explain any new regulatory mechanism to staff and partners
Civil society organizations	‣ Representing public and community interests in the process ‣ Promoting equity, and the interests of disadvantaged groups ‣ Negotiating public health standards and approaches ‣ Building policy consensus, disseminating information about laws or other forms of regulation ‣ Enhancing public support for a proposed approach

ACTOR	ROLE
Professional associations	▸ Provide information for the situation analysis ▸ Provide input on behalf of their members ▸ Help with the generation of solutions ▸ Help build consensus with their memberships about the use of law or other forms of regulation ▸ Help explain the requirement of new laws or other forms of regulation to their members
Donors	▸ Provide resources for the law-making/regulatory process ▸ Provide information for the situation analysis ▸ Contribute to work on the development of regulatory options
International partner agencies	▸ Provide independent guidance and advice about the use of laws and other regulatory approaches and solutions ▸ Provide technical assistance to support the process ▸ Act as a facilitator or coordinator in the process
The law-making body (e.g. legislature or executive government)	▸ Provide a forum for political debate on a proposed new law ▸ Provide a forum for stakeholder comment on a draft law ▸ Create a new law or changes to an existing law
The courts	▸ Provide guidance on the requirements of regulatory tools (especially laws) ▸ Make binding rulings on disputes ▸ Provide a means for people to enforce their legal rights ▸ Ensure that regulators follow due process when applying the regulatory approach ▸ Impose and enforce sanctions for breaches of new regulatory requirements
The media	▸ Provide information about the process to encourage participation by a range of the actors described above ▸ Help people understand the requirements of the new regulatory approach

A health planner should ensure consideration of the following issues: a checklist

- ✓ Health planners should understand any legal rules and requirements, both in relation to the preparation of a country's National Health Plan/Strategy and in relation to the country's budget process.

- ✓ Copies of relevant laws and guidelines should be reviewed (for example those about the process of making health strategies or plans and relevant laws about the budget cycle), and legal advice taken where necessary on how to meet any related obligations, to ensure that any legal requirements about making plans are complied with (such as specific consultation requirements).

- ✓ Planning processes and procedures should be designed and implemented so as to meet relevant legal requirements.

- ✓ Health planners should work closely with finance ministry officials to ensure that the requirements of a country's budget laws are understood and complied with.

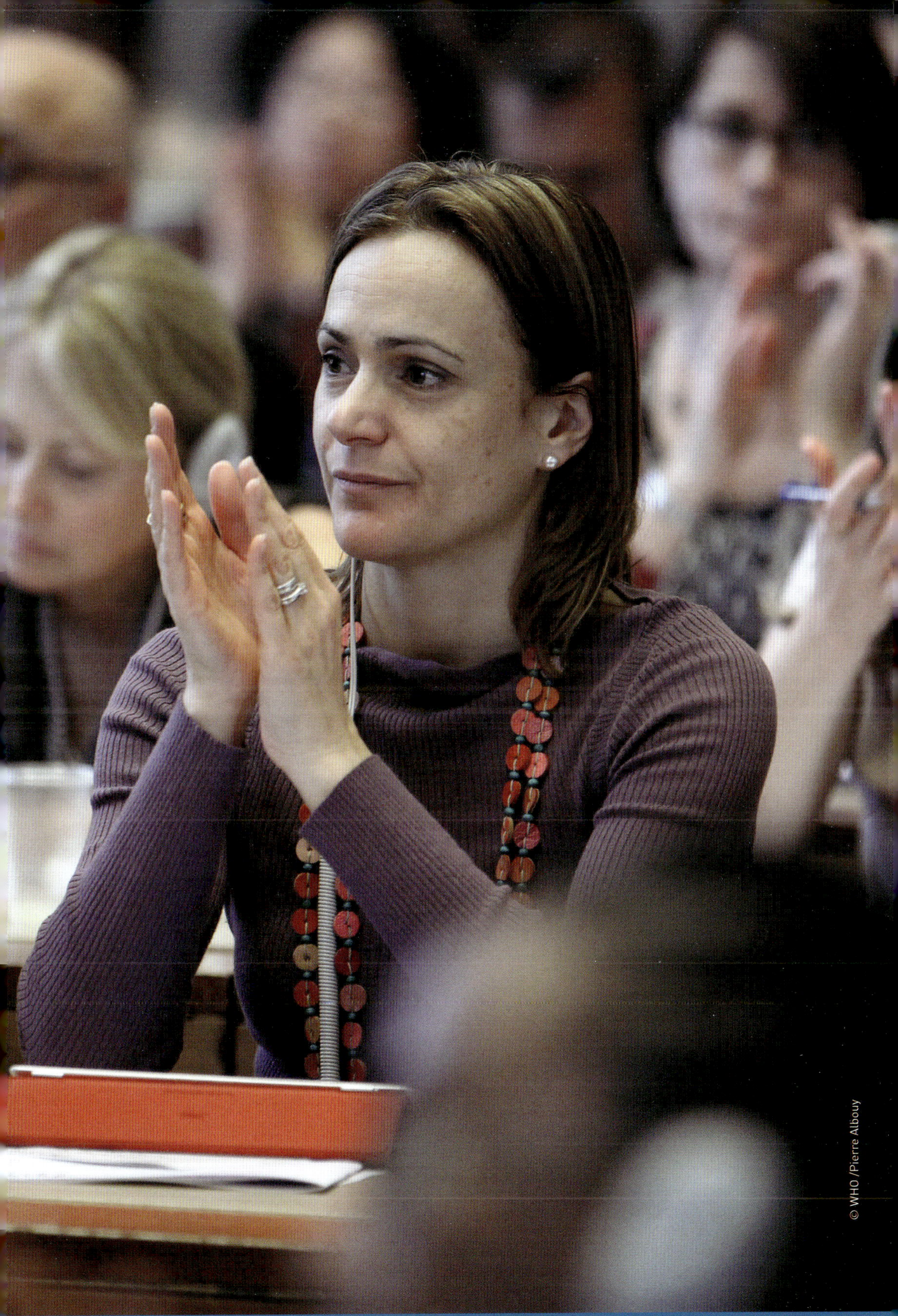
© WHO /Pierre Albouy

10.5 How do we go about work on law and regulation in the context of national health planning?

10.5.1 Specific law and regulation issues to consider during each stage in the national health planning process

Issues about legal/regulatory matters should be considered during these various stages:

Population consultation

There are two main ways that law and regulation are relevant to the population consultation stage of the national health planning process.

Some countries have legal rules about consultation.

First, there may be legal rules and requirements about consultation. For example, there may be rules about consultation in a law or established legal conventions, or duties about consultation that are enforced by the courts. The rules might apply to:

- who is to be consulted;
- how they are to be consulted;
- how long they have to respond;
- what should be done with any feedback from those consulted.

The second way that law or other forms of regulation relate to the consultation process is where they are proposed for use to give effect to a government's policy preferences or to help solve health system problems.

Here it might be necessary to consult the population on the details of the legal/regulatory proposals or issues under consideration. This is done to:

- inform people about the issue or problem and the government's objectives;
- gather required information to permit analysis of legal/regulatory options and to feed into work on the design of the law/regulation;
- facilitate collaboration and solution generation;
- gather information for a regulatory impact assessment (see the discussion below about stages 4 and 5 of the national health planning process);
- attempt to generate a consensus position/support for the legal/regulatory proposal.

Box 10.8

A Danish example of a law about consultation on health plans

The Danish Health Act 2005 provides for cooperation between municipalities and regions established in the form of mandatory regional health care agreements covering issues such as coordination of treatment, prevention, discharge and rehabilitation. The health care agreements are anchored in regional consultative committees consisting of representatives from the region, the municipalities within the region and private practitioners. The regional consultative committees are used to resolve disputes (e.g. about the service level, professional indications and referral criteria in the area of training) and to create the basis for a continuous dialogue about planning.

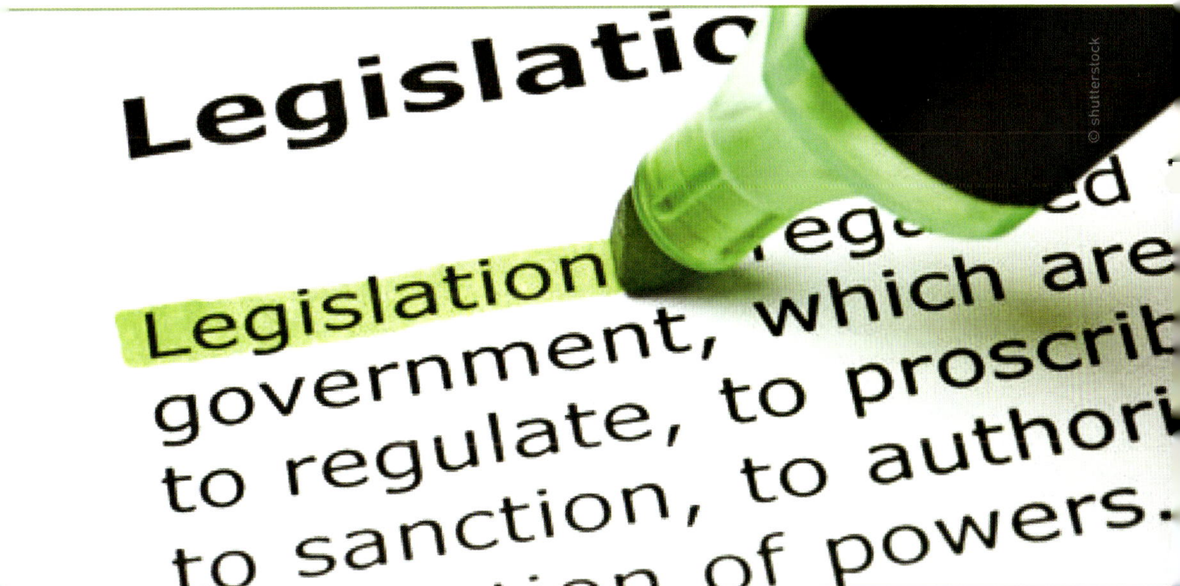

Box 10.9

An example of a legal framework for population consultation – Thailand's National Health Assembly

In 2007 Thailand enacted the National Health Act mandating the establishment of the National Health Commission and Office and the convening of an annual National Health Assembly. The Commission, chaired by the Prime Minister, has 39 members, evenly divided between and nominated from government, academia and health professionals, and civil society organizations.

The following diagram summarizes the process used by the National Health Assembly.

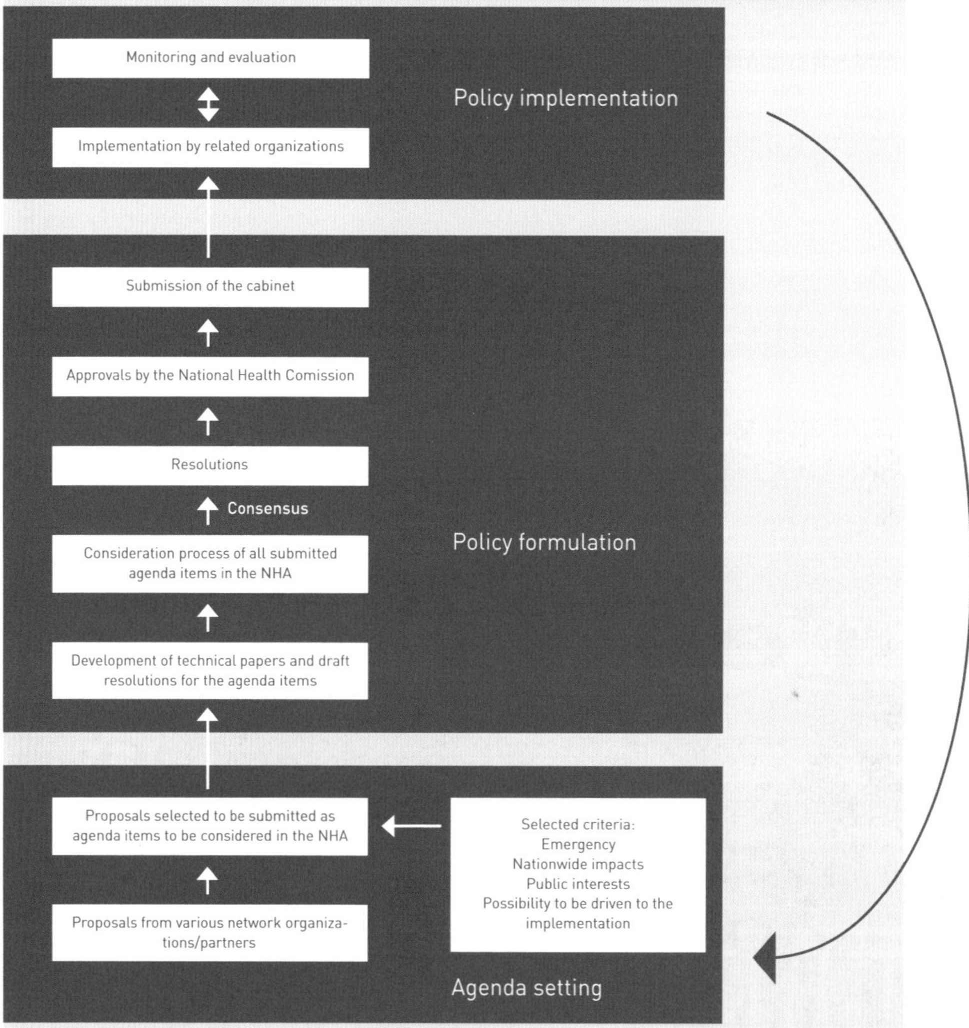

Legal issues to consider when preparing a population consultation

It is important to understand what the legal rules are about consultation in a particular country. The rules can be understood by examining relevant laws and guidance documents and by asking for advice from a specialist who understands the rules.

In the context of developing laws for the health sector, a population consultation can be carried out on a proposal for a new law, just as on any other topic.

When a population consultation is carried out on any health topic, possible related legal issues should be identified beforehand, and the population consultation methodology and questions adapted accordingly.

Decision-making on these issues is guided by the aim of the consultation process. For example, very different approaches may be required if you are consulting to simply inform people about a new law or consulting to encourage stakeholders to collaborate with government on finding feasible legal/regulatory solutions to particular health system problems.

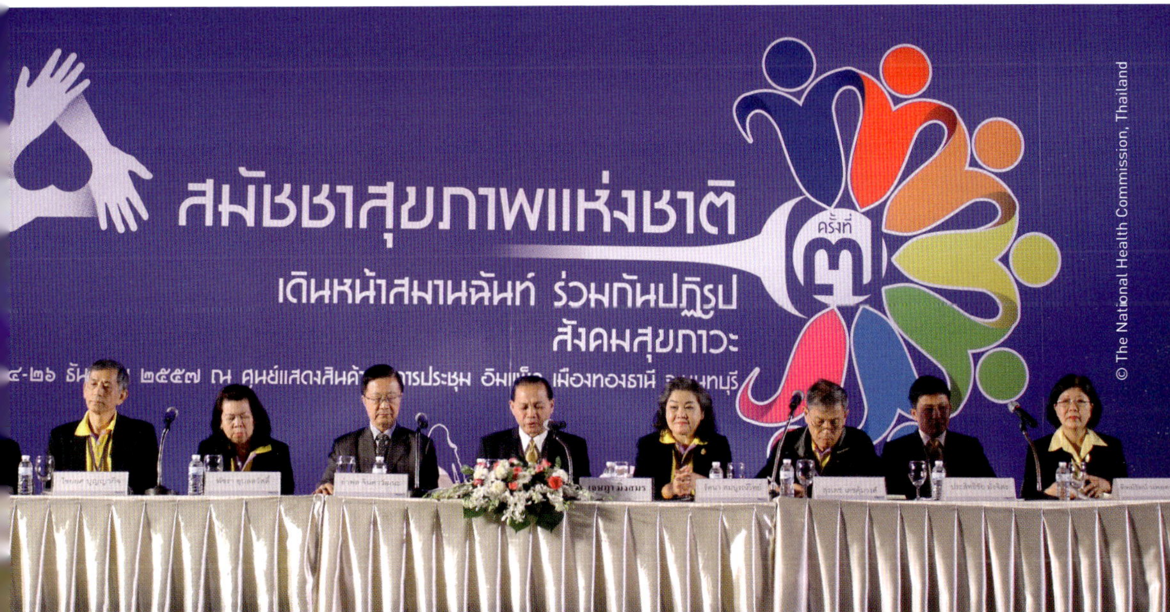

Situation analysis

Regulatory analysis should form part of a country's broader situation analysis. Regulatory analysis involves assessing a country's:

Regulatory analysis helps expose legal problems and constraints and supports regulatory reform efforts.

- existing laws and other regulatory mechanisms;
- regulatory actors, institutions and their capacities;
- binding international obligations that impact on the operation of the health system; and
- existing legal/regulatory systems; process and tools used in the country.

Why undertake regulatory analysis?

The purpose of looking at legal and regulatory issues as part of a country's situation analysis is twofold.

First, to look for legal constraints that might impact on a government's plans This is likely to involve analysing the country's laws (especially the health laws) and constitution to get a picture of any possible areas where existing laws may constrain the government's health plans.

Second, to inform any work on using legal/regulatory approaches to give effect to policy intentions or solve health system problems.

Legal issues to consider when preparing a situation analysis

The legal system (and how it works). Types of regulatory tools that are in use (laws and other tools).

The overall legal framework (constitution, laws, organic laws, traditional laws, administrative regulations, rules).

Any binding treaty obligations (for example, the International Health Regulations).

Effectiveness of current regulation tools in use (what has worked and what has not). The process for creating regulation (for example the legislation-making process and requirements).

Any legal constraints on regulation (for example, does the constitution affect or constrain regulation in any way).

The rule-of-law situation (issues of order and security, whether the legal system has legitimacy, whether there are checks and balances, whether it is applied fairly, the overall effective application of law).

Regulatory institutions, their role, capacity and funding (courts, law enforcement agencies, law schools, lawyers associations, public interest law groups, legal advocacy groups, legal NGOs).

The government's technical capacity to perform regulatory functions (set standards, monitor, evaluate and enforce);

Availability of trained regulatory personnel. Regulatory funding.

The results of a regulatory situation analysis should feed into a country's work on priority setting.

The assessment can clarify a number of issues for the priority-setting process.

- Some approaches might not be legally possible (e.g. because they are prohibited by the country's constitution, another law or by its international obligations).
- Other approaches might be legally possible but might not be legally practicable.
- The assessment can identify legal/regulatory approaches that are possible and promising and require further consideration during the identification of effective strategies phase.

Regulatory space

Regulatory space refers to the capacity of government to make and effectively implement regulation, and make choices between different regulatory tools. The regulatory space essentially sets the available parameters for work on regulation, including whether regulatory reform is actually possible. This involves looking at the acceptance (or degree of opposition to) the proposed reforms in a country, whether there is actual authority to proceed with reform (especially authority from key political decision-makers) as well as the practical ability to proceed with the planned reforms (e.g. the country has the resources to effectively implement the proposed law/regulation).[9]

Regulatory impact

An important analytical tool for the priority-setting stage (and also for the identification of effective strategies) is regulatory impact analysis (or RIA). RIA involves an assessment of the likely effects of any proposed new law or other regulatory change. It is a formal process that helps government officials to undertake regulation-making based on sound information and analysis.

Regulatory impact analysis (RIA) is a formal process for improving the quality of regulatory decision-making.

RIA aims to give clarity on whether a proposed law or other form of regulation will have the desired impact. It helps to reveal possible side-effects and hidden costs as well as possible alternatives. RIA quantifies the likely costs to citizens, businesses and government of new regulation. Typically, the outcome of a RIA will be a report summarizing the problem the regulation aims to address, the preferred options and the main impacts.

RIA is also an important tool in highlighting situations in which regulation is not appropriate or necessary.

RIA are commonly used in OECD countries.[10] There are, however, a number of challenges in using RIA in developing countries.[11]

Judicial intervention in health priority-setting

The other major way that legal issues might affect the priority-setting stage, involves countries whose constitutions, or other laws, confer a right to receive health services or products which can be enforced by a court.

Box 10.10

An example of an RIA process

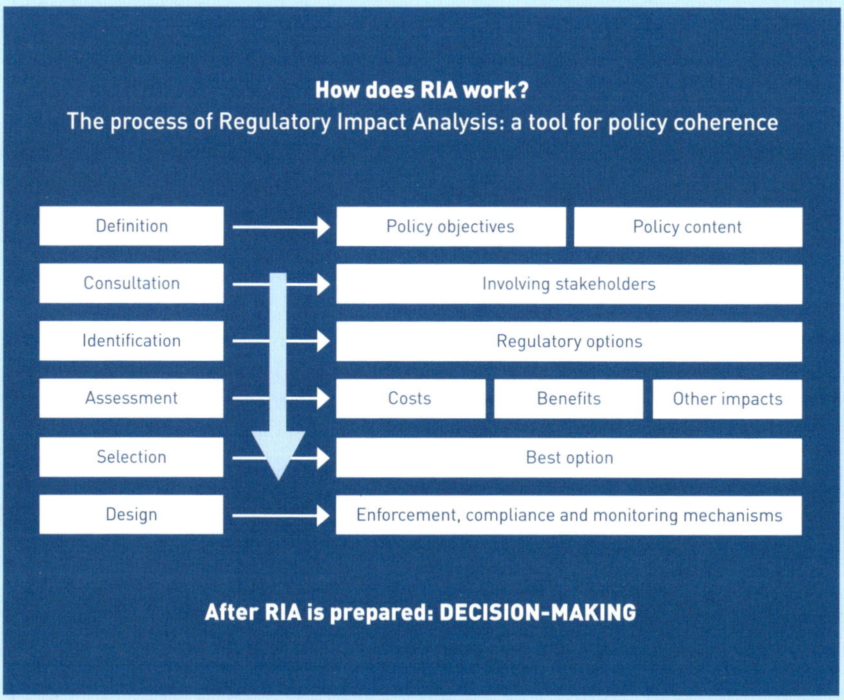

Box 10.11

An example of courts intervening to enforce a right to health

In recent years, several middle-income Latin American countries have seen a steep increase in the number of court cases litigating access to curative services and inputs. The basis for these claims is legal rights established by the country's constitution or other health laws. The claims are often about the right to access certain treatments or medicines. Some argue that these lawsuits are a mechanism for remedying widespread government failures in the delivery of health care in the affected countries.

On the other hand, public health administrators contend that lawsuits disrupt national and regional pharmaceutical distribution efforts, increase inequality in access, and encourage irrational drug use within the public health care system.[12]

Legal issues to consider during a priority setting-process

Understanding whether there are any legal/regulatory constraints that affect the process of prioritization. Information to make this assessment should have been generated during the situation analysis stage.

Understanding "the regulatory space" for any legal/regulatory work that might be required for a particular priority area.

For countries where priority-setting decisions can be challenged in court, ensure that the process followed and decision reached are objectively fair and evidence-based.

If there is a risk of court action about priority setting, take legal advice to ensure that legal requirements are complied with.

Transforming priorities into a national health plan

Work on laws and other forms of regulation started during stage 3 will continue during stage 4 to support the formulation of a country's national health plan.

During this stage it will be important to ensure compliance with any specific legal requirements that might apply to the process of constructing and finalizing the national health plan (for those countries with specific laws and requirements about national health plans).

Work may also continue on RIA where legal/regulatory approaches are needed to operationalize the plan.

Legal issues to consider when transforming priorities into a national health plan

Ensuring full compliance with any legal requirements related to the process of preparing and finalizing the national health plan.

Continuing work on RIA (as required) with a country's policy and legal advisors.

If a new law or regulation is needed, it will need to be implemented, maintained and reviewed.

Operational planning

During stage 5, the main focus of work on law and other forms of regulation depends heavily on what strategic direction is given by the NHPSP. If developing a new law or regulation is required to give effect to the national health plan, then implementation of these new laws need to be carefully planned.

There are two distinct phases to implementation of any new law or regulation:

- the initial phase when a new regulation is introduced; and
- the ongoing administration and review of the regulation.

The initial phase has distinct characteristics as it is at this point that historical behaviours are required to change in line with the expectations underlying the regulation. Behaviours are a function of both attitudes and capabilities. In addition, often, behaviours of more than one group need to change.

Behaviours that must change to achieve the objectives of the law are often path-dependent and can be deeply embedded, and it is important not to underestimate the effort required to effect change. Therefore, one needs to allow sufficient time for implementation, to adopt appropriate strategies to facilitate and manage the change process, and undertake sufficient ongoing monitoring and evaluation.

The questions below should be asked at the outset.

- What groups will be affected by this regulatory tool (key groups include providers, consumers, regulators, standards bodies, etc.)?
- What behaviours would we expect these groups to demonstrate if regulation is to achieve its intended objectives?
- What might act as barriers to behavioural change?
- What concrete activities are likely to work best to reduce these barriers?
- What incentives are in place to influence the behaviours of affected parties?
- What monitoring and evaluation strategy is required to identify and address emerging issues that are affecting the effective implementation of regulation?
- When considering the factors that influence the implementation of the regulation on an ongoing basis, it is important to note that interventions that do not deliver on their intended objectives may reflect poor strategy choice by the regulator rather than the rules themselves.

Issues to consider during the NHPSP operational planning

Making law and regulation to implement policy is not the end of the process – it is also important to plan for implementation.

Specific regulatory implementation considerations include:

Administration issues, such as which agency will implement and administer the regulation and how it will function.

Timing and transitional arrangements, for instance delayed or gradual introduction of new requirements and provision of interim assistance to affected parties, such as education about the new requirements.

Compliance costs minimization strategies, including what implementation strategies will be required, such as an education campaign, advisory services and testing with stakeholders, and if there exists regulation that can be reduced or removed to prevent overlap.

Implementation risks and their potential impact on the effectiveness of an option. Strategies for mitigating these risks should be explored.

Information that regulated parties will require in order to comply with the regulation, and how this will be provided (e.g. whether there is opportunity to rationalize or take advantage of existing information sources or methods of communication).

Enforcement strategy and how and who will enforce compliance.

The key legal/regulatory issues for stage 6 involve the costing of any legal/regulatory interventions, their implementation, supervision and enforcement.

Specific costing may be required in a number of categories.

Appropriate costing of regulation informs its feasibility.

- The human resource costs and costs of specific technical inputs (e.g. from legal and regulatory experts) for a law/regulatory reform process. These processes may range in complexity and scale from minor legislative changes to large-scale reform processes that may take several years and significant resources to complete.
- Ongoing administration costs of any new legal/regulatory scheme.
- In some cases a country may decide to establish a new regulatory agency to implement and supervise a new law or regulatory scheme. In such cases, the cost of establishing and operating such and agency will need to be determined.
- The costs of providing information to regulated parties about the new law or regulatory scheme to facilitate compliance.
- Costs associated with supervision and enforcement of the new law or regulatory requirements (for example the costs of maintaining an inspectorate to monitor compliance).

Box 10.12

An example from Thailand of the costs associated with establishing a regulatory agency

The National Health Security Act B.E. 2545 (2002) is the legal basis for the Universal Coverage Scheme (UCS) in Thailand. The Act stipulates the establishment of the National Health Security Office (NHSO) and the National Health Security Fund. The NHSO is an autonomous body with 13 regional offices which would govern the UCS. The establishment of the NHSO necessitated ongoing expenditure to meet its annual administrative cost. In 2013, the administrative cost of NHSO was 0.85% of the UCS.

This example demonstrates the importance of assessing and factoring in the cost of implementation when considering the feasibility of a new law.

Legal issues to consider during NHPSP costing

Ensuring full compliance with any legal requirements about the process of preparing and finalizing the national health plan.

Ensuring that work on law and other forms of regulation supports and is informed by the country's policy dialogue and is well aligned with the content and intent of the national health plan.

Continuing work on RIA (as required) with a country's policy and legal advisors.

Monitoring and evaluation

Any planned work to monitor and evaluate the impact of the NHPSP should (where legal/regulatory reform forms a key component or enabler of the NHPSP) include evaluation of the legal and regulatory reform itself. Legal and other types of regulation reform should be evaluated to do the following:

It is important to monitor the impact of regulation to ensure that it continues to deliver desired outcomes.

- Provide accountability to funders and stakeholders as to the value of the intervention.
- Increase knowledge and understanding about the intervention and its objectives, including knowledge of needs of potential beneficiaries and of effective practices.
- Contribute to the general body of knowledge on effective regulatory strategies and interventions.
- Measure the actual impact of regulation on the government's desired outcome(s).
- Governments need to establish indicators for measuring the impact of laws and other forms of regulation with respect to outcomes of concern. Through such measurements, conclusions can be reached about the extent to which law/regulation has actually brought about desired changes.[13]

Box 10.13

Learning practical lessons from evaluating regulation in low- and middle-income countries: an example

'Health system stewardship and regulation in Viet Nam, India and China' (HESVIC) was a multidisciplinary and multi-partner project implemented over a three year period (July 2009 to December 2012). Using maternal health as a critical case study, the project investigated regulation as it relates to wider governance in policy and practice of health systems in maternal health for Viet Nam, India and China. The study:

- examined the application of international standards in governance and regulation of maternal health activities - to the extent that such standards existed;
- outlined national standards for governance and regulation of maternal health activities in the three study countries; and
- explored the effects of governance and regulation of maternal health-care services and systems on equitable access to quality maternal health care, within and across each study country.

One of the key results of the project was the development of an integrated approach for the assessment of regulation. Applying this methodology, the project found that regulatory control is constrained under current conditions in low- and middle-income countries (LMIC) settings, with the possible exception of services that are centrally planned. The study also found that regulation-hampering mechanisms are related to historical, socio-political and administrative conditions in LMIC.

The study concluded that regulation should be nested in larger health policies for a number of reasons.

- Regulation is not very effective on its own, certainly under LMIC conditions.
- Regulations can yield undesirable effects. For instance, in Viet Nam, combined with the common perception that the quality of services is better at the provincial level than at district level, the emergency obstetric care regulation resulted in the overburdening of provincial hospitals.
- Health professionals cannot be motivated merely by material incentives and deterred by punishments, but also need non-financial incentives.
- Governments commonly are reluctant to ensure regulation for the private sector, but the private sector should be more involved in regulatory processes.
- Designing regulation in China, India, Viet Nam was carried out in a closed way by bureaucrats, politicians and government external advisers. Granting a voice to non-state actors – like health facility users and various socioeconomic groups – may help ensure that regulations better reflect the needs of these groups.[14]

Legal issues to consider during the monitoring and evaluation of an NHPSP

The key question is: how will the effectiveness of the regulatory changes be measured?

Plans should be made for monitoring, evaluating, and reviewing the performance of laws and other forms of regulation over time.

It is also important that any new law/regulation is monitored and periodically reviewed to evaluate whether the option is the preferred solution to the particular issue or problem over time. Such monitoring and evaluation helps to ensure that new laws/regulations are working as expected (delivering the anticipated benefits at expected costs), that there have been no unforeseen consequences and they continue to be necessary as circumstances change and evolve.

When new law or other regulatory options are being proposed, it is important to have a clear understanding of the channels through which the intervention is expected to generate the intended benefits. Analysis needs to consider how effectiveness will be measured: what indicators will be used; what data will be required; how this information will be collected, and by whom.

On-going or periodic consultation with stakeholders may be appropriate, in which case the arrangements for this should be agreed upon. It may be appropriate to establish a feedback mechanism (e.g. a way for stakeholders to ask questions or lodge complaints). Regular, public reporting on the effectiveness of the law/regulation may also be considered.

Plans should also be made for how and when the law/regulation will be reviewed. Agencies should consider committing to a periodic review of particular regulatory interventions. Reviews should be reported and consulted on with a view to ensuring that a law/regulation remains fit for its purpose. Reviews should consider the following issues:

- Is there still a problem (and is it the one originally identified)?
- Are the objectives being met?
- Are the impacts as expected? Are there any unforeseen problems? Are there any indirect effects that were not anticipated?
- Is intervention still required? Is the current intervention still the most appropriate, or would another measure be more suitable?

10.5.2 Legal impediments and constraints to consider in national health planning

On occasion, a country's pre-existing legal/regulatory framework might act as a constraint or impediment on a government's policy intentions. A health planner should be aware of and think through such constraints, and potentially seek legal advice or broach the subject at higher-level government meetings if it greatly impacts on a national health plan or any policy change to implement the plan.

Existing laws can support or block new policies and plans. It is thus important to identify relevant existing laws and their impact on what is being planned.

There are three main legal impediments a country may face in the health planning process.

1. First, there may be requirements in a country's constitution, laws or international obligations (e.g. binding legal commitments such as treaty obligations), which may either prohibit a particular policy or approach from proceeding or influence the way it is designed or implemented (and where it might not be possible or practical to change the constitution, amend the relevant law or treaty to make it consistent with the planned policy or approach). For example, a country with a decentralized health system may have a constitution which impacts on, or controls, how health services are funded/purchased at the national level. This would mean that the design of any national funding or purchasing system would need to be modified to comply with the constitution.

2. Second, where an existing legal/regulatory framework is not "fit for purpose", that is, it does not enable the proposed policy or approach because the legal/regulatory framework is out of date, out of step with the planned policy approach, or has gaps (and where it is possible to amend the law regulatory tool in question to make it consistent or to enable the planned policy or approach). For example, a country might want to require its health workers to comply with new requirements about how they provide services (for instance, to improve quality of care), but its existing law might not allow these standards to be imposed. This would mean that the law would need to be amended to address this gap.

3. Third, where the current legal/regulatory framework is consistent with the planned policy or approach, but the legal system is unable to support the planned policy or approach (because of problems with the capacity and/or capabilities of the regulatory actors, institutions or processes required to give effect to the planned policy or approach). For example, a country might want to set up a new scheme for contracting out the provision of health services to the private sector. It may have passed a law to allow this new policy to occur, but might lack the expertise or capacity to prepare and negotiate effective commercial contracts to give effect to its health objectives or to properly monitor the performance of contracted providers against the requirements of a contract.

However, even where a country lacks the capacity to make a commercial contract, it may be possible to adopt the use of what are known as relational contracts. In contracting terms "pure" commercial contracts and "relational" contracts are both categories of contract in the legal sense. The difference is that the first category, the detailed commercial contract, the detailed terms of the contract are important for its operation and the parties may go to court to enforce it in the event of a dispute. Contracts of this nature may, however, be difficult to establish in a context where monitoring the performance of, and enforcing the terms of, such contracts is difficult (because of the general lack of legal institutions).

A relational contract, on the other hand, is based on the parties' confidence that each will act in their mutual interest. Consequently, there is no need for the contract to be exhaustive and detailed; agreement on the main objectives of the relationship, the methods of work, and the means to be used to carry out the actions will suffice. The flexibility and cooperation characteristic of this type of contract are intended to secure not only its permanence, but also contractual efficiency.[15]

Box 10.14

An example from Cambodia of the use of relational contracts

A good example of the use of relational contracts is the health reforms in Cambodia. Prior to 1999, the health system was considered extremely weak and ineffective: mortality rates remained high, out-of-pocket payments dominated the total health expenditure of the country, despite the population being one of the poorest in the region, and shortages of drugs and medical supplies led patients to seek traditional care rather than that provided by the health system. Lack of regular salary payments was a major contributor to Cambodia's poor health system performance; health workers often provided informal and extra-legal[V] activities for more income, making health policies difficult to implement through existing regulatory channels. While some system weaknesses were addressed by instituting a new health coverage plan and establishing a minimum package of services, the guarantee of quality services had yet to be achieved. Legal and financial reforms were required to improve access to primary health services and create an effective and cost-efficient public health system.

In order to improve health system performance, a district contracting system was adopted, an approach largely favoured as a way to improve access to care for poor and underserved areas. Cambodian policy-makers experimented with different types of contracting for different districts, relying primarily on four-year relational contracts with NGOs. Some used contracting-out to private contractors, where the contractor would have complete control over staff and budget, while others used contracting-in of district management, where the private sector provided management services in a largely public health sector. The former method was considered more of a political commitment to district contracting, as full responsibility was placed on the contractor for service provision. By using the contracting-in method, the district governments had greater control over budgeting and regulation, including the start of a financial incentive programme for health workers to improve motivation to provide higher quality care.[16]

V Extra-legal activities are activities that are not authorized by government legislation; however, government authorities do not intervene to stop those activities for whatever reason. In this case it refers to government health workers opening their own private practices, laboratories etc. These are informal activities used to generate extra income because of the instability of government payments. Stakeholders accept this fact and understand that the government health workers need more money to live on, so any sort of legal action is not taken to prevent private informal business. In fact, health workers openly publicize and provide information about their activities to their employers.

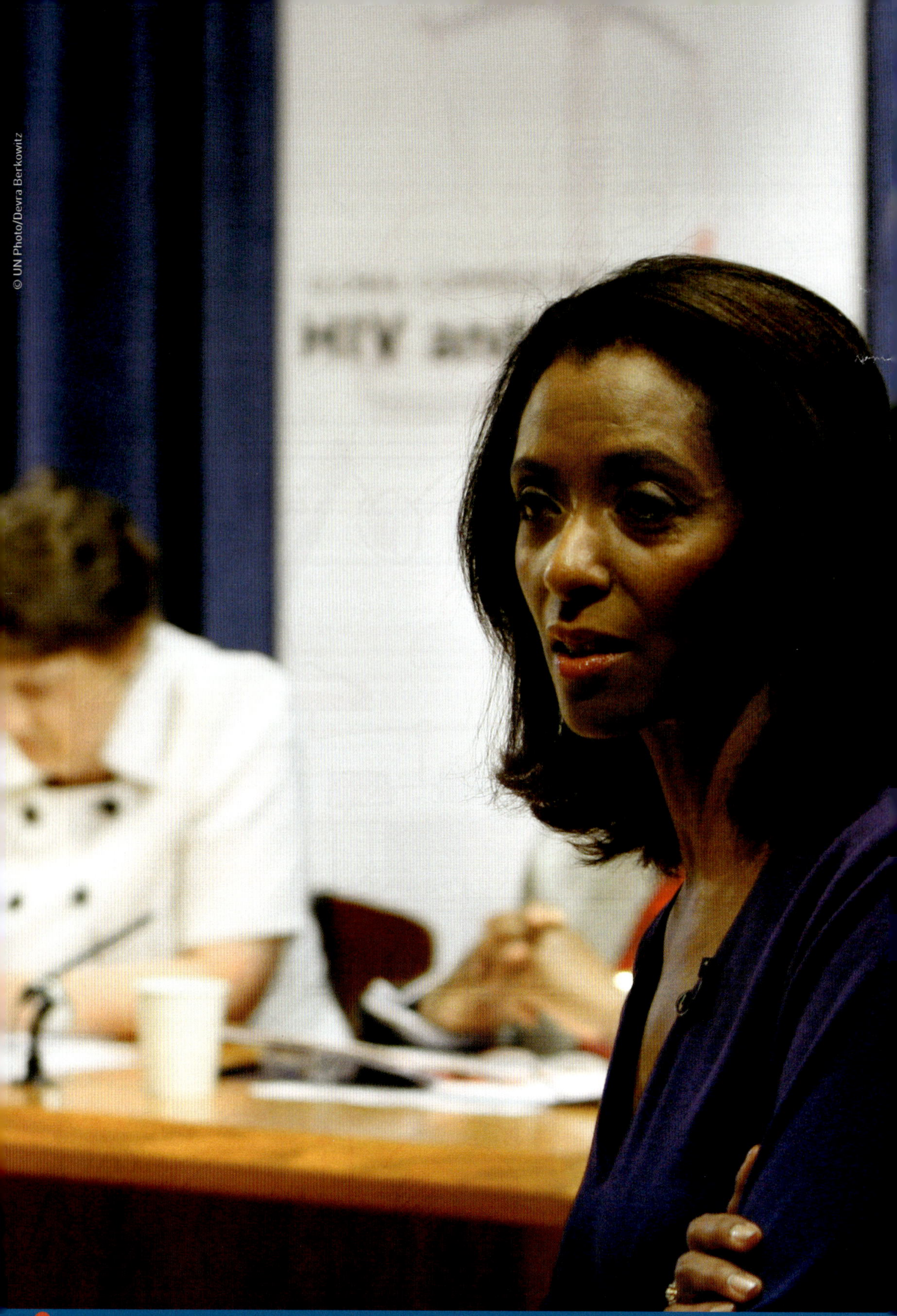

© UN Photo/Devra Berkowitz

10.6 Conclusion

This chapter explains the role and the importance of law and regulation for the national health planning process. It explains how law and regulation can:

- provide the structure and the rules for a country's national health planning process; and
- act as an important policy tool and lever for improving health system performance.

The key message from this chapter is that work on law and other forms of regulation should not be regarded as a separate process, but should form an integral part of a country's health policy dialogue engaging stakeholders from health, finance and other ministries, civil society, nongovernmental organizations, international agencies, academic institutions, professional associations, and communities. A similar approach should be taken when implementing law and regulation.

For planners and policy-makers, it is therefore essential to:

- understand any legal requirements that affect the national health planning process; and
- ensure that the task and inputs required for developing and implementing law and regulation are fully integrated into the national health planning process.

References

1 Akhtar A. Health care regulation in low- and middle-income countries: a review of the literature. Mebourne: Nossal Institute for Public Health; 2011 (Health Policy and Health Finance Knowledge Hub, Working Paper Series No. 14; http://community.eldis.org/.5b0c5e57/HPHF_Hub_WP_No_14_Health_care_regulation_in_low-and_middle-income_countries.pdf, accessed 1 March 2016).

2 Turkey marks progress in fight against noncommunicable diseases. World Health Organization; 2012 (http://www.who.int/features/2012/ncd_turkey/en/).

3 Lagarde M, Haines A, Palmer N. The impact of conditional cash transfers on health outcomes and use of health services in low and middle income countries. Cochrane Database of Systematic Reviews 2009, Issue 4; 2009.

4 Medical Council of India. The Indian MEdical Council Act, 1956. (http://www.mciindia.org/ActsandAmendments/TheMedicalCouncilAct1956.aspx, accessed 12 March 2016).

5 Morgan B, Yeung K. An Introduction to Law and Regulation. Cambridge: Cambridge University Press 2007.

6 National Health Service. The NHS in England: The NHS structure. (http://www.nhs.uk/NHSEngland/thenhs/about/Pages/nhsstructure.aspx, accessed 10 February 2016).

7 Office of the Auditor-General, New Zealand. Controller and Auditor-General. (http://www.oag.govt.nz, accessed 12 March 2016).

8 The legal framework for budget systems: an international comparison. OECD Journal on Budgeting. 2004;4(3):Special Issue (http://www.oecd.org/governance/budgeting/35933542.pdf, accessed 1 March 2016).

9 Odugbemi S, Jacobson T. Governance reform under real-world conditions: citizens, stakeholders, and voice. Washington (DC): WOrld Bank; 2008 (https://openknowledge.worldbank.org/handle/10986/6513, accessed 1 March 2016).

10 Regulation impact analysis. In: OECD/Directorate for public governance and territorial development/regulatory policy [website]. Paris: Organisation for Economic Co-operation and development; 2016 (http://www.oecd.org/gov/regulatory-policy/ria.htm, accessed 12 March 2016).

11 RIA in OECD countries. In: OECD/Directorate for public governance and territorial development/regulatory policy [website]. Paris: Organisation for Economic Co-operation and development; 2016 (http://www.oecd.org/gov/regulatory-policy/riainoecdcountriesand-challengesfordevelopingcountries.htm, accessed 12 March 2016).

12 Biehl J. Global Health Research: Right to Health Litigation. (http://joaobiehl.net/global-health-research/right-to-health-litigation/, accessed 12 March 2016).

13 Coglianse C. Measuring regulatory performance: evaluating the impact of regulation and regulatory policy. Paris: Organisation for Economic Co-operation and Development (OECD); 2012: 7 (Expert Paper No. 1; http://www.oecd.org/gov/regulatory-policy/1_coglianese%20web.pdf, accessed 10 March 2016) (OECD 2012).

14 Community Research and Development Information Service. HESVIC Report Summary. (http://cordis.europa.eu/result/rcn/57803_en.html, accessed 12 March 2016).

15 The Role of Contracting in Improving Health Systems Performance, Discussion Paper. World Health Organization. Discussion Paper Number 1 – 2004, Department "Health System Financing, Expenditure and Resource Allocation" (FER), Cluster "Evidence and Information for Policy (EIP). Geneva, Switzerland.

16 Robert Soeters and Fred Griffiths. Improving government health services through contract management: a case from Cambodia. Health Policy and Planning 18(1): 74-83. Oxford University Press 2003.

Further reading

Afifi NH, Busse R, Harding A. Regulation of health services. In: Harding A, Preker AS, editors. Private participation in health services. Washington (DC): Human Development Network; 2003: 221–344 (Health, Nutrition and Population Series; https://www.wbginvestmentclimate.org/toolkits/public-policy-toolkit/upload/Reading-Material-1.pdf, accessed 10 March 2016).

Baldwin R, Cave M. Understanding regulation: theory, strategy, and practice, 2nd edition. Oxford: Oxford University Press; 2011.

Bingham T. The rule of law. London: Allen Lane; 2011.

Consultation on strategic contracting in health systems: synthesis of the meeting, Geneva, 9–11 January 2008. Geneva: World Health Organization; 2008 (http://www.who.int/health_financing/documents/strategic_contracting_synthesis_en.pdf, accessed 10 March 2016).

The Fiscal Transparency Code. Washington (DC): International Monetary Fund; 2014 (http://blog-pfm.imf.org/files/ft-code.pdf, accessed 10 March 2016).

Hood CC, Margetts HZ. The tools of government in the digital age, 2nd edition. Basingstoke: Palgrave Macmillan; 2007.

The legal framework for budget systems: an international comparison. Paris: Organisation for Economic Co-operation and Development; 2004 (http://www.oecd.org/unitedkingdom/35933542.pdf, accessed 10 March 2016).

Morgan B, Yeung K. An introduction to law and regulation. London: Cambridge University Press; 2007.

Recommendation of the Council on Regulatory Policy and Governance. Paris: Organisation for Economic Co-operation and Development; 2012 (http://www.oecd.org/governance/regulatory-policy/49990817.pdf, accessed 10 March 2016).

Regulatory impact analysis handbook. Wellington: New Zealand Treasury; 2013 (http://www.treasury.govt.nz/regulation/regulatoryproposal/ria/handbook, accessed 10 March 2016).

Regulatory institutions and practices. Wellington: New Zealand Productivity Commission; 2014 (http://www.productivity.govt.nz/sites/default/files/regulatory-institutions-and-practices-final-report.pdf, accessed 10 March 2016).

The role of contracting in improving health systems performance. Geneva: World Health Organization; 2004 (http://www.who.int/health_financing/documents/cov-dp_e_04_1-role_contracting/en/, accessed 10 March 2016).

Saltman TB, Busse R, Mossialis B, editors. Regulating entrepreneurial behaviour in European health care systems. Buckingham: Open University Press; 2002 (European Observatory on Health Care Systems series; Saltman et al Regulating entrepreneurial behaviour in European health care systems, Open University Press 2002, accessed 10 March 2016).

Yeung K. The regulatory state. In: Baldwin R, Cave M, Lodge M (eds). The Oxford handbook of regulation. Oxford: Oxford University Press; 2010.

Chapter 11

Strategizing for health at sub-national level

Katja Rohrer

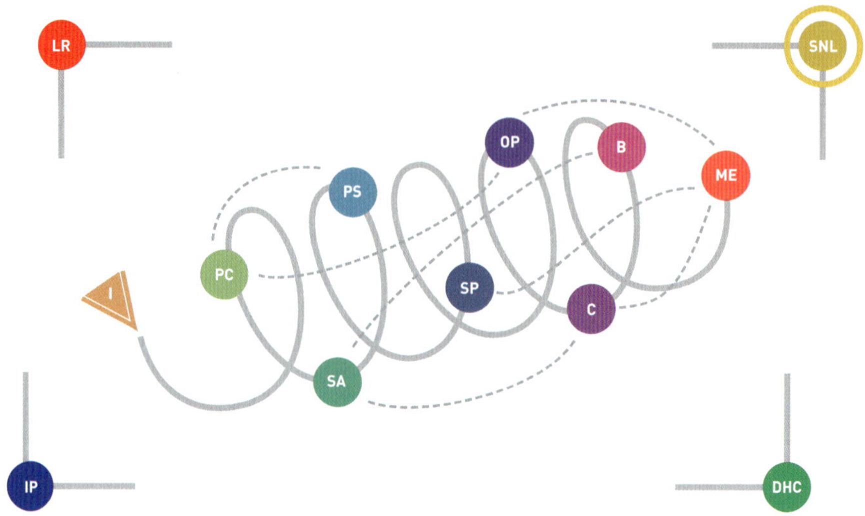

Cross-cutting topics relevant to national health planning

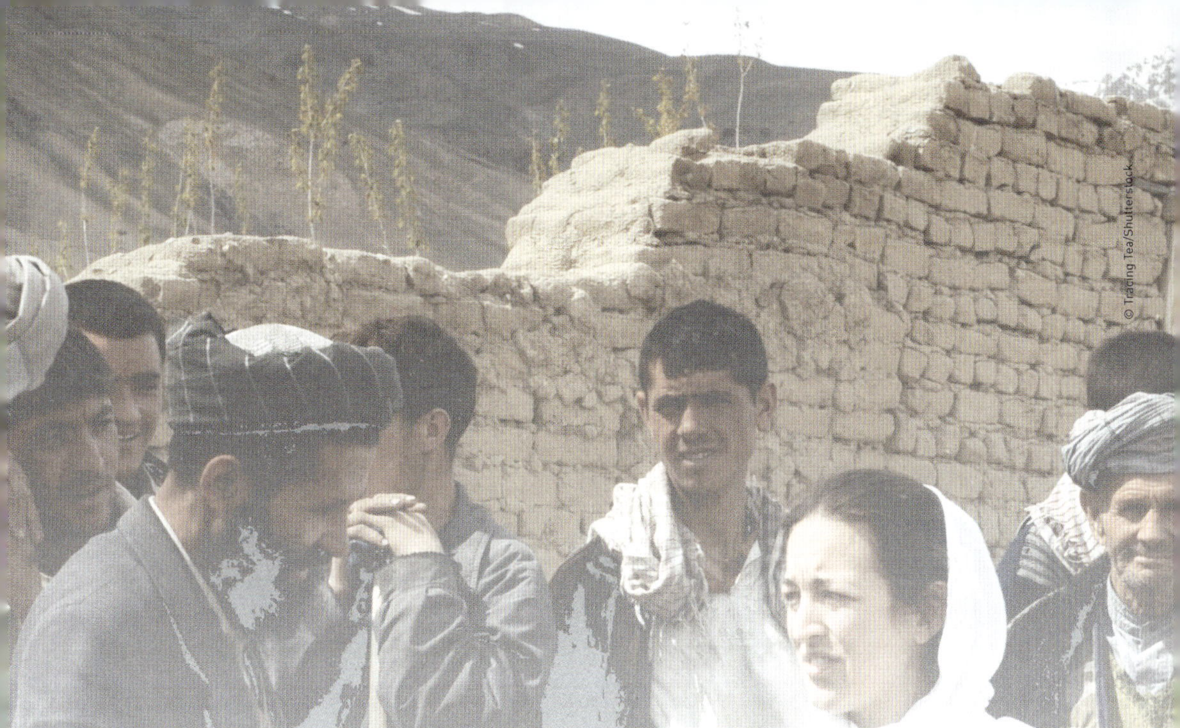

Overview

"Sub-national" describes any government entity below the national level, regardless of the political, financial and administrative design of the country. "Strategizing at sub-national level" refers to all systematic planning and programming as well as budgeting and resource allocation processes below the national level, i.e. at local, district or regional level. Moving the planning function to sub-national level, either through deconcentration, delegation or devolution (elaborated further in this chapter), can have positive impacts on the

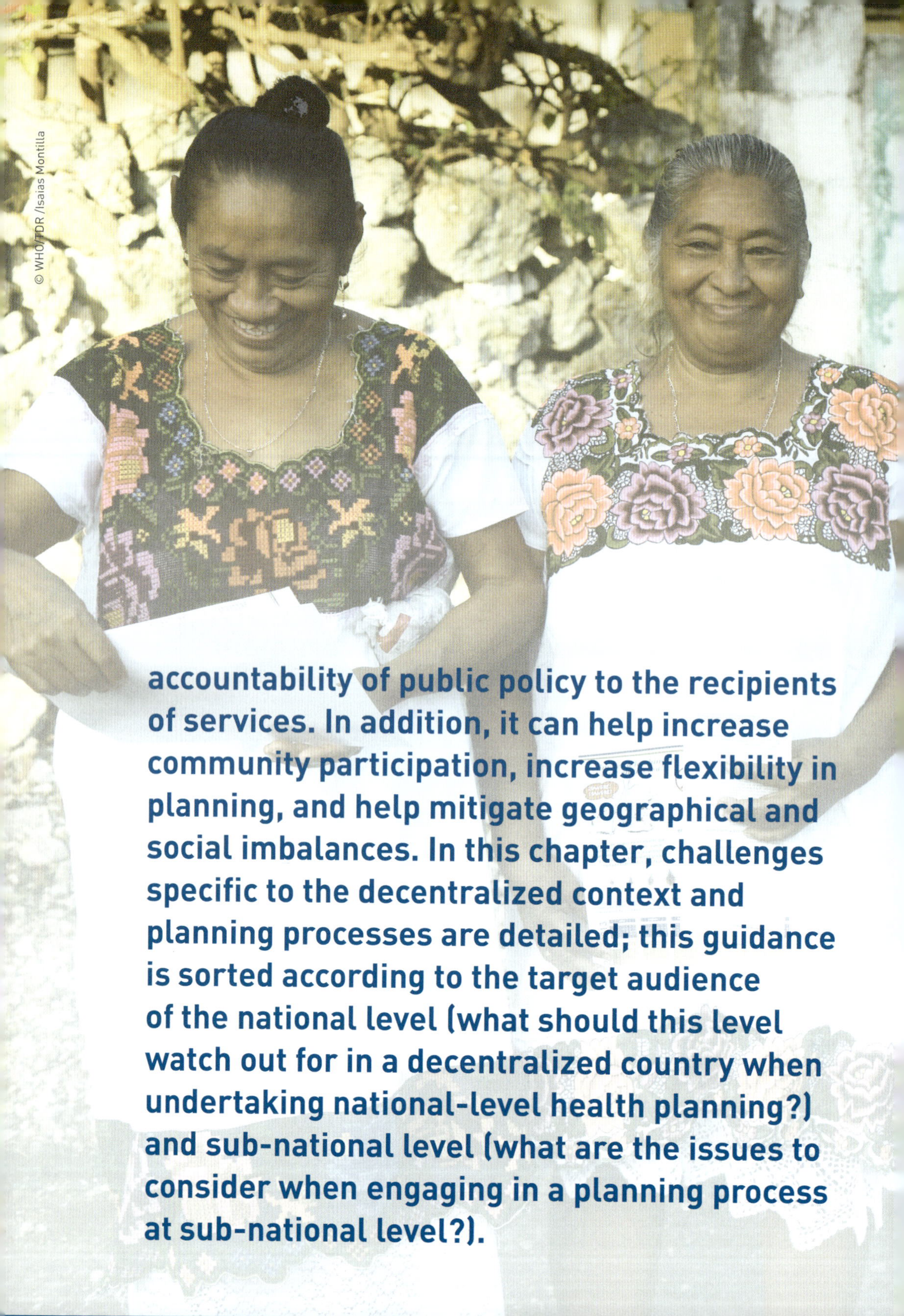

accountability of public policy to the recipients of services. In addition, it can help increase community participation, increase flexibility in planning, and help mitigate geographical and social imbalances. In this chapter, challenges specific to the decentralized context and planning processes are detailed; this guidance is sorted according to the target audience of the national level (what should this level watch out for in a decentralized country when undertaking national-level health planning?) and sub-national level (what are the issues to consider when engaging in a planning process at sub-national level?).

Summary

What is strategizing for health at sub-national level?

"Strategizing at sub-national level" refers to all systematic planning and programming as well as budgeting and resource allocation processes below the national level, i.e. at local, district or regional level. Sub-national planning is generally determined by the dimension and range of decentralization, as well as the degree of autonomy of the sub-national planning authority.

Why is strategizing for health at sub-national level important?

The features of decentralization have a strong influence on the structure, content, the different steps and the outcome of overall national health policies, strategies and plans (NHPSPs). In addition, Planning at sub-national level, either in deconcentration, delegation or devolution contexts (elaborated further in this chapter), can have positive impacts on the accountability of public policy to the recipients of services. In addition, it can help increase community participation, increase flexibility in planning, and help mitigate geographical and social imbalances. Furthermore, in some cases, it is simply a legal necessity, and not being aware of the consequences of decentralized planning is a missed opportunity.

When should sub-national planning be considered during the planning cycle?

National planning authorities must take sub-national planning into account throughout the policy and planning cycle. That being said, it is crucial that the arrangements and schedule for sub-national planning be carefully considered from the beginning in relation to the overall process of strategizing for health. Sub-national input is absolutely critical for shaping the overarching national health plan. At the same time, national-level collaboration in sub-national planning processes is necessary to ensure coherence across regions and sub-national structures, and to enable aggregation of data and information at national level.

Who should be engaged in sub-national planning?

All stakeholders involved in the national health planning process, be they within the ministry of health (MoH) or outside it, should be attentive to the decentralized health system structure and its consequences for sub-national and national planning. Nongovernmental actors or external partners (e.g. United Nations agencies, bilateral organizations) who are supporting planning processes should acknowledge the decentralized setting and act in accordance to its rules and regulations. The MoH has a special oversight function to provide guidance and capacity support to sub-national entities, ensuring overall coherence with the national health sector vision.

How to strategize for health at sub-national level?

Sub-national planning is relevant to each step of the policy and planning cycle. In this section, each such step is addressed in relation to planning at sub-national level per se, as well as in relation to national-level planning in a decentralized context. Concrete recommendations and special issues to consider are elaborated upon.

11.1 What is strategizing at sub-national level?

11.1.1 What do we mean by "sub-national"?

"Sub-national" and "national" define different organizational tiers of government. "Sub-national" describes any government entity below the national level, regardless of the political, financial and administrative design of the country. It therefore encompasses any intermediate (e.g. district, state, regional, provincial) and local governments as well as semi-independent government organizations (e.g. parastatals) at sub-national level.

- Most countries are equipped with a three-tier government system.
- The first tier is usually the national level, with the national – sometimes federal – MoH.
- The second tier is generally composed of a regional government. Examples are (federal) states (e.g. India, Germany, Nigeria), cantons (e.g. Switzerland) or regions (e.g. Mali).
- The third tier is usually the district (sometimes called "local health system" in the literature), a local administrative unit, with varying sizes and varying numbers of subunits (see Box 11.2, below). For example, in India, a district is a local administrative unit that is positioned immediately below the state level.

Hence, "sub-national" in this chapter and this handbook refers to any tier below the national level.

11.1.2 What do we mean by "strategizing at sub-national level"?

Strategizing at sub-national level, or sub-national planning, refers to all systematic planning and programming as well as budgeting and resource allocation processes (in essence, the full policy and planning cycle) below the national level, i.e. at local, district or regional level.

The degree of interaction between the national and sub-national level as well as the involvement of each in the other's planning processes is determined by the characteristics of decentralization and the degree of autonomy granted to each level of the health system. Sub-national and national-level planning are thus highly interconnected in terms of both hierarchical and functional relations. Consequently, understanding the dynamics of a sub-national planning process is essential for all health sector stakeholders, regardless of the level at which they function.

"Sub-national" describes any government entity below the national level, regardless of the political, financial and administrative design of the country.

Strategizing at sub-national level refers to all systematic planning and programming as well as budgeting and resource allocation processes below the national level.

Fig. 11.1 Strategizing for health at sub-national level

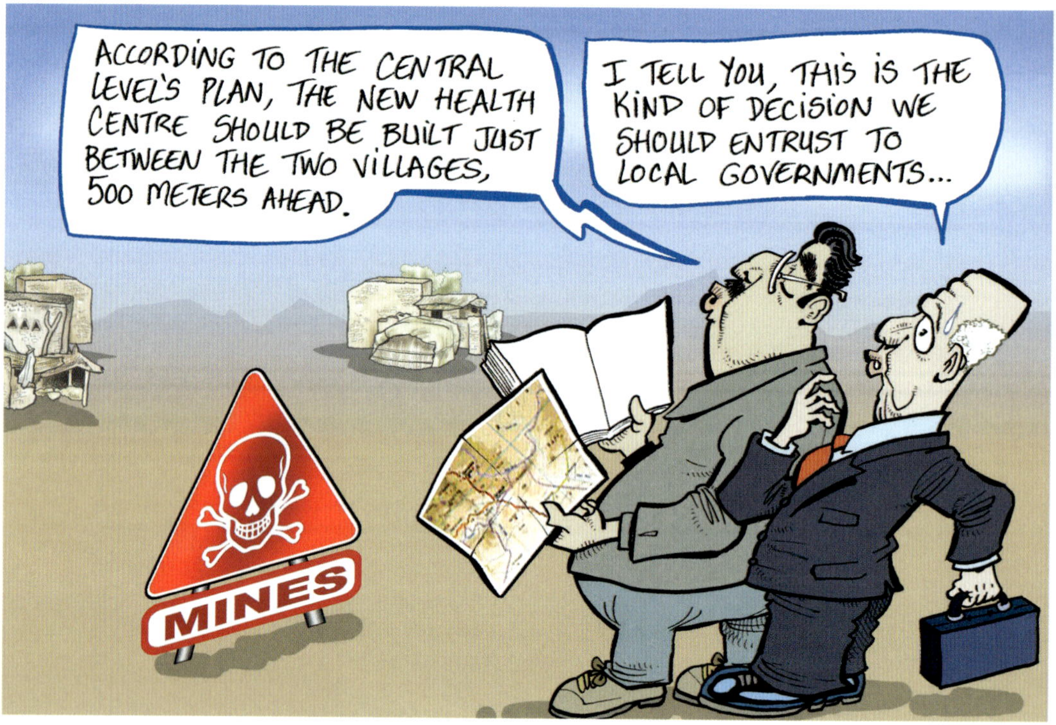
ACCORDING TO THE CENTRAL LEVEL'S PLAN, THE NEW HEALTH CENTRE SHOULD BE BUILT JUST BETWEEN THE TWO VILLAGES, 500 METERS AHEAD.
I TELL YOU, THIS IS THE KIND OF DECISION WE SHOULD ENTRUST TO LOCAL GOVERNMENTS...
MINES

Damian Glez; scenario by Bruno Meessen.

11.1.3 What do we mean by "decentralization"?

Decentralization manifests itself in practice in each country or setting in different ways, and heavily influences the arrangements of sub-national health planning.

Decentralization is "the transfer of formal responsibility and power to make decisions regarding the management, production, distribution and/or financing of health services, usually from a smaller to a larger number of geographically or organizationally separate actors".[1] Thus, a decentralized health system is one where responsibilities and decision-making power are transferred from the national level (i.e. MoH) to sub-national levels of government and administration.

Decentralization manifests itself in practice in each country or setting in different ways, and heavily influences the arrangements of sub-national health planning. The characteristics of decentralization as described in Box 11.1 thus determine the extent of deferral of power, responsibility, influence and accountability to sub-national levels.

Box 11.1

Characteristics of decentralization: dimensions, degrees and ranges[2,3,4]

Dimensions of decentralization (they can coexist and are not mutually exclusive):

- **Political decentralization:** political entities are run according to democratic rules: greater policy-making power for sub-national representatives.
- **Administrative decentralization:** administrative entities are run according to managerial precepts: greater role for sub-national level in service delivery.
- **Fiscal decentralization:** fiscal entities are run primarily as financial bodies: greater authority for sub-national institutions for collection and use of funds.

Degree of autonomy

- **Deconcentration:** shift of administrative responsibilities from national level to sub-national level. Authorities and responsibilities would be transferred from MoH at national level to sub-offices of the ministry at regional or local level.
- **Delegation:** transfer of defined administrative or policy initiation power to lower levels. Authorities and responsibilities would be transferred from MoH to entities that are not under the direct supervision of the ministry.
- **Devolution:** transfer of political power from national government to autonomous territory governments.

Range of decentralization

- **Number of sectors affected by decentralization:** all sectors of government or only specific sectors or functions.
- **Number of tiers of decentralization:** number of sub-national levels (e.g. federal level, state, district, municipal ...).

11.1.4 What does decentralization look like in practice? Some country examples

Given that different countries' health system features and characteristics vary across the globe based on historical and social patterns, decentralization in the health system is not a homogenous concept. A decentralized health system is the product of a multifaceted variety of factors specific to:[5]

- the national political, social and cultural context and circumstances;
- the way the national health system is organized;
- the characteristics of the functions that are decentralized; and
- the nature of institutions to which responsibilities are transferred.

Thus, "decentralization" and "centralization" are not two mutually exclusive concepts – they are rather two endpoints of a wide spectrum of possible elements and combinations.[6]

A decentralized health system is the product of a variety of factors such as: the national political, social and cultural context and circumstances; the organization of the national health system; the functional characteristics that are decentralized; and the nature of institutions to which responsibilities are transerred.

Hence, decentralized health systems can differ from country to country. In addition, in practice, there are no neat examples of a purely deconcentrated, delegated or devolved system. Instead, almost all systems are mixed, with a patchwork of different elements of decentralization, heavily influenced by the history, culture and politics of the specific setting. Just as an example, Canada´s health system is characterized by strong decentralization with autonomous sub-national levels – but the federal government remains responsible for health and pharmacy regulation and health financing. The principle responsibility for the provision of health services lies with Canada's 10 provinces. In Spain, based on historical developments, the degrees of decentralization vary across the different communities, especially in regard to fiscal responsibilities. Two communities (the Basque and Navarre Communities) are able to tax their population locally and use a portion of those funds for health, while all others are allocated a health budget by the national level.[7,8]

11.1.5 Sub-national planning in a decentralized environment

Since the specificities of sub-national planning are determined by the characteristics of health system decentralization (and the broader political context), it is important to understand the degrees of autonomy of sub-national institutions (see Table 11.1) as described below. These categories, while not so clear-cut and neat in reality, still contain essential elements which shape sub-national arrangements.

(a) Deconcentration: transfer of responsibility to a lower administrative level with much leadership and decision-making authority remaining at central level.

The national MoH shifts some of its authority and responsibility to (administrative) sub-national institutions responsible for health. Deconcentration enables the creation of sub-national management structures for health-related activities. Leadership is still embedded in the national level, but administratively executed through sub-national (e.g. local) offices of the national government:[9]

Portugal underwent a decentralization reform in the 1990s. To date, the national level is responsible for regulation, planning and administration. Thus, regional health administrative bodies report to the national MoH and oversee the administration of the health system at the regional level. Decisions concerning budget allocations to the regions as well as payment schemes for doctors and hospitals are taken care of at national level. Hospital management systems are thus run according to principles of deconcentration. The regional health administrative bodies oversee the administration of primary care as well as hospital management, while certain key decisions affecting the regional health system are taken at national level.[10]

(b) Delegation: transfer of responsibility to a lower organizational level.

Here, managerial and administrative functions and/or policy initiation power are transferred to the sub-national level, sometimes via a separate semi-independent parastatal (national or sub-national) entity. In essence, it refers to situations where authority and responsibilities are shifted from the national MoH to entities that may or may not be under the direct supervision of the ministry; control over those entities can only be executed indirectly.[11] More prominent examples of delegation come from settings where a transfer of power occurs from a governmental (national) to an independent (also national) institution. However, examples of delegation from national to sub national levels can be found in a variety of decentralized settings as well.

The following examples of the Ghana Health Service and Zambia demonstrate that the transfer of responsibility can imply delegation from the national to the sub-national level as well as from a national government institution to an independent (non-state) institution (which can operate at either national or sub-national level). Either way, the key principles remain the same.

Different categories of a decentralized environment—deconcentration, delegation, and devolution—shape how sub-national arrangements are made.

In 1996, Ghana passed the "Health Service and Teaching Hospital Act" that introduced decentralization in the health sector. This Act encompassed the fiscal decentralization of the health sector, including the delegation of health service delivery spending from the national MoH to an autonomous public institution. This institution is called Ghana Health Service (GHS) and is responsible for the implementation of national health policies. The GHS appoints regional and district administration offices. Even though the GHS is considered an independent institution ("executive agency"), it is still required to report to the MoH. Thus the GHS is supposed to implement policies that are approved through the MoH, such as increasing access to quality health services using assigned resources.

In the mid-1990s, Zambia also underwent a period of health sector decentralization, though the approach was slightly different from Ghana. Management responsibility of the health system at district levels was delegated to District Health Management Teams (DHMTs); however, their autonomy was limited, as the MoH maintained authority in the form of appointment of local board members and approval of plans and budgets. Delegation also occurred through the creation of the Central Board of Health (CBOH), a semi-autonomous institution. The CBOH was transferred major responsibilities for the day-to-day operations of the health system, in effect granting that body operational responsibility of the health system rather than local government.[12,13]

(c) Devolution: transfer of authority, including decision-making, to a lower political level

Devolution refers to the legal transfer of power and responsibility (authority) for decision-making, finance, and management from the national level to independent territory governments:[14]

The health systems of Northern Ireland, Scotland and Wales are separate from the English health system, following a devolution reform in the United Kingdom. Through this reform, the health systems became the full responsibility of the new democratic governments of the three regions: "Devolved politicians accountable to devolved voters gained responsibility for providing healthcare and the opportunity to enact reforms (...)".[15]

Uganda underwent a reform process in the 1990s and introduced political and administrative decentralization with huge implications for the health sector. Local governments received extensive political and administrative decision-making authority, including taxation power. As a first step, elected district representatives were made responsible for the management of all health services within their territory. As a second step, to further decentralize the districts, health sub-districts were created to further distribute responsibilities from district to sub-district level.[16]

Thus, the different functions of a health system – e.g. financing, service delivery – are taken over by different entities at different levels of the health system depending on the degree of and arrangements for decentralization.

Table 11.1 Characteristics of decentralization: degrees of autonomy and review

DEGREE OF AUTONOMY	TRANSFER OF...	THIS MEANS:
Deconcentration	... responsibility to a lower administrative level with much leadership and decision-making authority remaining at central level	▸ shift of defined authorities' responsibilities from national MoH to (administrative) sub-national institutions responsible for health; ▸ creation of sub-national management structures for health-related activities; ▸ overall leadership still with national level, but administratively executed through sub-national (e.g. local) offices of the national government.
Delegation	... responsibility to a lower organizational level	▸ shift of managerial and administrative functions and/or policy initiation power to sub-national levels – sometimes to semi-independent parastatal (national or sub-national) entity; ▸ shift of authority and responsibilities from national MoH to entities that may or may not be under the direct supervision of the ministry; ▸ control over sub-national entities can only be executed indirectly.
Devolution	...authority to a lower political level	▸ legal transfer of power and responsibility (authority) for decision-making, finance, and management from the national level to independent territory governments.

Decentralization is not static in practice. Instead, a dynamic relationship between the national and sub-national levels defines decentralization, with constant changes in the decision-making space of both (or more) levels. For purposes of sub-national planning, this means that the degrees of autonomy vary across the different tasks and decisions that a sub-national entity might need to make for the health system. In addition, a mix of those degrees might be observed within one country, which means sub-national planning might not be the same across different sub-national entities within the same country. Countries usually reflect a combination of the decentralization dimensions/ ranges and degrees of autonomy because of differing needs as well as specific political and historical contexts.[17]

Finally, it is useful to keep in mind that the degree of autonomy transfers certain policy and planning cycle steps from national to sub-national level. For example, deconcentration is more linked to operational planning and monitoring at operational unit level because all other policy and planning cycle steps are handled at central level. Delegation, on the other hand, transfers more strategic planning responsibilities to sub-national level. Devolution gives the full policy and planning cycle over to the sub-national level.

11.1.6 Sub-national planning in an unresponsive central environment

This chapter focuses on an institutionalized form of sub-national planning, i.e. it takes sub-national planning in relation to the existence of a (functioning) national level. Nevertheless, it is important to highlight that sub-national planning engagement can also occur in places where the national government is not "functioning" – for example, a fragile state or where simply central level is far-removed from sub-national levels and thus does not or cannot provide leadership or guidance. In this case, sub-national planning can be used as a way to substitute national engagement and to continue or to establish forms of public service provision. In effect, these are settings where a de facto decentralization has taken place, with the consequence that the health district can potentially take on the role of the principal functional operational unit in the health sector,[18] compensating for the lack of central-level normative power (see Box 11.2).

Sub-national planning can be used as a way to substitute national engagement and to continue or to establish forms of public service provision in fragile states or where the central level is far removed from sub-national levels.

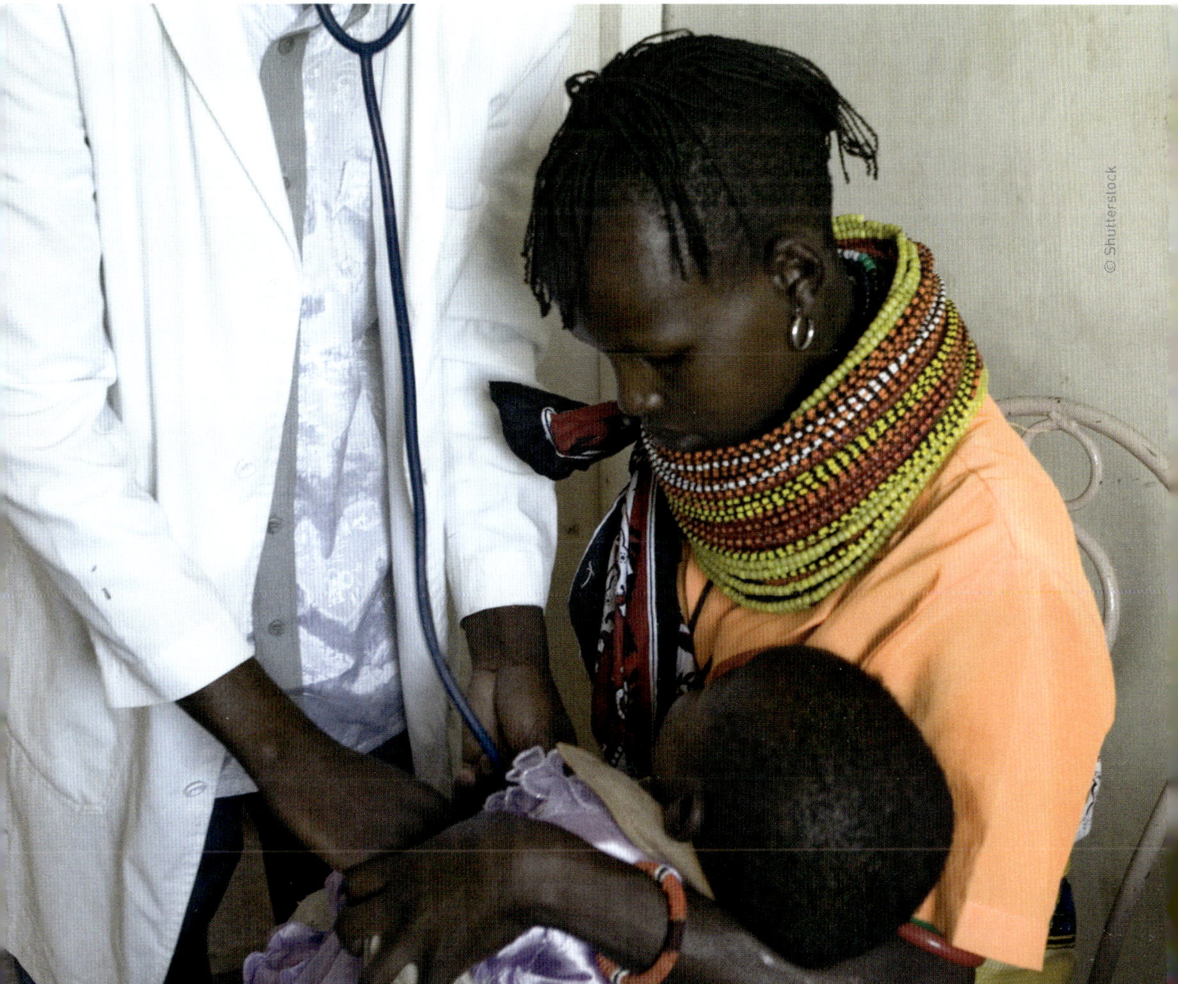

Box 11.2

District health systems

A district health system (DHS) is a specific example of a sub-national structure. It can be described as "existing and functional structures and managerial processes in the district that enable the provision of essential health care to the population".[19] DHSs are based on the principles of primary health care,[20] and include the involvement of local communities in the bottom-up planning and policy development processes. The DHS provides primary health care services, which includes curative and preventive care, responding to local needs and being in line with national policies.[21]

As an element of the national health system, the DHS covers one district, governed by elected district council members. Subject to the degree of decentralization, the council might hold the full responsibility for health care provision and policy implementation in the district. Often, the second tier (e.g. regional level) ensures national (health) policy implementation, training, quality control and coordination across districts.

The DHS includes not just public health service providers, but also private providers, nongovernmental organizations (NGOs), faith-based organizations and traditional healers that are active within the district.

An example of a district-based health system which has proven resilient and robust during a long period of conflict and unrest is the Democratic Republic of the Congo during the 1990s and 2000s.[22] During this period, economic, political and social stressors had a huge negative impact on health system performance, with a de facto non-existent central level when it came to sub-national affairs. Nevertheless, many districts continued to function with local infrastructure and local solutions, facilitated by a well-ingrained local district modus operandi. For example, Rutshuru health district in the North Kivu Province was able to continue providing health services through the height of conflict – not only to its own population but also to an unforeseen number of refugees from neighbouring districts and provinces, despite the absence of any real governance from central level.[23]

11.1.7 The social roots and political dynamics of decentralization

In most countries, decentralization is a consequence of historical, political, social and geographical differences between population groups within one country. Socioeconomic and cultural differences might create tensions between population groups and decentralization offers possibilities of local autonomy trying to counter those tensions. In some instances, decentralization might even be a legacy of colonial rule, and thus might have been introduced in state- and nation-building processes by external actors.

A formal, functioning decentralized (political and) health system might create the opportunity to officially acknowledge those differences. When it comes to strategizing for health, policy-makers should heed certain issues linked to the political economy of decentralization.

- Strategizing for health is about making choices based on regional or local priorities that might not reflect the priorities of the entire country.
- The national political context still ends up determining the institutional structure of decentralization (and its reform processes),[24] and thus the specificities of health planning, even at sub-national level.
- Health planning and resource allocation can become even more political in a decentralized country where population groups openly voice their differing needs.
- Legal and constitutional arrangements are important factors for determining roles and responsibilities during the planning process. They should be acknowledged and followed throughout the planning cycle.
- In some cases, the challenges of decentralization are not grounded in process or planning difficulties, but are part of the broader country context. For example:
  - *decentralized system* in a fragile environment: weak central government vs strong local government/governance;
  - *forced decentralization* due to geographical challenges: country divided by islands, territory divided by political restrictions (e.g. West Bank and Gaza Strip);
  - *decentralization* used as a means for other political purposes, such as marginalization of specific population sub-groups or through the creation of unlimited sub-units to increase financial dependency on national level and to lower the ability to execute responsibility and accountability of the sub-units.

In some cases, existing tensions and divergences between population groups can actually be mitigated through greater autonomy offered by decentralization. Nevertheless, tensions and conflicts between population groups or between sub-national and national levels might still be an intrinsic part of the political environment in some countries. The guidance and suggestions this handbook is proposing for sub-national planning are based on the assumption that communication and coordination are a supporting element of decentralized health planning. Thus, in highly conflictual circumstances, some of the guidance this handbook is proposing might not be realizable.

In most countries, decentralization is a consequence of historical, political, social and geographical differences between population groups within one country.

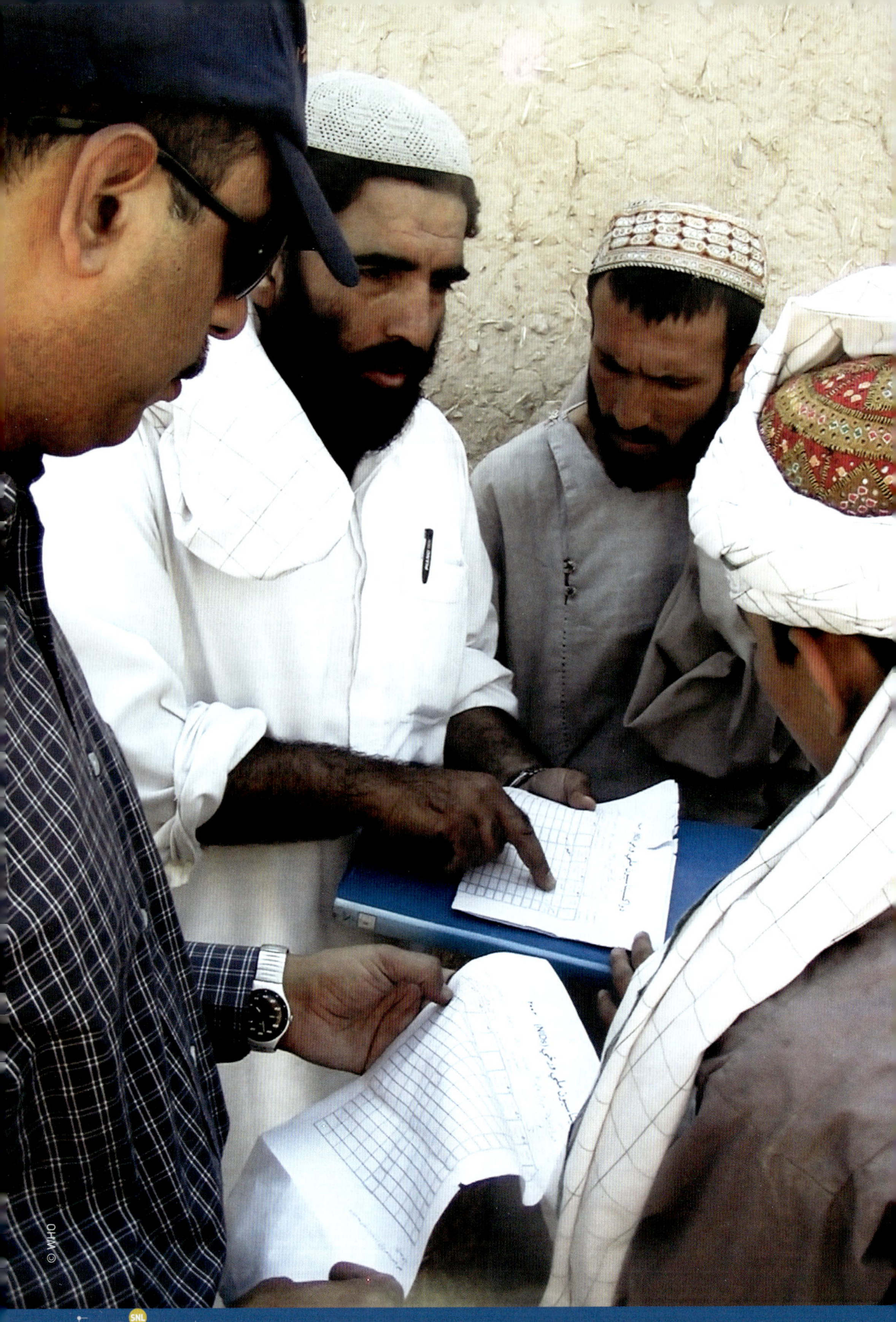

11.2 Why is strategizing for health at sub-national level important?

11.2.1 Positive impact on the accountability of public policy to the recipients of services

The degree to which decision-makers can be held accountable for their actions is linked to their ability to take decisions and thus achieve improvements in service delivery. Those decisions and actions are much closer together in terms of real time and chain of command at sub-national level. Studies have demonstrated that "downward accountability" can lead to greater equity and efficiency;[25] this "downward accountability" is rendered much more concrete at the sub-national level, where decision-makers are much closer to and integrated into the populations they serve. Consequently, the type and degree of decentralization will be a major determinant for decision-makers' ability to assume responsibility.[26] For example, pressure on sub-national governments might increase because citizens are able to evaluate local government's performance more easily than a central government's and directly assess the services provided to them. Thus sub-national planning can be used as an incentive to improve sustainable service provision.[27]

11.2.2 Increased (community) participation and engagement

Communities and the population are motivated to participate when decisions are close to home and the link to their daily lives is obvious. Those concrete health sector issues are debated at sub-national level, sometimes through formal participation mechanisms.[28] This community-level input is critical for strategizing for health in order to ensure a strong link between what people need and want and the country's vision for health.

Sub-national planning can be used as an incentive to improve sustainable service provision.

Sub-national planning can increase community participation through local inclusion mechanisms that can be tailored specifically to the local circumstances. Formal spaces are important for sustainable community participation and inclusion of population opinion in planning and political debate; a decentralized and close-to-people planning approach can offer those spaces more willingly.[I] A study on sub-national health planning in Maharashtra, India, has shown that it can ease the pathways for community-based evidence into health planning, and improve the soundness of planning by increasing responsiveness to local challenges, as well as improving the functioning of health facilities.[29]

The population is motivated to participate when decisions are close to home and the link to their daily lives is obvious; sub-national planning can increase community participation through local inclusion mechanisms tailored specifically to the local circumstances.

I For a discussion around population consultation, see Chapter 2 of this handbook.

11.2.3 Increased flexibility

Being closer to the realities and living conditions of the population is a huge advantage due to the ability to quickly adjust to local needs and expectations.[30] At the same time, strategizing for health at national level can benefit from the flexibility and adjustability to local contexts by close interaction with sub-national government entities.

Case studies show a positive link between strategizing at sub-national level and improved health outcomes, mostly linked to stronger local evidence and a more adapted reaction to problems.

A variety of case studies have shown that there is a positive link between strategizing at sub-national level and improved health outcomes.[31] These positive effects of decentralized planning are mainly linked to the local level possibilities in terms of stronger evidence if collected, analysed and contextualized at local-level and a swifter, more adapted reaction to problems.

11.2.4 Better mitigation of geographical and social imbalances

The fair allocation of resources, especially benefiting poorer areas, is more likely at sub-national level with administrative structures being close to the needs of the population.[32] Evidence suggests that one reason for improved pro-poor planning at sub-national level is due to the possibility for sub-national authorities to access and use additional information on the circumstances of beneficiaries, which the national level is not able to.[33]

Long-term improvements in access to health services for remote areas can be supported through national financial and capacity provision to the sub-national level, which has stronger information and incentives as well as responsibility to the local population.

The assessment of local health needs and the local response to these needs through a bottom-up approach are critical for national-level "allocative efficiency".[34] Local governments' interaction with their population on health issues helps shape a more realistic picture of the challenges to a nation's health.

11.2.5 Improved bottom-up intersectoral and multi-stakeholder collaboration

Through the transfer of responsibilities and authority to the sub-national level(s), the horizontal integration of health and other health-related services and sectors has the great potential to increase.[35] At sub-national level, the different sectors have fewer administrators involved, with collaboration often already taking place due to the close familiarity of the different actors with each other and with the communities. Thus, the coordination and collaboration with institutions, community networks and partnerships can be strengthened through the regionalization of decision-making power.

11.2.6 Legal necessity

In formally decentralized settings, sub-national planning might be stated in the constitution and thus be a legally binding requirement to the political set-up of the country.

Sub-national planning might be stated in the constitution and thus be a legally binding requirement to the political set-up of the country.

Additionally, certain political and economic arrangements cannot do without sub-national planning. For example sub-national planning might be a requirement in contexts with established fiscal decentralization. When the main source of funding for the health sector is through local taxation or revenues collected at decentralized level, one cannot but engage with sub-national levels and their planning processes in order to adequately manage the allocation and use of resources.

Box 11.3

Example of a decentralized health system: the development and design of the Brazilian health system

Historical development

Brazil's journey towards decentralization has been gradual. The Sistema Unico de Saude (SUS), Unified Health System, was created in 1990, based on the 1988 constitution which "enshrined health as a citizens' right and which requires the state to provide universal and equal access to health services".[36] The Sistema Unico de Saude formed a decentralized system for public health care, supplemented by private provision of services, where the federal government held responsibility for national policy-making and regulations and the municipalities were responsible for health planning and providing those services.[37] Before 1996, however, federal funds were allocated based on population and provider numbers rather than local needs.[38] As a result, the wealther, more populous municipalities had more providers and more funds, and consequently, better health service delivery, than poorer regions. The issuance of standards known as Normas Operacionais Basicas (basic operating norms) in 1996 adjusted for these inequalities by requiring municipalities to provide basic packages of services, called the Piso Assistencial Basico (PAB), to their populations and the federal government to financially support these services, with funds primarily coming from taxes at the federal, state, and municipal levels.[39]

Thus, fiscal decentralization[40] was combined with providing the states with the political and administrative autonomy regarding the management of public policies. This means that decision-making for health was transferred from national to sub-national levels.[41]

The current decentralized health system

Under the SUS, the federal government is primarily responsible for developing national health policies, in addition to monitoring and evaluation, managing private-public sector relationships, and providing financial support to devolved health sector administrations. The MoH at the national level has acting representatives, known as Secretariats, in place at the sub-national levels (each state and municipal level) to ensure health system functioning, particularly in relation to fiscal responsibility and resource management. While health planning is primarily a responsibility of the municipal level, national planning and allocation decisions occur every four years at National Health Conferences. Brazil's geographical infrastructure consists of 26 states, and within the states a total of 4390 municipal health councils, creating an extensive and widespread web across the country.[42] Municipal-level planning involves budget formulation and plans for resource allocation, in addition to human resource planning and administration.[43] Primary care delivery occurs through Brazil's Family Health Programme, which runs at the municipal level. The programme provides not only primary care via health professionals, but also has an outreach component in which the community is encouraged to play an active role. Decentralization of health care authority to the local level has thus increased resource mobilization and given municipal-level governments a more active role in service delivery.[44-46]

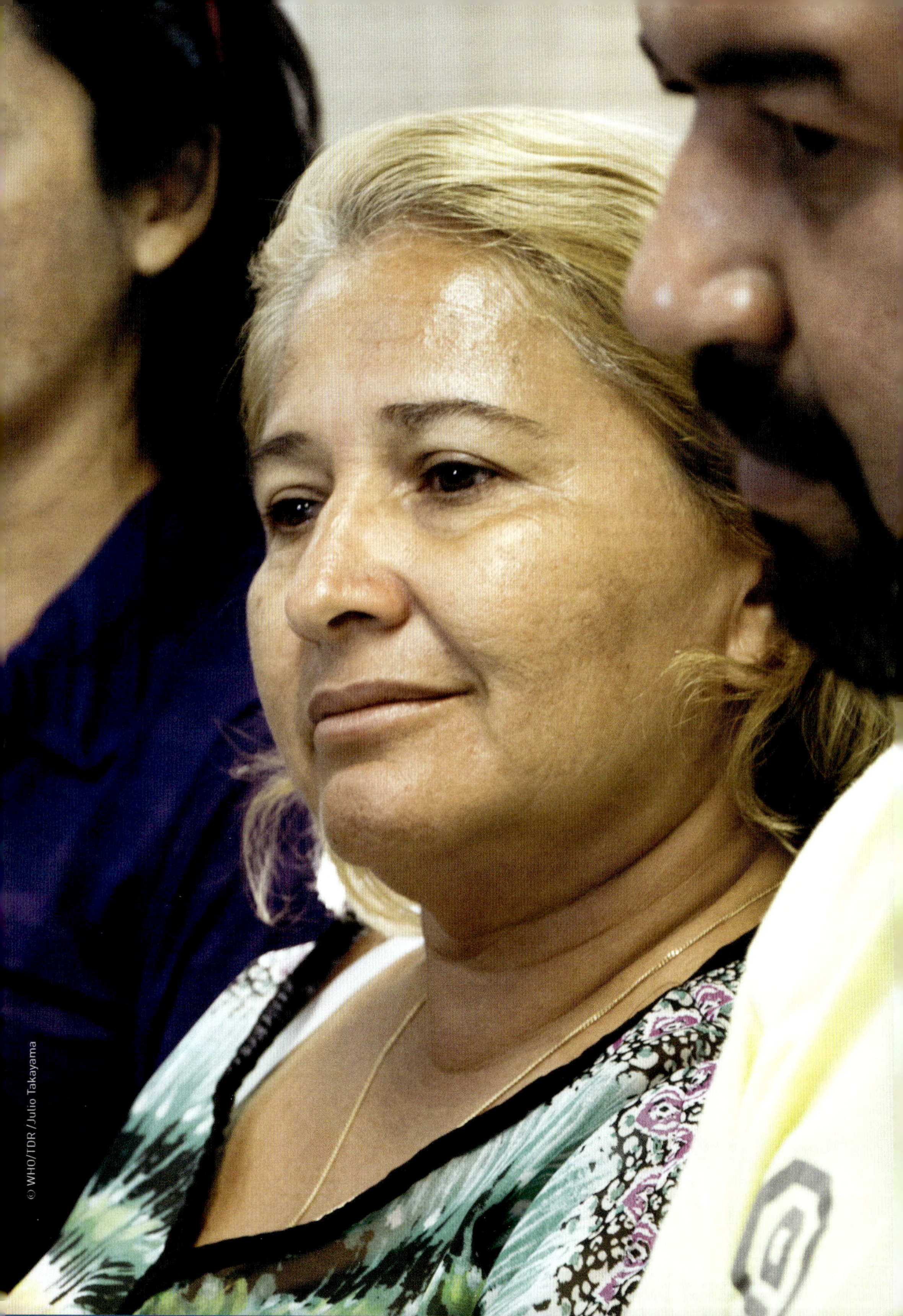

© WHO/TDR / Julio Takayama

11.3 When should sub-national planning be considered during the planning cycle?

National planning authorities must take sub-national planning into account throughout the policy and planning cycle. That being said, it is crucial that the arrangements and schedule for sub-national planning be carefully considered from the beginning in relation to the overall process of strategizing for health. Sub-national input is absolutely critical for shaping the overarching national health plan. At the same time, national-level collaboration in sub-national planning processes is necessary to ensure coherence across regions and sub-national structure, and to enable aggregation of data and information at national level.

The country's dimension and range of decentralization, as well as the degree of autonomy accorded to the planning entity, will be the key determining factors of sub-national planning arrangements, its timing and timeline. National and sub-national planning authorities should keep them in mind throughout the full planning cycle.

National and sub-national planning authorities should keep the country's dimension and range of decentralization, and the degree of autonomy according to the planning entity, in mind throughout the full planning cycle

11.4 Who should be engaged in sub-national planning?

All stakeholders involved in the national health planning process, be it within the Ministry of Health or outside, it should be attentive to the decentralized health system structure and its consequences for sub-national and national planning.

All stakeholders involved in the national health planning process, be it within the MoH or outside it, should be attentive to the decentralized health system structure and its consequences for sub-national and national planning (see Table 11.2). Nongovernmental actors or external partners (e.g. United Nations agencies, bilateral organizations) who are supporting planning processes should acknowledge the decentralized setting and act in accordance to its rules and regulations. This implies acknowledgement of not just national strategy documents (e.g. NHPSP) as a basis of programmes and interventions, but also sub-national plans, strategies and institutional structures. The MoH has a special oversight function to provide guidance and capacity support to sub-national entities, ensuring overall coherence with the national health sector vision.

Additionally, actors that may only exist at national (e.g. federal MoH, parliamentary groups, ministries of finance and planning, professional associations) or sub-national level (e.g. state MoH, grass-roots organizations, and professional associations) will need to be linked to the overall decentralized context of the country and included in dialogue processes across levels.

However, the specific roles as well as the type of actor that is relevant for decentralized planning depends on the country context and the type of decentralization (with an increased involvement, role and responsibility going from deconcentration to delegation, and ultimately to devolution). For example, the level of engagement, and thus the role in the planning process, of the national MoH varies according to the established degrees, ranges and dimensions of decentralization.

Table 11.2 Stakeholders and their roles in strategizing for health at sub-national level

ACTOR	LEVEL	ROLE
(Federal) MoH	**National level:** First tier	▶ Respect and enable constitutionally set decentralized health system structure and its consequences for sub-national and national planning ▶ If constitutionally foreseen and needed, provide control, oversight guidance and support to sub-national levels ▶ Act as bridge to other sectors at national level
Regional department of health	**Sub-national level:** Second and/or third tier	▶ Function as intermediary institution to support all tiers of government as well as interact with sub-nationally engaged non-state institutions to carry out their duties ▶ Resume responsibilities that were allocated to this level through the decentralization process ▶ Act as bridge to other sectors on sub-national level
International development partners (United Nations agencies, bilateral agencies, international NGOs)	**External:** Engagement possible at national (first tier) level and/or at sub-national levels (second and third tiers)	▶ Act and provide support in accordance with rules and regulations of decentralized environment ▶ Acknowledge national as well as sub-national strategic documents (e.g. district health plan) as the basis for any interventions
National[II] non-state institutions (e.g. private sector, NGOs, academic institutions, civil society organizations)	**Internal:** Engagement possible at national level (first tier) and/or at sub-national levels (second and third tiers)	▶ Respect the institutional arrangements for cooperation and coordination that are established through decentralization ▶ Provide support in accordance with rules and regulations of decentralized environment

II As opposed to international, not in regard to the layer of government.

11.5 How to strategize for health at sub-national level?

Sustainable and inclusive health planning is a matter of importance for all tiers of government. Thus, sub-national planning is relevant to each step of the policy and planning cycle. In this section, each such step is addressed in relation to sub-national planning, with concrete recommendations and issues to consider.

11.5.1 Population consultation

Undertaking a national population consultation in a decentralized context

There is nothing to stand in the way of a population consultation[III] in a decentralized context. The national constitutional background and legal framework of the broader political system will inform the feasibility and legal arrangements for a consultation, as well as potentially define the responsibilities of the different health system levels for a population consultation.

When undertaking a sub-national population consultation, it is important to involve the national level, realize that additional capacity and resource support may be necessary, and prepare for the sustainability of the consultation results at both national and sub-national level.

Involve sub-national levels and ensure tailored sub-national follow-up

A national population consultation can greatly benefit from decentralized planning structures. Sub-national engagement to a national consultation offers the possibility of closer interaction with the population. The design of the consultation should be more adapted to sub-national circumstances, specifically in regard to the inclusion of under-resourced and hard-to-reach contexts. In addition, the follow-up to the consultation should include working closely with sub-national authorities and decision-makers to provide specific feedback to sub-national levels on issues of relevance and interest to them.

III For a detailed discussion on population consultations, see Chapter 2 Population consultation on needs and expectations" in this handbook.

National authorities should take advantage of sub-national institutions' knowledge and awareness of local populations' living and health conditions. Therefore, local entities can help improve the design and follow-up of the consultation, as well as the NHPSP itself, based on the priorities identified through the consultation.

Remote and hard-to-reach areas as well as marginalized and vulnerable population subgroups should be integrated into a consultation through local actors who have built a relationship of trust with those subgroups. Sub-national planning structures need to be used in this regard, because they can offer a strong local and regional link to national institutions that may not have the same level of access to local population groups.

The chosen (national) methodological approach needs to be adequately translated and adapted to sub-national levels

In some countries the survey methods to be chosen have to fulfil requirements that need to be compliant with the legal and constitutional context of the country. For example, a nationwide referendum might not be legally possible, but other survey methods might be absolutely feasible. It is important to keep in mind that the chosen (survey) methodology:

- reflects clear roles and responsibilities between national and sub-national levels and all concerned levels, and ensures adequate representation during the preparation and follow-up to the consultation;
- accounts for the differing characteristics of the population – such as languages, living conditions, gender and access to services – that might be due to varying socioeconomic and cultural differences per region.

Special issues to consider when undertaking a sub-national population consultation

When undertaking a population consultation only at sub-national level, a few issues will need to be considered as well.

Involve the national level

The involvement of all levels of government is essential even at sub-national level. The national level can technically support, help coordinate, ensure coherence across sub-national entities and feedback into national planning processes. Well-managed coordination of involved stakeholders, both vertically (all levels of government) and horizontally (involved or conducting stakeholders)[47] is crucial, especially when the consultation is not carried out by the MoH directly. In contexts where tensions exist between national and sub-national levels, this involvement should be thought through and given great care, with clear terms of references agreed upon by all sides.

Box 11.4

Example of population consultation in Switzerland

A high degree of decentralization exists in Switzerland's health system. Cantons, or the sub-national level, have high levels of autonomy and are continually engaged in the political decision-making process at the national level.[48] Cantons are responsible for health care, including its financing, and regularly perform population consultations allowing for citizens to play a large role in health. Not only are citizens consulted, but referendums initiated by the people are regularly undertaken and citizens are called on to make health-sector decisions. In 2007 and 2014, for example, the population was called upon to decide whether to reform the health insurance system by abolishing private not-for-profit funds and introducing a single national government operated fund.[49] In both years the population voted against the reform, leaving it up to the cantons to manage insurance finance systems, demonstrating the influence of citizens in the decentralized state.[50]

Additional capacity and resource support may be necessary for a sub-national population consultation

For a population consultation undertaken only in one specific state[IV] or region, local government entities conducting the consultation might need to approach the national level to request human, financial and capacity resource backing to be able to conduct a well-managed and well-designed consultation.

Sustainability of the consultation results at both national and sub-national levels

The results of the consultation need to be made available to all concerned levels and stakeholders. Dissemination methods must make sure to adequately transmit the results in an understandable way, using simple language and no technical jargon. This includes clear communication in regard to the follow-up of the results and how they will be transformed into priorities that will feed into the planning process and create a demand-oriented plan.

Sub-national as well as national level are accountable towards the population regarding the results of the consultation, regardless of the level at which the consultation was undertaken. The consultation should preferably be seen as an entry point to credibly feed into regular national health sector reviews. Therefore, review processes at national level need to be designed in a way that allows for the results of sub-national consultation processes to be included, and vice versa.

IV The term "state" is used to describe sub-national governmental entities. For some countries another term might be more adequate (e.g. districts) – but for simplification purposes, this chapter uses the term "state". The varying political and administrative responsibilities that "states" have in different countries cannot be considered here.

11.5.2 Situation analysis

Undertaking a national-level situation analysis in a decentralized context

A situation analysis is a crucial step in any national health planning process.[V] However, for a situation analysis to be fully comprehensive and inclusive, especially in a decentralized environment, sub-national planning and its characteristics need to be taken into account. As with population consultations, a national-level situation analysis can profit enormously from the closeness to the population that sub-national planning can offer.

Improvement of national policies through sub-national evidence

A situation analysis undertaken at the sub-national level can have a positive impact on evidence-based policy and decision-making at national level. Sub-national approaches can address local concerns, include local information and data in policy design, priority-setting, and the allocation of resources, and thus render NHPSPs more adaptable to sub-national levels with a higher probability of good implementation. The results of a situation analysis can support all government levels in their planning and decision-making responsibilities through cross-linkages and information sharing.

Acceptance of situation analysis conclusions by all health system levels

Ensuring acceptance of the results of the national-level situation analysis by all levels is primarily an issue of adequate participation and representation of all levels (government and nongovernment stakeholders), in both the preparation as well as the follow-up of the situation analysis. Roles and responsibilities between national and sub-national stakeholders need to be clarified beforehand. Stakeholders who have a weaker negotiation power (e.g. due to a lack of capacity or because they are only represented in one state/region) can be given a more prominent role in the follow-up of the situation analysis.

V For a detailed discussion on situation analysis see Chapter 3 "Situation analysis of the health sector" in this handbook.

Special issues to consider when undertaking a sub-national situation analysis

A sub-national situation analysis should include input from national level

Even if the situation analysis might only be conducted at sub-national levels, the participation of the national level might be a constructive element and where possible needs to be ensured. Coordination and communication between the different tiers are important for the design of an adequate methodology and for input on issues that are relevant at sub-national level but where the expertise or information may lie elsewhere.

The opportunity to take into account the community's voice should not be missed

At national level, it is not easy to bring citizens' voices in a more individualized way into an aggregate planning process. At sub-national level, the opportunity and possibility to do so are much more real with the proximity of sub-national governments to the end-users of the health system. This opportunity should not be underestimated; making a concerted and targeted effort to ensure community leaders, families and patients a place in the local planning process can reap huge benefits in terms of health service utilization and patient satisfaction.[51] Doing so is more feasible and viable at sub-national level.

Box 11.5

Brazil and sub-national situation analysis

Brazil's Unified Health System places the responsibility of semi-annual and annual health planning primarily at the municipal level.[52,53] In the national health planning process—which takes place every four years to establish health guidelines, regulations, and make resource allocation decisions—results from situation analyses at municipal and state levels are a critical component.[54] The National Health Conference brings together representatives from Brazil's 26 states and 4,390 municipal health councils to review results from analyses and discuss specific health policy decisions. Conversations start at municipal-level committees during the conference then advance onto higher levels. Lower-level situation analyses in Brazil provide valuable results which allow local realities to be brought to the attention of state and national-level committees.[55]

At national level, it is not easy to bring citizen's voice in a more individualized way into an aggregate planning process. At sub-national level, the opportunity and possibility to do so are much more real with the proximity of sub-national governments to the end users of the health system.

11.5.3 Priority-setting[VI]

Undertaking a national-level priority-setting in a decentralized context

When it comes to making sense of the evidence and interpreting data to the local setting, sub-national planning authorities have the distinct advantage of local knowledge and understanding.

Especially when it comes to making sense of the evidence and interpreting data to the local setting, sub-national planning authorities have the distinct advantage of local knowledge and understanding.

A national priority-setting process should ensure tailored communication and dissemination strategies at sub-national level, especially when the chosen priorities are not relevant at a specific sub-national level. Communicating a country's health intervention priorities and strategic direction can best be done by sub-national actors who can package the information according to local interest and needs.

Vertical programmes

Vertical health programmes often have planning cycles that are different from the NHPSP cycle. This might mean that some priorities are already set, with resources already set aside, to priority vertical programmes before the overall health sector priority-setting takes place. This may play out most acutely at sub-national level, where priorities identified at national level for the health sector as a whole may be incongruous to the de facto priorities set at sub-national level by strong vertical programmes and funding flows.

The solution to this lies in better coordination between vertical programmes and national (cross-cutting) MoH departments, and with sub-national health authorities. The MoH at national level should take on a very strong coordination and facilitation role and promote integration and alignment between national, sub-national and programmatic cycles.

Identification of health demands and needs – differences between sub-national entities

Population demands and needs, and ensuing health priorities, might not be the same from one sub-national entity to another. Especially where the decentralization process was spurred on by sub-national cultural or social divisions, it is essential to keep in mind that generalizations, applicable at national level, should not be made based on a limited number of sub-national entities.

Special issues to consider when setting priorities at sub-national level

Striking a balance between national and sub-national priorities

Priorities should be set based on a robust local understanding of the health sector situation. In many cases, priorities have also been set at higher levels than a district, sometimes regionally, sometimes nationally, and sometimes transnationally or globally – but have an impact on the local-level priorities.

VI Please see chapter 4 'Priority-setting for national health policies, strategies and plans' in this handbook

A lengthy priority-setting exercise may not be useful if there is agreement at national level, with sub-national involvement, that certain activities will be given priority. As an example, an individual district will likely take part in global polio eradication efforts if the country and its health stakeholders have agreed to do so and have earmarked funding for it.

Close cooperation with national health planning authorities is thus vital during the priority-setting process. Differences in emphasis are needed when there are real differences in epidemiological patterns or in socioeconomic conditions. For example, there is no reason to include a hypothetical national priority such as schistosomiasis in an area where it does not occur.

Find adequate ways of follow-up communication

Given the complexity of priority-setting in regard to limited resources versus high demand, communication and responsible follow-up action is vital, especially at sub-national level where decision-makers and the population are closer together in a relationship of trust. People might not understand why health services in other parts of the country might be prioritized over their own demand. And in contexts with strong sub-national patriotism, competition between states or regions might exacerbate misunderstandings and false perceptions. Excellent communication of criteria for setting priorities and allocating resources and follow-up, should be given special attention in such situations.

Box 11.6

Uganda and sub-national priority-setting

In Uganda, nominated community members are recommended to represent the public on technical committees in health sector decision-making to ensure local priorities are adequately addressed in bottom-up planning.[56] In Uganda's decentralized system, participatory planning structures are strong and district-level representatives have decision-making powers to set priorities. Nevertheless, lingering concerns mainly centre around the degree of financial independence allocated to lower levels in setting priorities, the capacity of districts to absorb their increased roles in the process, and the resulting struggles to appropriately set priorities.[57] Efforts to improve communication between system levels and to increase public participation beyond representatives, such as by encouraging grassroots initiatives, have been discussed to combat these concerns and strengthen the translation of community needs into priorities.

11.5.4 Strategic planning

Strategic planning[VII] adopts an all-encompassing whole-of-sector perspective when identifying, sequencing and timing interventions.

Undertaking strategic planning at *national* level in a decentralized context

Sub-national plans and strategies need to be acknowledged

Sub-national plans (e.g. state plans or district plans) guide local decisions and implementation processes. These plans should not be ignored during the national planning cycle and should play a prominent role during the strategic planning phase when translating priorities into targets. For example, an analysis of all sub-national plans can be used as a basis for understanding sub-national and countrywide health needs and demands.

Consistency and communication between the different government tiers needs to be enforced

Communication between the different levels when undertaking strategic planning needs to be made explicit, must be accessible for all sides, and given due resources and investment.

The strategic planning process is usually not a linear exercise; instead it is often characterized by circular loops – going back and forth between demands and needs identified at local level and priorities and targets identified at national level. This will be the case in any setting: however, in a decentralized setting, there are more layers of decision-making power (at national and at sub-national levels), rendering the back-and-forth communication more complex (compared to a more centralized context where, in the end, the central authority makes the decisions). The means of communication to be used between the different levels during this planning phase thus need to be made explicit, must be accessible for both sides, and given due resources and investment.

Revisions to the national strategic plan might be more difficult to do in a decentralized setting

A revision of the strategic plan, for example, due to changing priorities during the course of the plan, is quite challenging in a decentralized setting. A revision might cause disruptions in service delivery at the local level or negatively affect the continuation of sub-national plans, e.g. state plans and district plans.

Thus, revisions, if really necessary, need to be orchestrated in an inclusive and participatory way, where all levels of health governance (and even actors beyond the health sector if necessary: e.g. officials from environment, transport, education etc.) will be included – resembling the initial strategic planning process of the plan.

Special issues to consider when planning strategically at sub-national level

True strategic planning at sub-national level takes place mainly in devolved settings with a strong federal structure. The national level may only give very rough orientations regarding an overarching health sector vision, leaving it up to the federal structures to define it further in practice. For example, in Canada, regional health authorities have a legal mandate to plan the coordination and continuity of care among a host of health care organizations and providers within a defined geographical area.[58] While a broad strategic direction is set by provincial health ministries, detailed planning and coordination is done at the regional health authority level. In

VII For a detailed discussion around strategic planning see Chapter 5 "Strategic planning: transforming priorities into plans" in this handbook.

India, the states undertake planning processes independently of the central level, covering key strategies and activities as well as budgetary requirements and health outputs and outcomes.[59]

Being aware of the available resources

Goals and targets for any strategic plan must be linked to the available budget. In a decentralized scenario, it might be more difficult to define what is "available". Sub-national levels might receive funds from the national level, collect their own revenues and/or receive external support. Being aware of the timing of the release of funds (especially from national level) as well as any restrictions and stipulations on funds can complicate the budget scene at sub-national level. It is important to be aware of this and plan in extra human resources and time within the overall timeline to ensure a solid overview of the available funds and disbursement timings.

In India, for example, the states submit a detailed plan to the national level. All of the states' plans are then collectively negotiated with the national level to decide about the resource envelope for each state. The resources are then disbursed to the states in chunks, depending on their utilization and spending rates.[VIII]

Linking the sub-national to the national level

Even though sub-national strategic planning might be a process that is undertaken completely independently from national processes, sub-national strategic plans need to be linked to the overall national health sector strategic plan – and vice versa. Harmonized and aligned timing and transparency of sub-national planning processes are therefore crucial (consistency and communication).

Box 11.7

United Republic of Tanzania: sub-national plans feed into national strategic planning process

Health Facility Governing Committees (HFGCs) and Community Health Service Boards in United Republic of Tanzania are instrumental organs in health planning at the community level in the country's decentralized health system.[60] HFGCs are the platform through which community members are involved in developing local plans.[61] This, in effect, allows for community needs to be raised and addressed. Once local health plans and budgets are determined, they are submitted to district councils for approval, as are local health progress reports for monitoring and evaluation. Devolution of health planning authority is laid out by the Local Government Reform Act (1998) and United Republic of Tanzania national health plans; local plans feed into the national strategic planning process through bottom-up planning and support of national goals such as poverty reduction, improvement of quality care and better health access.[62]

VIII WHO, India Country Office (personal communication).

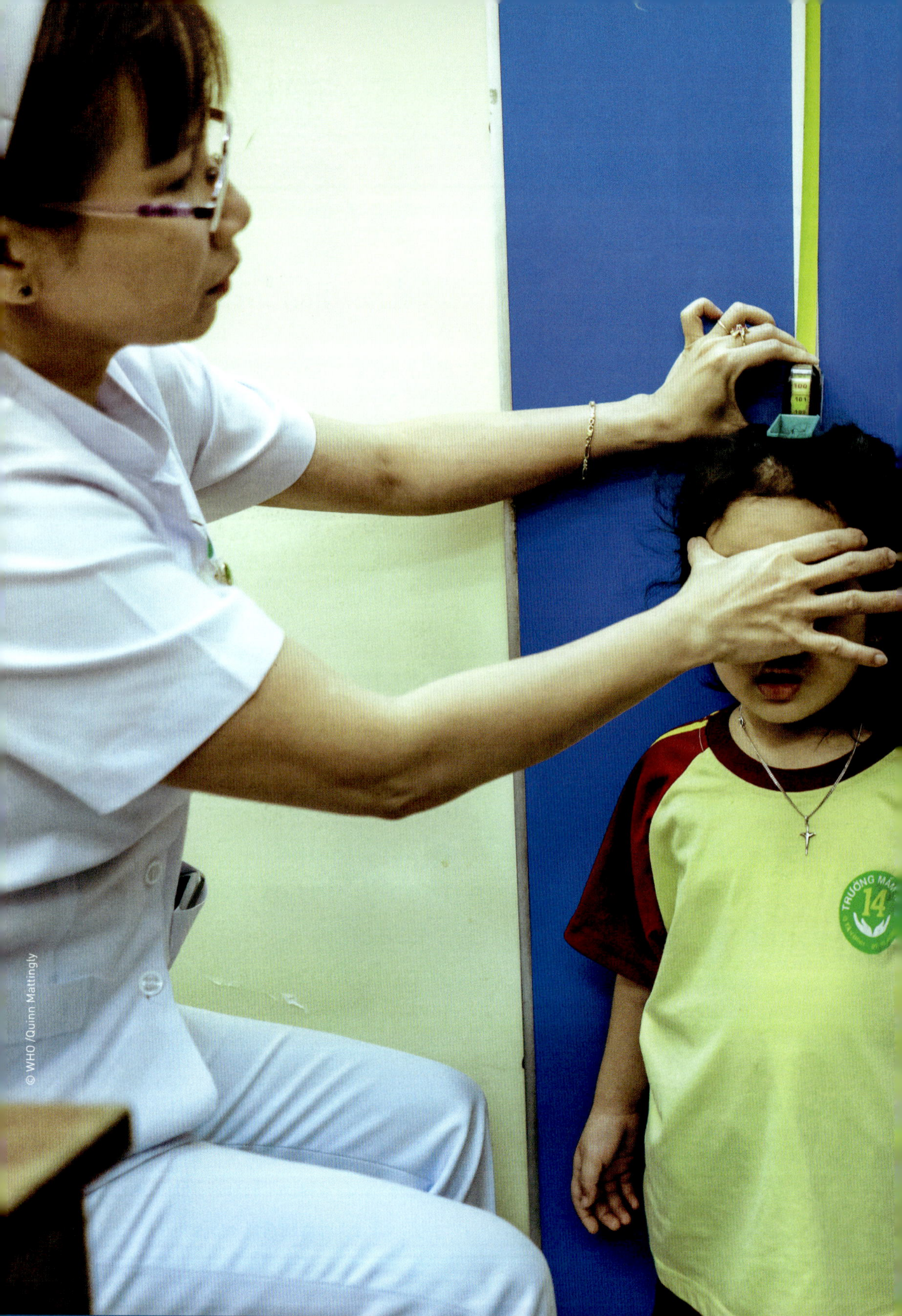

11.5.5 Operational planning in a decentralized context

Undertaking operational planning at national level in a decentralized context

Budget centres and operational units which are undertaking operational planning at national-level must consider sub-national needs depending on the institution's purview and scope.

Clarifying the source of funding

Where national-level entities cover sub-national-level activities, both levels of actors will be actively involved in the operational planning exercise for the national-level budget centre. In this case, it should be clarified beforehand where the resources for the process would be coming from. Especially for follow-up activities on recommendations, the source of the funds needed should be clearly identified (e.g. national budget or sub-national budgets/contributions).

Multiplicity of operational plans to be aligned to the national strategy

A national or state health strategy implies a variety of operational plans – at the national level, at the sub-national level and even at the local level. It is crucial to make sure that those sub-national and local operational plans are aligned with national operational plans and the NHPSP. Despite the levels and degrees of decentralization in the health system, the national MoH, where politically and constitutionally possible, might want to keep a guidance and oversight function to ensure alignment.

Special issues to consider when planning operationally at sub-national level

Managing complexities during the formulation of operational plans at local and sub-national levels

In (highly) decentralized settings, operational planning done at local and sub-national levels is circulated bottom-up to the next higher level for consolidation. The preparation and consolidation of these sub-national operational plans require intense human and financial resources and capacities. Sub-national and local levels might need to request extra capacity support from regional or national levels. Given the differences between the health issues in different states, each operational plan requires a specific knowledge and understanding of the context. The national level can do well in supporting the sub-national levels in the formulation and consolidation of the plans with technical expertise and facilitating functions, but accepting the final authority of the sub-national level on decisions.

Budget centres and operational units which are undertaking operational planning at national level must consider sub-national needs depending on the institution's purview and scope.

Coordinating sub-national operational plans with national budget line items

Preferably, the operational plan headings would correspond to the budget line items ("chart of accounts") of the financing authority, for example the ministry of finance at the national level and the district treasury office at district level. In actual practice, health planning stakeholders often find the headings from the national budget to be ill-suited for district purposes. A compromise is to do a "translation exercise" by adding another column to the operational plan matrix for the national budget line items.

11.5.6 Costing and budgeting in a decentralized context

Costing and budgeting[IX] both require a high level of expertise from all tiers involved in the process. The level and design of decentralization is especially relevant as described below.

Costing and budgeting at national level in a decentralized context

Unclear decentralization arrangements might jeopardize budgeting and costing exercises

Costing and budgeting both require a high level of expertise from all tiers involved in the process.

Advantages of proximity to local circumstances and context-specific information might be limited by unclear structures and distribution of roles and responsibilities. Ambiguity may lead to limited control and choice for sub-national authorities over expenditures, user fees, contracting, targeting and overall health governance. Also choices over major sources of revenues like local taxes might be challenged due to confused and mixed roles and responsibilities between the different government tiers.

Combining information and data that varies from state to state

A challenge in a decentralized setting is the different and heterogeneous data sets from the various sub-national levels. In this regard, the establishment of a national authority to provide guidance to homogenize costing, budgeting, and expenditure tracking methodology, aggregating country-wide data and producing national estimates might be an option to provide consistency across the country and produce comparable information.

Special issues to consider when costing and budgeting at sub-national level

Sub-national governments should make use of their understanding of local circumstances and access to context-specific information

Sub-national levels have the grand opportunity of ensuring that budget allocation decisions closely reflect local needs. Thus, supporting the sub-national level (capacity-building) to improve efficiency and effectiveness of spending at sub-national levels is crucial.

The more power and authority actually vested in local authorities, the more scope there is for rational costing and budgeting that is close to the real needs of the local population. Additionally, if there is a formalized fiscal decentralization, policy-makers should take revenue generation at different levels into account for improved and adequate fiscal space projections.

Raising resources at sub-national level

In many decentralized settings, local/sub-national entities are authorized to impose taxes (fiscal decentralization). However, in many cases, especially in low-income countries, the tax base might be quite weak. Strengthening community-level interventions and supporting budget analysis tools are effective ways to strengthen local governance capacity from national to sub-national levels. The outcomes of those (financial) capacity support interventions will increase technical efficiency through planning and management that is more aligned to local needs.

IX For a detailed discussion around costing and budgeting, see Chapter 7 "Estimating cost implications of a national health policy, strategy or plan" and Chapter 8 "Budgeting for health" in this handbook.

In a decentralized setting, being able to react quickly is also a distinct advantage: allocative efficiency and smart investments made with incremental funding might result in higher-quality services and better health.

Box 11.8

Costing and budgeting in a decentralized system

Costing and budgeting in Ethiopia's highly decentralized health system require alignment across all levels of the administration. Ethiopia's Health Sector Strategic Plan focuses on a "One-Plan, One-Budget, One-Report" approach to manage all health activities in the country. Made up of the nine regional states and two city administrations, "woredas" (a basic decentralized regional unit), and "kebeles" (lower-level local associations), the country requires an effective allocation system to transfer funds down the multiple levels of government.[63] Costing is performed at all levels of the health system, but may be most valuable at the woreda level as those offices have the strongest understanding of local health sector needs and costs.[64,65] The one-budget approach in which funds for health services are pooled relies on strong costing assumptions to consistently budget funds across the regionally diverse country.[66]

11.5.7 Monitoring and evaluation (M&E) in a decentralized context

The quality of M&E depends to a great extent on the quality of the M&E component of the national strategy and the sub-national strategies, the capacity of the involved people and institutions, and methods to collect data and ensure its quality.

The quality of M&E,[X] including review mechanisms, depends to a great extent on the quality of the M&E component of the national strategy and the sub-national strategies (alignment), the capacity of the involved people and institutions, as well as the methods to collect data and ensure the quality of the data.[67]

M&E at national level in a decentralized context

Alignment between national and sub-national strategies and plans

The NHPSP should identify and lay out a sound and comprehensive M&E element.[68] However, the design of this element, or framework, needs to be coordinated and translated to sub-national documents for coherence. Likewise, sub-national strategies should form the basis for the national M&E framework. A constant interaction between the national and sub-national levels is crucial for the success, repeatability and reproducibility of monitoring, evaluation and review mechanisms.

Review mechanisms and feedback loops should ensure accountability

The review mechanisms chosen should be comprehensive – not just in terms of sectoral and programme-related aspects, but also in regard to national and sub-national levels.

Thorough M&E activities require inclusive policy dialogue and systematic and regular assessments.[69] Those mechanisms – and the tools and methods to use them – need to be adapted to the formalized and non-formalized (especially in regard to dialogue processes) decentralization features that are prevailing in the country. Accountability towards the results of monitoring and evaluation need to be claimed at every government level.

Allowing reflections on the status of decentralization

When undertaking M&E in a decentralized context, it is important to consider the ways in which decentralization has been integrated and used in all the previous planning steps. As a consequence of the breadth of evaluation, process-related issues might be considered as well – apart from health-related issues. It might be beneficial for the planning process to establish a link between health outcomes and decentralization. For example, the set of indicators related to health outcomes could be complemented by political, administrative and fiscal indicators for M&E purposes of the performance of sub-national planning. Thus, routine data collection needs to be adapted, since those quantitative and qualitative indicators are not always part of the collection set in many countries.[70] As a consequence of including

X For a detailed discussion around monitoring and evaluation, see Chapter 9 of this handbook.

XI Hutchinson and LaFond (cited above) developed a "Conceptual Framework for Evaluating Decentralization" which offers a detailed guide for monitoring and evaluation of decentralization in the health sector, with an emphasis on conceptual questions and concrete options for action.

decentralization in the evaluation, current responsibility, authority and accountability arrangements might need to be adapted.[XI]

Monitoring sub-national regional inequalities

Monitoring health inequalities between sub-national levels can inform targeted health programmes and policies, especially if disparities are substantial. Summary measures of inequality can condense disaggregated data into concise outputs, which could be used to show trends and make comparisons.[71] The selection of appropriate summary measures to quantify sub-national inequalities should be carefully chosen to provide a good understanding of sub-national-level inequalities to policy-makers, partners and civil society, among others, and thus to facilitate targeting and deploying interventions to disadvantaged subpopulations.

Special issues to consider for M&E at sub-national level

Selection of tools and assessment methods

The analysis and assessment tools that will determine the success and validity of the M&E exercises as well as increase accountability towards its results need to be selected according to the features of the health system. It is important to ensure consistency and comparability across the different sub-national-levels and to support those levels (capacity and financial) to be able to analyse and use the data.

Sub-national M&E plans

Countries that have been going through devolution processes, such as Kenya, have created a new layer of sub-national government, with allocated resources and prescribed functions. Many of them choose to develop separate sub-national M&E plans. These plans spell out how sub-national level data will be used to monitor performance and how progress and performance of the sub-national health sector strategic and investment plans will be tracked. Central-level technical support may be necessary at the beginning. For example, Kenya has updated its national M&E roadmap to ensure that the M&E needs of its counties are identified and addressed through specific measures such as strengthening counties' data analysis, validation and synthesizing capacities.[72]

Table 11.3 Issues to consider when strategizing for health at sub-national level

	POPULATION CONSULTATION	SITUATION ANALYSIS	PRIORITY-SETTING
Benefits in a decentralized health system	▸ Formal and geographical closeness to needs and expectations of the population ▸ Better integration of marginalized communities	▸ Formal and geographical closeness to health needs and living conditions of the population ▸ National policies to profit from sub-national evidence	▸ Engagement of recognized sub-national actors to improve national priority-setting exercise ▸ Higher sensitization and participation due to decentralized information flows ▸ Quantity of stakeholders due to decentralized setting might increase – quality should not be affected
Issues to be aware of when undertaking...	▸ Involvement of all stakeholders at all levels ▸ Methodology of consultation to take decentralization and the different living conditions it might imply into account ▸ Feedback and follow-up scenarios to be built at sub-national level to be translated more easily to local contexts	▸ Involvement of all stakeholders at all levels ▸ Situation analysis conclusions to be accepted by stakeholders at all government levels ▸ Dissemination of outcomes of the situation analysis to all government tiers	▸ Clear roles and responsibilities are important ▸ Differences between sub-national entities (e.g. states) in demand and needs should be considered and communicated in a credible way ▸ Missing synchronicity between national, state and programme plans to be taken into account ▸ Methods, tools and approaches chosen to be in line with country context

STRATEGIC PLANNING	OPERATIONAL PLANNING	COSTING AND BUDGET	MONITORING AND EVALUATION
▸ Formal and geographical closeness to health needs and living conditions of the population can support all-encompassing perspective ▸ Increase legitimacy and inclusiveness of planning process	▸ Inclusiveness of actors and sub-national plans to increase legitimacy and adherence at sub-national level ▸ Formal and geographical closeness to health needs and living conditions ▸ Decentralization can strengthen operational planning process through link between sub-national health needs and national strategic views	▸ Better understanding of local circumstances and access to context-specific information ▸ Strengthened local government capacity for improved efficiency and local resource mobilization	▸ Closeness to the living conditions of the population and to the implementation of activities: data regarding coverage equity might be gathered more easily ▸ Status and quality of decentralized health system to be monitored and evaluated
▸ Involvement of all stakeholders at all levels ▸ Methods, tools and approaches chosen to be in line with country context ▸ Clear routes of communication between the different tiers ▸ Sub-national plans to be considered ▸ Revisions of national plan even more complicated in decentralized setting	▸ Multiplicity of operation plans to be aligned to national strategy ▸ Managing complexities during the formulation of operational plans at local and sub-national levels ▸ Revisions of sub-national operational plans to be communicated to national level and vice versa	▸ Well-done budgeting and costing depends on clear decentralization arrangements; ▸ Data that might vary from state to state to be combined at national level ▸ Reporting and transparency on money flows to be well-monitored through the different tiers	▸ Alignment between the M&E elements of national and sub-national strategies and plans ▸ Review mechanisms and feedback loops to be comprehensive and inclusive to ensure accountability ▸ Selections of tools and assessments methods to be adapted to decentralized health system context ▸ Clear roles and responsibilities

11.5.8 General issues to consider at sub-national level during all steps in the planning cycle

An unambiguous transfer of responsibilities is not always the reality

In a decentralized context, where different actors at different levels (inter-)act, clear coordination and communication is essential.

- The more clearly the different stages in the planning cycle are linked to clear (divisions of) roles and responsibilities, the smoother the planning can be organized. Contrarily, unclear roles as well as blurred responsibilities and lines of accountability between the different tiers might create unnecessary hiccups in the planning process. Especially when decision-making processes between national and sub-national level are not clearly regulated and outlined, there is a risk of blockages in decisions or reforms. The complementarity of roles of national and sub-national actors is one of the most important features of sub-national planning and should regularly be re-evaluated.
- The MoH usually does not have the sole monopoly of health service provision, be it in a centralized or a decentralized context. In many contexts, private sector and many other actors provide services as well (e.g. nongovernmental institutions, faith-based organizations). Many of them may only cater for a selected area or specific group of people.[73] Therefore, communication of roles and responsibilities between national and decentralized state institutions and the respective additional actors at each level is important to limit uncoordinated service provision.
- This is equally relevant in a situation where there is a separate national health service purchasing agency that pays local-level health providers (district hospitals, health centres) in addition to government budget allocations from the national to sub-national levels. This creates multiple funding flows arriving at the sub-national administrative level or directly at the provider level that are often pooled while requiring separate upwards reporting and creating multiple accountability lines. Critical issues with respect to providers are their level of autonomy to be able to coherently respond to incentives set by the separate purchasing agency's provider payment method as well as those by state sub-national units. A separate purchasing agency, e.g. a health insurance, should engage with sub-national authorities to work out funding flows and population needs in order to ensure appropriate procurement of drugs and other supplies, as well as proper planning for infrastructure and human resources. The challenge is that local governments end up handling both functions of purchasing and provision. Above all, when there is a purchaser-provider split, it raises questions on the actual division of labour between the stewards at national level, the separate purchasing agency(ies) and the sub-national units with respect to purchasing, provision, planning and regulation. Too often these are not sufficiently clarified.
- In some cases, development planning and administration might remain at the national level, while some sectors might be decentralized. In reality this turns into quite a difficult scenario with sometimes unclear rules and regulations for health. It is therefore essential to understand at what level(s) planning is actually done and how the different levels of planning are linked to each

Stakeholders involved in health planning need to be aware of existing inconsistencies and find a responsible and sustainable way to work with them – or if possible resolve them.

other. For example, if planning is only done at national level, how are the implications translated to sub-national levels? In some countries, even specific functions (e.g. drug regulation, hospital accreditation) remain at the national level while other functions are decentralized. Since both would be running in parallel, roles, responsibilities and lines of reporting need to be clear.

- Related to the last point are the inconsistencies in the broader political system, meaning that some functions and services might be centralized and others decentralized. This can pose additional burdens for planning in a decentralized (health) system. Some inconsistencies are enshrined in the health system and might be difficult to change. For example, a decentralized provision of services but a centralized accreditation system for facilities. Stakeholders involved in health planning need to be aware of existing inconsistencies and find a responsible and sustainable way to work with them – or if possible resolve them. The key here seems to lie in well-managed and harmonized horizontal (intersectoral) communication along the different involved sectors (especially finance) and vertical (within the health sector). Constant exchange between all involved actors can help find an agreement or workaround solution which enables complementarity and as little inefficiency and overlap as possible.

Box 11.9

New Zealand: clear roles and responsibilities in a decentralized system

The New Zealand Public Health and Disability Act of 2000 clearly lays out roles and responsibilities for the different levels of its health system. The law establishes the structure for public sector funding and organization of health and disability services in New Zealand. According to the law, at the federal level the MoH develops and reviews The New Zealand Health Strategy, negotiates Crown Funding Agreements to set relationships between the Crown and District Health Boards, and issues operational frameworks for funding and delivery of services.[74] At the district level, 21 District Health Boards (DHBs) are responsible for drawing up district strategic and annual plans. Parliament serves as an accountability partner, overseeing statements of intent and annual reports provided by both the MoH and DHBs. By directly setting out the duties and roles of key participants for the Health and Disability Act, each tier of New Zealand's decentralized health system stays accountable and organized through the planning, implementation, and evaluation processes.[75]

Transferring power to sub-national levels raises expectations

The different tiers in a decentralized context should complement each other in terms of roles and responsibilities. However, it is essential to manage expectations between the different levels of government.

- In some instances, sub-national entities, charged with highly-demanding responsibilities for planning and implementation, might have neither the time nor the capacity to meet the national government's expectations to satisfy the needs and expectation of the population (performance). Roles and responsibilities should therefore always go hand-in-hand with the capacities needed to fulfil those – thus, the national level has a special role in ensuring capacity support through to all levels.
- Additionally, there are cases where local structures do not match the expectations of the national level in terms of accountability. Even though it is recognized that accountability (and responsibility) could be enhanced through decentralized decision-making structures, a problem might occur where (historic) local leadership and power arrangements ("local power elites") do not reflect the expectations of the national level.[76] Addressing this sort of sensitive issues will involve extensive engagement with the communities in question over a longer period of time to ensure any change in power structures and improvements in accountability mechanisms to the local population. Allocating time and resources to this and collaborating with local structures (civil society organizations, community groups, etc.) should be envisaged and planned.

International engagement must be well-managed in a decentralized setting

International engagement is an additional factor for consideration when discussing decentralization in the health sector.

- Stakeholders involved in health planning should keep in mind that international actors (United Nations agencies, donor countries, Global Health Initiatives) might be acting only at certain levels (national level or only sub-national level), or in certain areas (only in specific states/regions) or on certain topics (e.g. child mortality in rural areas), which might create imbalances in service provision between different states/sub-national units. Being aware of these imbalances created by external service provision (that might not be obvious at first sight when planning is decentralized) will be relevant for planning purposes.
- International responsibilities of the national government (e.g. International Health Regulations, WHO, United Nations agencies, European Union) and their consequences for planning might need to be translated or adapted to sub-national levels, depending on the exact nature of the international engagement. For example, the International Health Regulations are signed and ratified at national level, but their impact needs to be translated to the sub-national levels.
- Supranational institutions (European Union, MERCOSUR, African Union) might add another layer of governance on top of the national level. Even though the characteristics and shapes of those supranational institutions vary greatly, it is important to understand what kind of implications, including opportunities, they might pose for the health sector and for sub-national planning.[77]

The distribution of wealth and financial resources should be carefully considered

In many countries, there are richer and poorer regions, each with potentially different tax rates and user fees.[78] An uneven distribution of access to health care by region might be the consequence, which can result in discussions on equity and financial compensation (equalization payments) from richer to poorer regions.[79] In some instances, the debate on equalization payments can be very challenging if there is an unwillingness of richer regions to support poorer regions.

When discussing the distribution of financial resources in a decentralized context, an additional issue to consider is whether the responsibilities of the sub-national units match their financial base and technical capacities and how those capacities can be increased of necessary.

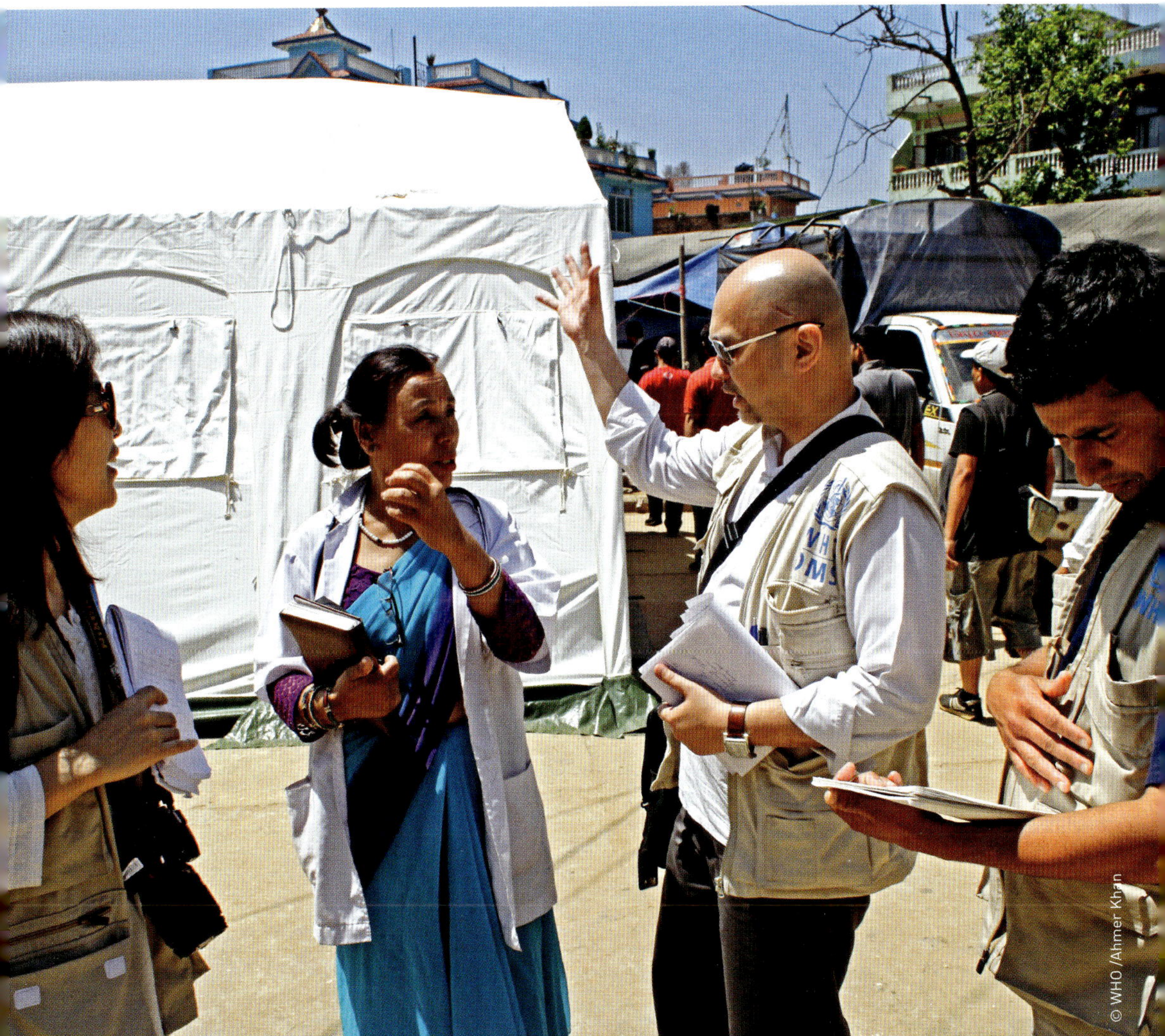

11.5.9 General issues to consider when putting in place sub-national planning structures during an on-going decentralization process[XII]

Many countries are currently in need of institutional reform, including a reduced role for the national level, especially in health service delivery,[XIII] based on the idea that smaller organizations are more flexible, more efficient and more accountable (in the health sector and beyond).

Clarifying the aims and objectives for increased sub-national level planning

It is important to keep in mind that sub-national planning and decentralization are to be seen as a means, not an end in itself. Decentralizing the health/political system in and of itself does not necessarily have a positive impact on health outcomes. Decentralization should rather be seen as a broad concept to improve planning and implementation processes with positive impacts on health outcomes. It should be regarded as a policy mechanism aiming to realize specific goals, such as increases in effectiveness and efficiency.

Hence, decentralization of health planning is not a solution per se. Before engaging in a decentralization reform process, it would be essential to clarify and acknowledge the problems and challenges the reform is intended to solve. Decentralization processes should therefore not be seen as a way to delegate responsibilities to other levels simply to get rid of them, but rather as a means to improve processes.

Preparing the ground before the decentralization reform process

Policy lessons drawn from existing case studies and analysis of decentralization processes suggest that capacity building at local/sub-national level is crucial prior to transferring responsibilities. Local/sub-national elected representatives need to be provided with capacity-building initiatives especially focused on planning in a decentralized health system. As there might be a higher turn-over through periodic elections at regional and local level, capacity-building should be conducted regularly and be formalized for flexible access for participants.[80]

- Implementation, monitoring and evaluation features and support modalities need to be specified for the sub-national level. It is essential to understand that the effects of a decentralization reform might be seen only in the long term; aspirations for short-term changes are likely to be disappointed.[81]
- Capacity-building should also be foreseen for the national level to ensure that the national level is capable of supporting sub-national levels with adequate planning, budgeting and logistical resources.

XII This is not a guide on how to decentralize the health sector/health planning. It is rather an attempt to discuss a few issues one should keep in mind during a political, fiscal and administrative decentralization process.

XIII Many countries (especially European countries) find themselves in a vicious circle of decentralizing – centralizing-redecentralizing, trying to find the right balance between responsiveness and efficiency (http://www.euro.who.int/__data/assets/pdf_file/0007/135664/EuroObserver13_1.pdf, accessed 25 Octpber 2016).

Box 11.10

Preparing the ground for decentralization in Pakistan

In Pakistan, the 18th Amendment of the Constitution in 2010 assigned only a limited set of functions to the federal level while other functions were devolved to the provinces. As a consequence, the Federal MoH was abolished and the remaining responsibilities for health at federal level were reassigned to other federal ministries. A number of problems arose from the implementation of the Amendment; these have generally been attributed to the unplanned abolition of the MoH and the transfer of responsibilities to the provinces without a transition period.[82,83] At federal level, there was a lack of clarity about the distribution of federal responsibilities in health among other ministries, and the capacity and motivation of these ministries to perform these health-related functions. The abolition of the federal MoH also resulted in the loss of health leadership at federal level and a fragmentation of decision-making processes with particular threat to areas such as health security and domestic and external resource mobilization.[84] At the provincial level, there was a general agreement among the provincial authorities that the provinces needed significant support and organizational restructuring to take on the responsibilities for the vertical programmes and other activities in information and regulation; these were previously federal responsibilities and were devolved after the 18th Amendment. Furthermore, variations in capacities across provinces were likely to further increase geographical disparities and inequities. Finally, unclear distribution of responsibilities between federal and provincial level further created areas of tensions. One example was the delay in the creation of a Federal Drug Regulatory Authority.[85] The newly elected democratic government endorsed the re-establishment of the federal Ministry of National Health Services Regulation and Coordination in 2013.

Designing a decentralized health system adapted to the country context

The overall context, in which a decentralization reform, usually an overall governance and government process, is embedded, has to be acknowledged. Especially the national political context may determine the institutional structure of the decentralization reform and consequently the impact and outcome of the decentralization process on the health sector.[86]

Opening communication channels from the population to local authorities during the design of the reform process takes full advantage of the benefits which decentralization has to offer. This is often only done once the major decisions with regard to decentralization have already been taken, missing a major opportunity for positive change.

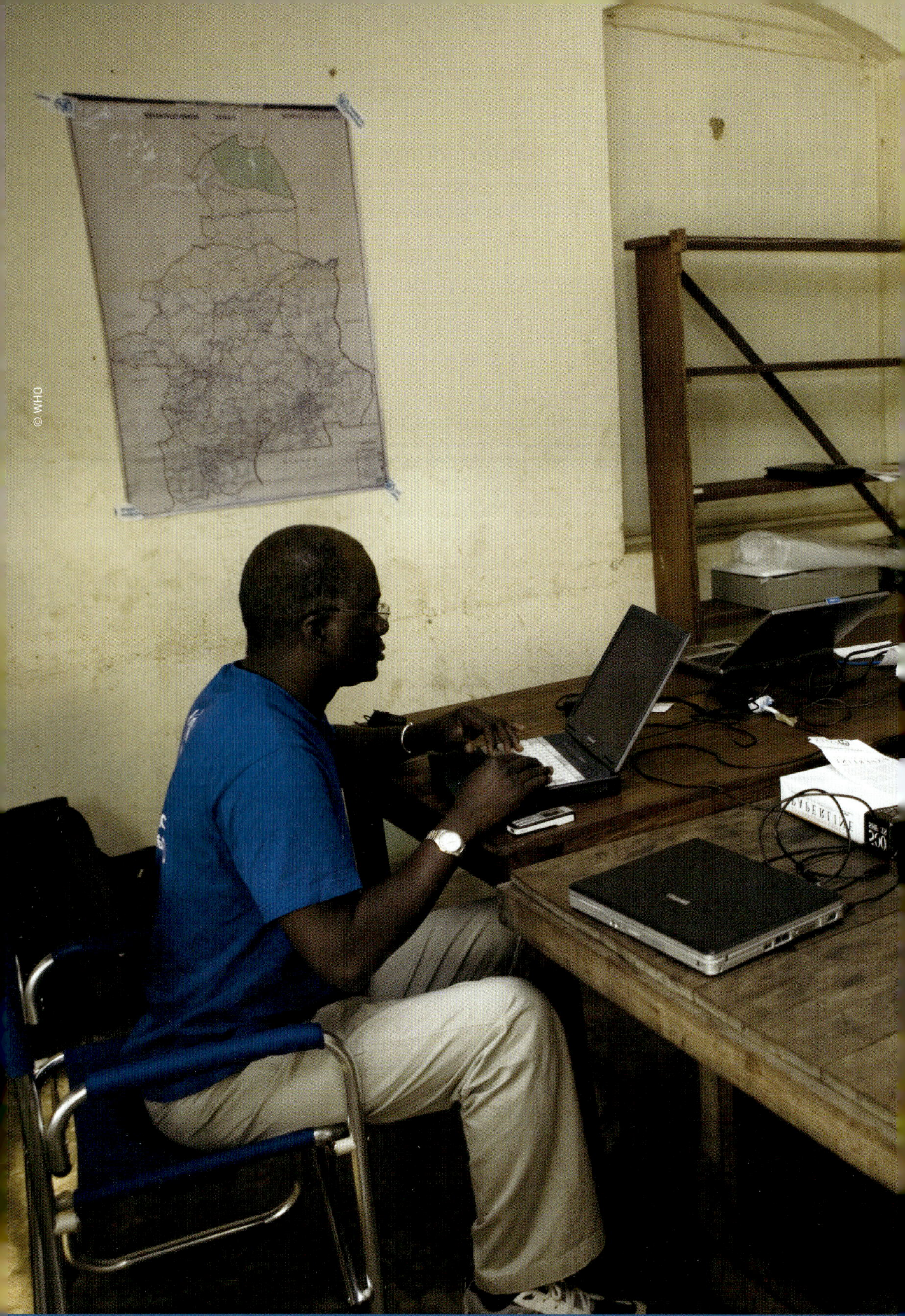

11.6 Conclusion

Sub-national planning is most often not a choice but a reality, a context to which the policy-maker has to adapt. But this situation actually offers a multiplicity of advantages and can be seen as a potential asset to national health planning. However, there are challenges that should be acknowledged and thought through in order to reap the benefits of planning that is closer to the population as beneficiaries and active actors. Many of the planning challenges discussed in this chapter arise because sub-national structures might not be adequately designed and in line with population needs; or because the lines of responsibility and accountability remain unclear. One major example is the lack of clarity in many countries regarding roles and responsibilities for health service purchasing, provision and regulation. Health sector planning at sub-national level cannot go far if such issues remain unresolved.

The conclusion to be drawn for health planning and policy-making processes in general is that broader institutional arrangements and functions need to be explicitly spelled out, and potential tensions clarified, when engaging in sub-national planning.

If planning and decision-making personnel are able to recognize and accept the complexities and inconsistencies that might accompany decentralization, it might be more effective to design an adequately tailored strategy or a policy.

This chapter proposes ways to leverage advantages of sub-national strategizing for health in order to deliver on better services and ensure responsiveness to the population's needs and expectations.

References

1 Vrangbaek K. Towards a typology for decentralization in health care. In: Saltman RB, Bankauskaite V, Vrangbaek K, editors. Decentralization in health care: strategies and outcomes. Maidenhead: Open University Press; 2007 (European Observatory on Health Systems and Policy Series; http://www.euro.who.int/__data/assets/pdf_file/0004/98275/E89891.pdf, accessed 21 October 2016).

2 Saltman RB, Bankauskaite V, Vrangbæk K, editors. Decentralization in health care. Maidenhead: Open University Press; 2007 (European Observatory on Health Systems and Policy Series; http://www.euro.who.int/__data/assets/pdf_file/0004/98275/E89891.pdf, accessed 21 October 2016).

3 Bremner J. The complexities of decentralization. EURO Observer. 2011;13(1):1–3 (http://www.euro.who.int/__data/assets/pdf_file/0007/135664/EuroObserver13_1.pdf, accessed 21 October 2016).

4 Paris V, Devaux M, Wei L. Health systems institutional characteristics: a survey of 29 OECD countries. Paris: OECD; 2010 (OECD Health Working papers No. 50, http://www.oecd.org/officialdocuments/publicdisplaydocumentpdf/?cote=DELSA/HEA/WD/HWP(2010)1&docLanguage=En, accessed 21 October 2016).

5 Mills A. Decentralization concepts and issues: a review. In: Mills A, Vaughan JP, Smith DL, Tabibzadeh I, editors. Health system decentralization: concepts, issues and country experience. Geneva: World Health Organization; 1990 (http://apps.who.int/iris/bitstream/10665/39053/1/9241561378.pdf, accessed 21 October 2016).

6 Ibid.

7 Lopez-Casasnovas G. Health care and fiscal decentralisation in Spain. 2003 (http://docplayer.net/985481-Guillem-lopez-casasnovas-prof-in-public-economics-director-of-the-center-for-health-and-economics-univ-pompeu-fabra-catalonia.html, accessed 21 October 2016).

8 Garcia-Milà T, McGuire TJ. Fiscal Decentralization in Spain: An Asymmetric Transition to Democracy. [Internet]. 2002 Mar 22 [cited 2016 Jan 25]:[about 15pp.]. Available from: http://crei.cat/people/gmila/fidespain.pdf Garcia-Milà T, McGuire TJ. Fiscal decentralization in Spain: an asymmetric transition to democracy. 2002 Mar 22 (https://repositori.upf.edu/bitstream/handle/10230/766/866.pdf?sequence=1, accessed 21 October 2016).

9 Saltman RB, Bankauskaite V, Vrangbæk K, editors. Decentralization in health care. Maidenhead: Open University Press; 2007 (European Observatory on Health Systems and Policy Series; http://www.euro.who.int/__data/assets/pdf_file/0004/98275/E89891.pdf, accessed 21 October 2016).

10 The management of health systems in the EU Member States: the role of local and regional authorities. European Union; 2012 (http://cor.europa.eu/en/documentation/studies/Documents/health-systems/health-systems-en.pdf, accessed 21 October 2016); Pita Barros P, Ribeirinho Machado S, de Alemida Simoes J. Portugal: health system review. Health Syst Transit. 2011;13(4) (http://www.euro.who.int/__data/assets/pdf_file/0019/150463/e95712.pdf, accessed 31 October 2016); Paris V, Devaux M, Wei L. Health systems institutional characteristics: a survey of 29 OECD countries. Paris: OECD; 2010 (OECD Health Working papers No. 50; http://www.oecd.org/officialdocuments/publicdisplaydocumentpdf/?cote=DELSA/HEA/WD/HWP(2010)1&docLanguage=En, accessed 21 October 2016).

11 Saltman RB, Bankauskaite V, Vrangbæk K, editors. Decentralization in health care. Maidenhead: Open University Press; 2007 (European Observatory on Health Systems and Policy Series; http://www.euro.who.int/__data/assets/pdf_file/0004/98275/E89891.pdf, accessed 21 October 2016).

12 Bossert T, Chitah MB, Simonet M, Mwansa L, Daura M, Mabandhala M, et al. Decentralization of the health system in Zambia. Bethesda (MD): Partnerships for Health Reform, Abt Associates; 2000 (Major Applied Research 6, Technical Report 2; https://www.hsph.harvard.edu/ihsg/publications/pdf/DecentralizationOfTheHealthSystemInZambia.pdf, accessed 15 September 2016).

13 Jeppsson A, Okuonzi S. Vertical or holistic decentralization of the health sector? Experiences from Zambia and Uganda. Int J Health Plann Manage. 2000;15(4):273–89 (https://www.researchgate.net/publication/12085252_Vertical_or_holistic_decentralization_of_the_health_sector_Experiences_from_Zambia_and_Uganda, accessed 21 October 2016).

14 Saltman RB, Bankauskaite V, Vrangbæk K, editors. Decentralization in health care. Maidenhead: Open University Press; 2007 (European Observatory on Health Systems and Policy Series; http://www.euro.who.int/__data/assets/pdf_file/0004/98275/E89891.pdf, accessed 21 October 2016).

15 Greer SL. Devolution and health: data and democracy. BMJ. 2014;(348) (http://www.bmj.com.ez.lshtm.ac.uk/content/348/bmj.g3096 [subscription required]). doi: 10.1136/bmj.g3096.

16 Tashobya CK, Ssengooba F, Cruz VO. Health systems reforms in Uganda: processes and outputs. London: Health Systems Development Programme, London School of Hygiene & Tropical Medicine; 2006 (http://r4d.dfid.gov.uk/pdf/outputs/healthsysdev_kp/uganda_book.pdf, accessed 21 October 2016).

17 Bossert T. Analyzing the decentralization of health systems in developing countries: decision space, innovation and performance. Soc Sci Med. 1998;47(10):1513–27 (https://www.hsph.harvard.edu/ihsg/pdf/science.pdf, accessed 25 October 2016).

18 Rajan D, Kalambay H, Mossoko M, Kwete D, Bulakali J, Lokonga JP, et al. Health service planning contributes to policy dialogue around strengthening district health systems: an example from DR Congo 2008–2013. BMC Health Serv Res. 2014;14:522 (https://www.ncbi.nlm.nih.gov/pmc/articles/PMC4224692/, accessed 21 October 2016).

19 Sambo LG, Chatora RR, Goosen ESM. Tools for assessing the operationality of district health systems: guidelines. Brazzaville: Regional Office for Africa, World Health Organization; 2003 . http://www.who.int/management/district/assessment/assessment_tool.pdf, accessed 21 October 2016).

20 Declaration on strengthening district health systems based on primary health care. Harare: World Health Organization; 1987 (http://apps.who.int/iris/bitstream/10665/61958/1/WHO_SHS_DHS.pdf, accessed 21 October 2016).

21 Görgen H, Kirsch-Woik T, Schmidt-Ehry B, editors. The district health system; experiences and prospects in Africa; manual for public health practitioners. 2nd edition Wiesbaden: Universum Verlag, 2004 (Schriftenreihe der GTZ; 276).

22 Rajan D, Kalambay H, Mossoko M, Kwete D, Bulakali J, Lokonga JP, et al. Health service planning contributes to policy dialogue around strengthening district health systems: an example from DR Congo 2008–2013. BMC Health Serv Res. 2014;14:522 (https://www.ncbi.nlm.nih.gov/pmc/articles/PMC4224692/, accessed 21 October 2016).

23 Porignon D, Soron'Gane EM, Lokombe TE, Isu DK, Hennart P, Van Lerberghe W. How robust are district health systems? Coping with crisis

and disasters in Rutshuru, Democratic Republic of Congo. Trop Med Int Health. 1998;3(7):559–65 (http://onlinelibrary.wiley.com/doi/10.1046/j.1365-3156.1998.00263.x/full).

24 Saltman RB, Vrangbæk, K. Drawing lessons for policy-making. In: Saltman RB, Bankauskaite V, Vrangbæk K, editors. Decentralization in health care. Maidenhead: Open University Press; 2007: pp. 77–84 (European Observatory on Health Systems and Policy Series; http://www.euro.who.int/__data/assets/pdf_file/0004/98275/E89891.pdf, accessed 21 October 2016).

25 Ribot JC. African decentralization: local actors, powers and accountability. Geneva: United Nations Research Institute for Social Development (UNRISD); 2002 (Programme on Democracy, Governance and Human Rights Paper No.8; http://www.unrisd.org/80256B3C005BCCF9/(httpAuxPages)/3345AC67E6875754C1256D12003E6C95/$file/ribot.pdf, accessed 21 October 2016).

26 Mitchell A, Bossert TJ. Decentralisation, Governance and Health System Performance: "Where You Stand Depends on Where You Sit". Development Policy Review. 2010;28(6):669–91.

27 Alves J, Peralta S, Perelman J. Efficiency and equity consequences of decentralization in health: an economic perspective. Revista portuguesa de saúde pública. 2013;31(1):74–83.

28 Shukla A, Khanna R, Jadhav N. Using community-based evidence for decentralized health planning: insights from Maharashtra, India. Health Policy Plan. 2014; 1–12 (http://heapol.oxfordjournals.org/content/early/2014/09/21/heapol.czu099.full.pdf+html, accessed 22 October 2016).

29 Ibid.

30 Bossert TJ, Beauvais JC. Decentralization of Health Systems in Ghana, Zambia, Uganda and the Philippines: a comparative analysis of decision space. Health Policy Plan. 2002;17(1):14–31.

31 Shukla A, Khanna R, Jadhav N. Using community-based evidence for decentralized health planning: insights from Maharashtra, India. Health Policy Plan. 2014;1–12 (http://heapol.oxfordjournals.org/content/early/2014/09/21/heapol.czu099.full.pdf+html, accessed 22 October 2016); Guanais FC, Macinko J. The health effects of decentralizing primary care In Brazil. Health Aff. 2009;28(4):1127–35. doi:10.1377/hlthaff.28.4.1127; Shukla A, Khanna R, Jadhav N. Using community-based evidence for decentralized health planning: insights from Maharashtra, India. Health Policy Plan. 2014;1–12 (http://heapol.oxfordjournals.org/content/early/2014/09/21/heapol.czu099.full.pdf+html, accessed 22 October 2016).

32 Bardhan P. Decentralization of governance and development. J Econ Perpect. 2002;16(4):185–205 (http://pubs.aeaweb.org/doi/pdfplus/10.1257/089533002320951037, accessed 22 October 2016).

33 Alderman H. Social assistance in Albania: decentralization and targeted tansfers. Washington (DC): World Bank; 1998 (Living Standards Measurement - Working Paper No. 134).

34 Bossert TJ, Beauvais JC. Decentralization of health systems in Ghana, Zambia, Uganda and the Philippines: a comparative analysis of decision space. Health Policy Plan. 2002;17(1):14–31.

35 Axelsson R, Marchildon GP, Repullo Labrador JR. Effects of decentralization on managerial dimensions of health systems. Saltman RB, Bankauskaite V, Vrangbæk K, editors. Decentralization in health care. Maidenhead: Open University Press; 2007:141–66 (European Observatory on Health Systems and Policy Series; http://www.euro.who.int/__data/assets/pdf_file/0004/98275/E89891.pdf, accessed 21 October 2016).

36 Jurberg C. Flawed but fair: Brazil's health system reaches out to the poor. Bull World Health Organ. 2008;86(4):248–9 (http://www.who.int/bulletin/volumes/86/4/08-030408/en/, accessed 22 October 2016).

37 Compare: Institutional structure [website] Washington (DC): Joint Learning Network for universal health care; 2016 (http://programs.jointlearningnetwork.org/programs/compare/structure/237, accessed 22 October 2016).

38 Health financing profile – Brazil.[online] Washington (DC): World Bank; 2014 (http://www-wds.worldbank.org/external/default/WDSContentServer/WDSP/IB/2014/05/29/000333037_20140529124205/Rendered/PDF/883440BRI0P1230l0final0January02014.pdf, accessed 22 October 2016).

39 Compare: Institutional structure [website] Washington (DC): Joint Learning Network for universal health care; 2016 (http://programs.jointlearningnetwork.org/programs/compare/structure/237, accessed 22 October 2016).

40 Mora M, Varsano R. Fiscal decentralization and subnational fiscal autonomy in Brazil: some facts of the nineties. Rio de Janeiro: Instituto de Pesquisa Econômica Aplicada; 2001 (Texto para discussão Nº 854; http://ipea.gov.br/agencia/images/stories/PDFs/TDs/td_0854.pdf, accessed 22 October 2016).

41 Pierantoni CR, Garcia ACP. Human resources for health and decentralization policy in the Brazilian health system. Hum Resour Health. 2011;9:12 (https://www.ncbi.nlm.nih.gov/pmc/articles/PMC3123266/, accessed 22 October 2016).

42 Compare: Institutional structure [website] Washington (DC): Joint Learning Network for universal health care; 2016 (http://programs.jointlearningnetwork.org/programs/compare/structure/237, accessed 22 October 2016).

43 Jha PC. Decentralization and Federalism in Brazil. The Indian Journal of Political Science. Jha PC. Decentralization and federalism in Brazil. The Indian Journal of Political Science. 2007;68(1):157–71 (http://www.jstor.org/stable/41858828, accessed 22 October 2016).

44 Compare: Institutional structure [website] Washington (DC): Joint Learning Network for universal health care; 2016 (http://programs.jointlearningnetwork.org/programs/compare/structure/237, accessed 22 October 2016).

45 Decentralization of Health Care in Brazil. Washington (DC): World Bank; 2003 (Report No. 24416-BR; http://documents.worldbank.org/curated/en/991401468741318246/Brazil-Decentralization-of-health-care-in-brazil, accessed 22 October 2016).

46 Jha PC. Decentralization and federalism in Brazil. The Indian Journal of Political Science. 2007;68(1):157–71 (http://www.jstor.org/stable/41858828, accessed 22 October 2016).

47 Mullins DR. Accountability and coordination in a decentralized context: institutional, fiscal and governance issues. Washington (DC): American University; 2004 (http://citeseerx.ist.psu.edu/viewdoc/download?doi=10.1.1.456.918&rep=rep1&type=pdf, accessed 22 October 2016).

48 Armingeon K, Linder W, Zohlnhöfer R. 2014 Switzerland report. Sustainable Governance Indicators. 2014 (http://www.sgi-network.org/docs/2014/country/SGI2014_Switzerland.pdf, accessed 22 October 2016).

49 De Pietro C, Camenzind P, Sturny I, Crivelli L, Edwards-Garavoglia S, SprangerA, et al. Switzerland: health system review. Health Syst Transit. 2015;17(4):1–288 (http://www.euro.who.int/__data/assets/pdf_file/0010/293689/Switzerland-HiT.pdf, accessed 22 October 2016).

50 Ibid.

51 Nannyonjo J, Okot N. Decentralization, local government capacity and efficiency of health service eelivery in Uganda. Journal of African Development. 2013;15(1):125–158 (http://www.jadafea.com/wp-content/uploads/2014/07/JAD_vol15_ch6.pdf, accessed 22 October 2016).

52 Decentralization of Health Care in Brazil. Washington (DC): World Bank; 2003 (Report No. 24416-BR; http://documents.worldbank.org/curated/en/991401468741318246/Brazil-Decentralization-of-health-care-in-brazil, accessed 22 October 2016).

53 Brazil: health systems and services profile: monitoring and analysis of health systems change/reform. Brasilia D.F.: Pan American Health Organization; 2008 (http://new.paho.org/hq/dmdocuments/2010/Health_System_Profile-Brazil_2008.pdf, accessed 22 October 2016).

54 Jha PC. Decentralization and federalism in Brazil. The Indian Journal of Political Science. 2007;68(1):157–71 (http://www.jstor.org/stable/41858828, accessed 22 October 2016).

55 Compare: Institutional structure [website] Washington (DC): Joint Learning Network for universal health care; 2016 (http://programs.jointlearningnetwork.org/programs/compare/structure/237, accessed 22 October 2016).

56 Bolsewicz Alderman K, Hipgrave D, Jimenez-Soto E. Public engagement in health priority setting in low- and middle-income countries: current trends and considerations for policy. PLoS Med. 2013;10(8):e1001495 (http://journals.plos.org/plosmedicine/article/asset?id=10.1371/journal.pmed.1001495.PDF, accessed 22 October 2016).

57 Kapiriri L, Norhein OF, Heggenougen K. Public participation in health planning and priority setting at the district level in Uganda. Health Policy Plan. 2003;18(2):205–13 (http://heapol.oxfordjournals.org/content/18/2/205.long, accessed 22 Octpber 2016).

58 Marchildon GP. Canada: Health System Review. Health Syst Transit. Copenhagen: WHO;2013 (http://www.euro.who.int/__data/assets/pdf_file/0011/181955/e96759.pdf, accessed 25 Jan 2016)

59 Framework for implementation: national health mission 2012–2017 New Delhi: Government of India Ministry of Health and Social Welfare (http://nrhm.gov.in/images/pdf/NHM/NHM_Framework_for_Implementation__08-01-2014_.pdf, accessed 22 October 2016).

60 Kilewo EG, Frumence G. Factors that hinder community participation in developing and implementing comprehensive council health plans in Manyoni District, Tanzania. Glob Health Action. 2015;8:26461 (https://www.ncbi.nlm.nih.gov/pmc/articles/PMC4452651/, accessed 22 October 2016).

61 Frumence G, Nyamhanga T, Mwangu M, Hurtig AK. Participation in health planning in a decentralised health system: experiences from facility governing committees in the Kongwa district of Tanzania. Glob Public Health. 2014;9(10):1125–38. doi:10.1080/17441692.2014.953563.

62 Kessy FL. Improving health services through community participation in health governance structures in Tanzania. Journal of Rural and Community Development. 2014:9(2);14–31 (journals.brandonu.ca/jrcd/article/download/826/179, accessed 22 October 2016).

63 Ethiopia Federal Ministry of Health. Health Sector Strategic Plan (HSDP-III) 2005/6-2009/10. Addis Ababa: Planning and Programming Department; 2005 (Ethiopia Federal Ministry of Health. Health Sector Strategic Plan (HSDP-III) 2005/6-2009/10, accessed 23 October 2016).

64 Federal Democratic Republic of Ethiopia Ministry of Health. Health Sector Development Programme IV: 2010/11–2014/15 Final draft. 2010 (http://phe-ethiopia.org/admin/uploads/attachment-721-HSDP%20IV%20Final%20Draft%2011Octoberr%202010.pdf, accessed 23 October 2016).

65 Savedoff WD, Grépin K. Health sector corruption in Ethiopia. In: Plummer J, editor. Diagnosing corruption in Ethiopia: perceptions, realities, and the way forward for key sectors. Washington (DC): World Bank; 2012:19–66 (https://openknowledge.worldbank.org/bitstream/handle/10986/13091/699430PUB0Publ067869B09780821395318.pdf?sequence=, accessed 23 October 2016).

66 Health care financing reform in Ethiopia: improving quality and equity. Washington (DC): USAID; 2012 (Health Systems 20/20; https://www.hfgproject.org/wp-content/uploads/2015/02/Ethiopia_Health_Care_Reform_Brief1.pdf, accessed 23 October 2016).

67 Monitoring, evaluation and review of national health strategies: a country-led platform for information and accountability. Geneva: World Health Organization; 2011 (http://www.who.int/healthinfo/country_monitoring_evaluation/1085_IER_131011_web.pdf?ua=1, accessed 23 October 2016).

68 Ibid.

69 Ibid.

70 See also: Hutchinson, PL, LaFond AK. Monitoring and evaluation of decentralization reforms in developing country health sectors. Bethesda (MD): The Partners for Health Reformplus Project, Abt Associates Inc.; 2004 (http://www.phrplus.org/Pubs/Tech054_fin.pdf, accessed 23 October 2016).

71 Hosseinpoor AR, Bergen N, Barros AJD, Wong KLM, Boerma T, Victora CG. Monitoring subnational regional inequalities in health: measurement approaches and challenges. Int J Equity Health. 2016;15(18) (https://equityhealthj.biomedcentral.com/articles/10.1186/s12939-016-0307-y, accessed 23 October 2016).

72 Communiqué on commitments to support One Monitoring and Evaluation Framework for Kenya. Kenya Ministry of Health; 2016 (http://www.healthdatacollaborative.org/fileadmin/uploads/hdc/Documents/Kenya_Final_One_ME_Communique.pdf, accessed 23 October 2016).

73 Mills A. Decentralization concepts and issues: a review. In: Mills A, Vaughan JP, Smith DL, Tabibzadeh I, editors. Health system decentralization concepts, issues and country experience. Geneva: World Health Organization; 1990 (http://apps.who.int/iris/bitstream/10665/39053/1/9241561378.pdf accessed 23 October 2016).

74 Controller and Auditor-General. New Zealand (www.oag.govt.nz, accessed 23 October 2016).

75 The New Zealand health and disability system: organisations and responsibilities: briefing to the Minister of Health. Wellington: New Zealand Ministry of Health; 2014 (https://www.health.govt.nz/system/files/documents/publications/new-zealand-health-and-disability-system-organisations-responsibilities-dec14-v2.pdf, accessed 23 October 2016).

76 Bardhan P. Decentralization of governance and development. Journal of Economic Perspectives. 2002;16(4):185–205 (https://www.aeaweb.org/articles?id=10.1257/089533002320951037, accessed 23 October 2016).

77 As an example, view: http://ec.europa.eu/health/index_en.htm, accessed 23 October 2016).

78 Jiménez D, Smith PC. Decentralisation of health care and its impact on health outcomes. Heslington (York): Centre for Health Economics, University of York; 2005: 1–51 (https://www.york.ac.uk/media/economics/documents/discussionpapers/2005/0510a.pdf, accessed 23 October 2016).

79 Alves J, Peralta S, Perelman J. Efficiency and equity consequences of decentralization in health: an economic perspective. Revista portuguesa de saúde pública. 2013;31(1):74–83.

80 Shukla A, Khanna R, Jadhav N. Using community-based evidence for decentralized health planning: insights from Maharashtra, India. Health Policy Plan. 2014; 1–12 (http://heapol.oxfordjournals.org/content/early/2014/09/21/heapol.czu099.full.pdf+html, accessed 22 October 2016).

81 Guanais FC, Macinko J. The health effects of decentralizing primary care In Brazil. Health Aff. 2009;28(4):1127–35. doi:10.1377/hlthaff.28.4.1127.

82 Nishtar S, Mehboob AB. Pakistan prepares to abolish Ministry of Health. Lancet (online) May 5, 2011 doi:10.1016/S0140-6736(11)60606-5.

83 Jinnah Institute. Devolution: provincial autonomy and the 18th amendment. Karachi: The Jinnah Institute 2014 (http://jinnah-institute.org/devolution-provincial-autonomy-and-the-18th-amendment/, accessed 23 October 2016).

84 Ibid.

85 Nishtar S. Drug regulation and beyond. The News International. 25 June 2011 (Heartfile Viewpoint No. 101; http://www.heartfile.org/pdf/101_DRUG_REGULATION_AND_BEYOND.pdf, accessed 23 October 2016).

86 Saltman RB, Vrangbæk, K. Drawing lessons for policy-making. In: Saltman RB, Bankauskaite V, Vrangbæk K, editors. Decentralization in health care. Maidenhead: Open University Press; 2007: pp. 77–84 (European Observatory on Health Systems and Policy Series; http://www.euro.who.int/__data/assets/pdf_file/0004/98275/E89891.pdf, accessed 21 October 2016).

Chapter 12

Intersectoral planning for health and health equity

Erik Blas

Nathalie Roebbel

Dheepa Rajan

Nicole Valentine

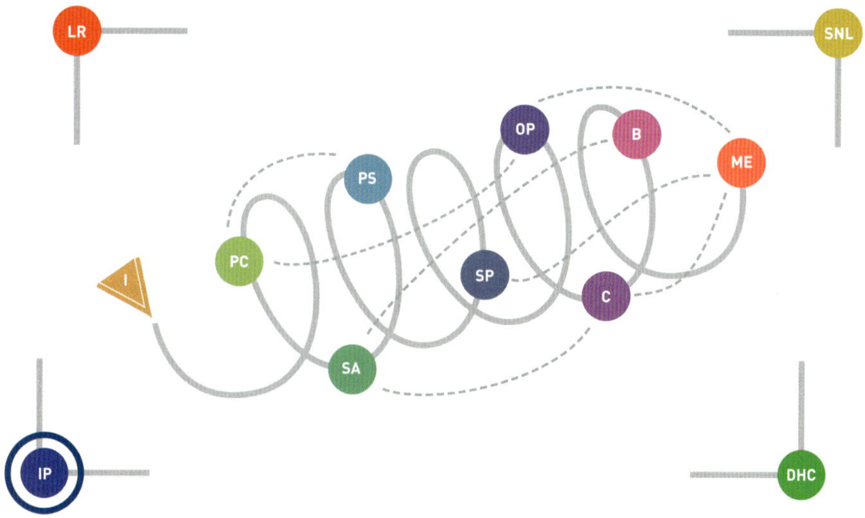

Cross-cutting topics relevant to national health planning

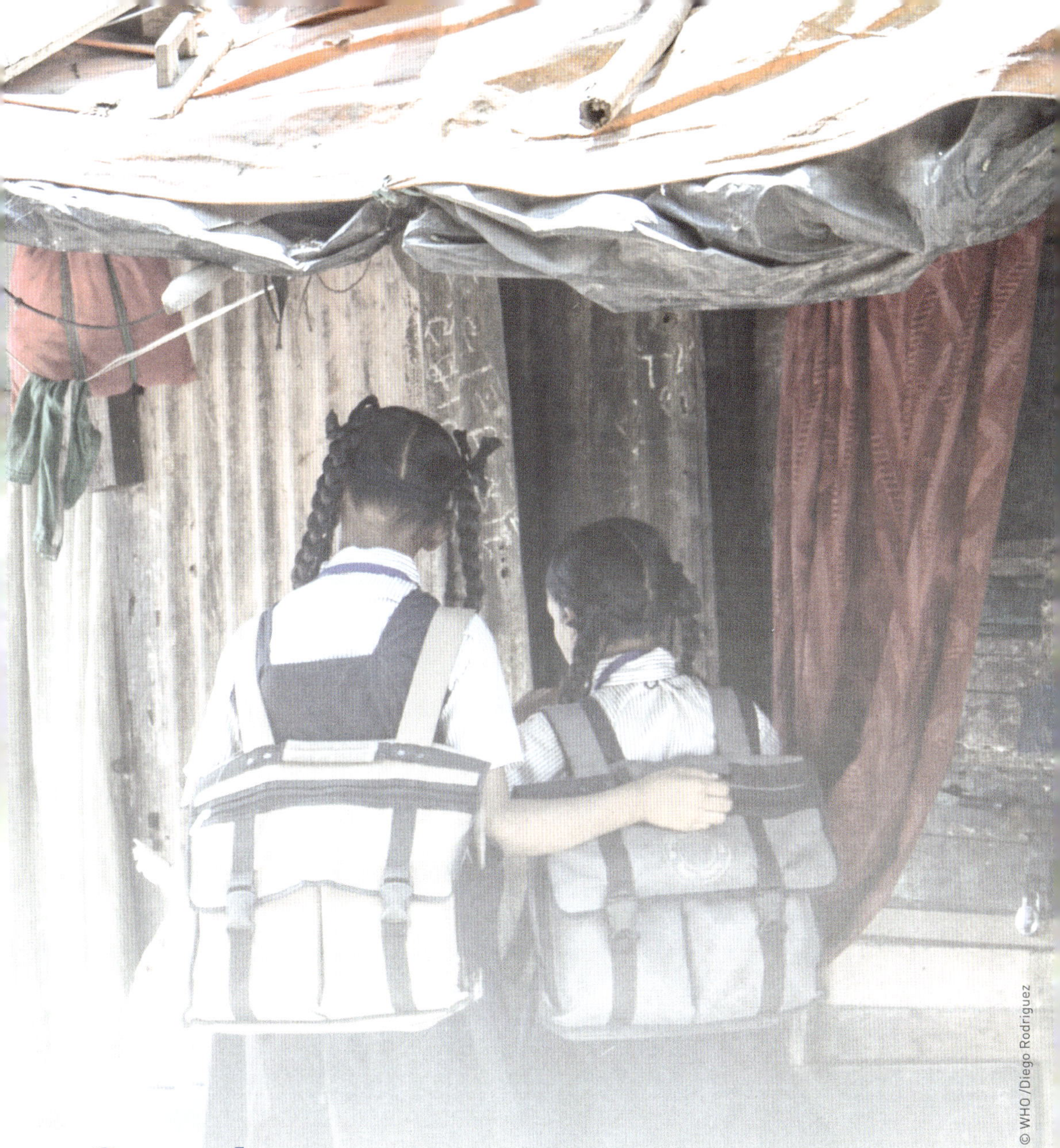

Overview

This chapter outlines the need and practical action for including intersectoral planning for health and health equity within the overall process of strategizing for health.

Summary

What is intersectoral planning for health and health equity?

Health equity is acknowledged as a critical component of the post-2015 sustainable development agenda, and is an essential element of any country's path towards universal health coverage (UHC). Intersectoral planning implies that governments and other stakeholders proactively address the determinants for health inequities by identifying and promoting intersectoral action as an integral and vital component of the national health planning process.

Why do we need intersectoral planning?

Intersectoral planning addresses determinants of health, alongside clinical services, in order to achieve greater sustainability of results through:

- determining and confronting risk factors of ill health in a concerted effort;
- increasing the level and equity in distribution of health within populations;
- supporting achievement of the SDGs.

When should we engage other sectors?

One should engage from the beginning of the national health planning process.

- However, intersectoral planning is not a linear process and thus several entry points exist.
- These different entry points find their correspondence in the approved SDGs.
- Intersectoral planning for health should be viewed as a multi-directional, continuous and constantly evolving process.

Who should be involved: roles and responsibilities ?

The health sector, and in particular the ministry of health, should lead and understand the different interests and roles of many other sectors.

- Partnerships with or sponsorships by levels of government that have responsibility across sectors (e.g. ministry of planning, prime minister's or president's office, etc.) should be sought.
- All sectors should be linked to the 17 SDGs.
- While all sectors can do something to improve the health situation, the mechanisms the different sectors have and their potential strength in influencing the top risk factors and the most important social determinants vary.

How should we plan for and implement intersectoral action?

Each country is different and needs to prepare and present its own case for intersectoral action on health inequities. It is important to:

- keep the target audience of non-health people in mind;
- find a common ground and build a common understanding between the health sector and all other relevant sectors;
- make good use of the situation analysis phase of the national health planning cycle;
- engage in policy dialogue and negotiation;
- link groups of indicators, including on social determinants, across dimensions of inequity and levels of results chains, as well as across different sectors.

12.1 What is intersectoral planning for health and health equity?

12.1.1 Health equity and social determinants of health – how do they relate to national health planning?

Health is a state of complete physical, mental and social well-being and not merely the absence of disease or infirmity. The enjoyment of the highest attainable standard of health is one of the fundamental rights of every human being without distinction of race, religion, political belief, economic or social condition.[1]

The above definition of health from the WHO Constitution indicates that some people might be deprived of their right to enjoy the highest attainable standard of health due to race, religion, political belief, economic or social condition, and that this is unjust. This definition inherently encompasses the concept of health equity by implying that the gold standard for health should be the same standard for all population groups, regardless of characteristics which are often the basis for discrimination or vulnerability – i.e. race, religion, political belief, economic or social condition. Indeed, despite major improvements in life expectancy and health outcomes globally, health inequities, i.e. differences in health status between more advantaged population groups and more disadvantaged population groups, therefore remain a significant – and in many cases growing – challenge. Indeed, even today, 70 years later, there are huge differences in health status across the world. For example, in Japan, life expectancy for women is 87 years but in Sierra Leone it is only 46 years. In Angola, out of 1000 children, 167 die before their fifth birthday; in Luxembourg it is only two.[2]

These health inequities – whether in relation to communicable diseases or noncommunicable diseases (NCDs), injuries, or resulting from new emerging risks like climate change – are rooted in the social determinants of health. The social determinants of health (SDHs) are the conditions in which people are born, grow, work, live and age, and the wider set of forces and systems shaping the conditions of daily life. These forces and systems include economic policies and systems, development agendas, social norms, social policies and political systems. The social and economic conditions, their effects on people's lives and the resulting differences in life expectancy and health status are also health inequities, because they are avoidable, unjust and unfair.[3]

Health inequities are rooted in the social determinants of health.

Health equity and SDH are acknowledged as critical components of the post-2015 sustainable development agenda, and are an essential element of any country's path towards universal health coverage (UHC). Intersectoral planning implies that governments and other stakeholders proactively address social determinants and health inequities by identifying and promoting intersectoral action as an integral and vital component of the national health planning process. In other words, reducing health inequities is pivotal to achieving the goal of UHC, one of the distinct strategic directions of many national health policies, strategies and plans (NHPSPs). Without intersectoral action as a fully integrated

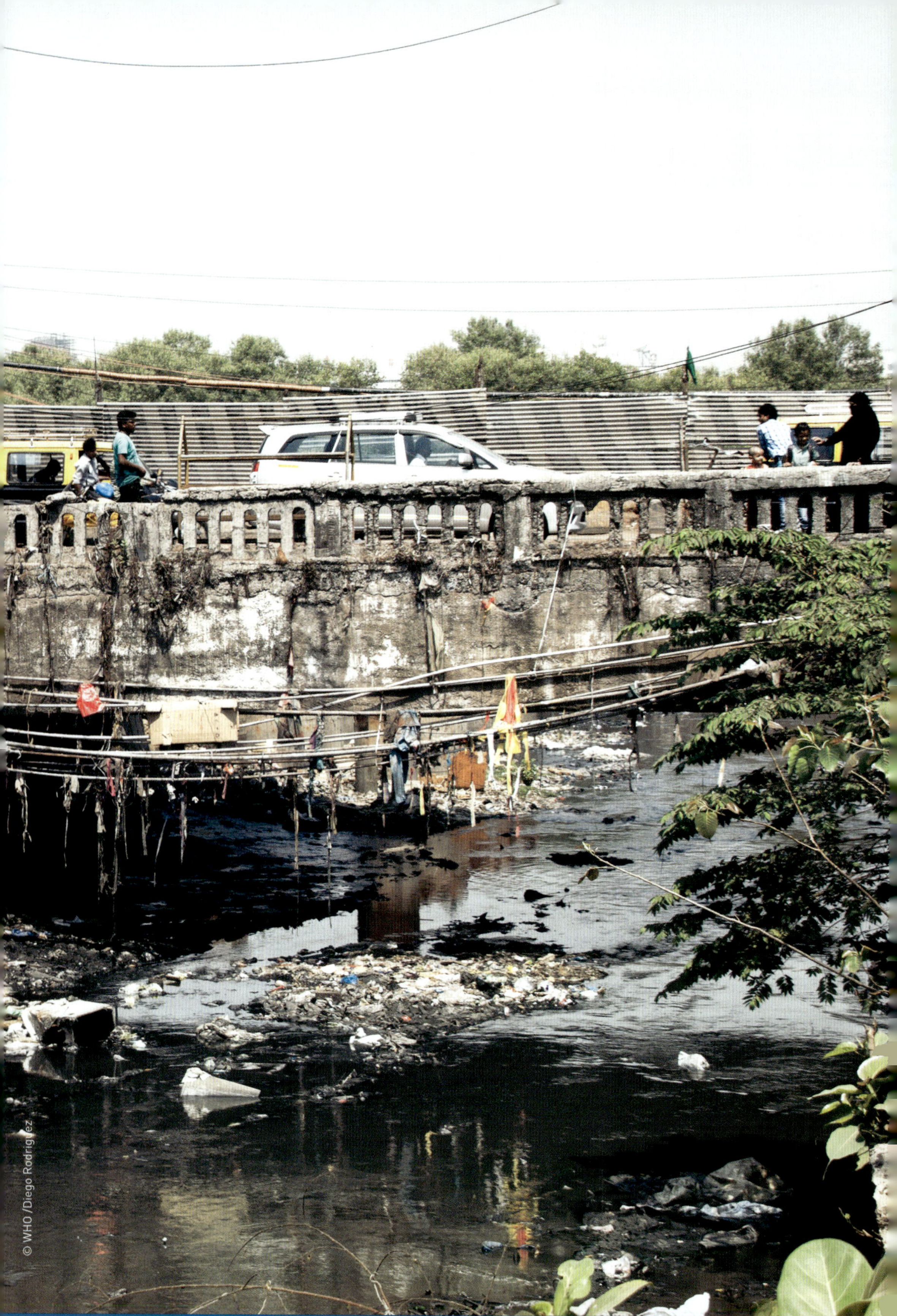

component – and indeed, mindset – embedded in the national health planning process, health inequities will likely persist, and as a result, the health of any nation's population will suffer.

In this regard, this chapter's objective is to describe the need and practical action for including intersectoral planning for health and health equity within the overall national health planning process. It discusses why and how to integrate other sectors into national health planning processes, with the objective of ensuring better health and health equity.

Box 12.1

Basic concepts[4]

What are health inequities or inequalities?
Health inequities are avoidable and unfair inequalities in health between groups of people within countries and between countries. These inequities arise from inequalities within and between societies. Social and economic conditions and their effects on people's lives determine their risk of illness and the actions taken to prevent them becoming ill or treating illness when it occurs.

What is meant by social gradient?
Within countries, the evidence shows that in general, the lower an individual's socioeconomic position, the worse is her or his health. There is a social gradient in health that runs from top to bottom of the socioeconomic spectrum. This is a global phenomenon, seen in low, middle and high income countries. The social gradient in health means that health inequities affect everyone.

What are the social "determinants" of health?
The social determinants of health are the circumstances in which people are born, grow up, live, work and age, and the systems shaping the conditions of life. These circumstances are in turn shaped by a wider set of forces: economics, social policies, and politics.

Intersectoral Action for Health:
"Coordination of health-related activities of the different sectors in order to achieve the highest attainable standard of health for every human being" according to the Alma Ata Declaration.

12.1.2 The Sustainable Development Goals (SDGs) – a marked accent on intersectorality

Since 1978 a number of different concepts, theories and frameworks have been designed and promoted to "achieve the highest attainable standard of health for every human being" through working across sectors. Examples include: Health for All,[5] Health Promotion,[6] Whole of government and whole of society,[7] Health in All Policies,[8] Human rights-based approaches,[9] Gender-based approaches,[10] and Social determinants approaches[11] to health. Each one of them has its own strengths and theoretical and ideological underpinning. However, all share a concern for health and health equity and require action by sectors other than health for their implementation – but, they also share the challenges of implementation.

Most major public health programmes have at one point or another considered intersectoral action in their global or regional strategies and some have produced multisectoral action frameworks. Just to mention a few: The global action plan for the prevention and control of noncommunicable diseases (2013–2020)[12] has multisectoral action as one of its overarching principles and has an appendix linking 21 different sectors to the main risk factors for NCDs. The UNAIDS 2016–2021 strategy On the fast-track to end AIDS has a whole section about HIV and the SDGs, calling for joint action and shared progress.[13] In 2013, the Roll Back Malaria partnership/United Nations Development Programme (UNDP) published a Multisectoral action framework for malaria;[14] and in 2014, the Reproductive, Maternal, Newborn and Child Health Programme published *A multisectoral policy compendium for RMNCH*.[15]

However, these examples all relate to individual public health programmes. Unfortunately, the past decades of global guidance on overarching national health planning have much less frequently included intersectoral action compared to programme-specific strategies (see Box 12.2). Only a very few countries have systematically and comprehensively integrated other sectors into their national health planning processes, e.g. Australia, Finland and New Zealand. This is quite remarkable as the collective work done by 16 public health programmes as part of the Commission on Social Determinants of Health found that most social determinants of health inequity are shared among the various public health conditions regardless of whether they are classified as communicable, maternal and neonatal, and nutritional disorders; noncommunicable diseases; or injuries.[16]

One explanation could be the perpetuation of the sectoral silo-thinking and fragmentation observed 30 years ago that include both health and other sectors (see Box 12.1). Managers and staff may want to stay within their familiar comfort zones. This might be due to budget allocation principles and accountability frameworks within governments that may not support multi-stakeholders and intersectoral collaboration. The single-sector focus of the Millennium Development Goals (MDGs) and donor financing mechanisms may also have contributed. However, the results are loss of opportunities for sustainably improving population health, and in the end higher health care costs and lower social and economic productivity in societies.

Box 12.2

Why is intersectoral planning missing in the planning process?[17]

"Recognizing the multisectoral character of health development, the Alma Ata Declaration called for the coordination of health-related activities of the different sectors...."

"There are several reasons why health strategies have not advanced far in this direction. Despite the new strategy for health, health planning has remained a more or less self-contained exercise within the health sector, carried out principally by health professionals, in relative isolation from other development processes. This isolation is reinforced by the tendency of most sectors to perceive health as comprising mainly medical services and their output. This pushes the health strategy back to a curative approach. In this context, other development sectors tend to regard intersectoral collaboration for health as a diversion of time and resources from their own sectoral priorities."

The Sustainable Development Goals (SDGs)[18] take a holistic multisectoral approach to development, compared to the selective single-sector approach of the MDGs. The SDGs differ from the MDGs in a number of ways. They are for all countries and are not just development assistance goals; they are concerned with equity, i.e. with specifying the need to disaggregate data and monitor achievement for different population groups, rather than just with average achievements; and they realize sustainable development can only be achieved by addressing all the goals at the same time – rather than selectively. By necessity, the achievements of the SDGs will require intersectoral action at global level, in each country, and within each country at sub-national levels. One extremely important way intersectoral action can take place at national level is through an intersectoral approach in the national health planning process, i.e. intersectoral planning, the subject of this chapter. The SDGs are thus a concern for all, whether national or local health planners or the international community.

By necessity, the achievements of the SDGs will require intersectoral action at global level, in each country, and within each country at sub-national levels.

12.1.3 Intersectoral planning made explicit: good examples from New Zealand and Norway

Some countries have already successfully integrated health equity and intersectoral action into their national health planning processes and documents and can be viewed as examples for health-specific strategies whose broad goals entail collaboration with other sectors.

There are examples of countries that to some extent have integrated health equity and intersectoral action into their national health planning processes and documents (see Boxes 12.5 and 12.7). Here, the New Zealand Health Strategy 2000 as well as the Norwegian Public Health Act of 2012 are highlighted, as they exemplify a health-specific strategy whose broad goals and specific objectives entail collaboration with or action by sectors other than health.

New Zealand is a country with three large ethnic population groups – Maori, Pacific and European – and a history of strong social welfare policy. A change of government in 1999 meant a shift in emphasis from a sole focus on economic growth as a measure of progress to achievement in social progress given equal weight. Comprehensive analyses were done as part of the strategic planning process for the Health Strategy 2000, e.g. on life expectancy by ethnicity and deprivation and on the distribution of risk factors such as tobacco smoking. The analyses showed huge inequities and the importance of tackling their root causes, i.e. the social determinants.[19]

The New Zealand Health Strategy 2000 thus set out the main aim to reduce the inequities between the three population groups and included tackling the broader determinant of health and reorienting health services. Some of the Strategy's 10 broad goals and 61 specific objectives require explicit intersectoral action. Other goals and objectives – such as improved access to health services, improved participation in health system decision-making and workforce by Maori and Pacific populations – were more directly within the remit of the health sector and its own institutions.

The roll-out of the Strategy was accompanied by an integration of social determinants of health and health inequity indicators into the social reports produced by the Ministry of Social Development. These social reports could follow medium- and long-term impact of policy initiatives and action, and thus have a potential to inform evaluation and design of public policy. However, one challenge highlighted by a study of the effectiveness of this approach was that government agencies concerned with economic development made negligible use of the reports. The study recommended anchoring the reports in the national legislation.[20]

By contrast, Norway's approach to a common framework for intersectoral monitoring was based on their Public Health Act of 2012,[21] which provided for a broad cross-government responsibility for health and health equity. It required much intersectoral work, between the launch of their Strategy to Reduce Social Inequalities in Health in 2007 and the development of the Public Health Act in 2012, to gain acceptance of this broader concept of health in the policy sphere.[22] The Public Health Act now forms the basis for reporting both on the status of public health and on the intersectoral public health policy work.

12.1.4 Intersectoral planning as the focus of this chapter

This chapter focuses on overarching national health and development planning rather than on health service and individual public health programme planning. Therefore, health inequities arising from differential access to and benefit from health services are, for example, only touched on very briefly. The chapter seeks to take a pragmatic rather than dogmatic approach. It realizes that there is no hard and fast blueprint for intersectoral action and health equity that will guarantee success. However, there are strong rationales and there are examples to be drawn on and inspired by.

There is no hard and fast blueprint for intersectoral action that guarantees success; this chapter, however, offers strong rationales for certain planning practices that can be used in different contexts.

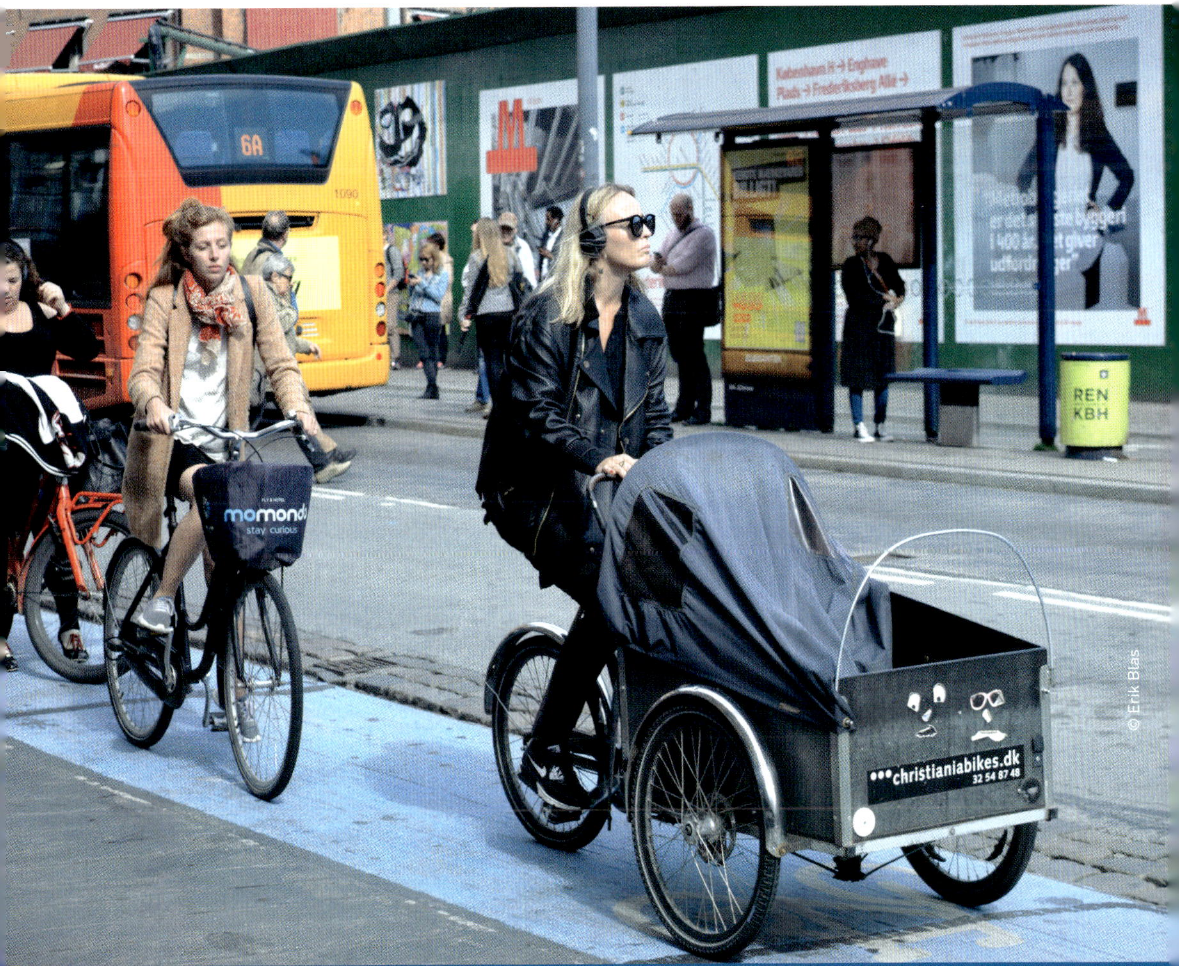

© Erik Blas

12.2 Why do we need intersectoral planning?

Endemic malaria has disappeared from most of North America and northern Europe with general social and economic development, including better housing, land drainage, less-crowded housing, closed windows and a reduced tendency for people to live close to their live-stock, and not as a result of direct vector or chemo-prophylactic control. However, while the time immediately after the First World War saw malaria epidemics spreading across Europe, these epidemics subsided or responded easily to control interventions, suggesting that strong health systems (i.e. for delivery of medications) and the improvement in overall socioeconomic conditions rather than changing the vector ecology were responsible for alleviating the problem. Transient resurgence of malaria in connection with war, population movements and associated disruptions has been seen in several places – including: Armenia, Azerbaijan, Italy, Spain, and Tajikistan – with a rapid return to the earlier situation once the societies recover. In contrast, when malaria control does not take into account broader development issues and is based solely on direct vector control and chemotherapy through local or global campaigns, resurgence with added virulence is often observed once the campaign measures are relaxed.[23]

Socioeconomic development and health systems development are mutually reinforcing; addressing determinants of health alongside clinical services leads to greater sustainability of results.

Another such example comes from the history of tuberculosis (TB) in Europe. TB death rates in Europe increased in the 17th and 18th centuries with industrialization and urbanization, when a rise in population density led to crowded living conditions and poor nutrition, contributing to the progression of the disease. With the subsequent economic growth, social reform, a gradual decline in the level of poverty and improved living conditions, the TB incidence had already declined about eight- to tenfold by the 1940s when chemotherapy first became available. Some have suggested that the decline until the end of the 1940s was almost exclusively due to improved nutritional status and living conditions. Others have argued that public health interventions such as isolation of infectious individuals and the pasteurization of milk to prevent bovine tuberculosis have also contributed to the decline. However, it seems clear that, on the one hand, the highest TB rates have been recorded in places where rapid urbanization was coupled with very poor living conditions for the disadvantaged. On the other hand, the most rapid declines in TB incidence and deaths have been recorded where economic growth was coupled with social and health sector reform and important medical advances.[24]

Both examples further suggest that there are strong links between general development and health development. They show that socioeconomic development and health systems development are mutually reinforcing and increase the chances for sustainable achievements. In other words, addressing the determinants of health (which intrinsically involves collaboration between sectors) concomitantly to addressing clinical services leads to sustainable results.

12.2.1 Burden of disease

There has been a remarkable reduction in the global burden of communicable diseases, maternal and neonatal conditions, and nutritional disorders from 1.18 billion disability-adjusted life-years (DALYs) in 1990 to 0.87 billion in 2010, i.e. a reduction of 26.6% (Fig. 12.1).[25] This success may be explained by a combination of factors. These include general poverty reduction; improved access to education, in particular for girls; improved access to clean water and sanitation; and improved access to selected health services. All these factors were specifically emphasized in the Millennium Development Goals and the action spheres of different sectors.

However, Fig. 12.1. also shows that the overall global burden of disease remained constant at about 2.5 billion DALYs over the two decades, i.e. the gains in communicable, maternal, neonatal and nutritional disorders were outweighed by increases in noncommunicable diseases (NCDs) and injuries. The NCDs increased by 25.3%, i.e. from 1.08 billion DALYs in 1990 to 1.34 billion in 2010; and injuries increased by 0.03 billion in the same period. Some of this increase might be explained by people living longer (life-expectancy at birth in 1990 was 64 years and in 2013 it was 71 years[26]). However, changes in lifestyles and exposures may also have contributed to the increase.

If nothing is done to halt the epidemic of NCDs, it is very likely that the overall global burden of disease in 2030 will be higher than it was in 1990. Halting the epidemic of noncommunicable diseases requires effectively addressing their risk factors and determinants. This can only be done through the health sector and a range of other sectors working together in a concerted effort, i.e. through comprehensive intersectoral NHPSP.

Fig. 12.1 The Global Burden of Disease (1990-2010)

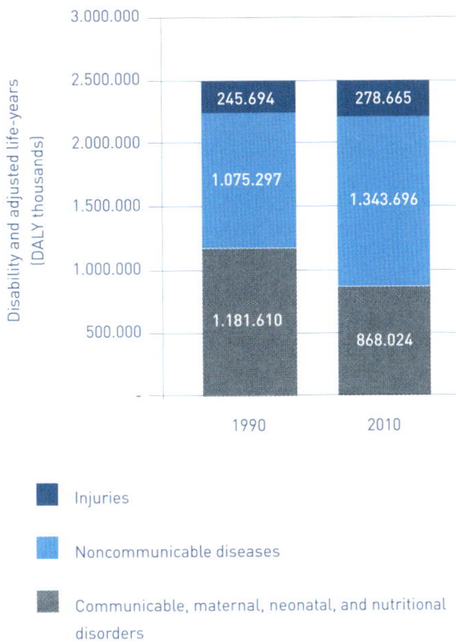

Halting the epidemic of noncommunicable diseases requires effectively addressing their risk factors and determinants – which in turn requires health and a range of other sectors to work together.

12.2.2 Social determinants

The overall global burden of disease numbers (Fig. 12.1) mask considerable differences across countries. Within countries, a disaggregation of national averages, e.g. by geographical location, wealth, ethnicity and sex, will almost always reveal considerable health inequities, as is the case in Suriname (Fig. 12.2).

Chronic kidney disease in Suriname is more than 2.5 times more prevalent in Saramacca district compared to Coronie district and diabetes II is about three times more prevalent among the poorest wealth quintiles compared to the richest. The HIV prevalence is much higher among the Creole and Maroon ethnic groups

Fig. 12.2 Examples of health inequities in Suriname[27]

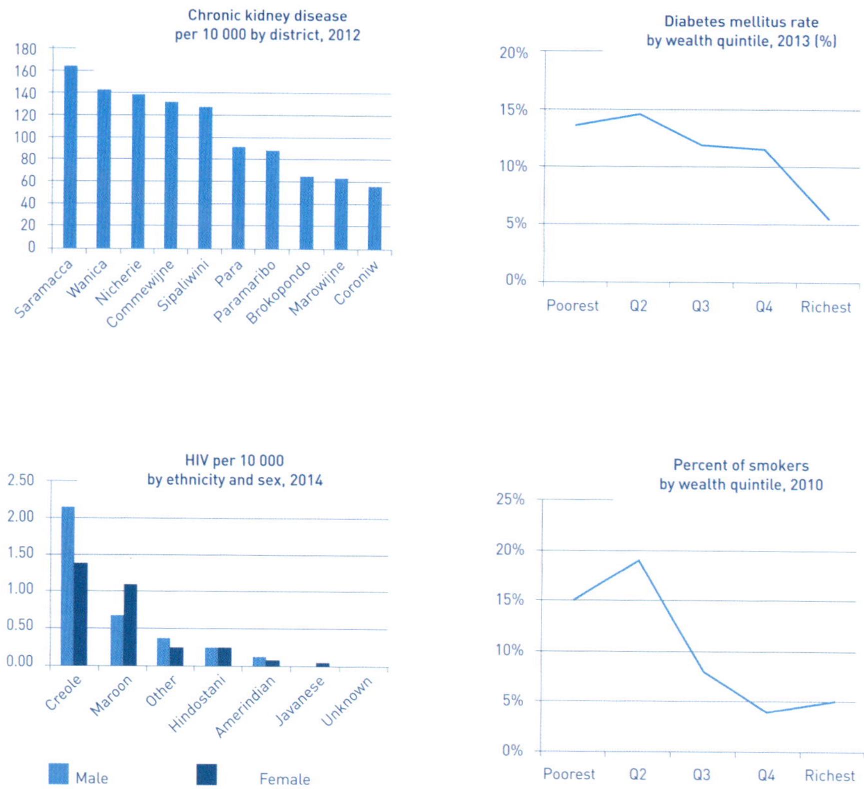

compared to other ethnic groups. However, it is interesting to note that the prevalence among Creole women is lower than among males, while for Maroons it is the other way round. Finally, smoking prevalence among the two poorest wealth quintiles was found to be three to four times higher than in the richest quintile. While the poorer wealth quintiles were found always to have higher disease and risk factor prevalence than the richer quintiles, the districts and ethnic groups that had the highest prevalence varied across diseases, conditions and risk factors. This raises the important question of what shapes the population health profile in a given society.

The effect that clinical care has on the health of populations is far smaller than commonly thought. A study across communities in the United States of America showed that access to and quality of clinical care explained only 20% of premature deaths in communities. Other factors together accounted for the other 80%, i.e. social and economic factors 40%; health behaviours 30%; and the physical environment 10% (Fig. 12.3).[28] However, both the health behaviours and the physical environment are in turn also shaped by social and economic factors. This means that about 80% of a population's health may be shaped by the circumstances in which people are born, grow, live, work and age, in other words, the social determinants of health.

Fig. 12.3 Factors affecting populations' health in the USA

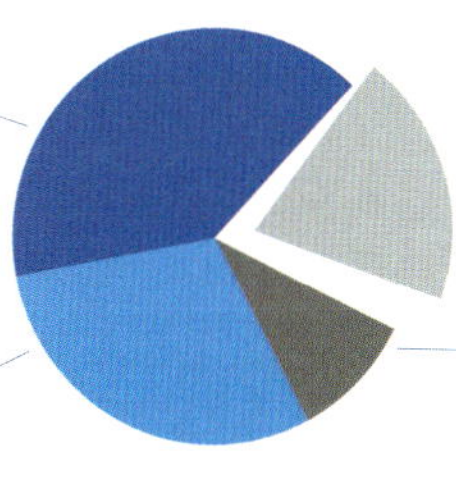

Equitable access to cost-effective quality clinical care should remain a fundamental right for all. However, effectively and sustainably improving the level and distribution of populations' health will require action across multiple sectors to address key risk factors related to exposures and behaviours, such as dietary risks; child and maternal malnutrition; tobacco use; air pollution; alcohol and drug use; unsafe water, sanitation and handwashing; unsafe sex; occupational risks; low physical activity; sexual abuse and violence; and other environmental risks of the global burden of disease.[29] It will further require action on those social determinants that create differential exposure and vulnerability across population groups and that are often grounded in societal context and in social, political and economic position.[30] The SDGs call for comprehensive action on these determinants and risk factors, by emphasizing equity across all goals and through the specific goal dedicated to equity (SDG 10), which underlines the dire need for data disaggregation (by income, gender, age, race, ethnicity, migratory status, disability, geographic location and other characteristics relevant in national contexts).[31]

80% of a population's health may be shaped by the circumstances in which people are born, grow, live, work and age, in other words, the social determinants of health.

Likewise, national health policies, strategies and plans thus need to be based on a thorough analysis of disaggregated data, and should put a distinct emphasis on and ensuring that the factors shaping population health are addressed. Ignoring these factors will mean that overall health status can only be marginally improved, at best. Addressing the social determinants of health means intersectoral action, and this approach must be embedded in the national health planning process.

Box 12.3

Early child development in Viet Nam – why improved intersectoral planning is sorely needed

Maternal education has long been considered an important determinant for maternal and child health status in many countries, including Viet Nam.[32] In Viet Nam's rural areas only 22.8% of mothers of children aged 0–8 years have completed secondary education, compared to 53.9% in urban areas. Health care seeking behaviour as well as utilization rates in Viet Nam are causally linked to educational levels.[33] Some suggest that this is due to limited knowledge of certain key childhood symptoms and the resulting health-seeking delays and a higher risk of adverse outcomes.

In the poorest Vietnamese income quintile, secondary school completion rate is 8.1%; it is 73.7% among the richest. Among the majority ethnic group of Viet Nam (Kinh population), the completion rate is 34.4%, but only 13.6% for ethnic minorities. 58.9% of children in the poorest quintile aged 36–59 months enjoy early childhood education, while for the richest it is 90.6%.[34] What a child experiences before eight years of age sets a critical foundation for her or his entire life, and there is a strong association between child survival and child development. The physical, social, emotional and language domains strongly influence basic learning, school success, economic participation, social citizenship, and health.[35]

These inequalities are part of a vicious circle of intergenerational inequity that can only be broken by appropriate action. This action must inherently be intersectoral in nature because it is at the intersections between education, local government, social welfare and health. Intersectoral action must be carefully planned for and embedded into NHPSPs. When intersectoral action is one-off and effectively isolated, it is unsustainable. Ensuring that intersectorality is an integral component of NHPSPs assures the longer-term collaboration necessary to bring about the kind of change needed in Viet Nam.

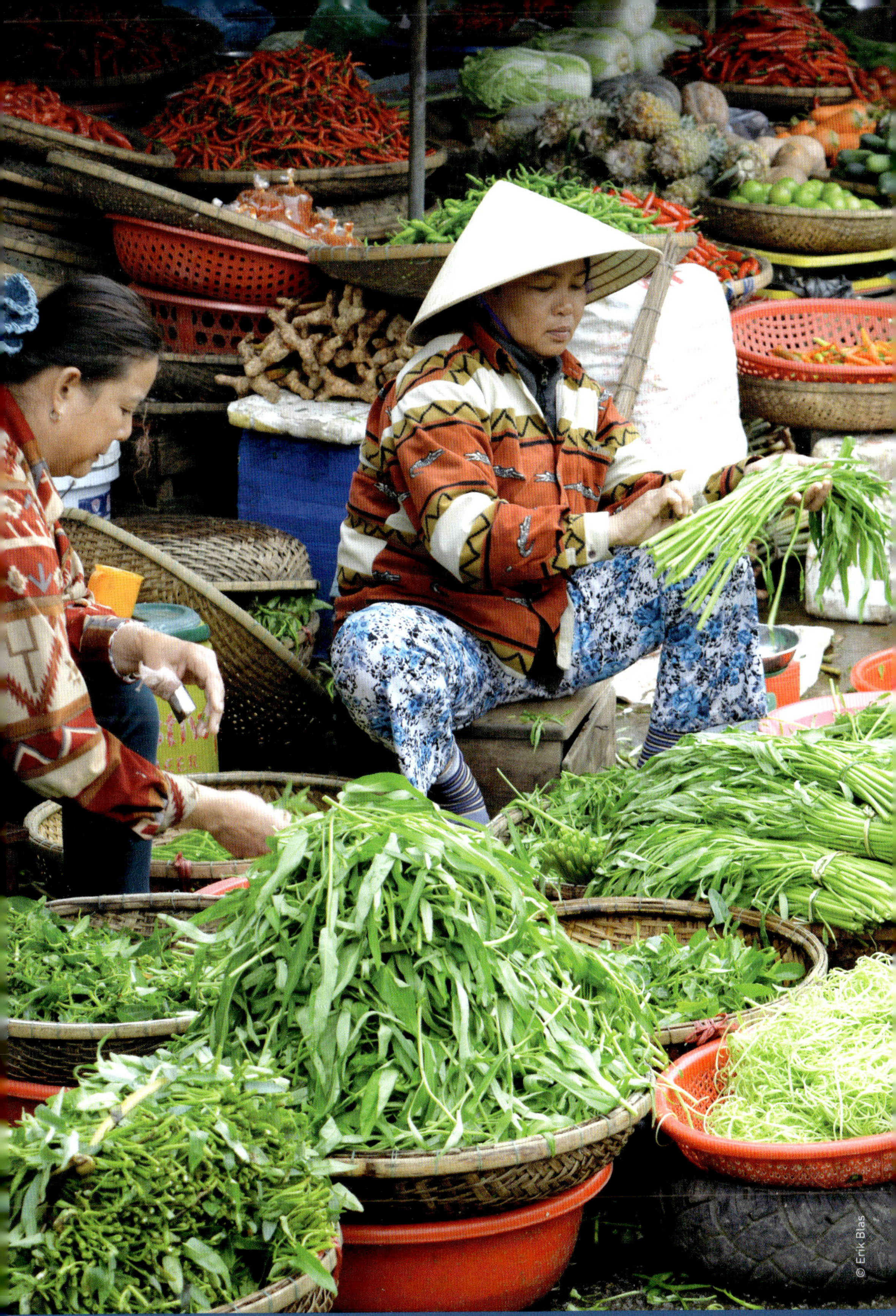

12.3 When should we engage other sectors?

Especially the situation analysis phase is an immense opportunity to ensure that the right questions regarding equity and the determinants of health are raised, and that those key issues are adequately assessed.

The short answer to the questionabove is "from the beginning". However, intersectoral planning, as part of the national health planning process, is not a linear process and thus several entry points exist, e.g. see Box 12.4. The situation analysis phase in particular is an immense opportunity to ensure that the right questions regarding equity and the determinants of health are raised, and that those key issues are adequately assessed. Actions may be undertaken all along the planning cycle; however, without the principal matters coming to the forefront during the situation analysis phase, these actions will not be slated in.

Box 12.4 summarizes eight entry-points for addressing health inequity and intersectoral collaboration in national health planning. For some of them, the health sector is both the leader and the implementer; for others, the health sector emphasis is on providing leadership; while for others again, the health sector may act primarily as a catalyst. These different entry points for tackling health inequalities find their correspondence in the approved SDGs, where health goes beyond Goal 3 (see Annex 12.1). Nearly all SDGs play a key role for health. Each entry point is briefly described with reference to three key SDGs in brackets. Please note that several of the analyses mentioned as entry points can be carried out during the situation analysis stage of the health policy and planning cycle.

Only the strongest links with other SDGs are indicated in Box 12. 4 – there are, of course, many more links of varying strengths (see Annex 12.1). Often the strength of a link between an entry point and an SDG will depend on national and local contexts. The many pieces of the analysis and action may in the end appear in different sectors' strategies and work plans. However, all the important ones should be mentioned in the NHPSP with reference to the sector and sectoral plan where the responsibility lies. All need to come together in a monitoring and accountability framework of the NHPSP as well as for the SDGs overall. In the following sections the specifics of the analysis, planning and monitoring will be elaborated.

Box 12.4

Eight potential entry points for reaching and sustaining greater health equity[36]

1. **Analysis of evidence on inequities and their causes.** Examine health data disaggregated as relevant to the country; review studies (including qualitative studies) conducted in subpopulations; explore the causes of inequity that require intersectoral action; and review reports by human rights bodies (SDG 5, SDG 10, and SDG 17).

2. **Analysis of and action on laws, policies, standards, protocols and guidelines.** Consider how equity, human rights, gender and social determinants are affected by the existing policy, legal, normative, programmatic and monitoring and evaluation frameworks, and how these issues could be addressed (SDG 5, SDG 10, and SDG 16).

3. **Analysis of and action on the causes of differentials** (social determinants at play) to identify the most relevant, including those that influence:

   - differential exposure to the physical environment, e.g. adverse workplaces and community settings, poor infrastructures, unhealthy and harmful consumables, etc. (SDG 6, SDG 8, and SDG 11);
   - differential exposure to the social environment, e.g. social norms that can undermine health, gender expectations and repression, ethnic and racial discrimination, unregulated marketing, etc. (SDG 5, SDG 10, and SDG 16);
   - differential community and individual vulnerability, e.g. poverty and unemployment, family and community dysfunction, poor knowledge, low levels of health literacy and care-seeking, alcohol abuse, food insecurity and malnutrition, etc. (SDG 1, SDG 2, and SDG 4);
   - differential access to health products and services, e.g. skewed availability, financial barriers, products and services with poor acceptability, etc. (SDG 1, SDG 10, and SDG 16);
   - differential benefit from health services, e.g. poor quality health services, discriminatory treatment and care, biased referral systems, services insensitive to needs, limited patient–provider interaction, poor adherence to advice and recommended treatments, etc. (SDG 5, SDG 10, and SDG 16); and
   - differential consequences of illness and disability, e.g. loss of income, impoverishment/catastrophic health expenditure, stigmatization or other forms of discrimination (SDG 1, SDG 10, and SDG 16).

4. **Analysis and allocation of resources.** It is not just a matter of the absolute level of resources – but also how they are distributed within societies and put to use. Skewed distribution of attention, resources and efforts in countries might prioritize outputs that increase rather than decrease inequity (SDG 1, SDG 10, and SDG 16).

5. **Analysis, strategies and actions to specifically address gender issues.** Gender-responsiveness should be promoted in all processes and in organizations and services (SDG 4, SDG 5, and SDG 16).

6. **Analysis and provision of means for civil society and individuals to participate in decision-making.** The right to health is best protected when individuals and concerned populations, including those marginalized or otherwise disadvantaged, are actively involved in decision-making on policy, health planning, and their individual health (SDG 4, SDG 10, and SDG 16).

7. **Transparency, accountability and keeping sectoral managers and services to task** are essential for reducing health inequities, together with safe mechanisms for reporting and addressing complaints whenever rights to health are threatened or violated, individually or collectively (SDG 5, SDG 10, and SDG 16).

8. **Ensuring gender balance and equity in organizational processes** through ensuring sex parity, appropriate gender representation, and inclusion of concerned population groups among staff, management and board members (SDG 5, SDG 10, and SDG 16).

12.4 Who should be involved: roles and responsibilities

Different sectors, and often also different health programmes, may have different planning cycles. Furthermore, in some countries, there may be an overall national development plan, again with its own cycle. The health sector's proactive coordination with all of them is paramount.

Intersectoral planning for health should be viewed as a multi-directional, continuous and constantly evolving process. It will be important to keep track of the different planning and monitoring cycles because they provide windows of opportunity to get health into the relevant sectors' plans and monitoring frameworks. From the perspective of the health sector, intersectoral planning means being engaged with other sectors on a regular basis, and being on the alert for crucial windows of opportunity where health needs to be part of the dialogue.

Opportunities that should not be missed for leading the engagement of other sectors are the preparation of the national development plan and the national health plan. This implies bringing in other sectors throughout the health planning process and bringing health into the other sectors' planning processes from the situation analysis, and priority-setting phases, for example.

A key role of the health sector and in particular the ministry of health is to lead and understand the different interests and roles of many other sectors actually or potentially influencing the risk factors and social determinants of health, and to facilitate the process (see e.g. the case of Estonia in Box 12.5). This requires technical capacity and knowledge as well as leadership considerably beyond the clinical aspects of health.[37] If this is not adequately available, consultants may be used and the capacity built during the process. The ministry of health will not be able to carry the responsibility alone. Partnerships with or sponsorships by levels of government that have responsibility across sectors (e.g. ministry of planning, prime minister's or president's office, etc.) will have to be sought. However, the health sector has to take the initiative for leading the process, and keeping it in motion and on track. Special attention should be given to ensuring it is based on facts and consensus, and to prevent it from being sidetracked by political agendas or particular interest groups.

Box 12.5

The National Health Plan 2009–2020, Estonia[38] links with a large number of strategies and development plans across different sectors

Ministry of Social Affairs

- Primary healthcare development plan (in preparation)
- Estonian Hospital Master Plan 2002
- Nursing Care Network Development Plan 2004–2015
- Strategy to Guarantee the Rights of the Child
- Development Plan for Prevention of Family Violence (in preparation)
- National Cancer Strategy 2007–2015
- National HIV and AIDS Strategy 2006–2015
- National Drug Addition Prevention Strategy until 2012
- National Tuberculosis Control Strategy 2008–2012
- National Strategy for Prevention of Cardiovascular Diseases 2005–2020
- Development Plan for Infertility Treatment 2007–2010

State Chancellery

- Estonia's European Union Policy 2007–2011
- Government Programme 2007–2011
- Ministry of Finance
- National Strategy Reference Framework 2007–2013

Office of the Minister Urve Palo

- Estonian Integration Programme 2008–2013

Ministry of Environment

- Estonian National Strategy on Sustainable Development 'Sustainable Estonia 21'
- Estonian Environmental Strategy until 2030
- National Radiation Safety Development Plan 2008–2017

Ministry of Culture

- Strategic Development Sports for All Programme 2006–2010

Ministry of the Interior

- Development Plan for Civic Initiative Support 2007–2010
- Regional Development Strategy of Estonia 2005–2015
- National Spatial Plan 'Estonia 2010'
- Internal Security Development Plan 2009–2013 (in preparation)

Ministry of Education and Research

- Youth Work Strategy 2006–2013
- General Education System Development Plan 2007–2013
- Bullying Prevention Programme 'Safe School' (in preparation)

Ministry of Agriculture

- Estonian Rural Development Strategy 2007–2013
- Development Plan for the Government Area of the Ministry of Agriculture 2009–2012

Ministry of Justice

- Development Plan for Reduction of Juvenile Delinquency 2007–2009
- Development Plan for Combatting Trafficking in Human Beings 2006–2009

Ministry of Economic Affairs and Communication

- Estonian Housing Development Plan 2008–2013
- Transport Development Plan 2006-2013
- Estonian National Traffic Safety Programme 2003–2015
- Estonian Information Society Strategy and Implementation Plan

To make a positive impact on a risk factor or social determinant of health, it is important first to map and understand who else shares a common interest in health and who is opposed to changes.

A first indication of which sectors to involve can be made based on Box 12.4 and the Annex that links the eight entry points to the 17 SDGs. While all sectors can do something to improve the health situation, the mechanisms the different sectors have and their potential strength in influencing the top risk factors and the most important social determinants vary. Furthermore, the interest of the different sectors to act may also vary. The interests may be categorized into:

Shared – this is the case where a sector shares the primary interest of health to make a positive change to a risk factor or a social determinant. For example, the education sector would likely share the interest to contribute making a dent on "clustering of disadvantages". This is because higher enrolment, lower drop-out and higher completion rates would be among the education sector's success criteria.

Different – in this case, the sector's interest will be different from health's interest without necessarily being opposed. For example, the primary interest of "urban planning and transport" might be to get the motorized road traffic flowing rather than providing easy, safe and preferred access to physical activity, including walking and cycling.

Opposed – there are, however, also cases where the interests of the other sector is directly opposed to the interest of health. For example, parts of trade and industry and others may be opposed to reducing marketing and access to tobacco and alcohol products, with a claim that it will directly affect their bottom line.

It is important to map who shares the primary interest of health in making a positive impact on a risk factor or a social determinant, who has a different interest and who is directly opposed to making changes. The reason is, of course, that it can have a major effect on the process and whether a particular component of the plan will be successfully implemented.

When interests are shared, the other sector would not need incentive or much negotiation to be convinced for action. However, when the interests are different, the sector in question might need some push and explanation of the health benefits to include relevant action. The primary focus should be on where there are potentially strong influences on the risk factor or the social determinant.

Special attention must be given to situations where a sector has opposing interests but exercises a potentially strong influence on a particular risk factor or social determinant. For the same risk factor or determinant, there might be other sectors with potentially very strong or medium-strong influence that share the interest with health or have different but not opposing interests. Forces can be joined with these, e.g. to change legislation and regulations or to strengthen enforcement of the same.

Table 12.1 briefly describes the roles and responsibilities of the ministry of health and other sectors and actors during three phases of planning and managing intersectoral action: analysis, negotiate and plan, and monitor and hold accountable. Details of these phases are provided in section 5.

Table 12.1 Roles and responsibilities

PHASE	MINISTRY OF HEALTH	OTHER SECTORS AND ACTORS
Analyse (see subsection 5.1)	▸ **Manage the process of knowledge gathering** – commission or take direct charge of getting all available knowledge together in a format conducive to decision-making ▸ **Lead analysis and consensus building** – involve the key stakeholders, experts and opinion leaders to have a common understanding of the causes of the burden of disease and the health inequity situation in the country ▸ **Inform and publicize** – to generate and nurture an evidence-based public debate and demand for action; ▸ **Identify knowledge gaps** – to encourage and direct future data collection and research	▸ **Prime minister's office, national planning, etc.:** sponsor, bring intersectoral action for health and health equity on cabinet agenda and into national development analysis ▸ **Researchers, bureau of statistics, information units of sectors, and civil society organizations:** provide data and participate in analysis ▸ **Politicians, opinion-makers, and media:** participate in consensus and dissemination process
Negotiate and plan (see subsection 5.2)	▸ **Set priorities for policy planning, design and implementation** – this may include bringing together all the parties and stakeholders in a consensus process ▸ **Identify and handle possible conflicts of interest and controversies** – this may include brokering and negotiating, proposing compromises, or mobilizing pressure for political or legislative decision ▸ **Train trainers** – to integrate health and health equity concerns into ongoing training programmes for different sectors and cadres ▸ **Move the political process** – bringing together the power of knowledge and evidence, the social power of civil society and the state power through accountable political leadership; and moving health higher on the political agenda ▸ **Appropriately link the national health plan with the plans of the relevant sectors** – to negotiate inclusion of relevant action into the plans of other sectors in formats that can be monitored across sectors	▸ **Prime minister's office, national planning, etc.:** sponsor, keep intersectoral action for health equity on cabinet agenda, and demand progress ▸ **Sectors, including civil society organizations:** participate in process, commit to action and results within their domains, and include in their own plans
Monitor and hold accountable (see subsection 5.3)	▸ Keep track of **activities in other sectors** that have bearing on health, including the policies and policy-results ▸ **Improve own data sources** with respect to completeness and possibility for disaggregation ▸ **Encourage, guide and support other data sources** to produce relevant disaggregated data, linking health with social determinants and risk factors ▸ **Analyse, disseminate and present information** in formats that are conducive to informing managerial action and political and public debates	▸ **Prime minister's office, national planning, etc.:** sponsor, keep sectors accountable for commitments and report to cabinet ▸ **Sectors, including civil society organizations:** report on committed actions and results, participate in reviewing progress, and commit to continued action and results within their domains ▸ **Politicians, opinion-makers, and media:** participate in evaluation, consensus and dissemination process

A question that sometimes comes up in connection with intersectoral planning is who pays for it. In the case of shared interest, it should obviously be the individual sector from its normal budget allocations. However, when the interests are different (non-opposing) it might impact on budgets, as sectors might have to do certain things additionally or differently in order to have a positive effect on health and health equity. This could mean that there has to be internal reallocation of budgets or that additional budget allocation will be required. However, as sectors will not be asked to do activities that do not fall within their mandates, implementation should be covered from within the sectoral budget – even if the ministry of finance will have to allocate additional resources, which could be generated, e.g. from public health taxes. Sectors that have opposing interests might be "brought to pay" in form of public health taxes, e.g. on tobacco, alcohol, unhealthy food, etc.[39] One activity that might be relevant to cover from the health sector budget would be capacity-building programmes for integrating health considerations into other key sectors' ongoing training programmes.

12.5 How should we plan for and implement intersectoral action?

Each country is different and needs to prepare and present its own case for intersectoral action on health inequities, based on its own data and analyses of the risk factors and social determinants that are causing the situation, in order to mobilize political attention and intersectoral commitment. When presenting the case, it is important to keep the target audience of non-health people in mind. They need to be able first to understand the message, second to see how the message is relevant to them, and third to be convinced why they should engage. There is the need to find a common ground and to build a common understanding between the health sector and all other relevant sectors.

A wide range of options and tools[40] exists for presenting data in tables and graphs in different formats (see, e.g. Fig. 12.2). It is important to link groups of indicators, including on social determinants, across dimensions of inequity and levels of results chains, as well as across different sectors. Tabular and graphic presentations frequently fall short; or might not be wholly understood by target audiences. It might therefore be useful to supplement tabular and graphic presentations by "telling the story", e.g. in short narratives specifically formulated with the relevant target audience in mind. In the Viet Nam case (Box 12.3), at least three sectors contribute directly to breaking the vicious circle of intergenerational inequity, i.e. education, local governments, and social welfare – while the underlying unfair distribution of resources is on the shoulders of finance, politicians and civil society. Other sectors, including the economic sectors, can recognize an interest in the results of action and indicator improvement – i.e. increased social and economic participation and reduced demand for health care.

Planning and implementing intersectoral action is unique for each country; planning must be based on its own data, analyses of the risk factors, and social determinants causing health inequities.

A parallel more comprehensive and more technical option is to pull all relevant information on each major disease in the country – prevalence, distribution across locations and population groups, and possible causes of the pattern – and present it in master sheets, one for each disease.[41] This option has the advantage of highlighting the causes of the diseases as well as identifying key knowledge and action gaps. Such an analysis is a good opportunity for engaging the scientific community as well as civil society organizations in preparing the case (see also subsection 12.5.1).

12.5.1 A good starting point: the situation analysis phase of the national health planning cycle

As explained earlier (Box 12.4), there are several analyses which can potentially be undertaken during the situation analysis phase of the planning cycle, with the view of integrating intersectoral planning for health and health equity into the overall national health planning process. Some countries may analyse data from existing monitoring systems containing good information on intersectoral factors influencing health equity (e.g. see Finland's compass system[l]). Others may start from broader survey analyses of the overall health situation and associated intersectoral priorities.[42]

Complementary to these analytical approaches, a concrete starting point could be the total burden of disease and its risk factors in the country, broken down by diseases and conditions and, where possible, disaggregated by the relevant dimensions of inequity in the country. This should be part and parcel of the situation analysis phase in the national health policy and planning cycle. The Global Burden of Disease Project produces updated profiles for each country.[43] The profiles provide ranking of the 25 largest contributors to premature death and DALYs, comparison between 1990 and 2010, and benchmarking with other countries of comparable levels of economic development.[44] Starting from the burden of disease profile, in particular the DALY components, will help to focus, prioritize, and overcome differences of interests. It can give appropriate weight to diseases and conditions that reduce social, mental and physical well-being without necessarily causing premature death. It will also help avoid falling into the trap of being led or misled by the availability of data or gaps in the same. The profiles also provide an overview of burden of disease driven by the 15 leading risk factors. This includes both those that are attributes, e.g. high blood pressure, high body-mass index, iron deficiency, etc. as well at those that are exposures, e.g. dietary risks, smoking, household air pollution, etc. Risk factors provide links to the social determinants and are the crux of the ill-health equation that cannot be addressed without true intersectoral action.

During the situation analysis (and at times, subsequent phases) of the health planning cycle, it will usually be sufficient to look at the largest 10–15 contributors to the burden of disease plus maybe one or two other diseases known to be focused in particular subpopulations or locations. The reason is that the same social determinants and risk factors are driving several diseases and their inequitable distribution.[45]

The burden of disease country profiles do not disaggregate the data as suggested for the SDGs by income, gender, age, race, ethnicity, migratory status, disability, geographical location and other characteristics relevant in national contexts.[46] To find such disaggregated data for the top diseases, conditions, and risk factors, one will have to look for locally-available information

l Finland has an intersectoral monitoring system that analyses population need and health and social service responses and is also used for national reporting, but less emphasis is placed on this data at the national level (http://www.hyvinvointikompassi.fi/en/web/hyvinvointikompassi/, accessed 26 May 2016).

from records, surveys, and studies; and data analysed in preparation for the national plan will need further scrutiny with respect to equity, risk factors, and social determinants in mind. More often, though, complete information will not be available. One of the results of a situation analysis phase can be to bring attention to the lack of information, and to stimulate dialogue on how to fill the gap in data generation.

However, even with data gaps, the inequity picture will generally come together like a mosaic, with the pattern showing up even if some of the pieces are missing. Once the pattern is beginning to show, it is time to start asking questions about what it means. Why do some districts have much higher prevalence of chronic kidney disease compared to others? Why do people in the lower income quintiles have higher prevalence of diabetes than those in the richer quintiles? Why do some ethnic groups have higher prevalence of HIV than others? Why do poor people smoke more than the richer? (see Fig. 12.2). And in those frequent cases where very little information is available, this should lead to an inclusion of inequality-monitoring mechanisms as a key discussion point during national health planning processes.

One challenge is that the disaggregated prevalence data – if they exist – are often scattered without any single source having the full overview. Another challenge is that the answers to the why-questions, i.e. the social determinants causing the observed inequities, are often country- and context-specific and come out only in planning processes that put effort into understanding root causes of bottlenecks. In order to overcome such challenges, planners could, for example, take an iterative Delphi method type approach as part of the situation analysis.[47] Other longer-term options include incorporating inequality data generation in routine health information systems, conducting regular surveys to measure progress on the determinants of health and inequalities, conducting focus groups with key informants in the health system, etc.

The Delphi method is particularly useful in revealing gaps in knowledge and in quickly reaching consensus on the situation, while longer-term efforts are made to improve the evidence base. It is thus elaborated upon here in more detail (in Box 12.6). A Delphi approach can expose and help overcome gaps in disaggregated data on diseases and risk factors, as well as the gaps in explaining causes for the inequities and, e.g. the higher levels of specific disease burden compared to the benchmarking countries. Approaches to cover gaps in knowledge and reach consensus should be a vital part of the policy dialogue around the national health plan, but also around the plans for other sectors.

Even in countries with data gaps, the inequity picture will generally come together like a mosaic, with the pattern showing up even if some of the pieces are missing. It is then time to start asking questions about what it means.

Box 12.6

The Delphi method for analysing key data for health planning

First Delphi round: a small number of people with access to data on the level and distribution of the diseases, conditions and risk factors to be focused on; product of the first round is data presented in a standardized format, e.g. as in Fig. 12.2.
Second round: an expanded number of participants to include people who could help interpreting data. While continuing to fill the data gaps, start asking the why-questions and ask people to provide available evidence (reports and studies) to support the answers they offer; product of the second round is a consolidated feedback.
Third round: Delphi panellist receives a questionnaire that includes the items and ratings summarized by the investigators in the previous round, and is asked to revise his/her judgments or "to specify the reasons for remaining outside the consensus".
Fourth round: In the fourth and often final round, the list of remaining items, their ratings, minority opinions, and items achieving consensus are distributed to the panellists; product of the fourth round should be a complete equity picture including key social determinants that shape the inequities.

This analysis can further support national health planning and be used to mobilize political will and publicity.

Each round should be reasonably short – e.g. one week to ten days – and provide full transparency in the return information, so that the participants can see their contributions reflected.

12.5.2 Policy dialogue and negotiation

Once the main risk factors and the social determinants that shape the population's health situation have been identified, the next step is to find out what should be done and who could potentially do something about it. This, in the first instance, does not mean the particular organization or individual – but which sectors are already in the field and in a position to influence the risk factors and social determinants, and what would be the mechanism and strengths of their potential influence.

The findings of the analysis, including on the level and distribution of health in the population and their root causes, need to be accepted and internalized by health and non-health sector actors, including public, private, and civil society. In some countries there are already forums that can provide platforms for discussion and consensus-building. Where platforms exist, they should be fully exploited to ensure dissemination of analysis results and an honest dialogue on the causes and consequences.

In countries where such forums do not exist, it might be necessary to conduct a national consensus workshop to confirm the analysis and agree broadly on action and on who is responsible. Briefings and consultations with the highest levels of government (prime minister, cabinet, and parliament) will help in mobilizing political will and support. In parallel, effective communication of the evidence revealed by the analysis will also be critically important to inform media, politicians and the public about what shapes the health of the country's population. The national health planning process is the ideal moment to bring attention to the vital issues of health inequities and social determinants of health so as to motivate stakeholders to propose agreements, offer concessions and reach compromises. The chosen negotiation strategies of the stakeholders will heavily influence the tone of the discussions and the potential agreements which can be reached. Various negotiation strategies and approaches exist for emphasizing the value of cooperative negotiating from the perspective of a Health in All Policies (HiAP) approach.[48]

Table 12.2 shows an illustrative example of how the top five risk factors in a country (according to the burden of disease profile) could match with two of the sectors in that country. There will of course be more sectors and possibly more risk factors depending on the local country context.

Once the main risk factors and social determinants that shape the population's health situation are identified, the next step is to find out what should be done and who (which sectors) could potentially do something about it.

Table 12.2 Illustrative examples of sector – risk factor match with mechanism and strength of influence – other than own staff (perceived strengths of influence are rated: ★, ★★, and ★★★)

SECTOR	Top-five exposure risk factors in the country (illustrative examples)				
	Dietary risks	Smoking	Physical inactivity	Alcohol use	Occupational risks
Urban planning and transport	Easy and preferred access to healthy food (★★)	Ban smoking in public places in- and outdoor (★★)	Easy and preferred access to physical activity, including for safe walking and cycling (★★★)	Regulate location/ opening hours of alcohol outlets (★★)	Plan placement of industry/business and provide public services (★)
Education	Educate on healthy diet – ban unhealthy food on premises/provide healthy food (★★★)	Inform, ban on premises, offer cessation aid (★★)	Inform, promote, provide opportunities and offer counselling (★★★)	Inform, ban on premises and offer counselling (★★)	Educate on risks and rights (★★)

All sectors can do something about all the population health risk factors. However, the type of mechanism they have at their disposal and their respective strengths of influence may vary. For example, in Table 12.2, "Urban planning and transport" is considered to have a potentially very strong influence on physical activity, medium-strong influence on dietary risks, smoking and alcohol use, and a weaker influence on occupational health. "Education", however, is considered having potentially strong influences on dietary risks, physical activity and medium-strong influence on smoking, alcohol use, and occupational risks. While the exact mechanisms and strengths may vary from one context to another, the onus for the intersectoral planning should be on those mechanisms where the sectors are seen to have a strong or medium-strong potential influence.

Table 12.3. shows some illustrative examples of five social determinants and two sectors – again with potential mechanisms and strength of influence. Only two sectors and five determinants are shown and there will be more depending on country context.

Table 12.3 Illustrative examples of sector – social determinants match with mechanism and strength of influence – other than own staff (perceived strengths of influence are rated: ★, ★★, and ★★★)

SECTOR	Most important social determinants in the country (illustrative examples)				
	Adverse social and cultural norms and gender roles	Lack of jobs and educational opportunities	Clustering of disadvantages	Marketing, pricing and availability of tobacco, alcohol and unhealthy food	Lack of social capital in families and communities
Urban planning and transport	Diversify settlements and plan for community centres (★★)	Plan for appropriate mix of employment, educational opportunities and residential areas; ensure safe, fast and easy public transport(★★★)	Plan for public services, diversify settlements, provide access to easy public transport and green spaces (★★★)	Marketing ethics not accepting advertisements of tobacco, alcohol and unhealthy food in public space and in or on transport means (★)	Plan for integrated public social and health services and community centres, allotment gardens, etc. (★★)
Education	Teach on social and cultural norms, gender roles, rights, participation, and respect for diversity (★★★)	Provide second-chance education, align education to labour market needs, etc (★★★)	Closely monitor and act on enrolment coverage, drop-out and completion rates for vulnerable locations and population groups (★★★)	Educate students and not accept advertisements or sponsorships from providers of tobacco, alcohol and unhealthy food products (★★)	Identify vulnerable students and work with social and health services to address their special needs and those of their families (★★★)

All sectors have the ability to impact all population health risk factors and social determinants with varying levels of strength and types of mechanisms.

All sectors can do something about all social determinants – however, to varying levels of strength. For example, in Table 12.3 "Urban planning and transport" is considered to have a very strong influence on "lack of jobs and educational opportunities" and on "clustering of disadvantages" while the influence on "lack of social capital in families and communities" is considered medium and with the potential influence on "social and cultural norms and gender roles" and "marketing, pricing and availability of tobacco, alcohol and unhealthy food" considered weaker. The foci of the intersectoral planning should be on those mechanisms where the sectors are seen to have a strong or medium-strong potential influence.

One challenge of intersectoral planning is that while it might be reasonably straightforward to agree on the goals (the desired impact and outcomes), it might be more difficult to agree on the outputs – policies and policy-results – and the source and allocation of necessary resources (financial and human). In addition to the variations in interests mentioned in section 12.4, different sectors often have different structures, employ staff of different educations and background and sometimes have different ways of measuring success. Another challenge is that intersectoral planning for health and health equity by definition will take place across several individual sectors' plans. If care is not taken, it could end up being too complex to be implemented.

Table 12.4 illustrates how the findings in Tables 12.2 and 12.3 could move forward to commitments by the individual sectors for action and how progress, i.e. policy-results could be measured. The commitments would be reflected in the intersectoral national health plan, while the detailed activities and inputs would be reflected in the individual sector plans. That is, unlike in logical framework systems, a lower-level result can contribute to more than one higher-level result, e.g. in the different sectors. Likewise, what may be deemed output in one sector may be regarded outcome in another.

Table 12.4 Illustrative example of results chain and commitments

IMPACT	OUTCOME	OUTPUT (individual sector commitments)	
Reduced burden of disease and reduced health inequity by key equity dimensions, e.g.: ▸ Geographic location ▸ Wealth ▸ Ethnicity/ gender	Reduction in risk factor prevalence and gradient, e.g. "physical inactivity"	Urban planning and transport (★★★)	**Policy:** All urban areas must provide easy access to physical activity, including safe walking and cycling
			Policy-result indicator: Proportion of urban areas that have easy access to physical activity, including safe walking and cycling
		Education (★★★)	**Policy:** All schools at all class-levels must provide opportunity for at least 60 minutes of moderate to vigorous intensity physical activity daily
			Policy-result indicator: Greater proportion of schools requiring 60 minutes of intense physical activity daily
	Reduction in adverse social determinants, e.g.: "clustering of disadvantages"	Education (★★★)	**Policy:** All school-districts must identify vulnerable locations and population groups and take appropriate action
			Policy-result indicator: Proportion of locations and population groups where enrolment and completion rates are higher than set thresholds
		Urban planning and transport (★★★)	**Policy:** All local urban areas must have adequate public services, with mixed housing opportunities, and provide access to easy public transport
			Policy-result indicator: New mixed housing opportunities available in urban areas with access to public services, increased number of public transportation options/lines to local urban areas

Those sectors identified in the analyses of Tables 12.2 and 12.3 as having a very strong influence on a risk factor or social determinant should be considered first. However, synergies of coordinated policy and implementation action between sectors will undoubtedly in many cases augment the strength of those considered in isolation as having medium-strong influence. Therefore, it makes sense to bring sectors together around individual or groups of risk factors and social determinants to decide who does what and when, and to commit for action and accountability for outputs.

All organizations, including public institutions and private firms, can act to positively influence the risk factors vis-à-vis their own staff. They can, for example, ban unhealthy food on their premises, and provide opportunities for healthy food instead. They can ban smoking during working hours and offer cessation services. They can also review work processes, inform, promote and provide opportunities for easy-choice physical activity and offer counselling to staff and their families; inform, ban alcohol during working hours and offer cessation and counselling to staff and their families. They can address stressful processes and other occupational risks in the work environment, and provide safe opportunities for reporting and dealing with such risks. Similarly, all organizations in all sectors can address the social determinants within their own settings and staff. For example, they can: emphasize social and cultural diversity and gender balance in their recruitment processes and equal career opportunities; provide decent employment conditions; provide employment opportunities in particular for young people; offer or refer to counselling services for staff members who are in vulnerable situations; keep marketing of tobacco, alcohol and unhealthy foods away from the work place; etc.

12.5.3 Monitoring and accountability

In the Rio Political Declaration on Social Determinants of Health,[49] heads of government, ministers and government representatives define health and health equity as a shared responsibility requiring engagement of all sectors of government and all segments of society. They further acknowledge that governance to address social determinants of health and health equity involves transparent and inclusive decision-making processes that give voice to all groups and sectors concerned. They also state the need for clear and measurable outcomes and for building accountability. The participating governments pledge to work across different sectors and levels of government, including through national development strategies, to enhance the accountability of policy-makers for health, while recognizing a leading role of health ministries for advocacy in this respect. Central to accountability is effective monitoring. For this, the availability of relevant data appropriately disaggregated is key. The 2030 Agenda for Sustainable Development Goals suggests that countries consider disaggregating data by income, gender, age, race, ethnicity, migratory status, disability, geographical location and other characteristics relevant in national contexts. Depending on which dimensions of inequity are relevant to monitor in a country, it will require smaller or larger changes to the sources of data collection in the country, e.g. surveillance systems, population-based sources (censuses, vital registration systems and household surveys), institution-based sources (resource records, service records and individual records), and ad hoc surveys and studies as well as the analysis, linking and communication of the resulting information. The need to strengthen countries' capacities in this respect is explicitly foreseen under "data, monitoring and accountability" in SDG 17.18 and SDG 17.19.[50]

In many countries, the monitoring and evaluation plan and platform is in place, although suffering from major weaknesses, in particular with respect to disaggregating data and cross-sectoral analysis. Monitoring of intersectoral action for health and health equity involves keeping track that what is planned is actually produced by different sectors and levels of society – from community to the highest levels of government – and that it has the desired effect. While the policies committed by the individual sector (e.g. "all school-districts must identify vulnerable locations and population groups and take appropriate action") can simply be counted, indicators will be required for monitoring if the policy-results, the outcomes (e.g. "reduced clustering of adverse social determinants") and the impacts (e.g. "reduced burden of disease and reduced health inequity by key equity dimensions") are achieved as planned (see Table 12.4). When selecting monitoring indicators of intersectoral planning for health and health equity, it must be taken into account that there will be many different sources and several types of data, including quantitative and qualitative data. Further, the use of the data as well as the accountability for delivery will be made at different points, e.g. communities; local area councils; district administrations and councils; sectoral managers at various levels, including institutions; and cabinet and parliament. These should be viewed in the context of their individual rights and their own needs, rather than just as part of a hierarchical system producing aggregated data. It may be useful to look at:

Technical feasibility – is concerned with how easy it is to acquire, analyse, and interpret the data required to monitor the impact and policy outcome indicators disaggregated by the relevant inequity dimensions and by the relevant data providers and users.

Technical reliability – relates to how the data sources can be relied on to provide accurate information at present and in the future. This means ensuring that methods and measures are scientifically sound and stable over time; level of errors and missing data is acceptable; processes are transparent with credible audits; data collection and analysis are free of political interference; the data collection cycle is shorter than or comparable to the expected pace of change; there are no upcoming regulations that could impede data collection and use; and that there is stable financing and local capacity present for continued data collection.

Technical validity – relates to how well the indicator captures the influence of social determinants and risk factors on the level (burden of disease) and distribution (inequity) of health in populations. In other words, it actually measures what it is supposed to measure; it is a reasonable proxy for a broader domain; it has scope for generalizing to the country as a whole. In short, it goes beyond what is directly measured by the indicator.

Programmatic feasibility – relates to whether the messages from the indicators are communicable and comprehensible by politicians, sectoral policy-makers and managers, media and civil society.

Programmatic relevance – is concerned with whether the messages from the indicators are useful for taking individual sector action, for intersectoral dialogue and action, and for informing the political and public debates.[51]

Monitoring is used to indicate whether policies, programmes, and practices are accomplishing what they are designed to achieve; results from monitoring can help shape eventual corrective action for policies, programmes, and practices which need improvement.

The purpose of monitoring is to indicate whether the policies, programmes and practices are accomplishing what they are designed to achieve. If they are not, then the monitoring should be able to inform eventual corrective action. Data from monitoring of intersectoral efforts need to be understood by often very diverse groups of people with different educational and professional backgrounds, different political observance, different interests, different levels of education and insight, etc.

Ultimately, monitoring and accountability are what will hold intersectoral action together and are closely linked to the governance of not only the national health plan but also of the national development plan and, internationally, the SDGs. Monitoring is part of a continuous process of adjustments and improvements in order to maintain the pace of progress to improve health and reduce health inequities. Monitoring of intersectoral action for health equity is also part of an accountability process that goes beyond just managerial accountability to cover political and moral accountability as well – and therefore moves out into the political and public space.

In Norway, the Directorate of Health has established a cross-governmental monitoring system. Drawing from this system their annual health report brings together all the indicators of the intersectoral action for reducing health inequities. The title Folkehelsepolitisk Report [Population Health Policy Report][52] underscores that the responsibility and accountability for reducing inequities is political rather than merely bureaucratic. As already mentioned, in New Zealand, indicators for social determinants of health and health inequity have been integrated into the comprehensive social reports produced by the Ministry of Social Development.[53]

The HiAP Monitoring Strategy of Suriname is rights-based, integrates and formalizes inclusiveness, transparency and accountability, and links with the political and public spheres. The monitoring process is set to include, for example, primary school children, ordinary citizens, civil society organizations, government and private sector staff, statisticians and other experts in various fields, as well as local and national politicians. A key tenet of the Strategy is that data should be analysed and used as close as possible to where action can be taken and where the people concerned are, as well as be appropriately consolidated for policy-making, and feedback. An annual population health report is presented to the National Assembly and an Annual National Health Forum is conducted (Box 12.7).

Once the format for the SDG reporting is established, this will provide a mechanism for national and international accountability, similar to the national accountability supported by the social reports in New Zealand. Words and concepts like "equitable access", "equal opportunity", "reduce inequalities", "inclusive", "universal", "equal", and "for all" appear in almost all the 17 goals. Also, the preamble to the UN General Assembly resolution (A/RES/70/1) on SDGs emphasizes that the implementation of the SDGs relies on a collaborative partnership.

Box 12.7

HiAP Monitoring Strategy Group[54]

Illustrative example of Suriname.

In Suriname the intersectoral planning and monitoring for health is coordinated by the HiAP Monitoring Strategy Group chaired by the Vice-president's Office and with the Ministry of Public Health as the Secretariat. This ensures a direct link to the day-to-day business of government, which is managed out of the Vice-president's Office. In addition, the HiAP Monitoring Strategy Group is charged to:

- prepare the Annual Population Health Report presenting the latest knowledge on the burden of disease, risk factors, inequity and social determinants at play, and policy action in Suriname – and, present it to the National Assembly;
- organize an Annual National Health Forum providing the opportunity for politicians, sectoral managers, researchers, private sector and civil society to review the newest knowledge, and policy and implementation progress, share experience; innovate and discuss the way forward.

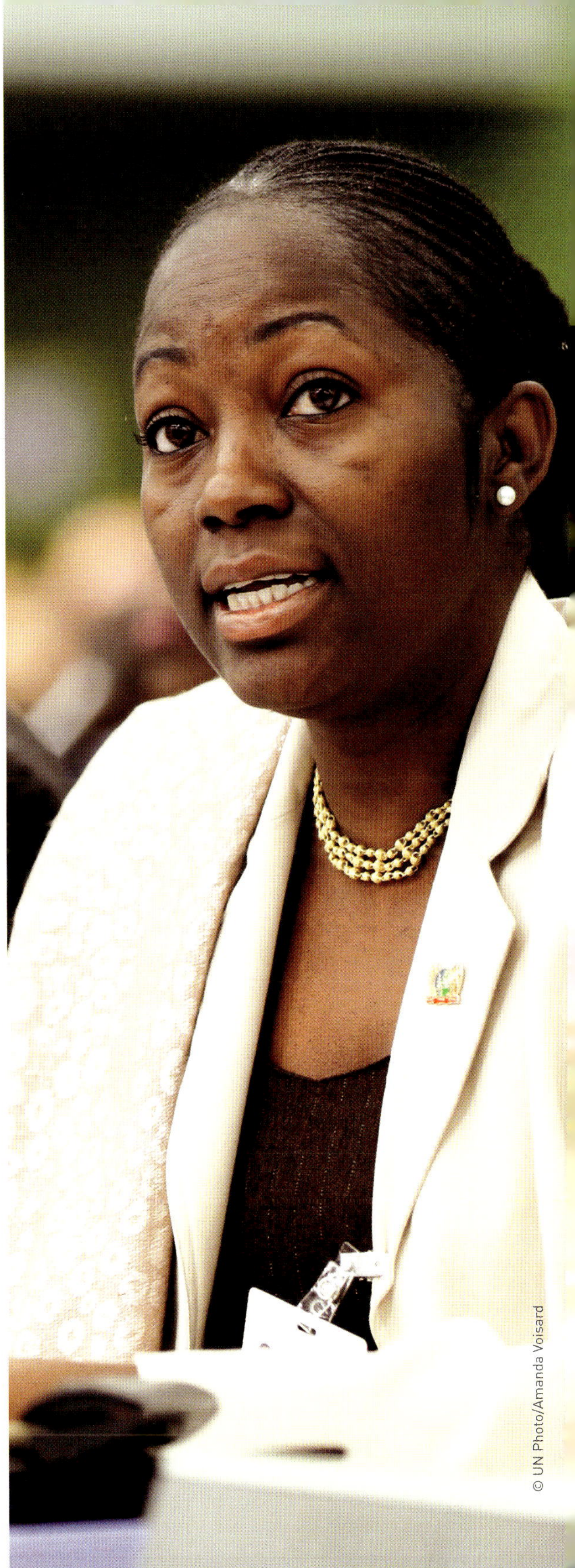

© UN Photo/Amanda Voisard

12.6 Conclusion

A national health planning process should be one of the entry points to address health inequity and social determinants of health. Intersectoral planning thus entails an explicit emphasis on health policy dialogue around intersectoral action.

Best practices exist, mainly from disease-specific or life cycle-specific programmes. The approaches these programmes adopted over the last decade to integrate intersectoral action in their global or regional strategies have resulted in multisectoral action frameworks and a better targeting of key health determinants. Many useful lessons-learned can be drawn from these experiences.

This chapter elucidates the various entry points for addressing health inequity and intersectoral collaboration in national health planning. For some of these entry points, the health sector is both the leader and the implementer; for some, the health sector emphasis is on providing leadership; while for others, the health sector may act primarily as a catalyst. These different entry points for tackling health inequalities find their correspondence in the approved SDGs, where health goes beyond Goal 3.

There is strong evidence demonstrating that socioeconomic development and health systems development are mutually reinforcing, increasing the chances for sustainable achievements. In other words, addressing the determinants of health (which intrinsically involves collaboration between sectors) needs to occur concomitantly with addressing clinical care services. This is not an impossible task. Examples from around the world show that other sectors can be successfully engaged in joint efforts for mutual benefit. However, it requires changes in the ways ministries of health usually work. New skill sets and approaches to analysis, planning, monitoring and accountability will have to be developed. These approaches will need to reach a wider audience that involves different sectors and professions as well as communities, higher levels of government, politicians and the public at large.

Some countries have already shown the way. However, there is no fast and easy blueprint and each country will have to find its own way – while learning from the experiences of others – in order to overcome lack of coherence across government policies. This lack of coherence has in the past led to one part of government working to improve health, while other parts of the government might promote trade and industrial development with initiatives that might be harmful to health and well-being.

One reason that these inconsistencies arise is because of a lack of understanding across sectors of the linkages between health and quality of life, on the one hand, and the social and economic determinants of health, on the other. Another reason they arise is because seemingly unrelated policies may have unintended impacts that go unmeasured and unaddressed.

This chapter provides some basic ideas and principles and encouragement for health planners to get started.

References

1 Preamble to the Constitution of the World Health Organization, as adopted by the International Health Conference, New York, 19–22 June 1946; signed on 22 July 1946 by the representatives of 61 States (Official Records of the World Health Organization, no. 2, page 100) and entered into force on 7 April 1948. Geneva: World Health Organization; 1948 (http://www.who.int/governance/eb/who_constitution_en.pdf, accessed 14 May 2016).

2 World Health Statistics 2015. Geneva: World Health Organization; 2015 (http://apps.who.int/iris/bitstream/10665/170250/1/9789240694439_eng.pdf, accessed 14 May 2016).

3 Whitehead, M. The concepts and principles of equity and health. Int J Health Serv. 1992;22(3):429–45.

4 Key Concepts. In: WHO/social determinants of health [website]. Geneva: World Health Organization, 2016 (http://www.who.int/social_determinants/thecommission/finalreport/key_concepts/en/).

5 Global strategy for health for all by the year 2000. Geneva: World Health Organization; 1981 (Health for All Series, No.3; http://apps.who.int/iris/bitstream/10665/38893/1/9241800038.pdf, accessed 14 May 2016).

6 World Health Organization, Ottawa charter for health promotion. Geneva; 1986 (http://www.phac-aspc.gc.ca/ph-sp/docs/charter-chartre/pdf/charter.pdf, accessed 18 May 2016).

7 Health 2020: a European policy framework and strategy for the 21st century. Copenhagen: WHO Regional Office for Europe, 2013 (http://www.euro.who.int/__data/assets/pdf_file/0011/199532/Health2020-Long.pdf, accessed 18 May 2016).

8 Health in all policies: training manual. Geneva: World Health Organization; 2015 (http://apps.who.int/iris/bitstream/10665/151788/1/9789241507981_eng.pdf, accessed 18 May 2016).

9 25 Questions and answers on health and human rights. Geneva: World Health Organization; 2002 (Health and Human Rights Publication Series, no. 1; http://www.who.int/hhr/information/25%20Questions%20and%20Answers%20on%20Health%20and%20Human%20Rights.pdf, accessed 18 May 2016).

10 Gender mainstreaming for health managers: a practical approach. Facilitators' guide. Geneva: World Health Organization; 2011 (http://apps.who.int/iris/bitstream/10665/44516/1/9789241501071_eng.pdf, accessed 19 May 2016).

11 Closing the gap in a generation: health equity through action on the social determinants of health. Final report of the Commission on the Social Determinants of Health. Geneva: World Health Organization; 2008 (http://www.who.int/social_determinants/final_report/csdh_finalreport_2008.pdf, accessed 19 May 2016).

12 Global action plan for the prevention and control of noncommunicable diseases 2013–2020. Geneva: World Health Organization; 2013 (http://apps.who.int/iris/bitstream/10665/94384/1/9789241506236_eng.pdf?ua=1, accessed 19 May 2016).

13 UNAIDS 2016–2021 strategy: on the fast-track to end AIDS. Geneva: UNAIDS; 2015 (http://www.unaids.org/sites/default/files/media_asset/20151027_UNAIDS_PCB37_15-18_EN_rev1.pdf, accessed 19 May 2016).

14 Blas E. Multisectoral action framework for malaria. Geneva: Roll Back Malaria Partnership and the United Nations Development Programme; 2013 (http://www.rollbackmalaria.org/files/files/resources/Multisectoral-Action-Framework-for-Malaria.pdf, assessed 19 May 2016).

15 A policy guide for implementing essential interventions for reproductive, maternal, newborn and child health (RMNCH): multisectoral policy compendium for RMNCH. Geneva: World Health Organization; 2014 (http://www.who.int/pmnch/knowledge/publications/policy_compendium.pdf, accessed 19 January 2016).

16 Blas E, Sivasankara-Kurup A, editors. Equity, social determinants and public health programmes. Geneva: World Health Organization; 2010 (http://www.who.int/sdhconference/resources/EquitySDandPH_eng.pdf, accessed 19 May 2016).

17 Intersectoral action for health: the role of intersectoral cooperation in national strategies for health for all. Geneva: World Health Organization; 1986 (http://apps.who.int/iris/bitstream/10665/41545/1/9241560967_eng.pdf, accessed 19 May 2016).

18 Transforming our world: the 2030 agenda for sustainable development (A/RES/70/1). New York: United Nations; 2015 (https://sustainabledevelopment.un.org/content/documents/21252030%20Agenda%20for%20Sustainable%20Development%20web.pdf, accessed 19 May 2016).

19 The New Zealand health strategy. Wellington: Ministry of Health; 2000 (https://www.health.govt.nz/system/files/documents/publications/newzealandhealthstrategy.pdf, accessed 25 August 2016).

20 Pega F, Valentine N, Matheson D. Monitoring social well-being to support policies on the social determinants of health: the case of New Zealand's "Social Reports/Te PĐrongo Oranga Tangata". Geneva: World Health Organization; 2010 (Social Determinants of Health Discussion Paper 3; http://www.who.int/social_determinants/corner/SDHDP3.pdf?ua=1, accessed 19 May 2016).

21 Norwegian Public Health Act. Oslo: Ministry of Health and Care Services; 2011 (ACT-2011-06-24-29; http://www.regjeringen.no/en/dep/hod/aktuelt/nyheter/2011/helse--og-omsorgsministeren-pa-who-konfe.html?id=660492, accessed 25 May 2016).

22 Strand M, Brown C, Torgerson TP, Giaever, O. Setting the political agenda to tackle health inequity in Norway. Copenhagen: WHO Regional Office for Europe; 2009 (Studies on social and economic determinants of public health, No.4; http://www.euro.who.int/__data/assets/pdf_file/0014/110228/E93431.pdf, accessed 25 May 2016).

23 Blas E. Multisectoral action framework for malaria. Geneva: Roll Back Malaria Partnership and the United Nations Development Programme; 2013 (http://www.rollbackmalaria.org/files/files/resources/Multisectoral-Action-Framework-for-Malaria.pdf, assessed 19 May 2016).

24 Lönnroth K, Jaramillo E, Williams B, Dye C, Raviglione M. Tuberculosis: the role of risk factors and social determinants. In: Blas E, Sivasankara-Kurup A, editors. Equity, social determinants and public health programmes. Geneva: World Health Organization; 2010:219–241 (http://www.who.int/sdhconference/resources/EquitySDandPH_eng.pdf, accessed 19 May 2016).

25 Murray CJL, Vos T, Lozano R, Naghavi M, Flaxman AD, Michaud C, et al. Disability-adjusted life years (DALYs) for 291 diseases and injuries in 21 regions, 1990–2010: a systematic analysis for the Global Burden of Disease Study 2010. Lancet. 2012;380:2197–223. (http://www.thelancet.com/pdfs/journals/lancet/PIIS0140-6736(12)61689-4.pdf, accessed 19 May 2016).

26 Life expectancy. In: WHO/Global Health Observatory (GHO) data [website]. Geneva: World Health Organization; 2016 (http://www.who.int/gho/mortality_burden_disease/life_tables/situation_trends/en/, accessed 19 May 2016).

27 Health in all policies Suriname. In: Health in all policies in the Americas [website]. Washington (DC): Pan American Health Organization; 2015 (http://www.paho.org/sur/index.php?option=com_content&view=article&id=494:health-in-all-policies-suriname&Itemid=0, accessed 3 June 2016).

28 Wisconsin Health Gaps Report. Madison: University of Wisconsin Population Health Institute; 2015 (http://www.countyhealthrankings.org/health-gaps/

wisconsin, accessed 19 May 2016).

29 Global, regional, and national comparative risk assessment of 79 behavioural, environmental and occupational, and metabolic risks or clusters of risks in 188 countries, 1990–2013: a systematic analysis for the Global Burden of Disease Study 2013. Lancet [online] 2015 (https://www.healthdata.org/sites/default/files/files/research_articles/2015/GBD2013_RiskFactors_TheLancet_0.PDF; accessed 19 May 2016).

30 Blas E, Sivasankara-Kurup A, editors. Equity, social determinants and public health programmes. Geneva: World Health Organization; 2010 (http://www.who.int/sdhconference/resources/EquitySDandPH_eng.pdf, accessed 19 May 2016).

31 Transforming our world: the 2030 agenda for sustainable development (A/RES/70/1). New York: United Nations; 2015 (https://sustainabledevelopment.un.org/content/documents/21252030%20Agenda%20for%20Sustainable%20Development%20web.pdf, accessed 19 May 2016).

32 Målqvist M, Hoa DT, Thomsen S. Causes and determinants of inequity in maternal and child health in Vietnam. BMC Public Health. 2012 Aug 11;12:641. doi: 10.1186/1471-2458-12-641.

33 Kaljee LM, Anh DD, Minh TT, Huu Tho L, Batmunkh N, Kilgore PE. Rural and urban Vietnamese mothers utilization of healthcare resources for children under 6 years with pneumonia and associated symptoms. J Behav Med. 2011 Aug;34(4):254-67. doi: 10.1007/s10865-010-9305-5. Epub 2010 Dec 3.

34 Van Minh H et al. Monitoring intersectoral factors influencing equity-oriented progress towards universal health coverage (UHC) and health equity - Vietnam case study. 2014. Unpublished.

35 Irwin LG, Siddiqi A, Hertzman G. Early child development: a powerful equalizer. Final report for the World Health Organization's Commission on the Social Determinants of Health. Geneva: World Health Organization; 2007 (http://www.who.int/social_determinants/resources/ecd_kn_report_07_2007.pdf, accessed 19 May 2016).

36 Adapted from: WHO handbook for guideline development, 2nd edition. Geneva: World Health Organization; 2014 (http://www.who.int/kms/handbook_2nd_ed.pdf, accessed 19 May 2016).

37 Drager N, McClintock E, Moffitt M. Negotiating health development: a guide for practitioners. Cambridge (MA)/Geneva: Conflict Management Group/World Health Organization; 2000 (http://www.who.int/trade/resource/en/Negotiating.pdf, accessed 19 May 2016).

38 National Health Plan 2009–2020. Republic of Estonia; 2008. (http://pns.dgs.pt/files/2010/03/pnsest.pdf, accessed 19 May 2016).

39 Pomeranz JL. Taxing food and beverage products: a public health perspective and a new strategy for prevention. U. Michigan J L Reform. 2013:46(3):299–1027 (http://repository.law.umich.edu/cgi/viewcontent.cgi?article=1011&context=mjlr, accessed 19 May 2016).

40 Handbook on health inequality monitoring: with a special focus on low- and middle-income countries. Geneva: World Health Organization; 2013 (http://apps.who.int/iris/bitstream/10665/85345/1/9789241548632_eng.pdf?ua=1, accessed 19 May 2016).

41 Health in all policies Suriname. In: Health in all policies in the Americas [website]. Washington (DC): Pan American Health Organization; 2015 (http://www.paho.org/sur/index.php?option=com_content&view=article&id=494:health-in-all-policies-suriname&Itemid=0, accessed 3 June 2016).

42 Ataguba, JE-O; Day, C; McIntyre, D. Explaining the role of the social determinants of health on health inequality in South Africa. Global Health Action 2015;8;2886. (http://www.globalhealthaction.net/index.php/gha/article/view/28865, accessed: 26 May 2016).

43 Institute for Health Metrics and Evaluation. Global burden of disease – country profiles 2013 [website] (http://www.healthdata.org/results/country-profiles, accessed 26 May 2016).

44 Institute for Health Metrics and Evaluation. Suriname; 2010 (www.health- data.org/suriname, accessed 26 May 2016).

45 Blas E, Sivasankara-Kurup A, editors. Equity, social determinants and public health programmes. Geneva: World Health Organization; 2010 (http://www.who.int/sdhconference/resources/EquitySDandPH_eng.pdf, accessed 19 May 2016).

46 Transforming our world: the 2030 agenda for sustainable development (A/RES/70/1). New York: United Nations; 2015 (https://sustainabledevelopment.un.org/content/documents/21252030%20Agenda%20for%20Sustainable%20Development%20web.pdf, accessed 19 May 2016).

47 Hsu C-C, Sandford BA. The Delphi technique: making sense of consensus. Practical Assessment, Research & Evaluation. 2007:12(10):1–8 (http://pareonline.net/pdf/v12n10.pdf, accessed 19 May 2016).

48 Health in all policies: training manual. Geneva: World Health Organization; 2015 (http://apps.who.int/iris/bitstream/10665/151788/1/9789241507981_eng.pdf, accessed 18 May 2016).

49 World Health Organization. Rio political declaration on social determinants of health. Geneva; 2011 (http://www.who.int/sdhconference/declaration/Rio_political_declaration.pdf, accessed 19 May 2016).

50 Transforming our world: the 2030 agenda for sustainable development (A/RES/70/1). New York: United Nations; 2015 (https://sustainabledevelopment.un.org/content/documents/21252030%20Agenda%20for%20Sustainable%20Development%20web.pdf, accessed 19 May 2016).

51 Blas E, Ataguba JE, Huda TM, Bao GK, Rasella D, Gerecke MR. The feasibility of measuring and monitoring social determinants of health and the relevance for policy and programme: a qualitative assessment of four countries. Global Health Action. 2016;9:29002 (http://www.globalhealthaction.net/index.php/gha/article/view/29002, accessed 19 May 2016).

52 Directorate of Health, Oslo Norway Folkehelsepolitisk rapport 2015. [Population health political report 2015] Oslo: Helsedirektoratet; 2015 (Rapport IS-2776; https://helsedirektoratet.no/Lists/Publikasjoner/Attachments/1130/Folkehelsepolitisk-rapport-2015-IS-2776.pdf, accessed 25 May 2016).

53 2010 the social report: te pÐrongo orange tangata. Wellington: Ministry of Social Development; (http://www.socialreport.msd.govt.nz/documents/the-social-report-2010.pdf, accessed 25 May 2016).

54 Health in all policies Suriname. In: Health in all policies in the Americas [website]. Washington (DC): Pan American Health Organization; 2015 (http://www.paho. org/sur/index.php?option=com_content&view=arti- cle&id=494:health-in-all-policies-suriname&Itemid=0, accessed 3 June 2016).

Further reading

Ashwill M, Saavedra-Chanduvi J, Narajan A, Tiwari S. Analysing the World Bank's goal of achieving "shared prosperity". Inequality in focus. 2013:2(3); 1–15 (http://www.worldbank.org/content/dam/Worldbank/document/Poverty%20documents/inequality-in-focus-october2013-v12.pdf, accessed 24 May 2016).

Blas E, Sivasankara-Kurup A, editors. Equity, social determinants and public health programmes. Geneva: World Health Organization; 2010 (http://www.who.int/sdhconference/resources/EquitySDandPH_eng.pdf, accessed 19 May 2016).

Drager N, McClintock E, Moffitt M. Negotiating health development: a guide for practitioners. Cambridge (MA)/Geneva: Conflict Management Group/World Health Organization; 2000 (http://www.who.int/trade/resource/en/Negotiating.pdf, accessed 19 May 2016).

Handbook on health inequality monitoring: with a special focus on low- and middle-income countries. Geneva: World Health Organization; 2013 (http://apps.who.int/iris/bitstream/10665/85345/1/9789241548632_eng.pdf?ua=1, accessed 19 May 2016).

Health in all policies: report on perspectives and intersectoral actions in the African region. Brazzaville: World Health Organization, Regional Office for Africa; 2013 (http://apps.who.int/iris/bitstream/10665/127848/1/9789290232445.pdf, accessed 25 May 2016).

Health in all policies: report on perspectives and intersectoral actions in the Western Pacific. Regional report. Manila: World Health Organization, Western Pacific Region; 2013. (http://www.wpro.who.int/topics/social_determinants_health/health_in_all_policy_report.pdf, accessed 25 May 2016).

Intersectoral actions for addressing the social determinants of health: report of a regional consultation WHO-SEARO, 23–25 August 2011. New Delhi: World Health Organization, Regional Office for SouthEast Asia; 2012 (http://apps.searo.who.int/PDS_DOCS/B4876.pdf, accessed 25 May 2016).

Leppo K, Ollila E, Peña S, Wismar M, Cook S, editors. Health in all policies: seizing opportunities, implementing policies. Helsinki: Ministry of Social Affairs and Health; 2013 (http://www.euro.who.int/__data/assets/pdf_file/0007/188809/Health-in-All-Policies-final.pdf?ua=1 accessed 19May 2016).

Transforming our world: the 2030 agenda for sustainable development (A/RES/70/1). New York: United Nations; 2015 (https://sustainabledevelopment.un.org/content/documents/21252030%20Agenda%20for%20Sustainable%20Development%20web.pdf, accessed 19 May 2016).

Annex 12.1

Entry points for intersectoral collaboration and SDG links

(Rating of links between entry point and SDG: very strong = ★★★; medium-strong = ★★, strong = ★; three of each per entry point – except for entry point 3 .– see also Box 12.4)

ENTRY POINTS		1	2	3
SDG		Evidence on inequities and causes	Laws, policies, standards, etc.	Causes of differentials
1	No poverty	★★	★★	★★★
2	Zero hunger			★★★
3	Good health and well-being			
4	Quality education	★★	★★	★★★
5	Gender equality	★★★	★★★	★★★
6	Clean water and sanitation	★	★	★★★
7	Affordable and clean energy			★★
8	Decent work and economic growth	★★	★★	★★★
9	Industry, innovation and infrastructure			★★
10	Reduced inequalities	★★★	★★★	★★★
11	Sustainable cities and communities	★	★	★★★
12	Responsible consumption and production			★★
13	Climate action			★★
14	Life below water			★★
15	Life on land			★★
16	Peace, justice and strong institutions	★	★★★	★★★
17	Partnerships for the goals	★★★	★	★★

4	5	6	7	8
Allocation of resources	Strategies for addressing gender	Participation of civil society and individuals	Transparency and accountability	Gender balance and equity in org. processes
★★★	★★	★★	★★	★★★
★	★		★	
★★	★★★	★★★	★★★	★
★★	★★★	★★	★	★★★
★	★★	★★		★
★★★	★★	★	★★	★★
★★				
		★★★	★★★	★★★
	★	★	★	★
★★★	★★★	★★★	★★★	★★★
★	★	★	★★	★★

Chapter 13

Strategizing in distressed health contexts

Enrico Pavignani
Sandro Colombo

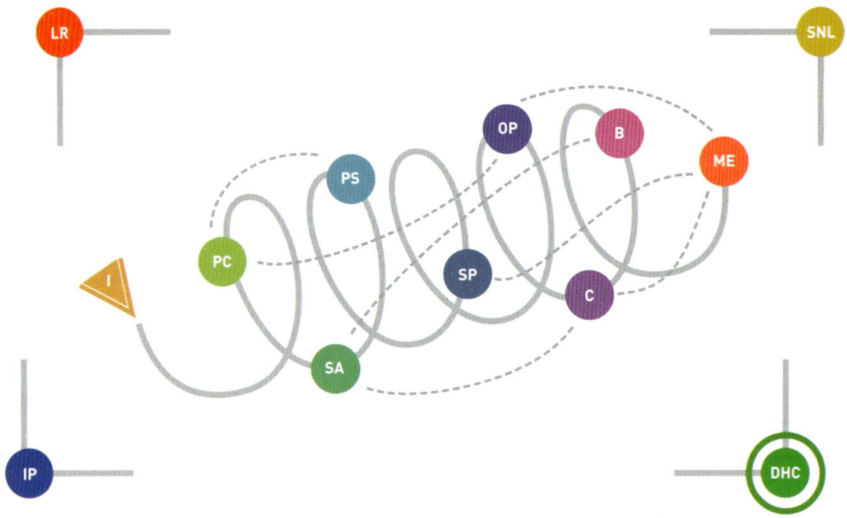

Cross-cutting topics relevant to national health planning

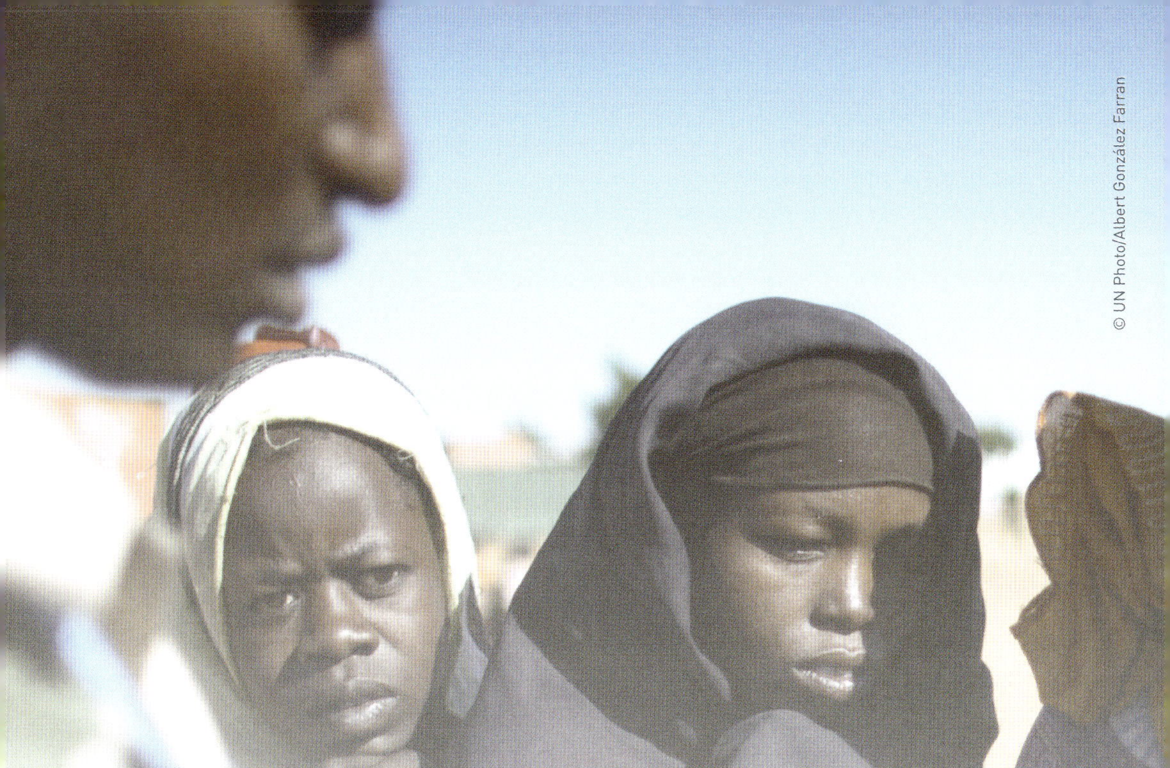

© UN Photo/Albert González Farran

Overview

This publication does not propose detailed instructions to be mechanically followed, nor does it attempt to simplify the issues at stake, in the firm belief that no blueprinted approach can produce satisfactory outcomes. The challenges posed by policy and strategy formulation and planning in health systems under stress are discussed, highlighting the main differences with these processes in more stable environments. Lessons learnt in "fragile" contexts are used to suggest adapted policy and planning approaches and to provide suggestions for avoiding the most common mistakes.

Summary

Section 1

Sets the scene, looking at how different situations of weakness, poverty and violence fit uneasily into the "fragile state" concept and category. The section introduces the main determinants of fragility and stresses their self-reinforcing nature. It emphasizes the need for understanding the context and its possible evolution before formulating strategies.

Section 2

Discusses aid in fragile states, an issue receiving renewed interest. The section looks at requirements and principles of aid management in fragile states, as well as at some of the most important donor agendas and instruments, arguing that current approaches are ill-suited to unstable contexts and new modalities are needed to improve aid effectiveness.

Section 3

Looks at those characteristics of fragile states that impact on health policy and planning and that require adapted approaches. It considers the dynamic and unpredictable context and the mix of actors within and outside of the health field. Performing a situation analysis in these settings, including assessing the capacity of key public and private health actors is critical, but challenging. Like in stable countries, strategy formulation and planning in fragile contexts are political, iterative and continuing processes, which require negotiation with the many stakeholders.

A strong monitoring and evaluation component is the link between strategy formulation and implementation. It provides indications about necessary adjustments to strategies and plans. To facilitate the tailoring of approaches to specific situations, a new empirical typology of situations is proposed, with suggestions about the possible courses of action. Critical aspects related to key subsectors (financing, human resources, medicines and infrastructure) are then discussed.

The chapter concludes with a selected annotated bibliography. Annex 13.1 presents criteria for appraising a policy or a strategy.

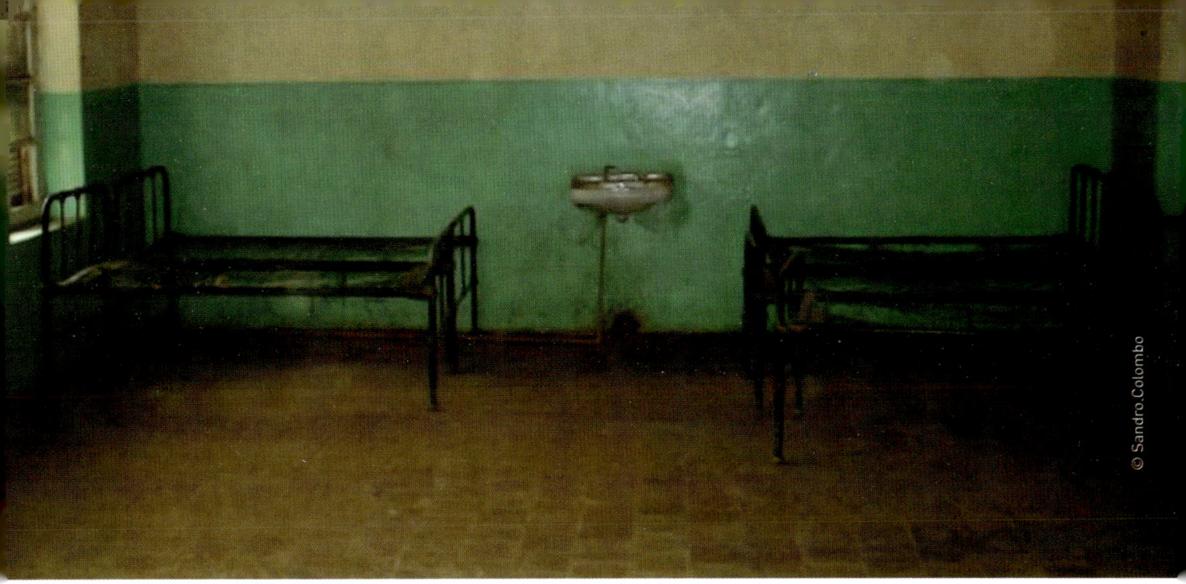

13.1 The context of "fragile" states

In this chapter, the term 'fragile states' is retained because of its widespread currency, despite its obvious inadequacy, which is discussed.

Terms to identify and classify weak states have evolved since the late 1980s, when policy-makers and scholars turned their interest to state failure.[1,I] More recently, the terms "fragility" and "situations of fragility" are being increasingly used, to highlight the need to look to non-state actors.[2] Yet, state fragility "remains an elusive concept".[3] Together with the evolution of the terms, typologies and indices of state fragility have multiplied: as a result, no agreement exists on a common list of actual fragile states. The various definitions converge towards a combination of dysfunctions in key governance dimensions: inability to protect populations from violence, failure to provide basic services, lack of legitimacy, often combined with human rights violations.

The label of fragile states is broad: not only are there differences in degrees, types and drivers of state weakness, but fragility varies substantially within the same country, as, for example, in the Democratic Republic of the Congo and Sudan. Further, fragile states tend to cluster geographically, as in the Great Lakes; the Horn of Africa; Afghanistan and Pakistan. Such regions are characterized by trans-border trade of legal and illegal goods, human trafficking and other criminal activities, and often provide havens to terrorist and rebel groups. Globalization enables, through communication technologies and market deregulation, the integration between informal and formal economies, and between state and non-state networks.

There is no agreement on a common list of fragile states.

Measuring state fragility is problematic: it requires not only defining some state model as a benchmark, but also choosing among ranking systems developed for different purposes and

I Quasi or pseudo states to least-developed countries, low-income countries under stress, collapsed, rogue, failed, failing, in crisis, poorly performing, in arrested development.

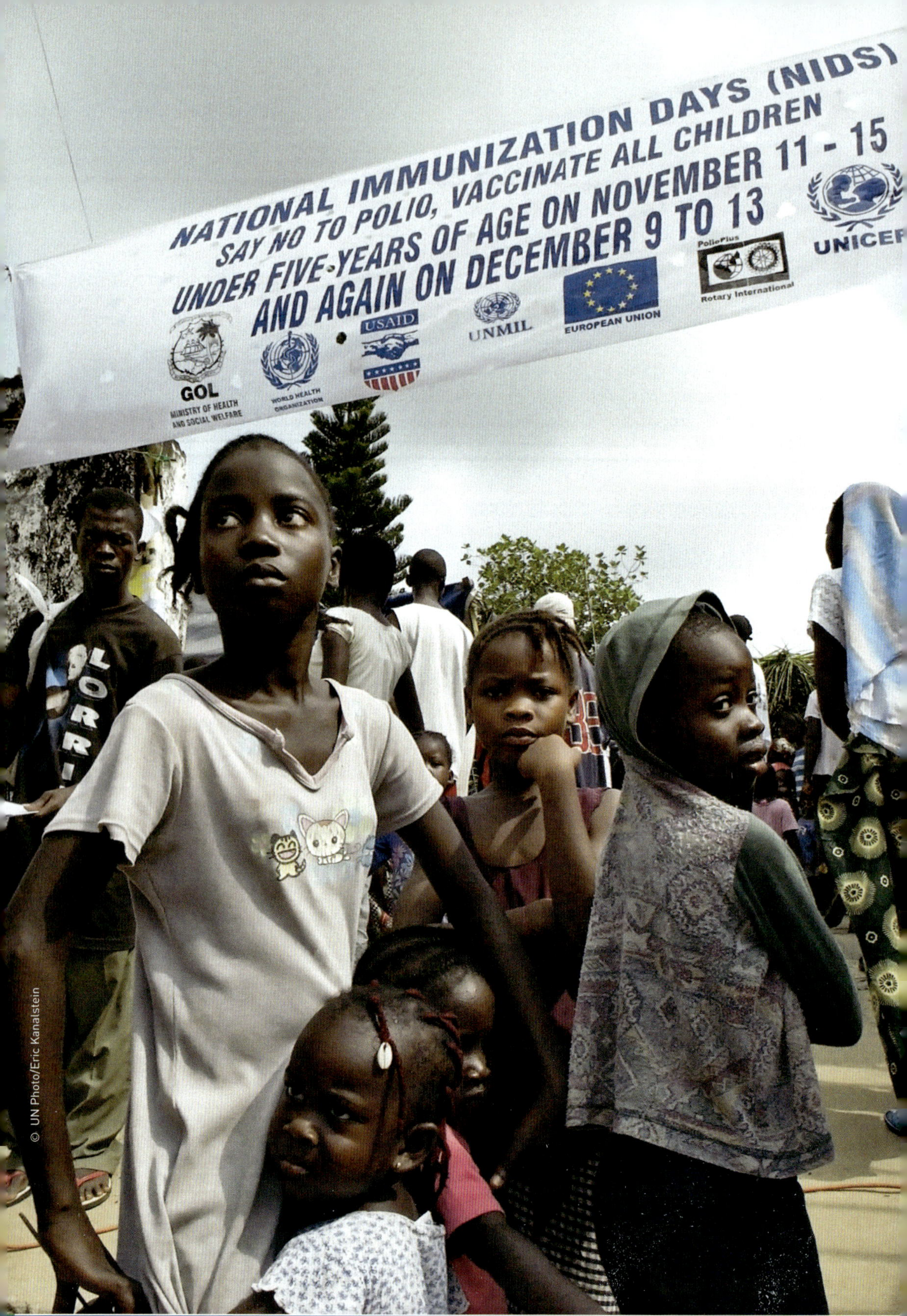
NATIONAL IMMUNIZATION DAYS (NIDS)
SAY NO TO POLIO, VACCINATE ALL CHILDREN
UNDER FIVE YEARS OF AGE ON NOVEMBER 11 - 15
AND AGAIN ON DECEMBER 9 TO 13
GOL
MINISTRY OF HEALTH AND SOCIAL WELFARE
WORLD HEALTH ORGANIZATION
USAID
UNMIL
EUROPEAN UNION
PolioPlus
Rotary International

based on different indicators, data sources and aggregation methods.

Determinants of fragility include conflicts, weak institutions, external shocks, poverty, disease and regional instability.[2,4] It is the interplay of these determinants that establishes the outcome; dynamics can vary from one situation to another, even when key characteristics of fragility look similar. Drivers of dysfunctional governance are often self- and mutually-reinforcing: as a result, the rapidly changing environments pose additional challenges to policy-makers, donors and practitioners.

Before formulating recovery strategies, stakeholders should consider what the main characteristics of the given crisis are, and what the future country context might look like.

- First, whether the present turmoil is structural or transient should be assessed. Indeed, the recent turbulent history of the Darfur region of Sudan or that of the Democratic Republic of Congo, once appraised in a perspective of the past 100 years, suggests the presence of structural stressors that are not likely to recede anytime soon.
- Second, the odds that a legitimate, benevolent, performing state administration will eventually emerge from the protracted crisis need to be realistically evaluated.
- Third, the chances of a country already fragmented by violence remaining intact must be assessed. Eritrea and South Sudan succeeded in their quest for internationally-recognized statehood, and there are regularly other political formations in the world that aspire for their own independent statehood.
- Fourth, the economic prospects, the recovery (or not) of livelihoods, and the resettlement of displaced people and refugees have to be appraised.
- Finally, the supranational landscape needs to be understood: for how long will external actors remain involved in domestic affairs? Will donors support transition and health system development? Will neighbouring countries recover, or contribute to perpetuating the crisis? Whereas the Guinea-Liberia-Sierra Leone crisis complex seemed to be on its way to recovery before the 2014 Ebola outbreak, the one constituted by the Central African Republic, Chad, and the Darfur region of Sudan offers no such hopes.

The first step in health strategy development and planning is to analyse the broad context, identify the main characteristics of the crisis, and understand likely political and economic evolutions.

In situations where facts are scarce but rumours abundant, simplified narratives may displace more insightful interpretations and strongly influence the identification of policy and strategy priorities, regardless of the reality on the ground. Autesserre illustrates how in the case of the Democratic Republic of Congo dominant "frames" about the country have had a profound influence on strategies and practices, with unintended consequences.[5]

The limitations of current definitions and typologies suggest that effective health policies and plans need a contextual understanding vastly deeper than the one of the conventional Fragile state approach. We propose, therefore, an empirical typology of situations for adapted approaches to health policy and planning. This characterization, to be discussed in section 3.5, considers the country context, the political and health actors, and their interactions in health policy and planning. Fragile states' health systems are typified according to the capacity and resources made available, the legitimacy and commitment of the government and other power holders, and the other key health actors: donors, charities, international agencies and programmes, private providers, etc.

13.2 Aid in fragile states

In the aftermath of the September 11 events in the United States of America in 2001, the discourse on dysfunctional states has taken centre stage: "The threat of an excluded South fomenting international instability through conflict, criminal activity and terrorism is now part of a new security framework",[6] a sharp turn from the previous doctrine that preached the rolling back of the state. Consensus is now that "resilient" states constitute a prerequisite for international security, stability and market liberalization.[7,8] Given the mounting awareness of the costs and consequences of instability, the risk of delivering aid to weak countries has been accepted. And, in fact, peacekeeping operations absorb larger resources than development assistance: for example, the cost of UN peacekeeping forces in Liberia and Sierra Leone was five times higher than aid flows.[9]

By conflating different situations, the fragile states agenda confounds rather than clarifies the issues at stake.

Discordant voices on the fragile states concept, however, claim that: "current donor interpretations of fragile statehood are flawed, serving ... [the] demand for simplistic forms of information and generalization that lead to technocratic 'solutions' to complex political problems".[10] By conflating different situations, the fragile states agenda confounds rather than clarifies the issues at stake. Moreover, by putting the onus of fragility on the troubled country, such an approach absolves donor states of their responsibilities. Indeed, the permanent turbulence of Afghanistan cannot be understood without considering the chronic intervention of external powers in its internal affairs, a factor sidelined by the fragile states discourse.[11]

Concomitantly with the new interest of donors in fragile states, more aid has been directed to these environments.[12] However, aid selectivity has been applied also to fragile states: Afghanistan and Iraq absorbed 34% of the total increase in aid to fragile countries between 2000 and 2008.[13] The need for changes in the volume of aid and the ways to deliver it in fragile contexts has reached the top of the agenda of the international community. Recognizing the special challenges presented by fragile states, the Organisation for Economic Co-operation and Development formulated, in 2007, a set of general principles for "good international engagement in fragile states".[14] Four years later, the "G7+" group was instrumental in the development of a "New Deal for Fragile States"[15] that was endorsed in Busan in 2011. As with other global commitments, however, this proclaimed awareness needs to be translated into actual changes in donor practice, an occurrence not to be taken for granted given the inherent conservatism of the aid industry.

Appropriate approaches wanted

Under- or misgoverned countries test to the extreme the way the aid industry is structured and performs. The role of aid in fixing structural problems, such as those plaguing fragile states, is limited, as Rogerson highlights: "Development processes are led by complex, uncertain, context-specific social and political dynamics and responses to national challenges. ... Aid is marginal to these dynamics in most country contexts unless, by fortunate positioning or even accident as much as good design, it happens to align with them. In the best of circumstances, it provides some positive reinforcement".[16]

Thus, the applicability of the main aid agendas and instruments must be seriously reconsidered. For instance, the basic enabling conditions for achieving the Millennium Development Goals (MDGs) – such as trust, predictability, adequate information, a controlled environment and sustained investment – are not present. A critic of the MDGs agenda claims that the MDGs may be, if the situation does not change, "another major failure of the prescriptive approach to strategy".[17]

The Aid Effectiveness Agenda, as defined by the Paris Declaration and Accra Agenda for Action,[18] needs to be adapted to distressed contexts, where political leaders often give primacy to short-term political needs, rather than to development goals.[19] In contexts where ownership is found mostly in its informal and fluid variety, at local level and with private institutions delivering public goods, aid effectiveness cannot be pursued through feeble governments. In fact, the blind application of the aid effectiveness principles to the complex settings of Afghanistan, where strong local constituencies oppose the strengthening of the central government, has had unwanted but predictable effects, such as undermining peace-building and state-building efforts and even obstructing the emergence of an inclusive national ownership.[20]

In addition, pursued policies can bear little resemblance to official documents: donors risk aligning their programmes to unused country strategies that have been conceived only to satisfy politicians and foreign agencies. The politicization of these environments clearly influences the degree of attainable consensus, inclusiveness and partnership. Alignment cannot be pursued in light of the precarious conditions of indigenous institutions, the increased role of non-state actors to fill the gap left by weak health authorities and the shaky developmental role played by recipient governments. Meanwhile, harmonization, stated commitments notwithstanding, remains elusive. Finally, in fluid contexts, rational programming and management by results must be questioned as realistic decision-making options.

Aid management in fragile contexts must adopt modest, politically-informed, context-specific, and tailor-made approaches.

Despite their appeal, the merits of multi-donor trust funds (MDTFs) in such contexts must be questioned. In several cases, the high cost of establishing these instruments, their slowness in disbursing funds, and poor response to unforeseen events have hampered their potential returns. Time and again "standards and procedures difficult for highly developed regimes to follow have been imposed upon young public administrations to the sole benefit of international financial firms".[21] The recent experience of the MDTF in South Sudan has confirmed the inappropriateness of such instruments.[22] Interestingly, Liberia (one of the most successful post-conflict recovery processes before the country was hit by the Ebola outbreak in 2014) has preferred to reject the MDTF model, opting for more modest sector arrangements.[23]

Another barrier to aid effectiveness is represented by the customary split between development and humanitarian aid, which is inappropriate in chronically-troubled settings, where acute crises are recurrent. Afghanistan, the Democratic Republic of Congo, Haiti, Somalia and South Sudan call for constant, open-ended aid flows, which sustain both developmental and humanitarian actions, according to the needs and opportunities.

"In countries in which donor funds contribute a significant proportion of public health expenditure, public sector failure must be regarded as 'donor and international agency failure' as well".[24]

In order to support dysfunctional states, donors must dramatically overhaul their understanding of the operating context and discard blueprinted solutions.

Donors must accept their expanded responsibility in contexts where health authorities are unable or unwilling to play their official role. Accepting their expanded role, and taking full responsibility for failures, implies a thorough redesign of the way donors intervene in under-governed environments, and evaluate their performance. In many distressed contexts, donors are already dominating the health policy process through the financing lever they control, without being willing to acknowledge it. In other situations, external assistance shapes the health field, without encouraging a productive policy process, with facts on the ground preceding intentions. For instance, in Haiti, performance-based financing (PBF) was initiated in 1999 by one nongovernmental organization (NGO); later on, all the NGOs funded by the same donor were using this scheme.[25] It was only recently, however, that PBF was piloted in public health facilities and was officially acknowledged as a guiding principle for health financing.

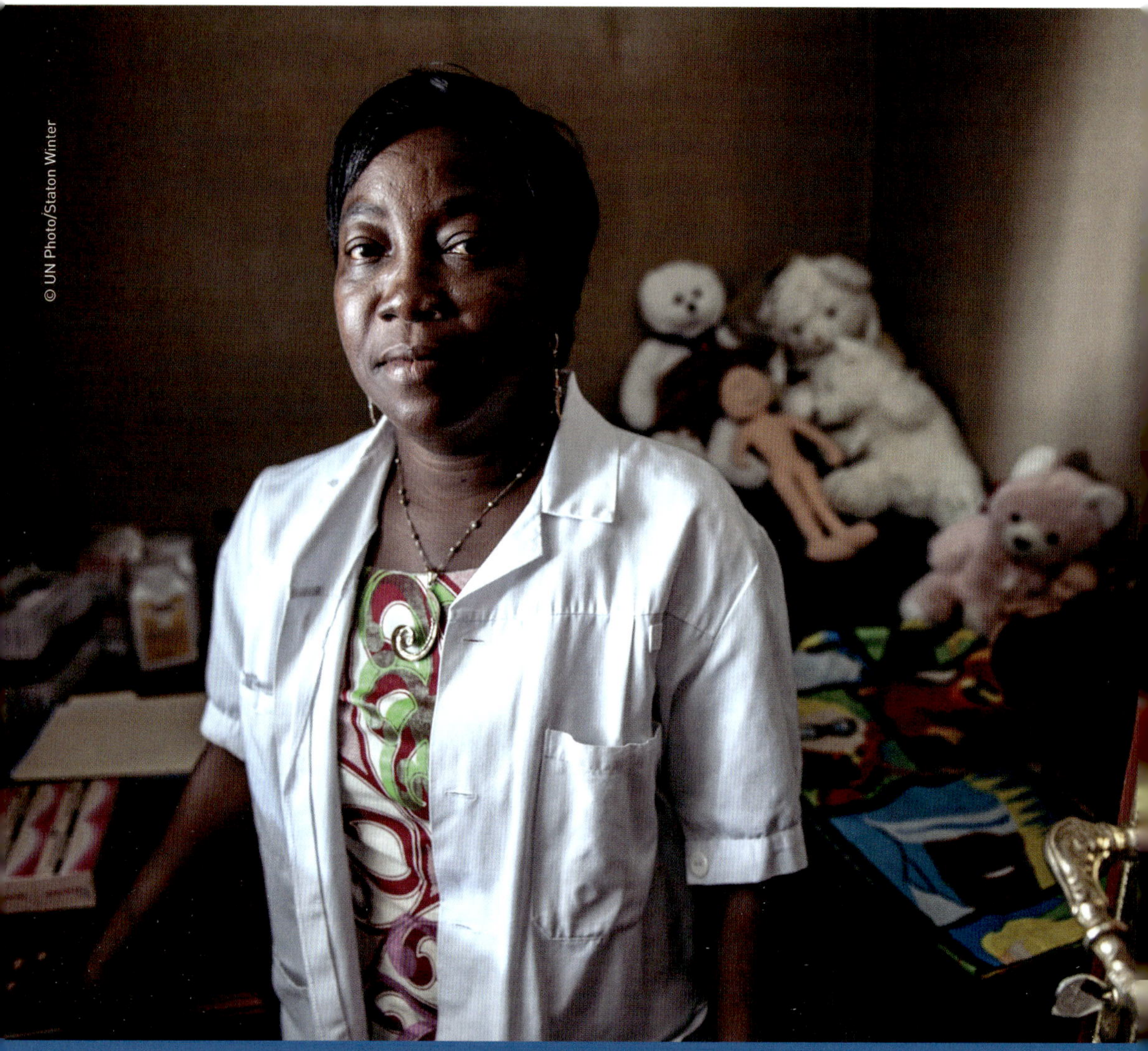

© UN Photo/Staton Winter

13.3 Health policies, strategies and plans in distressed settings

13.3.1 Context and actors

The analysis of the broad context of the crisis and its determinants – politics, economic and social aspects, and geography – is key to understanding which policies and strategies are feasible and have a chance of success. Fragile contexts are fluid, unpredictable, pluralistic, with huge variations within countries, and important trans-border links. In fact, the broader context shapes health care developments to an extent often unrealized by stakeholders. Thus, the neglect of social factors jeopardizes many health policy and planning efforts, as recognized with hindsight in Cambodia, where "it has most probably been the underestimation of the social impacts of transition that has been the 'missing piece' in recent national and regional policy analysis (which relies almost solely on epidemiological or technical health reference points)".[26] South Sudan's unravelling in 2013 provides a cautionary tale about investing in conventional health system development, without paying due attention to the precarious foundations on which the newborn state rested.

Among key contextual determinants, geography and the environment are frequently overlooked by health actors, despite their influence on events, and on the responses to them. Internal communications are as important as the links with neighbouring countries or regions. The Democratic Republic of Congo, with its poorly-connected populated peripheries and an empty core, is structurally fissiparous and opposed to centralized rule. Ecological factors, such as drought and desertification, alter established ways of living, and may extend or even perpetuate the crisis, as displayed in the Darfur conflict, which can be primarily read in environmental terms. Countries with a "difficult geography"[27] pose special challenges to state-builders, military commanders, revenue authorities and health planners.

Studying crisis complexes (e.g. the African Great Lakes and the Middle East), instead of single countries, provides a definite analytical advantage, in light of political, security, economic, ethnic, criminal and migratory links, which bind together countries officially separated by porous, arbitrary and often contested borders. Health services provision, too, is affected by supra-national factors, as people, germs, ideas, medicines, funds and health workers incessantly cross borders. The Ebola epidemic that ravaged West Africa in 2014 is a sober reminder of the inadequacy of a narrow focus on official state territories, rather than on populations. Unfortunately, most health management structures and health data are state-centric. Without additional analytical efforts "the geographical reorganization of health care within and across borders under conditions of war"[28] will be missed or misread.

Actors are an unruly mix of official and informal individuals and groups, enjoying different degrees of autonomy, entering and leaving the health arena, often playing multiple roles. Health authorities, state agencies, donors, international organizations, disease-control programmes, charities, NGOs, private entrepreneurs, health workers, professional associations, political parties, activist and opposition groups, all affect health care developments, sometimes explicitly but often quietly. Understanding their roles, links, networks, power and influences in the health system is critical; new approaches have been used to map out relationships between players.

The analysis of the context must be comprehensive, including all factors that can influence the development and then implementation of health strategies. This analysis requires analytical skills, a substantial investment in time and resources and a consultation process, whose modalities depend on the specific political context.

13.3.2 Information, the foundation of the policy and planning process

Since the picture is blurred and quickly changing, making sense of it and identifying trends is paramount. Assembling a reliable situation analysis entails adapted efforts, given the poor information base, the fluid context and the inadequate capacity of health actors to collect useful data, monitor trends and understand macro events and developments, both general and health-related. Penetrating messy realities requires deciding which data should and could be collected and analysed, their level of disaggregation, and their quality and limitations. The trends, patterns and relationships have to be understood, and the findings of the analysis shared in a meaningful and accessible way. Pre-crisis baseline indicators are often absent or too weak for a valid trend analysis; comparison with available data from relevant contexts becomes, therefore, crucial.

In many troubled health systems, the available information is quite rich, contrary to what is usually admitted.

In many troubled health systems, the available information is quite rich (contrary to what is usually admitted), but is dispersed among agencies, programmes and institutions and compiled in assorted formats according to narrow interests, such as disease control or population groups. Many participants hold a detailed knowledge of specific aspects, but lack an understanding of sectorwide characteristics and trends. Assembling the discrete pieces of information may go a long way towards producing a comprehensive picture, whose contours and internal relationships may have been missed even by the most informed actors. Keeping the picture updated is essential. Robust situation analyses have been produced in Afghanistan, Somalia, Sri Lanka, and in the Darfur region of Sudan, but the evolving context requires frequent revisions and adjustments.

A valid situation analysis helps to identify key issues of the health system to be addressed, and to choose between alternative courses of action. Health systems under stress exhibit recurring features, such as privatization and commoditization, urban and hospital biases, poor-quality care, a bloated but unproductive workforce, dysfunctional referral flows, and/or derelict infrastructure. These key issues must be clearly singled out by the situation analysis, and consistently tackled by any valid policy or strategy.

The process of building the situation analysis by putting together pieces of intelligence from different sources has to be iterative. Each round will produce a stronger analysis, single out new aspects to be investigated, and point to measures to be introduced. Once the main health policy and planning issues characterizing the health systems are recognized, the need must be determined for policy-oriented studies to help decision-makers appraise existing problems and options, and to bring attention to aspects that have been neglected. For instance, counterfeit medicines are reckoned to circulate freely in most under-regulated pharmaceutical subsectors. However, the evidence for this claim is frequently inconclusive. The severity of the problem should be assessed through a dedicated study, before corrective measures are discussed and introduced. In this way, a baseline would be set, and the relative weight of this issue would be appraised in comparison to other competing problems.

Common challenges in stable contexts – such as the changing environment, fragmentation, insufficient implementation capacity, extreme politicization, the actions of non-state actors, and the frequent turnover of players – are amplified in distressed environments, resulting in a disconnect between official policies and reality. For example, many countries give stated priority to primary health care, whereas in practice the bulk of the resources are absorbed by large hospitals. Analogously, even donor agencies that recognize the primacy of context in policy-making and planning, and the need to strengthen whole health systems, may direct their funding to vertical disease-control programmes despite their relative lack of importance at country level.

Furthermore, path dependency, i.e. how past health policy/strategy choices influence future options, has to be taken into account. Documenting past experiences may teach valuable lessons about approaches adopted and discarded, and later adopted again. For instance, many health systems have made repeated attempts with community health workers, each round looking strikingly similar to previous ones. Due to lost memory, continuous reshuffling of decision-makers and new international fashions, the same mistakes recur time and again. Analysing past health policies and strategies gives important clues,[29] including power relationships among key health actors and resistance (or receptiveness) of national authorities to change. In most health systems, the medical lobby enjoys a strong influence, which helps explain certain patterns, such as adopted service delivery models and financing mechanisms.

Conventional opposition terms, such as private/public, formal/informal, foreign/domestic, qualified/unqualified, traditional/modern, legal/illegal, look inapplicable and devoid of meaning in most circumstances. This calls for a redesign of the way data are collected and analysed. Many internationally-accepted data collection procedures are ill-suited to these environments and need to be adjusted. Adapted definitions are needed, so that data shed light on problems, rather than obscuring them. For example, the recognition that most health workers fall between the two poles of qualified and unqualified should help conceive definitions applicable in the majority of situations. Removing (or qualifying) value-laden concepts, such as corruption, from the analysis should in principle focus attention on actual patterns of health care provision, and their effects.

In distressed contexts, information must be assembled from different sources in an iterative process. Methods and approaches for data collection must be adapted to the often insecure and partly inaccessible context.

Routine information systems, even if they generate usable outputs, tend to neglect private, informal, illegal and folk health care provision, capturing only the small portion of the whole health system that is amenable to orthodox definition. Dedicated surveys applying specially tailored methods are needed to explore the large constituents of health services customarily missed. Otherwise, standard surveys carried out in troubled contexts will generate implausible findings, as happens frequently with National Health Accounts, or Demographic and Health Surveys. These surveys also have problems of representativeness, since some areas can be inaccessible for security or other reasons. Unless unconventional health care is brought to the fore, and its role(s) in the whole field understood, no meaningful sectorwide policy can be conceived, nor can a plan be successfully implemented.

Caution is in order about the soundness of situation analyses that may be based on incomplete and weak data, and fail to reflect true patterns and trends. Collected to satisfy the needs of agencies remote from the field, it is tempting for such analyses to portray the situation in convenient (when not misleading) terms, simplifying disorder and suggesting comfortable ways to deal with it. Fund-raising and reputation pressures encourage the production of reports claiming progress in the health field, amidst a deteriorating political and security situation (as in Afghanistan). To be truly helpful, a solid situation analysis should try to debunk any circulating "social facts", i.e. "things that are deemed to be 'true' because they are widely believed to be true".[30] Its factual foundations must be rigorously ensured, and their limitations acknowledged.

Recognizing diversity

Health systems development is impacted by long distances, poor communications, violence, market forces, demography, actors, climate and inadequate resources and capacity. The customary portrait of a "*national health system*" with a national health policy and strategy should be viewed with caution. Different patterns of health care provision are usually recognizable, if sufficient analytical efforts are made. Assorted local health care arrangements emerge and coexist, sometimes unnoticed (or reluctantly acknowledged) by official sources. In light of such spontaneous diversification, sectorwide analyses must be assembled bottom-upwards, by studying as many distinct local situations as possible, and refraining from countrywide generalizations, such as those based on average indicators, which can hide rather than reveal the variations existing on the ground. The health system under scrutiny has therefore to be seen as a constellation of differentiated regions, each evolving at its own pace and often in diverging directions. Strategies, interventions and service delivery models should be diversified to take advantage and respond to local needs, demands and opportunities. Likewise, "national" programmes should adapt to multiple under-governed environments. For example, different service packages need to be provided to high- and low-density communities, and to nomadic groups.

Strategies, interventions and service delivery models should be diversified to take advantage and respond to local needs, demands and opportunities.

Monitoring and evaluation

Monitoring and evaluation must be continuous, and feed decision-making in order to adjust strategies or plans in real time. Indeed, "a large part of the information needed for implementation is generated along the way, making it essential that plans are more adaptive to unfolding realities".[31] The resource implications of a strong and continuous monitoring system should be considered in the early phases of planning: "Less time and resources should be spent on upfront planning and more on processes to monitor and feed back learning from implementation".[32] Monitoring trends is essential to capture the progress registered in enforcing policies and implementing plans. Population figures are, in many settings, absent, volatile or vulnerable to manipulation. Trends would be more reliably monitored by using absolute output figures than through coverage rates or measures of impact.

A sectorwide perspective, which identifies and tracks unexpected events and processes as much as planned ones, must be adopted. In fact, certain important developments – such as private provision, dual practice, sub-standard goods and services and trans-border activities – may escape official recognition, despite their impact on service delivery.

Indicators are not only monitoring tools

They also may affect management decisions. Some services, or aspects of services, that are closely monitored by health authorities or international bodies (usually because they are easier to measure), are given more attention than others, regardless of their relative importance on the ground. Note also that the awareness of being monitored encourages cheating, particularly if reported figures are linked to incentives.[33] Indicators given special importance by central authorities may affect peripheral decisions. For example, the Sudanese Federal Ministry of Health (MoH) relies on ratios of health facilities to population to gauge the offer of basic services across the country. In the violence-plagued region of Darfur, this indicator cannot be relied upon, due to the lack of reliable census data, the displacement of large populations and the services provided by NGOs in IDP (internally displaced persons) camps. Furthermore, many facilities are substandard and frequently contiguous. In 2012, only one third of hospitals performed caesarean sections, while only one third of health centres had a laboratory; only a minority of health facilities had electricity and safe water.[34] The rational response to such shortcomings would be to close down redundant and underused facilities, in order to raise the capacity of the rest to acceptable levels. This move would improve actual access to services, but would also worsen population ratios. As such, it would not appeal to local managers keen to feed central health authorities with improving, rather than worsening, ratios.

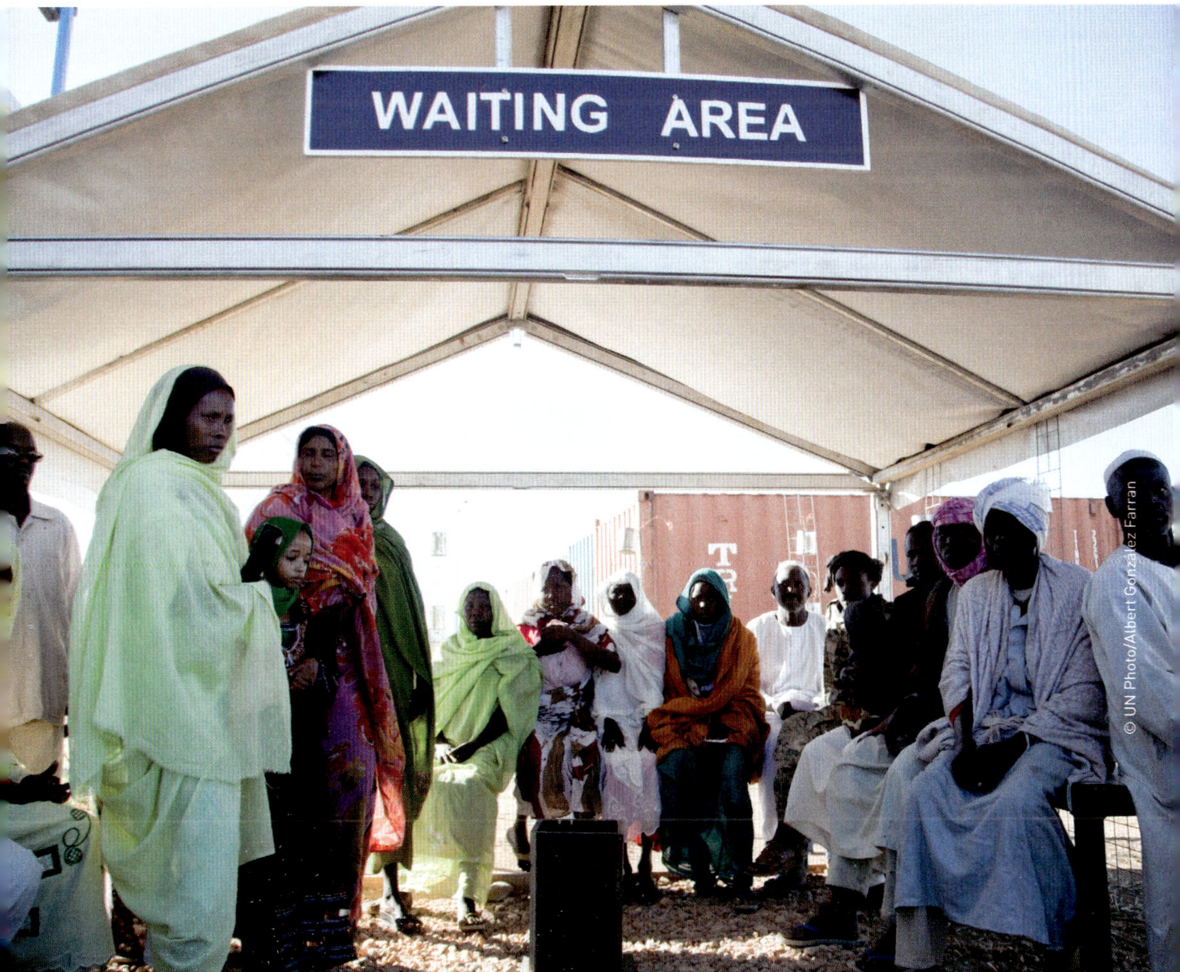

13.3.3 General principles

Negotiating health policies and plans

Successful strategies and plans cannot be imposed: they have to be negotiated with key health actors to have a chance of being successfully implemented. Flexible plans and learning from experience during their implementation allow for adaptation and adjustments.

Policy-making and planning in health systems under stress are "an inherently political process"[35] which involves negotiating realistic problem-oriented measures with autonomous stakeholders: "making and implementing strategy among a set of heterogeneous actors subject to a multitude of pressures and priorities is ultimately an act of continuous interpretation".[36] In these situations, it is not always easy to forge common goals; doing so can take up precious time and delay action, especially if tensions are high between stakeholders.

While policy papers and plans are written, facts on the ground are consumed, affecting the directions taken by health services. For example, many MoHs are keen to formulate idealized basic packages of care, while private and public facilities provide very different mixes of services. Or diaspora benefactors finance new health care outlets according to considerations other than rationalist planning criteria. Policies and strategies are often formulated without understanding the issues at stake, neglecting the feebleness of top-down controls and implementation capacity, and ignoring the action of other players, in settings where uncertainty and instability prevail.

Furthermore, overly optimistic forecasts of the outcomes of strategies and plans are common, driven by political factors or the desire to mobilize additional resources. "The world of strategy is full of disappointment and frustration, of means not working and ends not reached".[37] Policy-makers and planners deprived of resources and power in difficult environments for many years are invariably frustrated and cannot be the most innovative professionals. They must be supported and provided with financial and career incentives to regain confidence that policies and plans stand a chance of being successfully implemented.

In distressed settings, health system developments can be influenced, but not controlled: "by and large, strategy comes into play where there is actual or potential conflict, when interests collide and forms of resolution are required".[38] Some actors enjoy too much power and autonomy to be coerced into prescribed behaviours. Their collaboration must be obtained through compelling ideas based on sound information, coherent behaviour, and open negotiations about mutual benefits, using "the art of seduction. If you want to get others to accept your strategy, seduce them (so to speak)".[39] Policies, strategies, goals, procedures, approaches and indicators must evolve in accordance with the changing environment, while incorporating the experience acquired hands-on, and the fresh information generated by implementing the chosen measures.

Where central control is weak and formal strategy processes are marginally influential, strategies "emerge"[40] almost spontaneously, as a result of decisions taken at different levels of the health system, until a new pattern is recognizable and identified as a new strategy. For instance, the enhanced role of community health workers (CHWs) in service provision can be the result of training activities carried out by different actors at the periphery, until health authorities formalize the reality of these new "cadres". In the same vein, the famed Zone de Santé approach emerged in the former Zaïre, now the Democratic Republic of the Congo, as an effective ground-level response to a management vacuum, formulated by local actors endowed with capacity and resources.

Looking into the future

Crisis settings characterized by turbulence, unexpected discontinuities and uncertainty, amplify another inherent difficulty of policy and planning: to produce accurate forecasting of how the context will evolve and strategies and plans will unfold. Unforeseen changes in security, in donor priorities, in the price of commodities and thus in domestic revenues etc. can disrupt the implementation of strategies in ways impossible to predict when they were formulated. For example, the crisis in Mali at the beginning of 2012 was largely unexpected, as was its precipitous unfolding: the operating environment in the conflict-affected north changed overnight, and health care provision had to adjust to it.

As a result of the uncertainty, the temporal horizon of strategies in turbulent settings should contract, with proximate objectives and mechanisms for revising policies and strategies in place: "The more dynamic the situation, the poorer your foresight will be".[41] In particularly unstable situations, the absence of a prescriptive strategy can represent an advantage, allowing for more flexibility and easier learning and adaptation: "setting oneself on a predetermined course in unknown waters is the perfect way to sail straight into an iceberg. Sometimes it is better to move slowly, a little bit at a time, looking not too far away but very carefully, so that behaviour can be shifted on a moment's notice ... strategies are to organizations what blinders are to horses".[42]

Giving purpose to a fragmented field

Decision-makers must be opportunistic, focusing on the feasible, which is usually distant from the desirable: "plans should be light and imaginative, as they are primarily communication tools between involved actors".[34] Drawn-out, cumbersome formulation processes tend to exhaust participants through endless negotiations and the fruitless search for perfect configurations. Once approved, such policies and plans risk remaining on paper.

The challenge is to give a sectorwide purpose to assorted measures taken because they are considered feasible. Clarity of long-term goals must govern decisions that are in large part reactive rather than planned. Even modest success may attract other players, and generate the willingness to tackle more difficult issues. Partners should seek concrete responses to real problems, which bring benefits to the whole system and stand a chance of working even in a possible worst-case scenario. For example, the establishment of a non-profit pharmaceutical supply agency, able to import and distribute low-cost quality medicines would benefit the whole health care system, as was the case with ASRAMES (Regional Association for the Supply of Essential Medicines) in eastern Democratic Republic of Congo in its first years of life.

Crisis settings are characterized by turbulence, unexpected discontinuities and uncertainty.

Realistic policy-making and planning are premised on the appraisal of resource and capacity constraints. Maximizing the returns of finite resources and scarce capacity is the essence of sound practice. Conversely, trying to address all health needs, by definition infinite, without prioritization, is futile. Needs are usually invoked as the overarching criterion of many policy and planning efforts, but their satisfaction is negated by real-life constraints. Because of resource and capacity determinants, as well as donor interests, the costs of reconstruction of health systems produced by Post-Conflict Needs Assessments are vastly different, despite their intention.[43] In each assessment, the proposed interventions were envisioned according to the varying resource package expected to become available, not according to the health needs of the affected population, which would arguably differ less from one country to the other.

The formulation of delivery strategies for a health service never starts with a blank sheet of paper.

"The formulation of delivery strategies for a health service never starts with a blank sheet of paper. The present service exists, in whatever form that may be, and the MoH will want to maintain continuity wherever possible".[44] Recurrent funding tends to follow implanted capacity (i.e. investment decisions). Redistributive policies have to be pursued by applying different growth rates to competing health care components, within forecasted total resource constraints. A severe, protracted crisis, by crippling the old architecture of an affected health system, may offer opportunities to design a new one. At the start of the Liberia recovery process, the wrecked condition of the most sophisticated tertiary facility in the country gave health authorities room to invest resolutely on primary health care (PHC), unencumbered by the pressing capacity and resource demands the tertiary facility would have made if it were functioning.

Health systems in these contexts are fragile: they are not suitable to radical and rapid reforms.

Bottom-up planning focused on strengthening structures already in place, integrating them into a functional system, and establishing new ones as the case permits, is usually more valuable than labouring over a grand national plan with a distant time horizon (which may miss the internal diversity of the health system, and risks remaining on the drawing board). In many contexts under stress, the most promising level for pursuing the rationalization of health service delivery seems the provincial or local one. Here, at a pragmatically-decentralized level, information shortages can be addressed, political dynamics can be understood and taken into account, results can be monitored and informal management practices harnessed to positive effect.

Keeping a systemwide perspective

Even simple measures targeting one aspect of service delivery may have system-level effects, which have to be considered when they are conceived and later evaluated.[45] Changing one component of a complex system triggers a readjustment of its functioning. The new level attained may deliver the desired result, but with unexpected side effects or no recognizable effect. Thus, the effects of introducing a change in a subsector must be appraised across the whole health system. For example, physical investment impacts on the number and skill mix of human resources, the supply of medicines, the support systems and, last but not least, the future recurrent costs. Historically, there have been many examples of donor support to narrowly-conceived investments, without any consideration of their effects on the whole health systems, mainly in post-conflict reconstruction.

Questioning the conventional planning approach

Most strategy-formulation processes start by defining a vision, identifying objectives and then describing the ways and means to reach the end goals, but "a strategy that starts with objectives and works backwards is one that is likely to fail".[46] In fact, particularly if the strategy is for the long term, unexpected events will disrupt the envisaged path in its implementation. Freedman argues that "strategy is often expected to start with a description of a desired end state, but in practice there is rarely an orderly movement to goals set in advance. Instead, the process evolves through a series of states, each one not quite what was anticipated or hoped for, requiring a reappraisal and modification of the original strategy, including ultimate objectives".[47] Adaptation to the evolving context and learning from experience are key: "the more complex and elusive our problems are, the more effective trial and error becomes. Yet it is an approach that runs counter to our instincts, and to the way in which traditional organisations work".[48]

Enforcement and implementation

Enforcement and implementation are the most formidable phases for policies and plans. But they are also the stages of the whole cycle when more learning can be achieved. Resources, capacity and political attention are needed at this stage to a larger extent than during the formulation phase. A serious shortcoming recurring during the implementation of policies and plans is the inability of decision-makers to assess the actual results. Budget formats may impede the identification of allocative choices, administratively-aggregated data may hide inequitable outputs, and the prevailing fragmentation may blur sectorwide patterns, such as the deployment of the health workforce. Policies and plans must devote serious attention to the indicators to be collected in order to monitor their implementation, to the mechanisms needed to ensure such monitoring, and to making the necessary adjustments.

Building implementation capacity on the move

Policies and plans should deal not only with the features to be acquired by the health system, but also with the role of health authorities in the new political, administrative and financial settings, as well as the structures needed to play such role. A capacity assessment encompassing the whole health system must complement the situation analysis. In most cases, capacity will be regarded as inadequate if only official structures are considered. Expanding the scope of the assessment to cover private and informal operators will frequently modify the verdict. Realistic measures to boost capacity must be introduced across the constitutive elements of the health services provision system, to ensure that enacted policies are enforced and plans are implemented. Compelling plans may constitute powerful capacity-building enhancers.

Enforcement and implementation are the stages of the policy and planning cycle when more learning can be achieved.

Capacity-building traps should be avoided. State agencies are encouraged by international partners to acquire institutional capacity, by emulating the structure of their developed congeners.[49] This model usually translates into larger, structured institutions composed of many departments interacting through hierarchical rules. MoHs recovering from decades of disarray may see their premises, working tools and employees expand considerably. Their outputs, however, may not improve proportionally to the registered growth of their physical assets and to the related operating cost. In the Democratic Republic of Congo, such "institutional inflation"[50] was fuelled more by the lure of external assistance than by performance-enhancing considerations.

Everywhere, procedure-bound civil servants absorbed by internal activities or international events demonstrate a progressive loss of touch with reality. Ideally, a nascent or recovering MoH should be lean, responsive and competent. Given the degree of informalization and privatization attained in most settings, a problem-solving, task-oriented culture would be preferable to a rule-bound one. Some brains rather than many hands are needed to govern a health system under stress. High salaries delinked from civil-service rates must be paid to ensure a small group of highly-qualified and motivated cadres.

Prioritizing and sequencing

Prioritizing and sequencing the activities foreseen by a strategy or a plan is critical. Too many "strategic" documents are un-strategic in nature, presenting exhaustive lists of activities, without clearly prioritizing the order of interventions. No action ensues, as implementers are paralysed by the sheer quantity and difficulty of the actions included in such strategies and plans. Selecting the first steps to be taken, with added details about implementing practicalities and respective responsibilities, and setting realistic deadlines within a timeframe of 6–12 months, may trigger action, while offering indications about existing capacity and commitment. Clarifying priority actions may also help decision-makers react to unexpected shocks, such as funding cuts. For instance, if revitalizing referral capacity calls for the building and upgrading of 40 rural hospitals, choosing a subset of 5–10 vital facilities to benefit first will be useful in case of funding or implementation delays. The same rationale holds for human resources (HR) development: among the many categories of health workers to be trained, those most demanded by the services should be singled out by strategies and plans.

Prioritizing and sequencing first entails the scrutiny of the various actions included in the strategy or plan.

Prioritizing and sequencing entails first the scrutiny of the various actions included in the strategy or plan. Within their remit, some will logically precede others in the implementation. The sequence obtained in this way will have to be revisited in light of interventions already under way, some of which will mesh with the adopted strategy or plan, while others will not. Additionally, the funding in the pipeline must be explored, as some actions will materialize sooner than others. A round of negotiations with the actors involved will provide valuable indications for reformulating the original prioritization and sequencing. The resource and capacity implications of ongoing investments will have to be estimated, and budgets adjusted accordingly. For example, when the investments of agencies specialized in infrastructure and equipment have been decided apart from the sectorwide strategy, but are not at odds with it, modifying the latter to operationalize the former would make good sense. More demanding will be the handling of interventions impacting negatively on the adopted strategy or plan. In resource-poor settings, the typical occurrence is the building of a sophisticated facility, which would absorb or redirect most inputs and capacity, in this way enfeebling further the rest of the services. When negotiating a trade-off or a revision of the original decision is impossible, the only option may be to take a wait-and-see approach.

Planning for contraction

A special, largely neglected challenge is posed by a misalignment between health care supply capacity and the ability of a society to sustain it. A large supply capacity may have been planned in light of rosy economic forecasts, such as was the case in United Republic of Tanzania in the 1970s and 1980s. In other cases, the situation may have arisen spontaneously during years of laissez-faire, due to private initiatives. Or it may be due to oil-backed political expediency, as happened in Angola. Whatever the origins of an excess supply capacity, its correction is poorly served by orthodox policy and planning techniques (by nature, expansive), and clashes with inherently-conservative management habits.[51] Backing sensitive measures with credible information helps reduce the impact of the predictable backlashes. To contain political controversies, planning for contraction must be discreet; resource and capacity constraints can be artfully invoked to support downsizing measures. In this way, an oversized hospital may be "temporarily" rebuilt to half its original size, without attracting too strong objections.

Annex 13.1 proposes a simplified set of criteria for appraising a policy or a strategy.

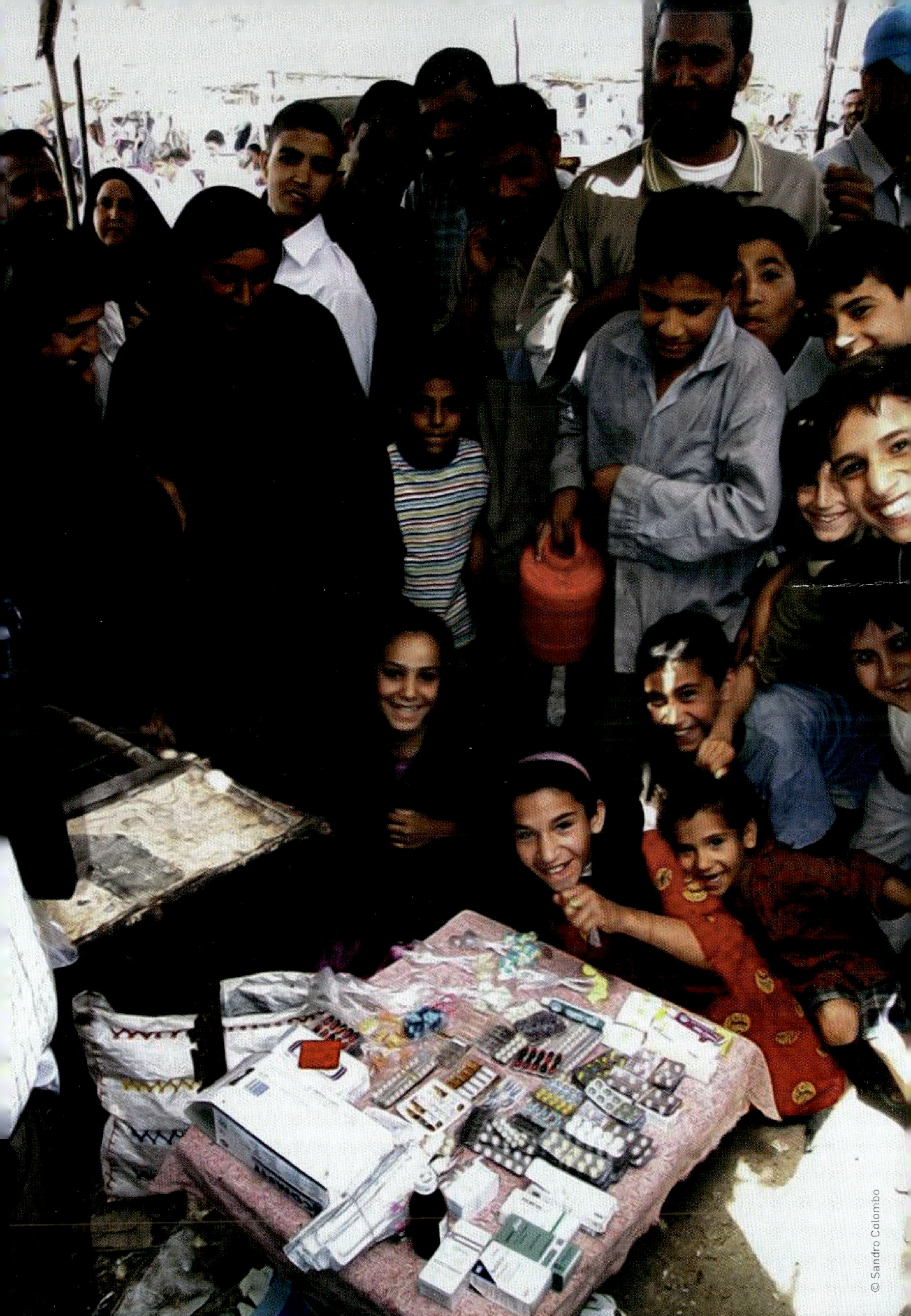

© Sandro Colombo

13.3.4 Learning from international experience

Radical reform approaches have a poor record in distressed contexts.

- Fast-changing environments offer opportunities for the testing of innovative approaches to health financing, delivery and regulation. But caution is in order: radical reform approaches have a poor record in distressed contexts. Newcomers are inclined to perceive the health space as open and advocate for hurried reforms, usually sold as unproblematic, easy fixes. This danger increases if the context improves and hopes of recovery start to be entertained by outsiders. Blueprinted, imported reforms are unlikely to take root in distressed health environments.
- Policy and planning standards borrowed from international models, usually premised on the assumption of stable and homogeneous contexts ruled by competent health authorities, appear inapplicable in light of the huge transformations caused by protracted conflict, state withdrawal and mass displacement. For instance, the accelerated and frequently forced urbanization of large rural populations is usually ignored by health policy and planning guidelines. The time-honoured operational district model is ill-suited to spontaneously-growing large cities, inhabited by mobile health customers with different purchasing power.
- Health authorities called to govern recovering health systems have often preferred to neglect their regulatory mandate, usually seen as thorny and unrewarding. Most have focused on direct health services provision, with lacklustre results. Health authorities willing to lead the sector might invest on regulation early, rather than contemplating its inadequacy later, when the stage has stabilized and introducing regulatory provisions would face even higher hurdles. Liberia deserves to be studied in its efforts to monitor and raise the service standards practiced in its facilities, through a quite sophisticated accreditation system.[52]
- Donor preferences, by stressing some components at the expense of others, are prone to distorting health service development. Proliferating "priorities" may overburden the health sector and undermine rational resource allocation. A review of "priority" areas must identify where efforts must be concentrated. Priority-setting is meaningful only when parsimoniously practiced. The purposeful collection of relevant information becomes a critical preventive strategy to ward off irrelevant "priorities".

- Donors do not generally transfer national ownership and leadership, unless they are proactively obtained by national health authorities. Successful takeovers, such as those witnessed in Liberia and Mozambique, have involved committed, realistic, coherent, open and frank national health authorities. On the other hand, genuine ownership may be manifested by indigenous choices, which may look unorthodox to international eyes, like the rejection of free-market pressures in Mozambique after the peace agreement, or the partial and temporary adoption of the performance-based financing model in Liberia during the transition to peace. If well justified, they may attract the support of true development partners. Ownership, as expressed by government bodies, should not be interpreted as popular ownership: global health policies adopted by national health authorities may be flatly rejected by a mistrustful population.
- In many post-conflict health systems, policy documents have been produced, with negligible impact on actual dynamics on the ground. Inadequate information, poor enforcement capacity and pressures from various interests can yield "decorative planning" or "planning as public relations".[53] Additionally, the merit of drawing up formal policies and plans in extremely informalized environments, such as Somalia, must be seriously questioned. Even no-nonsense, solid, context-grounded policy and strategy proposals may be ignored, if considered risky, unpalatable, or just unfashionable by the decision-makers concerned. All in all, investing scarce resources and capacity in writing elaborate policies and strategies, usually covering extended periods exceeding the decision-making and planning time horizon of most stakeholders, may be unwise. Conversely, an open-ended policy process may be more conducive to progress than a sequence of one-off policy papers: "strategy could never really be considered a settled product, a fixed reference point for all decision-making, but rather a continuing activity, with important moments of decision".[54]

In many post-conflict health systems, policy documents have been produced, with negligible impact on actual dynamics on the ground.

- After decades of profound disorder, the temptation of rebuilding a large public health care system is usually very strong. Several health recovery processes were guided by the assumption that a well-designed, adequately-funded and competently-run public health system would reclaim its traditionally-dominant role vis-à-vis private competitors who had expanded their share of the market during the crisis. The assumption applies to an even larger degree if the publicly provided services are geographically and financially accessible. Yet such a sensible rationalist assumption has been found wanting in a number of health systems already advanced in their recovery trajectory, such as Afghanistan and Cambodia. Private provision, far from shrinking as expected due to the resurgence of its public competitor, has thrived.[55]

Table 13.1 Proposed typology of health systems under stress

Countries in crisis require health strategy and plan approaches tailored to their dynamic context.

TYPE
Politically-legitimate but technically-weak government, with a ministry of health willing to lead health care developments
Absent, disinterested or resourceless government leaving both policy formulation and health care provision to other actors
Stable / peaceful but poor and vulnerable country, with health authorities unable to play a leading role in the health care field (despite their legitimate mandate)
Recognized central government, formally in charge of the health care field, but with contested regions and opposed by powerful donors on political or human-rights grounds
Permanent turmoil, with contested government, competing power holders, unresolved conflicts

13.3.5 Specific situations, calling for tailored approaches

Whereas most of the general principles covered in the previous sections apply to these situations, each of them demands dedicated approaches. The goals set and the methods adopted must be fine-tuned to match the respective contexts, the demands expressed, the risks incurred and the opportunities offered. This characterization (summarized in Table 13.1) is necessarily fluid, with countries moving from one group to another, and frequently back. In 2005–2007, Liberia changed, quite suddenly and to the surprise of many observers, in a favourable direction. Devastated by the Ebola outbreak, its health system has been pushed back. On the other hand, Syrian Arab Republic, for long considered a paragon of stability, has been engulfed in a vicious civil war whose end is not in sight, with a severe impact on its health system.

Politically-legitimate but technically-weak government, with a MoH willing to lead health care developments (e.g. Mozambique 1990–2000)

This privileged situation occurs only rarely. In many other countries, the hopes nurtured at the beginning of a perceived transition from turmoil to stability have been rudely frustrated. In Afghanistan, the unravelling of the political and military situation has jeopardized the advancement attained in the health systems. Elsewhere, a misreading of the picture by over-optimistic international partners has induced premature investments in MoHs not ready or interested in assuming a leadership role (beyond ritual but shallow gestures).

Working on the formulation of policies and plans can reveal the extent of the commitment of new or recovering institutions to play a constructive role in health care provision.[56] Signs of commitment would be the active participation of apprentice policy-makers and planners in discussions, arguments over competing priorities, curiosity in relation to alternative options, awareness of the field conditions in which plans would have to be implemented, concerns with the political implications and the technical challenges of the proposed measures. When these signs are recognizable in some key actors, a renewed effort in policy formulation and planning is warranted. Otherwise, a reappraisal of the whole health system is needed: perhaps the MoH is not (yet) the place where health care developments can be promoted and take shape.

Working on the formulation of policies and plans can reveal the extent of the commitment of new or recovering institutions to play a constructive role in health care provision.

A committed MoH is a necessary but insufficient determinant of progress in the health field. Other players influencing health systems development must be engaged, starting with powerful government agencies, such as the ministry of finance and the civil-service authority. Influential international bodies, like the International Monetary Fund and the World Bank, determine events to an extent frequently unrecognized by health stakeholders. For instance, if the number of public employees is part of an agreement conditioning debt relief, it is likely to be honoured regardless of health service needs. Global health initiatives tend to rely on their financial clout and proceed on their own, paying little attention to overarching policies and plans. To these official players, private ones must be added.

If progress is registered, thanks to sensible policies and plans, effective leadership and generous donor support, there is a real risk of the health field being overwhelmed with proposals, projects and pilots pushed by international agencies. The aid industry loves success stories, which are rare and usually oversold. Both Liberia and Mozambique quickly became "donor darlings", partly

The locally-embedded health systems that may have emerged in response to protracted stress should be supported with incentives and technical inputs.

due to the convincing policies and plans they formulated. Large aid flows followed, spurring an impressive growth, which vastly exceeded the modest original expectations. In both cases, developments diverged markedly from the planned goals.

Absent, uninterested or resource-less government, leaving both policy formulation and health care provision to other actors

(e.g. Somalia since 1991)

Such situations create room for experimenting with alternative approaches. Intelligence from the field should inform discussions among decision-makers, in order to identify encouraging approaches and/or to avoid the replication of less successful models in the absence of serious evaluations. Ideally, policies and plans should aim to harness spontaneous events by apportioning tailored incentives. These in turn should be continuously adjusted, in light of the effects detected in the health system.

However, such a sensible, down-to-earth approach is rarely adopted. Without government oversight, different approaches are applied by external agencies at the periphery, without learning from their implementation and open discussion of the results at country level, and only positive findings are published in scientific journals. In these situations, policy transfers pushed by strong agencies — such as PBF in the Democratic Republic of Congo — can give unsatisfactory results because, contrary to other countries where they have been relatively successful, key enabling factors are simply not in place.[57] But, as observed in Haiti, lack of positive evidence is not enough for a powerless MoH to reject a strongly-advocated and generously-funded approach.

In most cases, the overall situation will remain precarious: fragmented health management arrangements with inefficient operations will result in unequal access to poor-quality health care. Given the likelihood of protracted turmoil, health services should maintain a degree of redundancy (to withstand recurrent shocks). For example, several mid-sized hospitals might be better adapted to an open-ended crisis than a large and sophisticated referral one, which would be more vulnerable and less accessible. Moreover, health services need to maintain some autonomy from the state, itself a source of troubles. Private management with a public-good orientation may constitute a sensible alternative: in northern Uganda in the 1970s and 1980s, faith-based facilities provided most of the health services. The locally-embedded health systems that may have emerged in response to protracted stress should be supported with incentives and technical inputs.

Stable/peaceful but poor and vulnerable country, with health authorities unable to play a leading role in the health care field

(despite their legitimate mandate)

In the absence of financial means to develop health services provision, nor to shoulder the future recurrent expenditure generated by such development, health policy and planning may play a crucial role, provided they are sensibly practiced. Credible policies and plans that are actually used to make decisions may influence partners' behaviour and provide negotiating levers with other influential government bodies. They may give credibility and leverage to otherwise powerless health authorities, and reassure donors about their good faith and commitment. External funds may in this way be tapped, sometimes surpassing both expectations and absorption capacity. By attracting competent international professionals, acted-upon policies and plans may help the health sector acquire badly-needed skills.

A feeble MoH might improve its reputation and clout by investing its scarce capacity in policy and planning, rather than in administration. Such an institution might lead by superior knowledge and a compelling vision, even without harnessing sufficient funds, nor enforcing capacity. These enlightened health authorities should remain aware of their future limitations, and avoid burdening themselves with excessive duties. Donors, too, would be wise to refrain from shouldering unsustainable investments. In a country vulnerable to shocks, financing and management responsibilities should be distributed among public and private actors, mostly assumed at local level, in order to inject flexibility and resilience in the health care provision system. Financial squeezes, epidemics, natural disasters, refugee inflows, and/or social upheavals will certainly strike: the stronger, more responsive and distributed the future system becomes, the more it will be able to react successfully.

Whatever the wisdom of adopted policies and plans, it may prove difficult for them to withstand pressure from various concerned parties. The modest goals praised on technical grounds may be criticized, and the unmet needs of the population may be invoked to launch ambitious programmes. That such forward leaps failed in the past to attain their goals and were not sustained is usually ignored by domestic, as well as foreign, actors. Producing reliable information in formats understandable to different stakeholder groups may help defuse some negative reactions. In the end, vested interests, ideology, convenience or fashion will regularly overrule decisions suggested by available evidence.

To withstand frequent shocks, financing and management responsibilities should be distributed among public and private actors, mostly assumed at local level.

Recognized government, formally in charge of the health care field, but opposed by powerful donors on political or human-rights grounds

(e.g. Myanmar until 2012)

Policy and strategy formulation in these contexts tend to be a domestic affair. For political reasons, donors usually refrain from being involved in these processes, when they are not barred from them. With aid channelled to NGOs mainly for relief and/or using separate management instruments, limited resources reach government health services. The formulation of humanitarian and recovery strategies is usually managed by the UN, with a formal, but token participation of the government. Coordinating aid-supported health care provision is even more difficult than in other settings.

Policy-making and planning are essentially window-dressing processes, with vision, goals and principles often detached from reality, or referred to privileged parts of the country. Strategies aim at conveying the sense of central control, even in a federal system like Sudan, where decentralization has been more the result of "laissez-faire" unwritten policies and practices than design. On the other hand, the low status assigned by the government to health care provision gives some room for manoeuvering (to be discreetly and ambiguously enjoyed) to the players engaged.

In sensitive contexts, such as Darfur, state authorities and aid agencies are forced to cohabitate in tense, awkward terms marked by mutual distrust. Heavy restrictions, imposed by government, donors, rebels, militias and criminals curtail the actions of health care providers. Activities on the ground depend more on their feasibility (once all the restrictions are taken into account) than on official policies and plans.

Activities on the ground depend more on their feasibility (once all the restrictions are taken into account) than on official policies and plans.

Independent research is hampered by danger and restrictions. Such weak grasp of actual features, events and trends in the health care field undermines policy discussions, which tend to become theoretical rather than factual. The fear of eliciting negative responses inhibits frank debates, while valuable data are not circulated as they should be. Thus, monitoring and evaluating health care developments is all the more arduous. Without an appraisal of the effects of the introduced measures, new mistakes will follow old ones, and go unrecognized.

Myanmar has long presented a peculiar pattern of segregated health services, induced by its political geography. On the one hand, the central valley was served by flourishing private health services, with limited public contributions and a constrained role for aid agencies. Meanwhile, humanitarian agencies based across the borders were offering health care to refugees, and supporting mobile health workers inside the country. Facts on the ground prevailed over policies and plans. Furthermore, while health services provision inside Myanmar was poorly documented, humanitarian cross-border health services were studied in detail. A similar split of health services provision across political and military frontlines was recognizable in Afghanistan during the Soviet intervention, in southern Sudan before the peace agreement and the ensuing secession, and in the West Bank and Gaza Strip (with the unique characteristics of this permanent crisis).

Protracted turmoil, with contested government, competing power holders, unresolved conflicts

Classical policy formulation and planning sit uneasily in such contexts. On the one hand, even the best-intentioned policy proposals (a rare occurrence in such circumstances), once issued by a contested government will be rejected by the opposition, or viewed with suspicion by mistrustful constituencies. UN agencies collaborating with such governments (as they must in light of their charter) may find themselves in an awkward position, as occurred in Darfur in 2006, when the UN were blamed for conducting a recovery-oriented needs assessment in the midst of increasing violence and political crisis, or in Syrian Arab Republic in 2014, where the World Health Organization (WHO) was criticized for its conduct in responding to the polio outbreak.[58] In these situations national and international agencies would need strong communication skills to manage perceptions and rumours fuelled by the prevalent mistrust in official

III and the twin Post-Disaster Needs Assessment, applied in natural disasters.

bodies. Many authoritarian states fare poorly in this respect.

On the other hand, the capacity of an embattled government to access territories and populations, to enforce any policy or plan, to allocate funds to the sector, to coordinate external agencies and to deliver services, is necessarily limited. With the emergence of regional or local governance arrangements de facto autonomous from the state administration, separated health policy and planning domains may take root (when the respective power holders are interested in health care provision). In some settings, such as in Iraq and the West Bank and Gaza Strip, costly trans-border referrals of large contingents of patients (in part financed by the public purse) have become established practice, by necessity if not by design.[59] Such a development is instructive of the gap that may open between conventional policy and planning habits and on-the-ground responses to shifting contextual determinants.

Even in the face of such constraints, abandoning any pretence of formulating policies and plans and falling back exclusively on pure humanitarian assistance, is unsatisfactory. The humanitarian response is needed to address immediate needs, but its drawbacks are well-known. If relief operations are left to provide health services without direction, fragmentation of services, inequality, egregious waste, high costs, inefficiencies and unstable delivery will follow. The aid system has formulated approaches intended to give coherence to its interventions, such as the post-conflict needs assessments.[III] Such exercises are nominally conducted jointly by the government and international agencies, but in practice are usually run by the latter. They have generated recovery strategies that have been at best only partially implemented, and in some cases not at all. Their main unstated purpose has been largely limited to raising political attention and funds for reconstruction. Indeed, many hoped-for peace processes have stalled, political interest has soon faded away and donor support has not materialized as expected; as a result, plan documents have been promptly shelved and forgotten. In some cases, the proposed recovery strategies were probaby too impractical to implement anyway.

A solid, continuously-updated situation analysis, understood in its implications, can encourage informed decision-making, and in turn foster some planning coherence.

In such trying circumstances, the stakeholders concerned cannot hope to unify an inherently fragmented field, but can attempt to encourage informed decision-making, so that some policy and planning coherence is fostered by converging interventions. For instance, autonomous players made aware of the comparative service deprivation of a certain region may opt for addressing such an objective gap. A solid, continuously-updated situation analysis, widely disseminated and discussed in its contents and strategic and operational implications, is perhaps the best result to be aimed for. To induce actors to design adapted, long-term responses, such analysis must factor in the enduring turmoil, rather than assuming unlikely turnarounds towards peace.

13.3.6 Essential aspects to be considered in relation to some subsectors

Health care financing

The chosen or – in many health systems under stress – the spontaneously established financing mechanisms affect all aspects of health care provision. The common occurrence of health professionals setting plans related to service delivery, while economists debate financing strategies, should be avoided.

In many settings, health expenditure reaches surprisingly high levels (for the assumed severity of poverty).

In many settings, health expenditure reaches surprisingly-high levels (for the assumed severity of poverty). Larger-than-expected private expenditure, remittances from abroad and aid inflows add together to attain quite respectable totals. In response to dwindling or absent public financing, private health spending is large in every situation where estimates were produced, be it Afghanistan, Liberia or the Darfur region of Sudan. The ability to pay for health care becomes the main determinant in a deregulated market. Inequities of access and inefficiencies of service production ensue.

Health expenditure figures are of dubious accuracy, and never complete. Gathering information on finances requires particular skills when national health accounts and expenditure reviews are not available, incomplete or unreliable. The study of aid flows to the health sector in Somalia is illustrative of the significant challenges encountered when analysing a complex health aspect in a complex environment.[60]

Expenditure levels appear to be rising everywhere. The mix of factors pushing expenditure upwards differ from one country to another, and even within the same country. Disease-control programmes, multiplying practitioners, easy access to medicines, the prominence of curative care, high-tech choices, referrals abroad (like in Iraq or the West Bank and Gaza Strip), and expensive humanitarian operations contribute to health spending inflation. Lebanon offers precious lessons about out-of-control health expenditure: "[The hospital] sector has been characterized by unplanned expansion and high-cost coverage, arising not out of health need but in order to maximize revenue. [...] the public sector, through its contracting arrangements, foots the largest share of the health bill".[61]

Public health financing is paltry in most under-governed health systems. Crippled public financial management systems thwart the spending of budgeted funds, particularly in insecure, remote regions lacking roads, banks, safes and telecommunications. When they are known, actual health expenses regularly diverge from budgeted amounts.

In many health systems under stress, official external assistance accounts for a sizeable proportion of total health expenditure – although not as dominant as perceived in aid circles, if private spending is taken into account. Aid flows support health services provision, through the formal financing of health activities, as well as informal resource transfers to indigenous entrepreneurs. The latter phenomenon (inadequately studied) helps explaining the buoyancy of the commercial segment of certain health care markets, such as those of Afghanistan and Somalia.

Private benefactors make in the aggregate a large contribution to health financing, using a variety of intermediaries: charities, foundations, international agencies, solidarity groups and political parties. The extreme dispersion and informality of many charitable transactions makes exploring their aggregate patterns labour-intensive and technically demanding. In contexts with a large diaspora, this sustains health services through direct initial investment, the recurrent support provided to facilities, donated equipment and goods, as well as voluntary short-term work. Remittances are also critical to enable destitute patients to buy health services that would otherwise be unaffordable. In most cases indistinguishable from profit-oriented operations, diaspora investments are prone to generate redundancies as well as gaps in health care provision.

Key considerations in relation to health care financing are summarized below.

- Discussions in this area tend to assume ideological tones, and to end inconclusively with pitting alternative options rarely appraised for their merits and drawbacks. Such options are often invoked in abstract terms, without considering their applicability to a given context. Thus, user fees may be banned without introducing alternative funding means; or a social health insurance may be recommended in the absence of the basic enabling conditions. Furthermore, market forces shaping the health systems are often overlooked when financing options are debated.
- Estimating the total future resource envelope likely to be allocated to health is the first step to be taken to ensure meaningful policy and planning discussions. Once a credible figure has been obtained, it has to be conveyed to the policy-makers concerned in such a fashion that they grasp the way it has been computed, its meaning and implications. In light of the enormous uncertainty of every forecast, boundaries can be set for future financing levels. Planning scenarios consistent with low- and high-level financing can then be sketched. These can be used as fund-raising levers, as well as to assuage excessive expectations. If additional resources are attracted in this way, the best-case planning scenario can be adopted; otherwise much more modest goals are preferable.
- In light of the large private expenditure characterizing many health care markets, a devoted study ranks among the most useful initiatives at the beginning of a policy and planning cycle.
- Service delivery costs need to be estimated, with a view at projecting the outputs to be produced for certain financing levels. Different delivery models should be considered in their different resource implications, together with the financial impact of high-tech approaches.

The dispersion and opacity of financing flows in these contexts makes studying their aggregate patterns and trends technically difficult.

Pharmaceuticals

The benefits of successful policies and interventions in the pharmaceutical area justify the risks incurred in addressing its main distortions and inefficiencies.

Where estimates of expenses on pharmaceuticals are available, they are consistently large, mostly shouldered by households, and account for a fat share of total health expenditure. Medicines are commoditized, with profit or affordability taking precedence over therapeutic indications. Self-medication is widespread. Substandard and counterfeit medicines circulate freely in most health systems, due to poor regulatory and management capacity.[62] Medicines play a central role in sustaining underfunded health services, frequently constituting the largest source of income for health workers officially earning meagre salaries.

Many countries under stress present thriving, if under-regulated, pharmaceutical markets. These are, however, poorly studied despite the visibility of import-export dealers, selling outlets and street vendors in most derelict settings. The informality of such pharmaceutical markets combines with their illicitness to cause challenges to researchers. The precarious conditions of many long-suffering states make the resuscitation of their border, law enforcement and regulatory functions unlikely. Depending on geography, under-governed pharmaceutical markets may acquire regional dimensions, with unchecked and unrecorded medicines supplying neighbouring (and sometimes distant) countries. This aspect is missed by most studies, which restrict their remit to national borders, despite the permeability of such borders to agents, money, goods, and diseases. Pharmaceutical policies and plans tend to suffer from the same flaw.

Public and private not-for-profit schemes have been set up to improve the situation, with questionable success. Revolving drug funds, central supply stores, and essential drug programmes have sooner or later run into trouble, sometimes inflicted by health authorities. Fragmented procurement and supply channels tend to prevail, with predictable effects on prices, availability and quality of medicines. The competitive edge of private for-profit dealers and vendors may be so strong that even public operators prefer to place their pharmaceutical orders with them. In some instances health authorities have interests in the commercial deals they are supposed to regulate. Furthermore, the highly informal operating environment, with its prevailing incentives, puts formal public schemes at a disadvantage.[63] In reality, the pressure to sustain health services through the sales of medicines encourages adoption by public providers of business-oriented practices akin to those of their private colleagues.

Understanding the characteristics, business models and the rules governing these pharmaceutical markets would greatly help public policy-makers in their quest for ways to regulate them. The intersections between multilateral, bilateral and private procurement and distribution have to be explored before realistic policies and plans are conceived and negotiated with the stakeholders affected by them. Realistic ways to manage the danger to public health caused by the unregulated supply and consumption of medicines, as well as to tap the potentials represented by this market, must be conceived, tested and adopted.

Formulating enforceable policies and implementable plans in these pharmaceutical areas is forbiddingly difficult. Some considerations should be kept in mind when engaging in this field.

- Given the interests involved, some political clout is needed to intervene with any chance of success. On the other hand, the benefits that successful interventions can induce in the pharmaceutical area are huge, thus justifying the risk incurred. Indeed, a hands-off stance should not be adopted, due to its ominous consequences for the whole health system: rising and inequitable health expenses, severe market distortions and potentially-dangerous health outcomes.
- Borrowing the models developed in more affluent countries is futile, as they presume substantial capacity, resources, and enforcement procedures. Most poor countries have imported pharmaceutical policies without the ability to enforce regulations; this often promotes corruption.
- The advanced privatization registered in many settings is probably irreversible. This market can be harnessed through positive incentives, rather than coerced. Effective incentives have to be negotiated with the operators concerned, so that mutually-acceptable trade-offs are struck. Informing the public, accreditation and franchising rank among the strategies to be considered.
- Every alteration in the economy of health services provision (salary levels, user fees, incentives, subsidies, financial management) affects the way medicines are traded and used. Measures targeting pharmaceuticals must be considered in a sectorwide perspective. Conversely, many interventions not directly related to medicines have an impact on their access, quality, and use.

Health facilities

The health care network is deeply affected by violence, under-resourcing, mismanagement and the reshaping of societal patterns, including altered livelihoods and population movements. Thanks to investments shouldered by charities, aid agencies, local entrepreneurs, politicians and the diaspora, it may expand in an unplanned and often undocumented way. Small, lightly-equipped facilities may come to dominate the landscape, as seen in Lubumbashi, Democratic Republic of Congo.[64, 65] Booming cities, such as Nyala in Darfur, present quite large health care networks, with sizeable hospitals. Clusters of redundant facilities can be found in comparatively-privileged areas, in contrast to investment-deprived ones. Underutilization is a recurrent pattern, due to a variety of factors deterring customers: user fees, poor quality of care, absent staff, unavailable medicines, lack of diagnostic capacity, competition among facilities, limited opening times, lack of transportation and insecurity.

Small, lightly-equipped health facilities may come to dominate the landscape in distressed contexts.

Inventories compiled by assorted agencies usually present grossly-diverging counts. Particularly at primary level, many ghost or derelict facilities may be included. Misclassification is a regular occurrence, for several reasons. Atypical health facilities diverging from the standards set by health authorities usually escape inclusion. Privately-owned facilities not subjected to regulatory criteria tend to evolve organically, adding revenue-fetching equipment and services whenever the opportunity arises. Their nomenclature varies, regardless of the services actually provided. Similarly, publicly-owned facilities fail to adhere to the standards implied by their official classification. Vertical programmes contribute to the diversification of health facilities, by strengthening selected services while ignoring others.

The health care network may look more akin to an archipelago than to the referral pyramid postulated by health authorities. In fact, proper referral paths may be negated by political and military barriers, by geographical, financial, and transportation obstacles, by misconceived guidelines, by perverse incentives, by violence, sectarian/ethnic mistrust and by partisan partition. In the end, referral flows depend more on customer opportunities and preferences than on provider decisions. In most distressed settings, health care is consumed locally, or conversely far away thanks to the mobility of its users.

Oddly, violence-affected locations may be better served than peaceful ones, owing to aid-backed investments: eastern Democratic Republic of Congo, Mogadishu and the Gaza Strip are instructive examples. Frequently, trans-border health-seeking movements account for a large if inadequately-quantified share of the health care market. Health statistics confined to officially-administered territories regularly miss, or misinterpret, actual service uptake on both sides of the border. Additionally, mutually-segregated health networks have emerged in some conflicts (Angola, Myanmar and South Sudan). This poses distinctive challenges to policy-makers and planners on each side of the frontline, who tend to ignore the events taking place beyond it.

Health care networks in fragile states should not be considered homogeneously; they present different mixes of services, staffing, ownership, utilization, and financing modalities across different regions.

Studying and planning the health care network as a homogeneous set is a common fallacy. In reality, it presents different mixes of services, staffing, ownership, utilization and financing modalities across different regions. When considering the public-private mix, different aspects must be considered before classifying a health facility: its ownership (official and de facto), its management, its financing and its modus operandi (health- or profit-oriented). Given the different combinations that are recognizable in the field, few facilities belong exclusively to one or the other category. In any case, as public and private health facilities tend to respond to similar commercial imperatives, the distinction becomes blurred.

Main considerations to be taken into account in relation to managing and planning health care facilities are listed below.

- The health care network can be meaningfully studied only through the formulation of empirical classification criteria that manage to capture non-standard facilities. Adopting functional criteria may dramatically modify the outlook of the whole health system. Interventions should be conceived starting with the actual situation on the ground, rather than with idealized patterns, such as basic packages of services.
- Rationalizing a fragmented health care network requires sustained efforts backed by flexible investments. Usually, it is preferable to start by supporting the functional recovery of favourably-located health facilities. Building of new facilities should be postponed until peripheral security improves, displaced populations resettle, and reliable demographic data become available.
- Maximum efforts should be made to ensure the accreditation and contracting of existing private health facilities, so that they are induced to provide public goods. Adequate funding modalities have to be introduced by governments and donors alike.
- Raising capital for investment is usually easier than covering the subsequent financing of recurrent costs.[66] Ensuring that adequate resources and capacity are deployed to

operate upgraded or new health facilities should rank among the top concerns of decision-makers.

- Big hospitals tend to remain the largest component (in terms of absorbed resources) of most health systems, stated policies notwithstanding. They are usually able to attract resources and capacity, therefore fuelling their own growth. Containing this spontaneous tendency is crucial to the development of a balanced health system, but is made difficult by several factors: political (prestige of local administrators), economic (due to the large investments implied), financial (opportunities for health workers to raise additional income) and expectations of local communities.

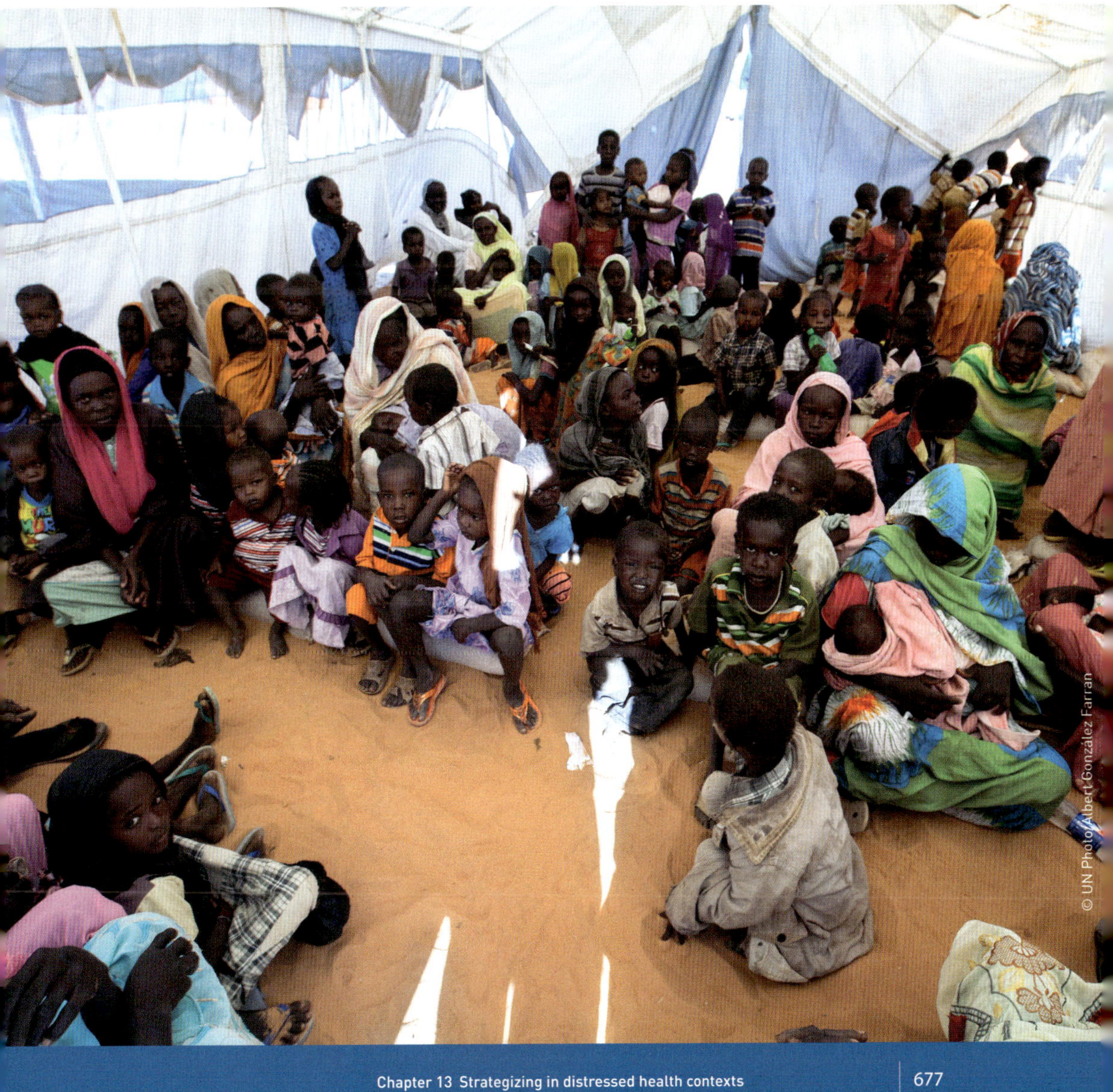

Human resources for health (HRH)

Human resources respond to stressors, individually as well as by professional groups. Coping strategies take precedence over other concerns. Looking for security, health workers move to safer areas. Public employees complement their shrinking earnings with private practice. Average productivity usually decreases due to reduced demand, overstaffing of secure health facilities, absenteeism, inadequate working tools and environment, poor or absent supervision, and low salaries. Professional skills across the workforce deteriorate, whereas they may improve in aid-supported secure spots. The number of unemployed professionals is usually unknown, but it is 'believed to be high in most cases.

Normative planning based on absolute needs should be abandoned in favour of contextualized criteria taking resource and capacity constraints into due account.

The workforce may contract due to death and outward migration, particularly where health workers have become political targets, as witnessed in Iraq and Syrian Arab Republic. Conversely, the over-production of under-skilled health professionals is recognizable in many under-governed health systems. In the Democratic Republic of Congo, this phenomenon has reached an extreme degree, with myriads of training institutions churning out crowds of job-seekers holding a health degree backed by precarious skills. In most under-regulated settings, training institutions largely financed by student fees offer courses demanded by applicants, rather than those needed by health services. A surplus of medical doctors and a shortage of nurses and midwives is the predictable outcome.

Public sectors hire large numbers of health workers, trying to absorb new entrants into the labour market, regardless of health service needs. Creating new positions and raising the funds needed to pay the related salaries appears to be one of the most pressing concerns of health authorities keen to gain political leverage and ensure loyal supporters. This trend is visible in many settings, with varying intensity depending on the financial position of public employers. In this way, an expanding workforce may absorb most of the scarce public funding for health.

Professional job titles tend to multiply, leading to overlapping, inconsistent categories. Civil-service payrolls give a very misleading picture of actual staffing patterns in public health facilities. On the one hand, ghost and absentee employees may constitute a large portion of the official ranks. On the other hand, many health workers without formal jobs may join their officially-employed colleagues, a frequent observation in the Democratic Republic of Congo. Personnel inventories are plagued with flaws, in most cases underestimating the actual number of active staff. In fact, not all practising health workers hold recognized qualifications. Some went through informal training initiatives, or formal programmes unrecognized by health authorities. Workers posing as qualified professionals, holding fake diplomas, or no papers at all, are common.

In some countries, health training programmes have been developed to satisfy the requirements of foreign labour markets. A health care career abroad is increasingly seen as an appealing prospect, given the scarcity of job alternatives in the home market. In countries with large diasporas, many health professionals have been trained abroad, and may return home to stay, or commute from and back to the country of settlement.

A gender bias may skew the production of health workers in favour of males. Once trained, the scarce female health workers are less likely to be deployed to hardship posts; in conflict-affected areas, the incurred danger curtails further the availability of female health workers, with severe effects on service provision. Such a staffing flaw is difficult to correct, due to a shortage of female candidates to health care training programmes, and cultural restrictions on the employment of women, common in many traditional societies.

Aid agencies have encouraged the training of community health workers (CHWs) in many contexts, despite the doubts about their effectiveness and cost, generated by past experiences. Reliance on these cadres appears questionable, given the limited support that weak formal health systems can ensure to these grassroots providers and the attrition caused by the lack of career and financial perspectives.

When formulating HRH-related policies and plans, some considerations are worth noting.

- Most health professionals surviving a protracted crisis need intensive and sustained retraining and skill upgrading. But before launching training initiatives, the actual job practice of assorted health workers, who cannot in most cases be barred from the health care market, needs to be empirically assessed.
- The management and regulation of HRH need as much attention as training.[67] Deployment, fulfilled tasks, workloads, terms of employment, incentives and career prospects rank among the key aspects to be assessed by HRH managers as well as by planners.
- A certification programme open to assorted health workers is one of the first steps to be taken in the resuscitation of a distressed workforce, as done in Cambodia and later in Afghanistan.[68] In the process, categories can be merged and upgrading training programmes introduced, in this way reducing the existing fragmentation. This exercise will generate a wealth of information useful for later HRH planning.
- The accreditation of health training institutions deserves adequate attention. In an open health care market, a reputable accreditation system may induce operators to abide by norms otherwise ignored. Where it cannot be enforced by feeble health authorities, a voluntary process can be offered. If the state is mistrusted or contested, an international body could be assigned this role.
- Normative planning, whereby the health workforce is projected to expand according to absolute needs, should be abandoned in favour of contextualized criteria taking resource and capacity constraints into due account. Indeed, different service models and health care networks have different HR requirements, whatever the served population is. Forecasted financing levels offer a much better guidance to HRH development than international norms (themselves the result of averaging vastly diverse situations).

Normative planning guided by absolute needs and international ratios should be abandoned in favour of contextualized criteria taking resource and capacity constraints into due account.

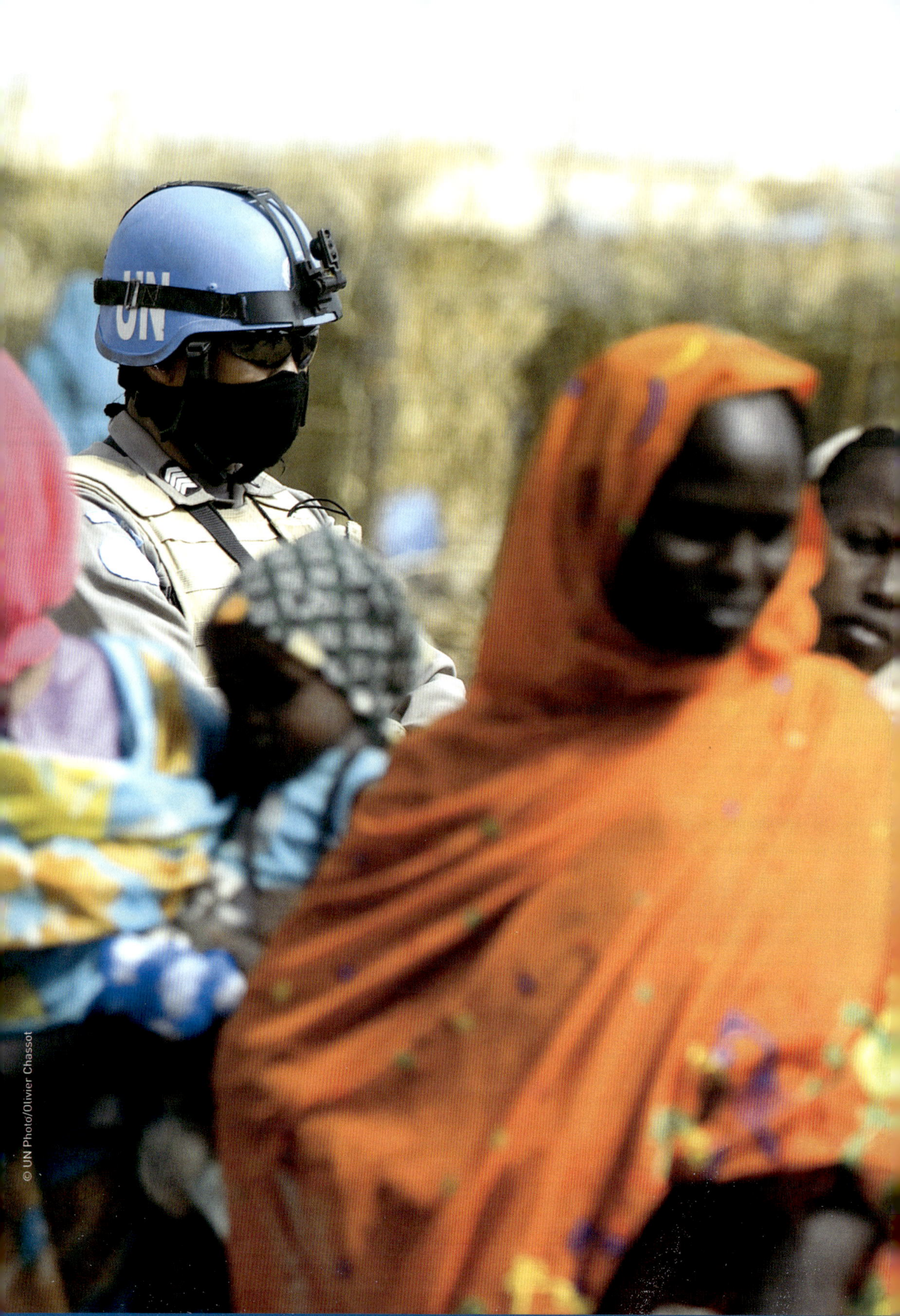

© UN Photo/Olivier Chassot

13.4 Conclusion

As repeatedly stressed in this chapter, fragile contexts present policy-makers and planners with complex and diverse challenges requiring innovative, flexible and incremental approaches.

- Many of the issues discussed are not exclusively relevant to fragile environments, but apply equally well to more stable health systems weakened by underfunding and poor management. However, the need for formulating and implementing realistic, feasible policies and strategies is higher where the duration and intensity of the crisis have damaged the health system and eroded the legitimacy and capacity of the government to a much larger extent. Addressing such gaps is arduous, and cannot be achieved through conventional approaches.
- A sound analysis of the context, focused on the determinants of the crisis, its historical evolution, the constraints posed and the opportunities offered, should be at the basis of any engagement in dysfunctional contexts. An investment in intelligence, related to both context and health care, must be associated with profound changes in the way decisions are taken. Moving closer to the service delivery point is a necessary step towards informed choices.
- Conceptual distinctions, such as the role of state vs non-state actors in health systems and service delivery, humanitarian vs development aid, formal vs informal policy processes, public vs private sector are not useful in distressed contexts. Traditional conceptual distinctions should be disregarded where the multiplicity of actors, the weakness of the government, the presence of different settings in the same country, the coexistence of humanitarian and development needs, the interplay of factors, and the emerging local strategies blur traditional dichotomies.
- Where uncertainty is pervasive, risks of mistakes and wasted resources can be reduced, but not eliminated. Shorter planning horizons, more modest goals, and stronger monitoring permit readjusting and adapting strategies and plans to unanticipated events, constraints and errors.
- The formulation of top-down, countrywide strategies is ineffective in situations of central government weakness, fragmentation of health system and diversity of situations. The alternative line of conduct is shifting the focus to the local level; supporting and documenting promising approaches that can be transferred to other areas of the country; and addressing concrete problems.
- Strategy development and planning are inherently political processes, even more in turbulent, politicized contexts; negotiation with the different key players is crucial. Trade-offs need to be made, to reduce the risk of resistance when policies and strategies will be implemented.
- Blueprint approaches and policy transfers from other contexts have proved ineffective time and again. No prescriptive guidelines can be issued for fragile contexts, as Zoellick claims: "...the worst thing the development community could do is develop a step-by-step handbook for dealing with fragile states".[69]

References

1 Francois M, Sud I. Promoting stability and development in fragile and failed states. Dev Policy Rev. 2006;24(2):141–60. doi:10.1111/j.1467-7679.2006.00319.x.

2 Mcloughlin C. Topic guide on fragile states, updated version. University of Birmingham, UK: Governance and Social Development Resource Centre; 2012 (http://www.gsdrc.org/docs/open/CON86.pdf, accessed 11 November 2015).

3 Carment D, Prest S, Samy Y. Determinants of state fragility and implications for aid allocation: an assessment based on the Country Indicators for Foreign Policy Project. Helsinki: United Nations University World Institute for Development Economics Research; 2008 (Project Research Paper No. 2008/46; https://www.ciaonet.org/attachments/911/uploads, accessed 11 November 2015).

4 Di John J. Conceptualising the causes and consequences of failed states: a critical review of the literature. London: Crisis States Research Centre; 2008 (Working Paper No. 25; http://www.lse.ac.uk/internationalDevelopment/research/crisisStates/download/wp/wpSeries2/wp252.pdf, accessed 11 November 2015).

5 Autesserre S. Dangerous tales: dominant narratives on the Congo and their unintended consequences. Afr Aff (Lond). 2012;111/443:202–22 (http://afraf.oxfordjournals.org/content/early/2012/02/09/afraf.adr080.abstract [subscription required]).

6 Duffield M. Global governance and the new wars: t. The merging of development and security, 2nd edition. London/New York: Zed Books; 2014.

7 Ibid.

8 Ghani A, Lockhart C, Carnahan M. Closing the sovereignty gap: how to turn failed states into capable ones. London: Overseas Development Institute; 2005 (ODI Opinions 44; http://www.odi.org/sites/odi.org.uk/files/odi-assets/publications-opinion-files/670.pdf, accessed 12 November 2015).

9 Overseas Development Institute. Getting better results from assistance to fragile states. (Briefing paper 70, 2011; http://www.odi.org/sites/odi.org.uk/files/odi-assets/publications-opinion-files/7297.pdf, accessed 12 November 2015).

10 Barakat S, Larson A. Fragile states: a donor-serving concept? Issues with interpretations of fragile statehood in Afghanistan. Journal of Intervention and Statebuilding. 2014;8(1):21–41.

11 Ibid.

12 Kharas H, Makino K, Jung W. Overview: An agenda for the Busan High-Level Forum on Aid Effectiveness. In: Kharas H, Makino K, Jung W, editors. Catalyzing development: a new vision for aid. Washington (DC): Brookings Institution Press; 2011:1–37 (http://www.brookings.edu/~/media/events/2011/6/28%20development%20aid/catalyzingdevelopment_chapter.pdf, accessed 12 November 2015).

13 Bertoli S, Ticci E. A fragile guideline to development assistance. Dev Policy Rev. 2012;30(2):211–30. doi:10.1111/j.1467-7679.2012.00572.x.

14 Organisation for Economic Co-operation and Development. Principles for good international engagement in fragile states and situations; 2007. (http://www.oecd.org/dacfragilestates/43463433.pdf, accessed 12 November 2015).

15 New Deal Document. g7+; 2016 (http://www.g7plus.org/new-deal/document/, accessed 12 November 2015).

16 Rogerson A. What if development aid were truly 'catalytic'? Overseas Development Institute; Background note; 2011 (http://www.odi.org/sites/odi.org.uk/files/odi-assets/publications-opinion-files/7373.pdf, accessed 12 November 2015).

17 Ramalingam B. Aid on the edge of chaos. Rethinking international cooperation in a complex world. Oxford: Oxford University Press; 2013: p.57.

18 Organisation for Economic Co-operation and Development. http://www.oecd.org/dac/effectiveness/34428351.pdf, accessed 2 September 2016.

19 Booth D. Aid effectiveness: bringing country ownership (and politics) back in. London: Overseas Development Institute; 2011 (ODI Working Paper 336; http://www.odi.org/sites/odi.org.uk/files/odi-assets/publications-opinion-files/6028.pdf, accessed 12 November 2015).

20 Goodhand J, Sedra M. Who owns the peace? Aid, reconstruction, and peacebuilding in Afghanistan. Disasters. 2010;34(S1):S78–S102. doi:10.1111/j.1467-7717.2009.01100.x

21 Barakat S. The failed promise of multi-donor trust funds: aid financing as an impediment to effective state-building in post-conflict contexts. Policy Studies. 2009;30(2):107–26. (http://www.researchgate.net/publication/248966341_The_failed_promise_of_multi-donor_trust_funds_Aid_financing_as_an_impediment_to_effective_state-building_in_post-conflict_contexts, accessed 12 November 2015 [downloadable]).

22 Larson G, Ajak PB, Pritchett L. South Sudan's capability trap. Building a state with disruptive innovation. Helsinki: United Nations University; 2013 (WIDER Working Paper No. 2013/120; https://www.wider.unu.edu/publication/south-sudan%E2%80%99s-capability-trap, accessed 12 November 2015 [downloadable]).

23 Hughes J, Glassman A, Gwenigale W. Innovative financing in early recovery: the Liberia Health Sector Pool Fund. Washington (DC): Center for Global Development; 2012. (CGD Working Paper 288; http://www.cgdev.org/content/publications/detail/1425944, accessed 12 November 2015).

24 Global Health Watch. Health care systems and approaches to health care. In: Global Health Watch 2005–2006. An alternative world health report. London/New York: Zed Books; 2005: 55–99 (http://reliefweb.int/sites/reliefweb.int/files/resources/AF558D1E144DAD0BC1257130005C9B60-medico.pdf, accessed 12 November 2015).

25 Zeng W, Cros M, Wright KD, Shepard DS. Impact of performance-based financing in primary health care services in Haiti. Health Pol Plan. 2013;28(6):596–605 (http://heapol.oxfordjournals.org/content/28/6/596.long, accessed 12 November 2015).

26 Grundy J, Khutb QY, Oumc S, Annear P, Ky V. Health system strengthening in Cambodia: a case study of health policy response to social transition. Health Policy. 2009;92:107–15. doi:10.1016/j.healthpol.2009.05.001.

27 Herbst J. States and power in Africa: comparative lessons in authority and control. Princeton(NJ): Princeton University Press; 2000 (Princeton Studies in International History and Politics).

28 Dewachi O, Skelton M, Nguyen V-K, Fouad FM, Abu Sitta G, Maasri Z et al. Changing therapeutic geographies of the Iraqi and Syrian wars. Lancet. 2014;383:449–57. doi: 10.1016/S0140-6736(13)62299-0.

29 Paton C. Health policy: overview. In: Carrin G, Buse K, Heggenhougen HK, Quah SR,editors. Health systems, policy, finance and organization. Oxford: Academic Press; 2009: p.12.

30 Andreas P, Greenhill KM. Sex, drugs and body counts. The politics of numbers in global crime and conflict. Cornell University Press 2010.

31 Hummelbrunner R, Jones H. A guide for planning and strategy development in the face of complexity. London: Overseas Development Institute; 2013 (ODI Background Note; http://www.odi.org/sites/odi.org.uk/files/odi-assets/publications-opinion-files/8287.pdf, accessed 12 November 2015).

32 Ibid.

33 Sandefur J, Glassman A. The political economy of bad data: evidence from African survey and administrative statistics. Washington (DC): Center for Global Development;2014 (Working Paper 373; www.cgdev.org/sites/default/files/political-economy-bad-data.pdf, accessed 29 August 2016).

34 Hummelbrunner R, Jones H. A guide for planning and strategy development in the face of complexity. London: Overseas Development Institute; 2013 (ODI Background Note; http://www.odi.org/sites/odi.org.

uk/files/odi-assets/publications-opinion-files/8287.pdf, accessed 12 November 2015).

35 Paarlberg LE, Bielefeld W. Complexity science: an alternative framework for understanding strategic management in public serving organizations. Int Public Manage J. 2009:12(2):236–260. doi:10.1080/10967490902868523.

36 Schmidt A. Coordinating development in conflict states: donor networks in Somalia. IDS Bulletin. 2013:44(1). doi: 10.1111/1759-5436.12007.

37 Freedman L. Strategy: a history. New York: Oxford University Press; 2013.

38 Ibid.

39 Liedtka J. Strategy and the art of seduction. In: Mintzberg H, Lampel J, Ahlstrand BW, editors. Strategy bites back. It is far more and less, than you ever imagined. Harlow/New York: Financial Times & Pearson Prentice Hall; 2008: 198–201.

40 Mintzberg H. The rise and fall of strategic planning: reconceiving roles for planning, plans, planners. New York: The Free Press; 1994: 25.

41 Freedman L. Strategy: a history. New York: Oxford University Press; 2013.

42 Mintzberg H. Adapted from: The strategy concept II: Another look at why organizations need strategies. In: Mintzberg H, Ahlstrand B, Lampel J, editors. Strategy bites back. It is far more and less, than you ever imagined. Harlow/New York: Financial Times & Pearson Prentice Hall; 2008: 30.

43 Pavignani E, Colombo S. Analysing disrupted health sectors. Geneva: World Health Organization; 2009 (http://apps.who.int/iris/bitstream/10665/44299/1/9789241599269_eng.pdf, accessed 11 November 2015).

44 Segall M. Health sector planning led by management of recurrent expenditure: an agenda for action research. Int J Health Plann Manage. 1991;6(1):37–75.

45 De Savigny D, Adam T, editors. Systems thinking for health systems strengthening. Alliance for Health Policy and Systems Research, World Health Organization, 2009 (http://apps.who.int/iris/bitstream/10665/44204/1/9789241563895_eng.pdf, accessed 12 November 2015).

46 The Economist. Why a strategy is not a plan; 2013 (http://www.economist.com/news/books-and-arts/21588834-strategies-too-often-fail-because-more-expected-them-they-can-deliver-why, accessed 12 November 2015).

47 Freedman L. Strategy: a history. New York: Oxford University Press; 2013.

48 Harford T. Adapt: why success always starts with failure. London: Abacus; 2012: 35.

49 Ottaway M. Rebuilding state institutions in collapsed states. Dev Change. 2002;33(5):1001–23 (http://archives.cerium.ca/IMG/pdf/Ottaway_Rebuilding_Collapsed_States.pdf, accessed 12 November 2015).

50 République Démocratique du Congo; Ministère de la Sante. Stratégie du renforcement du système de santé; 2006. http://www.nyankunde.org/documentation/SRSS%20VERSION%20FINALE.pdf, accessed 12 November 2015).

51 Cumper G. Should we plan for contraction in health services? The Jamaican experience. Health Pol Plan. 1993;8(2):113–21 (http://heapol.oxfordjournals.org/content/8/2.toc [subscription required]).

52 Sondorp E, Coolen A. The evolution of health service delivery in the Liberian health sector between 2003 and 2010: a policy analysis. 2012 (http://adhscourse.org/assets/grocery_crud/texteditor/plugins/filemanager/files/Health_Service_Delivery_study_Liberia_final_2012b.pdf, accessed 12 November 2015).

53 Mintzberg H. Planning as public relations. In: Strategy bites back. It is far more and less, than you ever imagined. Harlow/New York: Financial Times & Pearson Prentice Hall; 2008: 30.

54 Freedman L. Strategy: a history. New York: Oxford University Press; 2013.

55 Meessen B, Bigdeli M, Chheng K, Decoster K, Ir P, Men C et al. Composition of pluralistic health systems: how much can we learn from household surveys? An exploration in Cambodia. Health Pol Plan. 2011;26(1):i30–i44 (http://heapol.oxfordjournals.org/content/26/suppl_1/i30.full, accessed 12 November 2015).

56 Beesley M, Cometto G, Pavignani E. From drought to deluge: how information overload saturated absorption capacity in a disrupted health sector. Health Pol Plan. 2011;26(6):445–52 (http://heapol.oxfordjournals.org/content/26/6/445.long, accessed 12 November 2015).

57 Fox S, Witter S, Wylde E, Mafuta E, Lievens T. Paying health workers for performance in a fragmented, fragile state: reflections from Katanga Province, Democratic Republic of Congo. Health Pol Plan. 2014;29(1):96–105 (http://heapol.oxfordjournals.org/content/29/1/96.long, accessed 12 November 2015).

58 Coutts AP, Fouad FM. Syria's raging health crisis. New York Times. 1 January 2014 http://www.nytimes.com/2014/01/02/opinion/syrias-raging-health-crisis.html?_r=0, accessed 12 November 2015).

59 Dewachi O, Skelton M, Nguyen VK, Fouad FM, Abu Sitta G, Maasri Z et al. Changing therapeutic geographies of the Iraqi and Syrian wars. Lancet. 2014;383:449–57 (http://www.thelancet.com/journals/lancet/article/PIIS0140-6736%2813%2962299-0/fulltext , accessed 12 November 2015 [registration required]).

60 Capobianco E, Veni N. A review of health sector aid financing to Somalia. Washington (DC):World Bank; 2008 (Working Paper No.142, Africa Development Series; http://elibrary.worldbank.org/doi/pdf/10.1596/978-0-8213-7517-4, accessed July 12, 2014 [subscription required]).

61 Sen K, Mehio-Sibai A. Transnational capital and confessional politics: the paradox of the health care system in Lebanon. Int J Health Serv. 2004;34(3):527–51. doi:10.2190/6X2V-GE4T-9BQF-WYXB.

62 Caudron JM, Ford N, Henkens M, Mace C, Kiddle-Monroe R, Pinel J. Substandard medicines in resource-poor settings: a problem that can no longer be ignored. Trop Med Int Health. 2008;13(8):1062–72 (http://citeseerx.ist.psu.edu/viewdoc/download?doi=10.1.1.488.1222&rep=rep1&type=pdf, accessed 12 November 2015).

63 Ensor T, Witter S. Health economics in low income countries: adapting to the reality of the unofficial economy. Health Policy. 2001;57:1–13. pmid:11348690.

64 Chenge M, Van der Vennet J, Porignon D, Luboya N, Kabyla I, Criel B. La carte sanitaire de la ville de Lubumbashi, République Démocratique du Congo. Partie I: problématique de la couverture sanitaire en milieu urbain congolais. Global Health Promot. 2010;17(3):63–74. doi:10.1186/1472-6963-14-173.

65 Chenge M, Van der Vennet J, Porignon D, Luboya N, Kabyla I, Criel B. La carte sanitaire de la ville de Lubumbashi, République Démocratique du Congo. Partie II: analyse des activités opérationnelles des structures de soins. Global Health Promotion. 2010;17(3):75–84. doi:10.1177/1757975910375174.

66 Segall M. Health sector planning led by management of recurrent expenditure: an agenda for action-research. Int J Health Plann Manage. 1991;6(1):37–75. PMID:10113548.

67 Pavignani E. Human resources for health through conflict and recovery: lessons from African countries. Disasters. 2011,35(4).661–677. doi.10.1111/j.1467-7717.2010.01236.x.

68 Smith J. Guide to health workforce development in post-conflict environments. Geneva: World Health Organization; 2005 (http://apps.who.int/iris/bitstream/10665/43243/1/9241593288_eng.pdf, accessed 13 November 2015).

69 Zoellick RB. Fragile states: securing development. Survival: Global Politics and Strategy. 2008–2009;50(6):67–84. doi:10.1080/00396330802601859.

Further reading: a selected annotated bibliography

Buse K, Mays N, Walt G. Making health policy, 2nd edition. Maidenhead: Open University Press; 2012.

An updated development of the classic: Walt G. Health policy: an introduction to process and power. London: Zed Books; 1994. This book, drawing on different disciplines and theories, helps the reader to understand the role of actors, as well as of political, economic and contextual factors in shaping policies and strategies that directly affect how a particular health system performs. The importance of understanding the processes through which policies are developed and implemented is discussed. Real-life examples illustrate the difficulties and intricacies of analysing the health policy process, at the same time pointing to issues that are relevant in an emergency context, such as the role and influence of international agencies and institutions in the policy arena. Activities, intended to stimulate the participation of the reader and to encourage the exploration of well-chosen topics, punctuate the text.

Freedman L. Strategy: a history. New York: Oxford University Press; 2013.

This important book reviews the concept of strategy and its applications over recorded human history, covering the most diverse domains, from zoology to politics, war, the corporate world and social science. To a curious reader Freedman distils many propositions and examples that are useful also for health policy-makers and planners. Rational choice in policy and strategy making is wishful thinking; strategy is rather bound up with intuition, deliberation, persuasion and the "rationality of irrationality", a concept that fits well with most health systems under stress.

The book suggests that "as a practical matter, strategy is best understood modestly, as moving to the 'next stage' rather than to a definitive and permanent conclusion. The next stage is a place that can be realistically reached from the current stage". The authors of this chapter could not agree more with Freedman when he claims that "the picture of strategy that should emerge from this book is one that is fluid and flexible, governed by the starting point and not the end point". Thus, "the realm of strategy is one of bargaining and persuasion as well as threats and pressure, psychological and physical effects, and words as well as deeds ... strategy is the central political art".

Green A. An introduction to health planning for developing health systems. Oxford: Oxford University Press; 2007.

Now in its third edition, this is a classic textbook, clear, comprehensive and readable, which offers the best available comprehensive review of the field, thoroughly balancing techniques with real-world concerns and constraints. Green provides a fair appraisal of the most influential ideas that have shaped health systems world-wide, examining their strengths and weaknesses, as well as the assumptions and values they are built upon. In spite of portraying the difficulties of planning health care in developing countries and admitting its unsatisfactory record to date, the book nonetheless succeeds in conveying the necessity of supporting decision-makers with rational, evidence-based approaches, stripped of ideological elements and wishful thinking. Worthwhile reading for every practitioner interested or already involved in health planning. Even if the book does not address the specific features of fragile contexts and the additional constraints posed by them, it provides a wealth of general insights and instruments, against which crisis-adapted approaches can be developed.

Mintzberg H. The rise and fall of strategic planning: reconceiving roles for planning, plans, planners. New York: The Free Press; 1994.

A classic that does not show its age. Despite being directed to business organizations, from which it draws its examples, this book is an important resource for everybody engaged in policy-making and planning. Full of provocative statements, it debunks a lot of myths in strategy development and planning, pointing out the numerous fallacies and flaws of the rationalist approach to strategic planning. Mintzberg claims that "most organizations enter into planning with little understanding of the definitions and various purposes of planning", a statement that has not lost its validity twenty years after it was made.

Due to this lack of understanding and the adoption of bureaucratic approaches, only a few strategies are successfully implemented. The failure of strategies and plans that look too far ahead to identify discontinuous changes impacting on the organization explains in part their poor performance. Instead, Mintzberg proposes a more flexible approach, one that is more "simultaneous, holistic, and relational than linear, sequential and orderly.... No amount of elaboration will ever enable formal procedures to forecast discontinuities, to inform managers who are detached from their operations, to create novel strategies". Discontinuous changes are defining aspects of fragile contexts, hence the need to heed Mintzberg's cautionary words, and to follow his advice in the pursuit of alternative approaches.

Noormahomed AR, Segall M. The public health sector in Mozambique: a post-war strategy for rehabilitation and sustained development. Geneva: World Health Organization; 1994 (Macroeconomics, health and development series no. 14; http://whqlibdoc.who.int/hq/1994/WHO_ICO_MESD.14.pdf; accessed 15 January 2016).

One of the very few examples of successful post-conflict health recovery strategy, it was developed before the end of the war in 1992 by the MoH of Mozambique, with limited external assistance. Resulting from three years of studies and discussions and largely conceived by insiders, this document provided a roadmap for sector reconstruction, planning what was at the time considered affordable in the long term; it managed to rally considerable donor support. Despite its age, it is a recommended reading to every practitioner involved in a recovery process.

Pavignani E, Colombo S. Analysing disrupted health sectors. Geneva: World Health Organization; 2009 (http://apps.who.int/iris/bitstream/10665/44299/1/9789241599269_eng.pdf, accessed 15 January 2016)

A modular handbook covering the main areas relevant to the study of health systems in crisis and offering practical advice, experiences from the field, references and suggestions for further study. The handbook is essentially practical and action-oriented, based on the long experience of the two authors in countries affected by crises, mainly conflicts. Common flaws in the analysis of the context and health care provision are discussed, together with their effects on strategies and plans. Most of the issues covered in this chapter can be found, expanded and complemented with examples, tools and references, in the handbook.

Ramalingam B. Aid on the edge of chaos: rethinking international cooperation in a complex world. Oxford: Oxford University Press; 2013.

Everybody interested in the debate on aid effectiveness should read this original book. Drawing on complexity theory and systems thinking, Ramalingam provides a scathing critique of aid policy and practice, characterized as they are by the fact that "there is far more policy-based evidence than evidence-based policy". Simplifications, mechanical models and assumptions, and standard tools and prescriptions on which aid is built are inadequate, if not damaging in complex and dynamic environments: "Some problems are so complex that you have to be highly intelligent and well informed just to be undecided about them". The root problem is the common belief among many aid experts and agencies that there are technical and often simple solutions to underdevelopment. As a result of this misconception, effort and money are spent finding "ways to do the wrong thing righter". For example, discussing the inadequacy of the logframe for monitoring complex development interventions, Ramalingam quotes a donor arguing that: "We don't pretend that it matches reality, but we still find it useful". No aid tenets or myths are spared by the critique: MDGs, PRSPs (Poverty Reduction Strategy Papers), 'bestpracticitis', or the excessive focus on results.

The introduction to complexity theory is brilliant: the reader can not only appreciate its principles, but also its relevance to development and humanitarian work, including strategy formulation. Aid adaptive strategies are needed in the face of complexity: "different solutions need to find their niche in an evolving landscape ... the development strategic toolkit ... needs to find a dynamic balance between no strategy at all and the rigidness of blueprints. Effective aid strategies are those adaptively positioned between order and chaos". New approaches, based on the 'new science' of complex adaptive systems can make aid more relevant and effective, as experiences of practitioners who have put these principles into practice have shown. Wisely, the book does not provide clear-cut recommendations. Maybe to pre-empt criticism, the author argues that aid practitioners "should move from being people who know the answers to people who know what questions to ask".

Republic of Liberia, Ministry of Health and Social Welfare. Country situational analysis report. Monrovia: 2011 (http://www.indiana.edu/~cehls/2011%20Country%20Situational%20Analysis%20Report_Liberia.pdf, accessed 15 January 2016).

The product of an inclusive national health policy and planning exercise started in 2010, this frank, complete and thorough analysis of the health system highlighted both its post-conflict impressive achievements and the departures from the planned track. The evolution that occurred during the period 2006–2010 was not only described, but understood in its fundamental characteristics. A wealth of data and insights dispersed across programmes, institutions, publications and subsectors were blended to an unprecedented extent into a clear picture. The impact of the National Health Policy and Plan formulated in 2006–2007 was appraised, and the reasons behind the recorded divergences from the original goals were unpacked. Events taking place in the health system were read within the broader political and economic context.

Particularly valuable is the discussion of the choices made in 2006–2007 against the dearth of relevant information affecting the policy discussion at the time, revisited in light of the stronger understanding of patterns and events gained afterwards. Whereas the preparation of such an analysis in 2011 offered to decision-makers an excellent starting point to steer the health system through another planning cycle, the magnitude of the detected problems offers a reminder of the need to make sense of events continuously, or at least more frequently than at 5-year intervals. Many of such problems, if identified earlier, would have been more easily addressed.

This brilliant work should offer inspiration to participants to future health recovery processes, who will find in it plenty of valuable insights, related to methodological issues as well as policy and planning aspects.

Segall M. Health sector planning led by management of recurrent expenditure: an agenda for action-research. Int J Health Plann Manage. 1991;6(1):37–75.

This almost historical paper offers a clear, insightful overview, firmly grounded in direct experience, of what health planning is all about: the making of informed choices between alternative allocative options, within political, financial and managerial constraints. The logical steps to be taken and the frequent hurdles to be overcome for a progressive, redistributive policy such as primary health care (PHC) to materialize, are discussed. Both the poor reputation health planning has suffered from in recent times and the mediocre results registered in implementing PHC in many health sectors may be ascribed to a certain degree to the prevailing neglect of the rational, realistic approach presented in this classic paper. No reference is made to the additional, specific constraints affecting war-torn health sectors. However, most if not all of the considerations offered by the author hold in these settings as well, at least at the conceptual level.

Annex 13.1

Assessing the usefulness of a health policy/strategy/plan

- **Degree of contextualization**
  If the policy or plan could easily be applied to other settings, it scores low in this respect. The extent the conflict, or other societal stressors, is/are factored into the proposed actions is revealing.
- **Plausibility of the assumptions adopted (explicitly or otherwise)**
  For instance, is the stabilization of the political landscape likely to occur, as assumed by many recovery plans? Will the economy take off, and tax extraction improve, so that planned health services will become affordable?
- **Value for decision-making**
  Guidance to managers facing difficult choices in uncertain conditions should be offered by the policy/strategy/plan under scrutiny. To that effect, its content has to be related to concrete decisions with tangible effects.
- **Appropriateness of the adopted time frame**
  While the decision-making horizon is necessarily short, large investments are slow to materialize and have long-term effects.
- **Appraisal of costs, capacity implications, risks and side effects**
  A thorough appraisal suggests solid technical work, a broad perspective and readiness to address problems as they emerge.
  A policy/strategy/plan extolling only the benefits of the proposed measures is dangerous, as it may lead to misinformed decisions.
- **Integration of monitoring and evaluation tools into the policy/strategy/plan, with explicit reformulation/updating mechanisms included**
  The fluid context imposes the frequent revisiting of the original documents. Otherwise, when left untouched during years of rapid change, they cease to offer valuable guidance for decision-makers. In many cases, they were never appropriate, which explains their oblivion.
- **Extent of prioritization and sequencing of the proposed actions**
  When every proposed action is given the same weight and is expected to take place at the same time, implementation is likely to be incoherent, or will stop.
- **Accessibility (in terms of language, technical contents and cultural meanings) for the different stakeholder groups affected by the policy/strategy/plan**
  Proposals resonating only with health actors will be neglected or misunderstood by other influential parties.
- **Consistency between stated ends and the means (resources, capacity and political clout) made available**
  Discrepancies may be due to technical flaws, political expediency or external factors.
- **Receptivity of the main actors to the measures proposed by the policy/strategy/plan**
  Where the relationships between the parties concerned, say government and foreign agencies, are adversarial, not much implementation can be expected, whatever the merits of the proposal.

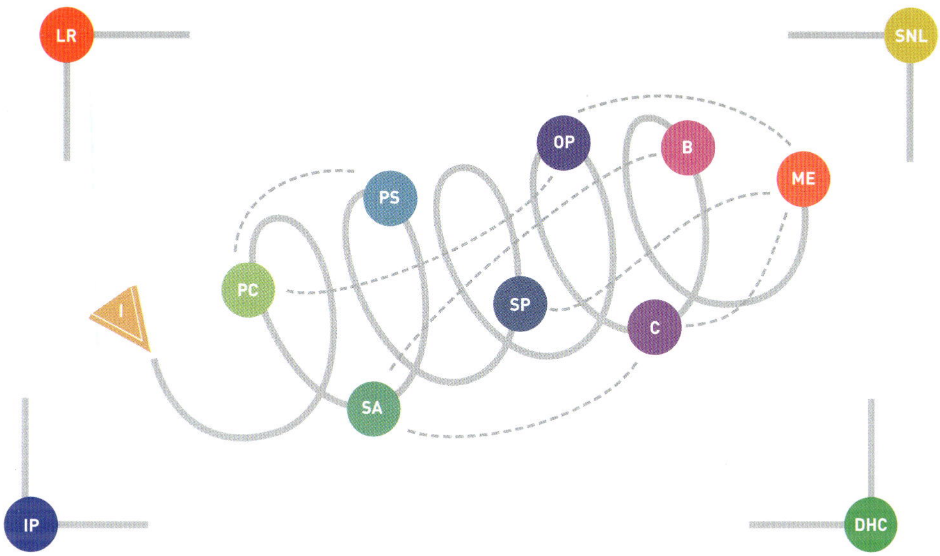
LR
SNL
OP
B
ME
PS
PC
I
SP
C
SA
IP
DHC